Diagnostic Imaging of Drug Resistant Pulmonary Tuberculosis

Pu-Xuan Lu • Hong-zhou Lu • Yong-xiang Yi
Editors

Diagnostic Imaging of Drug Resistant Pulmonary Tuberculosis

PMPH
PEOPLE'S MEDICAL PUBLISHING HOUSE

Springer

Editors
Pu-Xuan Lu
Diagnostic Imaging
Shenzhen Center for Chronic Disease Control
Shenzhen, China

Hong-zhou Lu
Infectious Disease
The Third People's Hospital of Shenzhen
Shenzhen, China

Yong-xiang Yi
Hepatobiliary Surgery
Nanjing Drum Tower Hospital
Nanjing, China

ISBN 978-981-99-8338-4 ISBN 978-981-99-8339-1 (eBook)
https://doi.org/10.1007/978-981-99-8339-1

This Springer imprint is published by the registered company Springer Nature Singapore Pte Ltd.
The registered company address is: 152 Beach Road, #21-01/04 Gateway East, Singapore 189721, Singapore

Printed on acid-free paper

Preface

As indicated by WHO Global TB Report 2022 [1], the estimated global increase of newly diagnosed tuberculosis (TB) patients was 10.6 million in 2021. Patients in the 30 high-burden TB countries accounted for 87% of all cases in the world, and those in 8 highest-burden TB countries, including India (28%), Indonesia (9.2%), China (7.4%), the Philippines (7.0%), Pakistan (5.8%), Nigeria (4.4%), Bangladesh (3.6%), and the Democratic Republic of Congo (2.9%), accounted for more than 2/3 of total patients in the world. Based on the estimates by WHO [1], there were 450,000 newly diagnosed cases of rifampicin-resistant pulmonary TB (95% CI: 399,000–501,000) in 2021, showing an increase of 3.1% from 437,000 cases (95% CI: 390,000–483,000) in 2020. The main reason for the increase of cases with drug-resistant TB was the overall rise of the incidence of TB from 2020 to 2021 [2]. In 2021, the estimated number of deaths in TB patients was 1.4 million among the HIV-negative population, and one of the main causes of death is the increased incidence, compounded by difficulties in diagnosis and treatment of drug-resistant TB. In 2012, the WHO clearly pointed out that successful prevention and control of three major challenges in TB epidemics, including drug-resistant TB, HIV and Mtb dual infection, and migration of populations with TB, would help achieve global TB control targets within the next 20 years. Confronted with one of three major challenges in drug-resistant pulmonary TB, we specifically organized and compiled this monograph entitled *Diagnostic Imaging of Drug Resistant Pulmonary Tuberculosis* to summarize our latest experience and achievements in the prevention, diagnosis, and treatment of drug-resistant TB. We aimed to provide suggestion and guideline for improving the precision diagnosis and treatment for drug-resistant TB and contribute to the grand goal of "end the global TB epidemic" by 2035 endorsed by WHO, through presenting classic cases and comprehensively elaborating on results of the latest research.

This book was written by more than 80 experts in China and abroad, who are directly involved in the fields of prevention, diagnosis, treatment, and basic research of drug-resistant TB. Divided into 17 chapters, the book consists of an overview, detection of drug-resistant TB and its epidemics, laboratory examination for drug-resistant tubercle bacillus, pathogenic mechanism of drug-resistant TB and its diagnosis, differential diagnosis, treatment, prevention and prognosis of drug-resistant pulmonary TB. This book focuses on providing information on classic cases of drug-resistant TB, including mono-drug-resistant cases (including Rifampicin resistance, etc.), multidrug-resistant cases, poly-drug-resistant cases, extensively drug-resistant cases (pre-extensively drug-resistant), drug-resistant bronchial TB, and pediatric drug-resistant cases, as well as AIDS complicated with drug-resistant TB, and the diagnosis and treatment of drug-resistant cervical TB lymphadenitis. We also provided a comprehensive description and in-depth analysis for each selected case and a systematic explanation for latest cutting-edge issues, such as dynamic changes in images during the treatment of drug-resistant TB as well as the research and application of artificial intelligence in diagnosing drug-resistant TB, to further inspire our readers.

Full of details and excellency in both pictures and literacy, this book includes valuable typical TB cases and more than 600 images carefully collected from large TB hospitals in China. The process for diagnosing and treating each of these collected cases is the fruit of continuous exploration and investigation by professional medical practitioners, reflecting their dedication, persistence, and intellect. This book also presents many clinical characteristics, image manifestations, and the process of diagnosis and treatment for different types of drug-resistant TB in a vivid and systematic manner using both pictures and texts, focusing on each type of drug-resistant TB, so as to provide readers with a comprehensive understanding of the clinical characteristics of this disease and its typical image findings in its different pathological stages. Therefore, this book can be used as vital and important guidelines for the disease diagnosis, differential diagnosis, treatment, and assessment of response to treatment. This book has also provided important and valuable references for medical practitioners engaged in research and clinical practice including the prevention, diagnosis, and treatment of drug-resistant TB, government administrators, and medical students, both in China and abroad.

References

1. World Health Organization. Global TB report 2022[EB/OL]. https://www.who.int/teams/global-TB-programme/tb-reports/global-TB-report-2022.
2. Song Min, Lu Puxuan, Fang Weijun, et al. The global TB report 2022: key data analysis for China and the global world[J/CD]. Electron J Emerg Inf Dis 2023;8(1):87–92.

Shenzhen, China Pu-Xuan Lu
Shenzhen, China Hong-zhou Lu
Nanjing, China Yong-xiang Yi

Contents

About the Editors

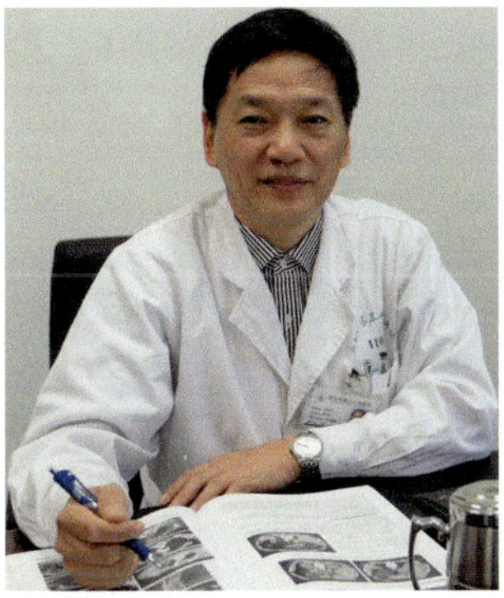

Pu-Xuan Lu is a Chief Medical Specialist of Shenzhen Center for Chronic Disease Control, Shenzhen Institute of Pulmonology; first-level chief physician of the Third People's Hospital of Shenzhen; a professor and graduate supervisor of Guangdong Medical University.

His academic titles include chief editor of *Electronic Journal of Emerging Infectious Disease*; deputy chair, Radiology of Infectious Disease group at the radiology branch of Chinese Medical Society; deputy chair, Radiology of Infectious Disease group at Chinese Radiology Society; deputy chair, Radiology branch of Chinese Sexually Transmitted Disease and HIV/AIDS Society; deputy chair, Beijing Diagnostic Imaging Technology Innovation Alliance; deputy chair, Radiology branch of Provincial Health Management Society of Guangdong, China; and editorial committee member of the *Journal of Radiology of Infectious Disease*.

His research fields include diagnostic imaging and differential diagnosis of emerging infectious diseases, such as SARS, MERS, AIDS, human infected avian influenza, tuberculosis, hepatitis, and other infectious diseases as well as clinical and basic sciences of emerging infectious diseases.

Professor Lu has edited or co-edited more than 20 academic treaties. *Diagnostic Imaging of Emerging Infectious Diseases* has been published by Springer in November 2015, which obtained national key award for book output in May 2017 by the General Administration of News and Publishing, China. In 2020, he co-edited *Tuberculosis Control in Migrating Population* published by Springer and won the third Springer Nature: China New Development Award in September 2021.

In the last 25 years, he has directed and finished five national and provincial as well as international collaborative research projects. Pu-Xuan Lu has published more than 180 papers, 43 of which were published in SCI-indexed journals. He received 12 awards from Chinese Medical Society, Chinese Preventive Medicine Society, Guangdong provincial government, and Shenzhen city government.

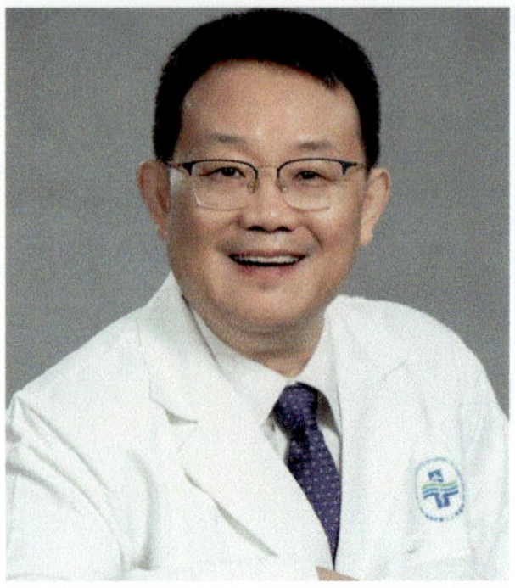

Hong-zhou Lu, MD, PhD, is the director of Shenzhen Third People's Hospital, a world-renowned scholar of infectious diseases, World's Top 2% Scientists in 2021 (Stanford University), winner of the Charpak Dubousset Prize of the French National Academy of Medicine, and a fellow of the American Academy of Microbiology.

Prof. Lu has long been dedicated to the basic research and clinical practice of infectious diseases. During the influenza A (H1N1, H7N9) and COVID-19 pandemics, he led the early treatment efforts and pioneered clinical and basic research on related diseases in Shanghai, making essential contributions to the prevention of disease epidemics in China. Professor Lu's work has been supported by the National Science and Technology Major Project of the Ministry of Science and Technology of China (n = 3), the National Natural Science Foundation of China (n = 7), the Bill & Melinda Gates Foundation, and the National Institutes of Health. He has published more than 500 research papers in international journals, including *Nature, New England Journal of Medicine,* and *Cell Research.* He is involved in the editorship of national and international journals, including *AIDS* Chinese Edition, *Infectious Diseases Radiology*, and *Journal of Antivirals & Antiretrovirals*, the executive editor of *Drug Discovery and Treatment, Chinese Medical Journal*, *Emerging Microbes & Infections*, *Bioscience Trend*, *Infection International*, and *Global Health and Medicine.* He also is a frequent ad hoc reviewer for prestigious journals such as *New England Journal of Medicine, JAMA Internal Medicine, Lancet, Lancet Infectious Diseases, Journal of Clinical Microbiology,* and *mBio.*

Professor Lu has an exceptional record of teaching and mentoring. He has successively served as an adjunct professor at Fudan University and Southern University of Science and technology; Doctoral Advisor of Internal Medicine, Nursing, and Public Health Management; Master Advisor of Law in Public Health; Head of the Post-Doctoral Stations; the Co-Director of the WHO Collaborating Centre for Clinical Management, Training, and Research on Emerging and Re-emerging Infectious Diseases and is a member of the Clinical Expert Group of WHO; the chairman of the Tropical and Parasitic Diseases Branch of the Chinese Medical Association; the leader of the AIDS Group and deputy leader of the AIDS Professional Group of the Infectious Diseases Branch of the Chinese Medical Association; the deputy director of the Public Health Management Branch of the Medical Institutions of the Chinese Preventive Medicine Association; the deputy Chairman of the China Association of Integrative Medicine Medical Infectious Diseases Professional Committee, Hagiology Branch of Shanghai Prevention Medical Association; and the leader of the Shenzhen Public Health Expert Group on Epidemic Prevention and Control.

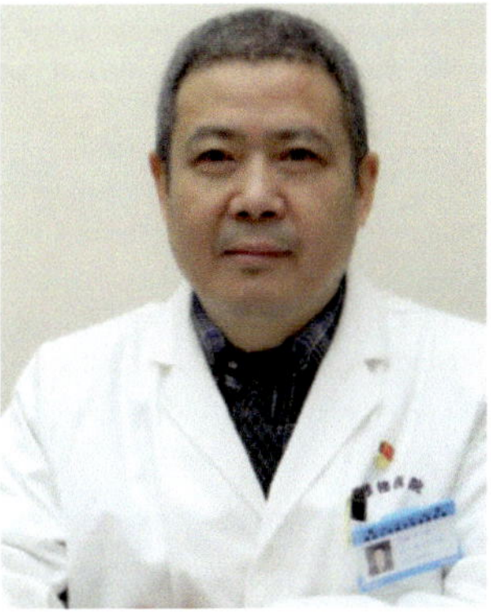

Yong-xiang Yi, MD, serves as the Vice President of Nanjing Drum Tower Hospital. He is a Distinguished Professor and a Ph.D. Supervisor of Nanjing University of Chinese Medicine. He is also the president of National Excellent Hospital and has been recognized as an expert with special government allowances from the State Council. Additionally, he holds the position of Vice Chairman at the Infectious Disease Hospital of the China Hospital Association and Vice Chairman of the Liver Disease Committee of the Chinese Association of Research Hospitals. He is the Leader of the Liver Cancer Group and serves as the Chairman of Infectious Disease Hospital of Jiangsu Hospital Association. Furthermore, he is the Vice Chairman of the Jiangsu Anti-Cancer Association, the Chairman of the Infectious Diseases of Jiangsu Association of Traditional Chinese Medicine, and the Vice Chairman of the Liver Disease Committee of Jiangsu Medical Association. He is a Member of the Standing Committee of the Cancer Committee.

He has been engaged in general surgery for more than 30 years and has long been committed to the research of various complicated liver diseases, gallbladder and pancreatic tumors, and intestinal microbiota. He has conducted multiple national, provincial, and municipal scientific research projects, published more than 60 SCI papers, written 7 professional books, and published 2 international patents.

About the Associate Editors

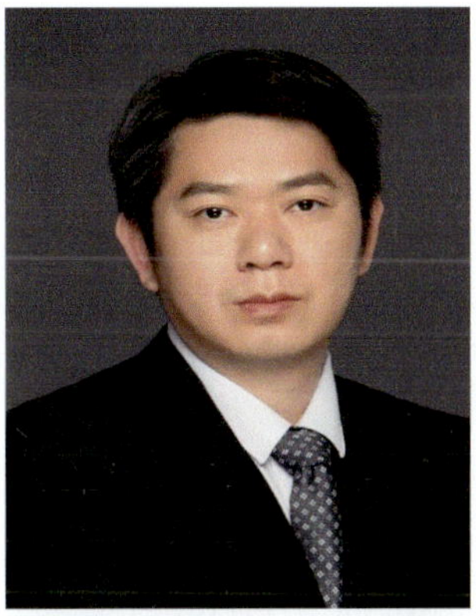

Weijun Fang Professor

Director of the Department of Imaging of Guangzhou Chest Hospital

Chairman of Guangzhou Hospital Association Committee of Radiological Medicine

Councilor of Radiation Branch of Guangdong Medical Association

Member of the standing committee of the 12th Imaging branch of Chinese Antituberculosis Association

Member of the standing committee of the 18th Phthisiology branch of Chinese Medical Association

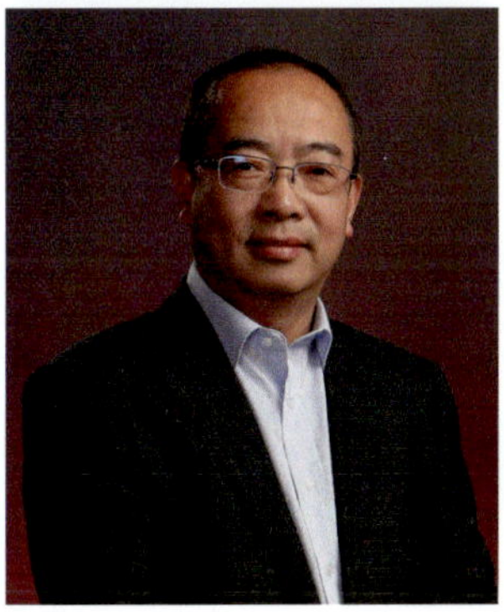

Ru-ming Xie Professor

The chief physician, the chief of the imaging center of Beijing Ditan Hospital, Capital Medical University

The editorial board member of *Chinese Journal of Antituberculosis* and *Electronic Journal of Emerging Infectious Diseases*

The vice chairman of the imaging special committee of the tuberculous branch of the Chinese medical association

The vice chairman of the multidisciplinary diagnosis and treatment branch of the Chinese Antituberculosis Association

The vice chairman of the medical imaging quality management committee of the medical quality management association

The standing committee member of the infection imaging committee of the China Association for the Prevention and Control of AIDS and VD, and the standing committee member of clinical medicine committee of the Chinese Antituberculosis Association

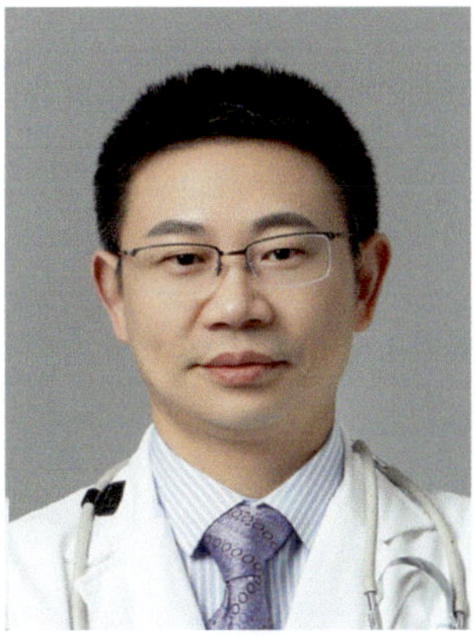

Guofang Deng Professor

Chief of the Department of Tuberculosis of Shenzhen Third People's Hospital

Director of the Tuberculosis and Diabetes Branch of Chinese Anti-Tuberculosis Association

Vice-Director of Tuberculosis Branch of Shenzhen Medical Association

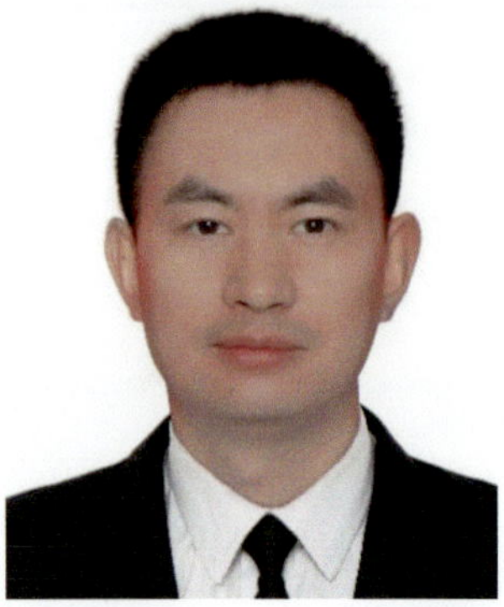

Chun-hua Li Professor

Chief Medical Specialist and research team leader of Chongqing Public Health Medical Center, Department of Radiology

Member of the Infectious Diseases Group of the Radiology Branch of the Chinese Medical Association, Imaging Professional Branch of the China Anti-Tuberculosis Association, Radiology branch of Chinese Sexually Transmitted Disease and HIV/AIDS Society, Beijing Diagnostic Imaging Technology Innovation Alliance, Infection and Inflammatory Radiology Professional Committee of the Chinese Research Hospital Association

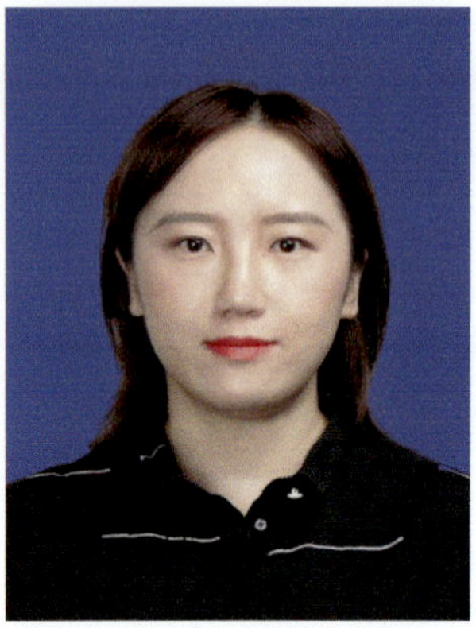

Qi An Deputy Division Head of General Planning Division (Secretariat of Municipal City Planning Committee), Planning and Natural Resources Bureau of Shenzhen Municipality (Municipal Ocean and Fisheries Bureau, Municipal Forestry Bureau)

Ph.D. Candidate, Urban Planning Department, Faculty of Architecture, Harbin Institute of Technology (Shenzhen)

Planner in the field of Urban Medical Facilities spatial planning

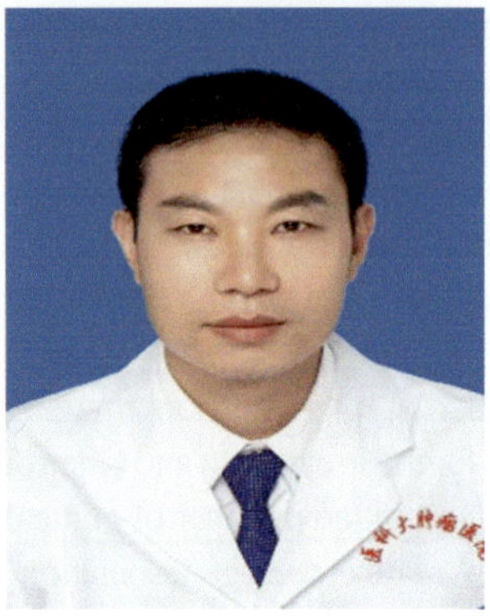

Guan-qiao Jin Professor

Chief of Medical Imaging Center, Department of Teaching and Research, Affiliated Tumor Hospital of Guangxi Medical University

Chief of Guangxi Key Laboratory of Tumor Molecular Imaging Research (Cultivation)

Standing member of the Cancer Imaging Committee of Chinese Anti-Cancer Association

Standing member of the Cancer Imaging Diagnosis Committee of Chinese Research Hospital Association

Member of the Head and Neck Committee of the Radiology Society of Chinese Medical Doctor Association

Member of the Imaging Branch of China Medical Association

Chairman of the Tumor Imaging Professional Committee of Guangxi Anti-Cancer Association

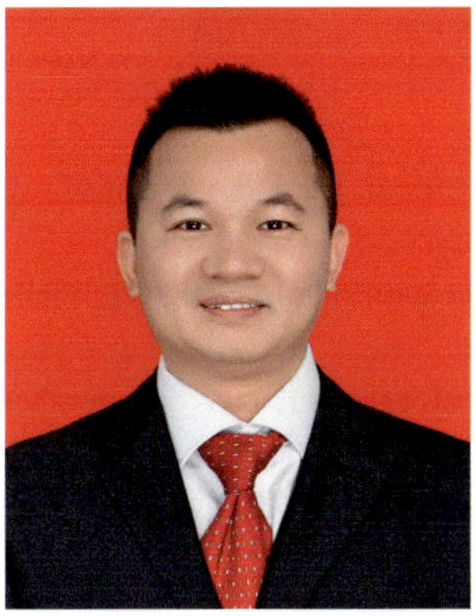

Yibo Lu Professor

Director of Radiology Department, Director of Ultrasound Department, and Director of Medical Imaging Teaching and Research Office at the Fourth People's Hospital of Nanning City. Expert in formulating imaging diagnostic standards for statutory infectious diseases by the National Health Commission

Academic Part time: Chairman of infectious diseases Imaging Professional Committee of Guangxi Preventive Medicine Association; Vice Chairman of Infectious Radiology Professional Committee of China AIDS and STD Prevention Association; Vice Chairman of Nanning Radiological Society and Deputy Director of Nanning Radiological Diagnosis Quality Control Center

Editorial board member of the *Electronic Journal of Emerging Infectious Diseases*, *Radiology of Infectious Diseases*, and *Radiology Science*, and co-edited 16 monographs.

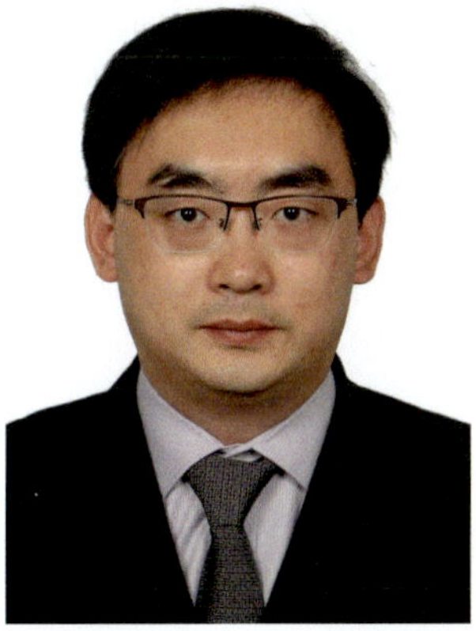

Yufeng Xu, MD Deputy Chief Physician of the Department of Radiology, Peking University First Hospital

Deputy Chairman of Tumor Medical Imaging Professional Committee of China Association for Promotion of Health Science and Technology

Deputy Head of the Endocrinology and Rheumatology Group of the Radiology Branch of Beijing Medical Association

Member of Imaging Group of Rheumatology Society of Chinese Medical Doctor Association

Member of Hematology Oncology Group of Tumor imaging Special Committee of Chinese Anti-Cancer Association

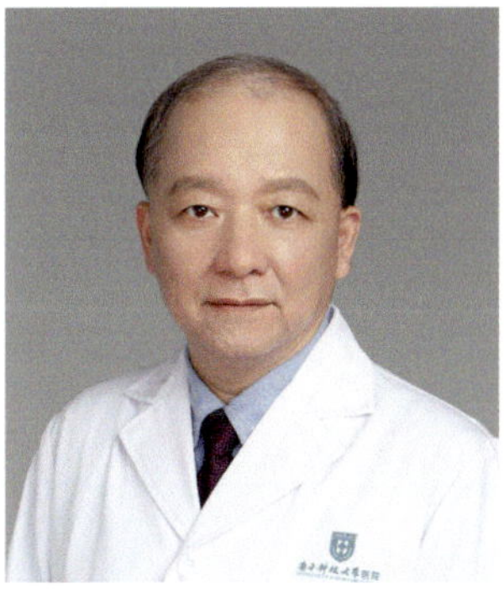

Zhun Yu Professor

Deputy Director of the Health Management Professional Committee of the Shenzhen Medical Association

Standing Committee Member of the Cardiovascular Internal Medicine Professional Committee of the Shenzhen Medical Association

Deputy Director of the Cardiovascular Prevention and Rehabilitation Professional Committee of the Shenzhen Physicians Association

Vice Chairman of the Shenzhen Geriatrics Association, Deputy Director of the Shenzhen Geriatric Health Management Association

Deputy Editor-in-Chief of *Electronic Journal of Emerging Infectious Diseases*

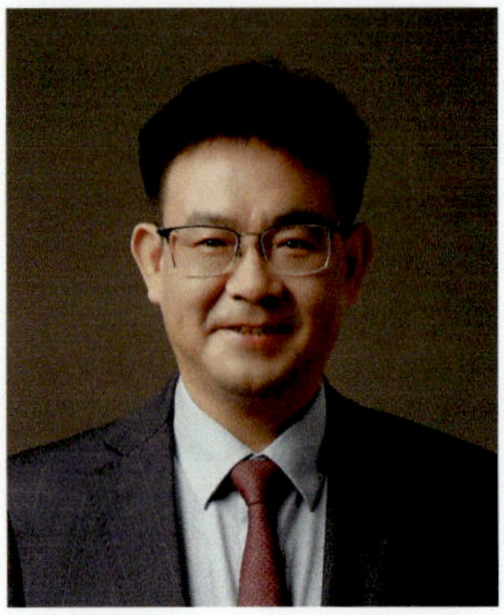

Liang-geng Gong Professor, Doctoral supervisor

Director of Radiology, the 2nd Affiliated Hospital of Nanchang University

Director of the Intelligent Medical Frontier Technology Research Center of Nanchang University

Young and middle-aged experts with outstanding contributions to health in Jiangxi Province

Member of the China Group of International Society for CMR (SCMR)

Member of the China Group of Society of Cardiovascular Computed Tomography (SCCT)

Chairman of Jiangxi Society of Radiology

Vice Chairman of the Infection and Inflammation Committee of the Chinese Research Hospital Association

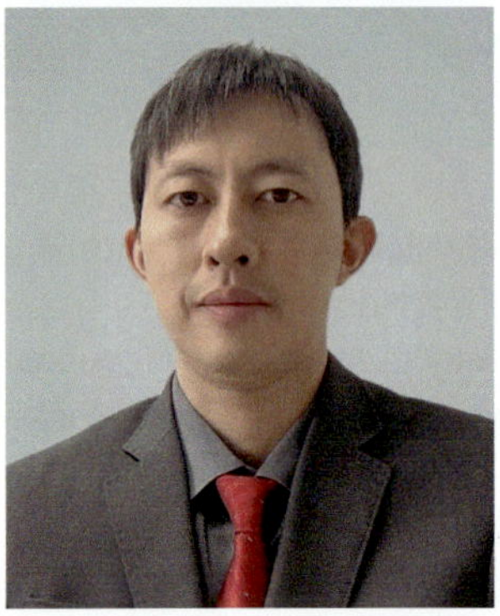

Nu Zhang, MPharm Deputy Director of Pharmacy Department of Shenzhen Center for Chronic Disease Control

Member of Shenzhen Pharmaceutical Association

Member of Pharmaceutical Management Professional Committee of Guangdong Health Economics Association

Member of Therapeutic Drug Monitoring Professional Committee of Shenzhen Pharmaceutical Association

Editorial Board Member of *Chinese Journal of Medical Instrumentation*

Member of Hospital Architecture Equipment Engineering Branch

Editors and Contributors

Chief Editors

Pu-xuan Lu Diagnostic Imaging, Shenzhen Center for Chronic Disease Control, Shenzhen, Guangdong, China

Hong-zhou Lu Infectious Disease, The Third People's Hospital of Shenzhen, Shenzhen, Guangdong, China

Yong-xiang Yi Hepatobiliary Surgery, Nanjing Drum Tower Hospital, Nanjing, Jiangsu, China

Associate Editors

Wei-jun Fang Department of Radiology, Guangzhou Chest Hospital, Guangzhou, Guangdong, China

Ru-ming Xie Department of Radiology, Beijing Ditan Hospital, Capital Medical University, Beijing, China

Guo-fang Deng Department of Tuberculosis, The Third People's Hospital of Shenzhen, Shenzhen, Guangdong, China

Chun-hua Li Department of Medical Imaging, Chongqing Public Health Medical Center, Chongqing, China

Qi An Urban Planning Department, Faculty of Architecture, Harbin Institute of Technology, Shenzhen, Guangdong, China

Guan-qiao Jin Department of Medical Imaging, The Affiliated Cancer Hospital of Guangxi Medical University, Guangxi, China

Yi-bo Lu Department of Radiology, The Fourth People's Hospital of Nanning, Nanning, Guangxi, China

Yu-feng Xu Department of Radiology, Peking University First Hospital, Beijing, China

Zhun Yu Department of Cardiovascular, Southern University of Science and Technology Hospital, Shenzhen, Guangdong, China

Liang-geng Gong Department of Radiology, The Second Affiliated Hospital of Nanchang University, Nanchang, China

Nu Zhang Department of Pharmacy, Shenzhen Center for Chronic Disease Control, Shenzhen, Guangdong, China

Contributors

Bu-dong Chen Department of Radiology, Beijing You'an Hospital, Capital Medical University, Beijing, China

Chao Chen Department of Tuberculosis, The Third People's Hospital of Shenzhen, Shenzhen, Guangdong, China

Gen-Ming Chen Department of Radiology, Baoan central Hospital of Shenzhen, Shenzhen, Guangdong, China

Qiu-qi Chen Department of Tuberculosis, The Third People's Hospital of Shenzhen, Shenzhen, Guangdong, China

Rong Chen Tuberculosis Prevention and Control Department, Shenzhen Center for Chronic Disease Control, Shenzhen, Guangdong, China

Ying-ying Deng Department of Radiology, Yantian District People's Hospital, Shenzhen, Guangdong, China

Liang Fu Department of Tuberculosis, The Third People's Hospital of Shenzhen, Shenzhen, Guangdong, China

Xiao-li Gu Department of Radiology, Luohu Hospital of Traditional Chinese Medicine, Shenzhen, Guangdong, China

Lin Guo Shenzhen Zhiying Medical Co., Ltd., Shenzhen, Guangdong, China

Yuan-yuan Han Department of Radiology, Guangzhou Chest Hospital, Guangzhou, Guangdong, China

Wei He Department of Medical Imaging, Beijing Chest Hospital, Capital Medical University, Beijing, China

Yu-lin He Department of Radiology, The First Affiliated Hospital of Nanchang University, Nanchang, Jiangxi, China

Dai-lun Hou Department of Radiology, Beijing Chest Hospital, Capital Medical University, Beijing, China

Fang-xiang Hu Department for Tuberculosis Control and Prevention, Bao'an Chronic Diseases Prevent and Cure Hospital, Shenzhen, Guangdong, China

Ya-nan Hu Department of General Practice, ZiWei Community Health Care Service Center of Longgang District People's Hospital, Shenzhen, Guangdong, China

Hua Huang Department of Radiology, The Third People's Hospital of Shenzhen, Shenzhen, Guangdong, China

Kui Huang Infectious Diseases Department, Chest Hospital of Guangxi Zhuang Autonomous Region, Liuzhou, Guangxi, China

Ying-yu Huo School of Electronic Information Engineering, Foshan University, Foshan, Guangdong, China

Stefan Jaeger National Institutes of Health/National Library of Medicine, Bethesda, MD, USA

Feng-li Jiang Department of Radiology, Zhongda Hospital, Medical School, Southeast University, Nanjing, China

Hong-jun Li Department of Radiology, Beijing You'an Hospital, Capital Medical University, Beijing, China

Lin Li Department of Radiology, Lin Yi People's Hospital, Shandong, China

Tong-xia Li Department of Tuberculosis, Qingdao Chest Hospital, Qingdao, Shandong, China

Hou-ming Liu Department of Clinical Laboratory, The Third People's Hospital of Shenzhen, Shenzhen, Guangdong, China

Jing-zhe Liu Department of Medical Imaging, The First Hospital Of Tsinghua University, Beijing, China

Miao-na Liu Department of Pharmacy, The Third People's Hospital of Shenzhen, Shenzhen, Guangdong, China

Pei-ying Liu Department of Radiology, Lin Yi People's Hospital, Shandong, China

Xin-jiang Liu Department of Radiology, Fudan University Pudong Medical Center, Shanghai, China

Xian-rong Long Department of Medical Imaging, Foshan Fourth People's Hospital, Foshan, Guangdong, China

Kun-zhen Lu Editorial Department of the Electronic Journal of Emerging Infectious Diseases, Shenzhen, Guangdong, China

Shui-hua Lu Department of Tuberculosis, The Third People's Hospital of Shenzhen, Shenzhen, Guangdong, China

Yong-yi Lu Bloomberg School of Public Health, Johns Hopkins University, Baltimore, MD, USA

Jie-qi Luo Department of Radiology, The Third People's Hospital of Shenzhen, Shenzhen, Guangdong, China

Wei-Jun Luo Department of Medical Imaging, Shenzhen Center for Chronic Disease Control, Shenzhen, Guangdong, China

Zhe-huang Luo Department of Nuclear Medicine, Jingxi Provincial People's Hospital, The First Affiliated Hospital of Nanchang Medical College, Jingxi, China

Fleming Lure Shenzhen Zhiying Medical Co., Ltd., Shenzhen, Guangdong, China

Sheng-xiu Lv Department of Medical Imaging, Chongqing Public Health Medical Center, Chongqing, China

Yan Lv Department of Medical Imaging, Beijing Chest Hospital, Capital Medical University, Beijing, China

Wei Ma Department of Radiology, The Third People's Hospital of Longgang, Shenzhen, Guangdong, China

Jin-zhou Mei Department for Tuberculosis Control and Prevention, Bao'an Chronic Diseases Prevent and Cure Hospital, Shenzhen, Guangdong, China

Li-ai Peng Department for Tuberculosis Control and Prevention, Bao'an Chronic Diseases Prevent and Cure Hospital, Shenzhen, Guangdong, China

Wan-shui Shan Clinical Laboratory, The Third People's Hospital of Shenzhen, Shenzhen, Guangdong, China

Yu-xin Shi Department of Radiology, Shanghai Public Health Clinical Center, Shanghai, China

Min Song Department of Radiology, Guangzhou Chest Hospital, Guangzhou, Guangdong, China

Wei-guo Tan Tuberculosis Prevention and Control Department, Shenzhen Center for Chronic Disease Control, Shenzhen, Guangdong, China

Feng Wang Department of Medical Laboratory, Shenzhen Center for Chronic Disease Control, Shenzhen, Guangdong, China

Hai-jiang Wang Department of Thoracic Surgery, The Third People's Hospital of Shenzhen, Shenzhen, Guangdong, China

Luo-lin Wang Department of Gastroenterology, Shenzhen People's Hospital, Shenzhen, Guangdong, China

Yi Xiang J. Wang Department of Imaging and Interventional Radiology, Faculty of Medicine, The Chinese University of Hong Kong, New Territories, Hong Kong SAR

Yun-xia Wang Department for Tuberculosis Control and Prevention, Bao'an Chronic Diseases Prevent and Cure Hospital, Shenzhen, Guangdong, China

Fang-jun Wei Department of Radiology, The Third People's Hospital of Shenzhen, Shenzhen, Guangdong, China

Xin-nian Wen Department of Medical Imaging, Chest Hospital of Guangxi Zhuang Autonomous Region, Liuzhou, Guangxi, China

Ji-li Wu Department of Medical Imaging, The Fourth People's hospital of Taiyuan, Taiyuan, Shanxi, China

Jin-ping Wu Department of Radiology, Third People's Hospital of Changzhou City, Changzhou, Jiangsu, China

Wen-feng Wu Jiangxi JF Healthcare Limited Company, Nanchang, Jiangxi, China

Chuan-jun Xu Department of Radiology, The Second Hospital of Nanjing, Nanjing University of Chinese Medicine, Nanjing, China

Gen-dong Yang Department of Radiology, The Third People's Hospital of Shenzhen, Shenzhen, Guangdong, China

Qin Yin Editorial Department of the Electronic Journal of Emerging Infectious Diseases, Shenzhen, Guangdong, China

Dong Yu Department of Prehospital Care, Shenzhen Center for Prehospital Care, Shenzhen, Guangdong, China

Ming-yuan Yuan Department of Radiology, Affiliated Zhoupu Hospital, Shanghai University of Health and Medicine Science, Shanghai, China

Fan Zhang Department of Tuberculosis Prevention and Control, Shenzhen Nanshan Center for Chronic Disease Control, Shenzhen, Guangdong, China

Hui Zhang Department of Radiology, The Third People's Hospital of Shenzhen, Shenzhen, Guangdong, China

Juan-juan Zhang Department for Tuberculosis Control and Prevention, Bao'an Chronic Diseases Prevent and Cure Hospital, Shenzhen, Guangdong, China

Qian-qian Zhang Magnetic Resonance Room, Zhoukou Central Hospital, Zhoukou, Henan, China

Guang-ping Zheng Department of Radiology, The Third People's Hospital of Shenzhen, Shenzhen, Guangdong, China

Jian Zheng Department of Pharmacy, The Third People's Hospital of Shenzhen, Shenzhen, Guangdong, China

Qiu-ting Zheng Department of Medical Imaging, Shenzhen Center for Chronic Disease Control, Shenzhen, Guangdong, China

Yong Zhong School of Electronic Information Engineering, Foshan University, Foshan, Guangdong, China

Jie Zhou Department of Tuberculosis, Foshan Hospital of Traditional Chinese Medicine, Foshan, Guangdong, China

Yun Zhou Department of Radiology, The Third People's Hospital of Shenzhen, Shenzhen, Guangdong, China

Yu-mei Zhu Department of Medical Laboratory, Shenzhen Center for Chronic Disease Control, Shenzhen, Guangdong, China

Overview of Drug-Resistant Pulmonary Tuberculosis

1

Yun-xia Wang, Juan-juan Zhang, Li-ai Peng, Fang-xiang Hu, Jin-zhou Mei, and Pu-Xuan Lu

1.1 Definitions

1.1.1 Definition of Mycobacterium Pulmonary Tuberculosis Drug Resistance and Its Classification [1]

Drug resistance in Mycobacterium pulmonary tuberculosis is defined as in vitro tests that confirm that Mycobacterium pulmonary tuberculosis has developed resistance to one or more antituberculosis drugs. Drug resistance in Mycobacterium pulmonary tuberculosis can be classified into four types based on laboratory bacteriology and the causes of drug resistance.

1. Primary drug resistance

   Mycobacterium pulmonary tuberculosis is resistant to one or more antituberculosis drugs in patients with tuberculosis who have never received antituberculosis drugs. It includes drug resistance due to the spread of drug-resistant Mycobacterium tuberculosis strains and susceptible Mycobacterium pulmonary tuberculosis strains undergoing a genetic mutation in patients body resulting in drug-resistant.
2. Acquired drug resistance

   Mycobacterium tuberculosis is susceptible at the beginning but develops drug resistance in the course of antituberculosis drugs treatment. Acquired drug resistance is mostly due to inappropriate treatment and other factors that kill the original sensitive main flora, and a few drug-resistant mutant strains become the dominant flora, resulting in drug resistance.
3. Initial drug resistance

   Mycobacterium tuberculosis is known to be resistant to one or more antituberculosis drugs in patients with tuberculosis, but the patients treatment history is unknown. This includes primary drug resistance and a proportion of unproven acquired drug resistance.
4. Natural drug resistance

   It is a genetic mutation of Mycobacterium tuberculosis infected by a patient with tuberculosis prior to exposure to the drug, resulting in drug resistance. The process of its formation is a minority drug-resistant strain of Mycobacterium tuberculosis produced by the wild strain of Mycobacterium tuberculosis during its continued proliferation. This resistance is also a type of primary drug resistance, which also referred to a kind of wild-type drug-resistant mutant strains.

1.1.2 Definition and Classification of Drug-Resistant Pulmonary Tuberculosis

The definition and classification of drug-resistant tuberculosis are constantly changing and being updated. The current definition and classification of drug-resistant tuberculosis are based on the World Health Organization's (WHO) Definition and Reporting Framework for Tuberculosis (2013 revision), and cases are classified into the following categories [2] based on the results of drug sensitivity testing of clinical isolates of Mycobacterium tuberculosis.

1. Monoresistance

   Resistance to one first-line antituberculosis drug only.
2. Polydrug resistance

   Resistance to more than one first-line antituberculosis drug (other than both isoniazid and rifampicin).
3. Multidrug resistance (MDR)

   Resistance to at least both isoniazid and rifampicin.
4. Extensively drug resistant (XDR)

Y.-x. Wang (✉) · J.-j. Zhang · L.-a. Peng · F.-x. Hu · J.-z. Mei
Department for Tuberculosis Control and Prevention, Bao'an Chronic Diseases Prevent and Cure Hospital, Shenzhen, Guangdong, China

P.-X. Lu
Diagnostic Imaging, Shenzhen Center for Chronic Disease Control, Shenzhen, China

P.-x. Lu et al. (eds.), *Diagnostic Imaging of Drug Resistant Pulmonary Tuberculosis*,
https://doi.org/10.1007/978-981-99-8339-1_1

Resistance to any fluoroquinolone and at least one of the three second-line injectable drugs (capreomycin, kanamycin, and amikacin), in addition to multidrug resistance.

In October 2020, meeting report of the WHO Expert Consultation on Extensively Drug-Resistant Tuberculosis proposed a definition of Pre-XDR tuberculosis and revised the definition of XDR tuberculosis [3].

Pre-XDR: Fulfilling the definition of MDR/RR and also resistance to any fluoroquinoloneXDR: fulfilling the definition of MDR/RR and also resistance to any fluoroquinolone and at least one additional group A drug (including levofloxacin or moxifloxacin, bedaquiline, and linezolid).

5. Rifampicin resistance

   Resistance to rifampicin detected using phenotypic or genotypic methods, with or without resistance to other anti-TB drugs. It includes any resistance to rifampicin, whether monoresistance, multidrug resistance, polydrug resistance, or extensive drug resistance.

   These categories are not always mutually exclusive. For example, when enumerating rifampicin-resistant tuberculosis, multidrug-resistant tuberculosis and extensively drug-resistant tuberculosis are also included. Although the practice to date has been to limit the definition of monoresistance and polydrug resistance to first-line drugs, future treatment regimens may make it important to classify patient based on their strain resistance patterns to fluoroquinolones, second-line injectables, and any other antituberculosis drugs for which reliable drug sensitivity testing can be performed.

   In 2018, WHO Treatment Guidelines for Isoniazid-Resistant Tuberculosis introduced the concept of isoniazid-resistant tuberculosis, which refers to Mycobacterium tuberculosis strains with resistance to isoniazid and susceptibility to rifampicin confirmed in vitro [4].

1.2 Brief History of Drug-Resistant Pulmonary Tuberculosis

1.2.1 Causes of the Emergence of Drug-Resistant Pulmonary Tuberculosis

Drug-resistant tuberculosis is caused by microorganism, clinic and incorrect antituberculosis treatment.

1. Microbiological factors [1]
   (a) Inherently resistance, a wild strain that has never been exposed to a drug is inherently resistant to it, and the cause of which is not known.
   (b) Natural drug resistance, which refers to the natural mutations of Mycobacterium tuberculosis in the process of proliferation can lead to the emergence of a small number of drug-resistant bacteria.
   (c) Primary drug resistance, where Mycobacterium tuberculosis strains are resistant to one or more drugs before receiving antituberculosis treatment. It is caused by spread of drug-resistant Mycobacterium tuberculosis.
   (d) Initial drug resistance, defined as drug resistance that occurs on patients whose previous drug use is unknown or previous antituberculosis drug use duration is less than 1 month. This includes primary resistance and partially acquired resistance that occurs on patients whose drug use history is missing or concealed.
   (e) Acquired drug resistance, which occurs after antituberculosis drugs have been used for a period of 1 month or more, is called acquired drug resistance. The sensitive subject population is killed due to the factors such as inappropriate treatment, and a few naturally resistant mutant strains become the dominant population.
2. Clinical and planning factors [5]

   Inadequate or incorrect treatment regimens result in drug-resistant mutant bacteria becoming dominant in TB patients. Table 1.1 summarizes the common causes of incorrect treatment [5, 6]. Short courses of chemotherapy can cause patients with tuberculosis infected with drug-resistant strains to become more serious resistant to the drugs they used. This phenomenon has been defined as

Table 1.1 Reasons for incorrect antituberculosis treatment

Health service providers Incorrect regimens	Drugs Incorrect supply/quality	Patient Incorrectly taking medication
1. Incorrect guidelines 2. Guidance not followed 3. No guide 4. Inadequate training 5. Lack of treatment monitoring 6. Inappropriate management of drug adverse reactions 7. Poorly organized or underfunded planning for tuberculosis control	1. Poor quality of drugs 2. Lack of certain drugs (insufficient stock or interruption of supply) 3. Poor drug storage conditions 4. Wrong dose or combination of drugs 5. Poor drug administration	1. Poor adherence (or poor DOT implementation) 2. Lack of information 3. Lack of funding (free treatment cannot be provided) 4. Lack of therapeutic support (lack of transportation, lack of food, etc.) 5. Adverse reaction 6. Social problems 7. Drug malabsorption 8. Drug abuse/dependence

the "amplification effect" of short courses of chemotherapy. The spread of drug-resistant strains in the population is also an important source of primary drug-resistant patients.

1.2.2 Strategies for the Prevention and Control of Drug-Resistant Pulmonary Tuberculosis

Drug-resistant TB control strategies are integrated into global TB control strategy. From the perspective of the evolution of the global TB control strategy, drug-resistant TB control is playing an increasingly important role in global TB control.

1. TB control strategy based on directly observed treatment, short course (DOTS strategy)

   Due to the resurgence of tuberculosis in the early 1990s, the relevant WHO tuberculosis bodies began to re-evaluate tuberculosis control strategies. At the 46th World Health Assembly in 1993, WHO declared a "global tuberculosis emergency" and mobilized and requested governments to intensify tuberculosis control efforts to contain the tuberculosis crisis. In 1995, WHO launched the Directly Observed Treatment Short-course (DOTS) strategy, a global TB control strategy with the following five elements [7].

   (a) Government policy, financial and work capacity commitment to national TB control planning to guarantee the implementation of TB control measures.
   (b) Case detection among symptomatic patients self-reporting to health services, utilizing sputum smear microscopy.
   (c) Free treatment for sputum-smear-positive tuberculosis patients with the standard short-course chemotherapy, and direct observation of treatment must be administered in full or at least for the first 2 months of the course.
   (d) Establishment of a system of regular drug supply of all essential antituberculosis drugs.
   (e) Establishment and maintenance of a standard recording and reporting system allowing assessment of treatment.

2. DOTS-Plus strategy

   While the DOTS strategy can cure most TB patients, short-course chemotherapy regimens cannot completely cure patients with multidrug-resistant TB. Therefore, a considerable number of multidrug-resistant TB patients are chronically infectious. To achieve the goal of preventing the spread of multidrug-resistant TB, the WHO proposed a DOTS-Plus strategy in 1998.

   The DOTS-Plus strategy is an extension and complement of the DOTS strategy and is a comprehensive management strategy that includes the five essential elements of the DOTS strategy [8]. However, the DOTS-Plus strategy also takes into account issues that require special attention in areas where multidrug-resistant TB is severely prevalent, such as the use of second-line anti-TB drugs, individualized treatment regimens, etc. The DOTS-Plus strategy differs from the DOTS strategy as follows:

   (a) Treatment regimens should be individualized, not standardized.
   (b) There should be a laboratory capable of performing culture and drug sensitivity testing, not just sputum smear microscopy.
   (c) The need for continuous supply of reliable and affordable second-line antituberculosis drugs.
   (d) To carry out the necessary studies with practical applicability for the revision of the control plan.
   (e) In addition to the support of local governments, there should be more support from international organizations and developed countries.

3. Stop TB strategy

   On March 17, 2006, in order to significantly reduce the global burden of TB and achieve the United Nations Millennium Development Goals, WHO and the Stop TB Partnership proposed a new Stop TB Control Strategy based on an analysis of the successes of DOTS implementation over the years and the identification of new problems. The strategy addresses the current challenge faced by countries: how to continue strengthening TB control activities and also address TB-HIV co-infection and the spread of MDR-TB. It recognized the critical challenges of TB/HIV and multidrug-resistant TB based on the successful implementation of the DOTS strategy while. It also reflects constraints of the DOTS strategy implementation, its equity and quality, with the goal of ensuring all TB patients can access diagnosis and treatment and reaching the 2015 TB Millennium Development Goals and reducing the global TB burden.

   The Stop TB Strategy has six principal components [5]:

   (a) Pursuing high-quality DOTS expansion and enhancement: Political commitment with increased and sustained financing; strengthening government commitment to ensure sustained and increasing funding; case detection through quality-assured bacteriology; standardized treatment with supervision and patient support; effective drug supply and management system; monitoring and evaluation system and impact measurement.
   (b) Addressing TB/HIV, MDR-TB, XDR-TB, and other challenges by implementing collaborative TB/HIV actions, preventing and controlling of drug-resistant tuberculosis (including XDR-TB), addressing pris-

oners, refugees, and other high-risk groups and situations.

(c) Enhancing the strength of the health system: Collaborating with other health care projects and public services, such as by mobilizing necessary personnel resources and financial resources available for implementation and effect assessment, sharing and applying the achievements in TB control and new achievements in other fields.

(d) Mobilizing the participation of all health service providers (including public, non-governmental, and private): Ensuring the international standards for TB care are followed by continuously strengthening the cooperation of public and private institutions, with a focus on the poorest and most vulnerable groups.

(e) Arousing the initiative of TB patients and communities: Participate in TB patients care activities through advocacy, communication, and social mobilization.

(f) Enabling and promoting research to improve program performance and to develop new drugs, diagnostics, and vaccines. In 2006, WHO published Guidelines for the Programmatic and Management of Drug-Resistant Tuberculosis [9], which provide standardized technical operational methods of the detection, diagnosis, and management of drug-resistant tuberculosis for areas with different epidemics and planning characteristics worldwide. In 2008, an emergency revision was developed, and the new guidelines focus on providing uniform and updated recommendations for the diagnosis and management of drug-resistant TB in different geographical, political, economic, and social regions. Meanwhile, multiple factors were also considered, including the administration of culture and drug sensitivity testing to all suspected drug-resistant TB patients. Recommendations for effective treatment are drawn from the many experiences of drug-resistant TB treatment, and the emphasis on drug-resistant TB and HIV infection is strengthened [5].

In 2010, WHO released the Global Action Plan to Stop TB (2011–2015) [10], which sets out goals and recommendations for countries to combat drug-resistant TB, including:

(a) Expand the first-line anti-TB drugs drug resistance screening for ordinary PTB patients;
(b) Expand the second-line anti-TB drugs resistance screening, and diagnosis of HIV/AIDS testing for MDR-TB patients;
(c) Expand the evaluation of treatment effectiveness for drug-resistant TB patients;
(d) Improve infection control for MDR-TB in hospital and outpatient department;
(e) Strengthen drug-resistant TB surveillance, including registration and reporting;
(f) Through global mobilization and policy guidance, improve the national management for drug-resistant TB.

4. End TB Strategy (ETS) [11].

In May 2014, Governments at the World Health Assembly accepted the WHO's proposal *WHO Global Strategy to End Tuberculosis beyond 2015*. The objective of this strategy is to "end the global tuberculosis epidemic," with three high-level overarching targets, associated targets (the year 2030 and 2035, indicators related to sustainable development) and milestones (the year 2020 and 2025). The three indicators are: (1) the number of TB deaths per year; (2) the annual incidence of TB; (3) the percentage of TB-affected family facing catastrophic expenditures due to TB (Table 1.2).

The end tuberculosis strategy has three pillars:

(a) Patient-centered comprehensive treatment and prevention: Carry out early diagnosis of TB, including universal access to drug sensitivity testing and systematic screening for contacts and high-risk groups; treat all TB patients including drug-resistant TB patients, and patients holding services should also be considered; conduct TB/AIDS cooperation activities, and manage TB combined with AIDS dual infection groups; provide preventive treatment for high-risk population and vaccination against TB.

Table 1.2 Indicators of the strategy to end tuberculosis

	Milestones		Targets	
Indicators	2020	2025	2030	2035
Percentage reduction in the absolute number of TB deaths (compared with 2015 baseline)	35%	75%	90%	95%
Percentage reduction in the incidence rate of tuberculosis (compared with 2015 baseline)	20%	50%	80%	90% <10/100,000
Percentage of tuberculosis affected households facing catastrophic costs due to tuberculosis (level in 2015 unknown)	0	0	0	0

(b) Strong policy and support system: Political commitment and sufficient resources should be provided for TB care and prevention; community, civil society organizations, and public and private health service providers participate in the TB control activities; establish national health coverage policy and case reporting regulatory framework frame, population dynamic registration, drug quality and rational use, infection control; improve measures for social security, poverty alleviation, and other determines the actions for TB.

(c) Strengthen research and innovation: New tools, interventions, and strategies should be discovered, developed, and quickly adopted; optimize implementation and effectiveness; and promote innovation through research.

5. The magnitude of the problem of drug-resistant pulmonary tuberculosis

Looking at global tuberculosis control strategies, it is clear that the control of drug-resistant tuberculosis has become increasingly crucial. Despite significant success in the control of drug-resistant tuberculosis in several countries with the improvement of tuberculosis control strategies, drug-resistant tuberculosis is still a critical public health threat.

The WHO released the 2021 Annual Global TB Report [12], which showed that 71% (2.1/3 million) of TB patients with positive etiological diagnosis received rifampicin resistance test in 2020, which was higher than 61% (2.2/3.6 million) in 2019 and 50% in 2018 (1.7/3.4 million). And a total of 157,903 MDR/RR-TB, pre-XDR-TB or XDR-TB cases were found (132,222 MDR/RR-TB cases and 25,681 pre-XDR-TB or XDR-TB cases), significantly lower than 201,997 cases in 2019 with a decrease of 22%. The burden of MDR/RR-TB was stable in the past decade, with the proportion of MDR/RR-TB among the newly diagnosed TB patients and among previous diagnosed patients maintaining at 3%–4% and 18%–21%, respectively. A total of 150,359 MDR/RR-TB patients were registered for treatment in 2020, which was only equivalent to one-third of the incidence of MDR/RR-TB, with a 15% decrease from 177,100 in 2019.

The success rate of drug-resistant TB treatment remains low, with a global average of 57%. In 2019, the annual number of MDR/RR-TB deaths is approximately 182000 [13]. Regarding this situation, urgent action is needed to further improve the coverage and quality of diagnosis, treatment, and care for people with drug-resistant TB. As of August 2021, there are 14 vaccine candidates in clinical trials, including candidates to prevent TB infection, prevent the development of TB, and improve TB patients outcomes [12, 14]. Efficacy can be expected in the future with the use of new effective vaccines in the clinic.

1.2.3 Major Journeys in the Diagnosis and Treatment of Drug-Resistant Pulmonary Tuberculosis

The prevalence of the drug-resistant TB has increased since the first application of streptomycin for the treatment of TB in 1943. In the 1970s, the widespread use of rifampicin led to the emergence of MDR-TB, which prompted the use of second-line antituberculosis drugs. With the widespread use of antituberculosis drugs, incorrect antituberculosis treatment exacerbated the emergence and spread of XDR-TB, leading to strains resistant to isoniazid, rifampicin and at least one fluoroquinolone and one injectable.

The diagnosis of drug-resistant tuberculosis plays an important role in the development of standardized treatment of tuberculosis. Bacteriological diagnosis and molecular biology diagnosis are the most widely used methods to diagnose drug-resistant tuberculosis in the world. Bacteriological diagnosis mainly includes isolation and culture of Mycobacterium tuberculosis and drug susceptibility test, among which, drug susceptibility test (DST) is currently the main tool to determine drug-resistant tuberculosis and is also a major diagnostic tool to determine whether antituberculosis drug resistance has developed. With the widespread use of molecular biology in the field of medicine, the principles of molecular biology have been applied to the diagnosis of drug-resistant tuberculosis and drug resistance monitoring. Molecular biology diagnosis has been increasing widely used in the diagnosis of drug-resistant tuberculosis because of its efficient and convenient. Currently, the main techniques of molecular biology diagnosis include molecular linear probe assays, gene Xpert MTB/RIF methods, and gene microarray technology, other methods such as DNA sequencing, dideoxy fingerprinting, heterologous double-stranded conformation, denaturing gradient gel electrophoresis, fluorescent quantitative PCR, and thermostatic amplification assays. The companion handbook to the WHO guidelines for the programmatic management of drug-resistant tuberculosis published in 2014 from WHO highlighted the important value of molecular biology methods in the drug-resistant TB diagnosis [15], which can shorten the time for pathogenic diagnosis and drug resistance surveillance. Molecular biology diagnosis is also recommended for rapid diagnosis of MDR-TB in high-risk populations in order to detect drug-resistant TB patients earlier, prevent further transmission of TB, and control the drug-resistant TB epidemic.

In terms of treatment, a comprehensive treatment strategy is usually advocated for drug-resistant tuberculosis, which mainly includes chemotherapy, interventional therapy, surgery, immunotherapy, traditional Chinese medicine, and nutritional support therapy, among which chemotherapy is currently the most important means of treating drug-resistant tuberculosis. When formulating a treatment plan, a comprehensive determination should be made to select the appropriate treatment drugs, considering the patient's drug use history, drug resistance, and the prevalence of drug-resistant strains in the region. In 2006, the first edition of the WHO Guidelines for the Programmatic Management of Drug-Resistant Tuberculosis (2006) was prepared [9], and an emergency revision was published in 2008 [5]. The emergency revision provides common treatment strategies for drug-resistant tuberculosis, drug groupings, and the design and recommendations of treatment regimens. The emergency revision states that the course of treatment is based on negative sputum cultures and recommends at least 18 months of treatment following negative sputum cultures, unless there is evidence to support a conclusive reduction in the course of treatment. The recommended duration of treatment for "chronic patients" with extensive lung lesions was extended to 24 months. The recommendations for regimen composition have been updated in 2011 update of Guidelines for the programmatic management of drug-resistant tuberculosis [16]: (1) Include at least four second-line antituberculosis drugs likely to be effective as well as pyrazinamide during the intensive phase of treatment; (2) No evidence found to support the use of more than four second-line antituberculosis drugs in patients with extensive disease. Increasing the number of second-line drugs in a regimen is permissible if the effectiveness of some of the drugs is uncertain; (3) The regimen should include pyrazinamide, a fluoroquinolone, a parenteral agent, ethionamide (or prothionamide), and cycloserine, or else PAS if cycloserine cannot be used; (4) Ethambutol may be used but is not included among the drugs making up the standard regimen; (5) Group 5 drugs may be used but are not included among the drugs making up the standard regimen. In the treatment of patients with MDR-TB, an intensive phase of 8 months is suggested for most patients, a total treatment duration of 20 months is suggested for most newly diagnosed patients with MDR-TB, and the duration may be modified according to the patient's response to therapy. Afterwards, WHO published Companion handbook to the WHO guidelines for the programmatic management of drug-resistant tuberculosis in 2014 [15] and again published the Updated Planning and Management Guidelines for Drug-Resistant Tuberculosis in 2016 [17] and proposed the short-course chemotherapy regimen. In 2018, WHO published "Rapid Communication: Key Changes to Treatment of Multidrug and Rifampicin-Resistant Tuberculosis (MDR/RR-TB)" [18], which changed the classification of major drugs in the long-course MDR-TB regimen based on the latest evidence-based medical evidence. The Guidelines for Isoniazid-Resistant Tuberculosis were published in the same year [4], outlining treatment regimens for isoniazid resistance.

1.3 Major Diagnostic and Treatment Advances in Drug-Resistant Pulmonary Tuberculosis

1.3.1 Advances in the Diagnosis of Drug-Resistant Pulmonary Tuberculosis

Currently, the diagnosis of drug-resistant TB relies heavily on DST, which in turn is based on a positive culture of Mycobacterium tuberculosis. Therefore, traditional techniques for the diagnosis of drug-resistant TB, such as absolute concentration method, proportional method, Bact/Alert 3D liquid culture system, BACTEC MGIT 960 detection technique, direct observation of drug sensitivity by microscopy, etc., often have the disadvantages, such as long reporting time, high technical requirements for laboratory operation, and biological hazards to the operating environment and personnel, which can hardly meet the demand for early diagnosis of drug-resistant TB [19].

In recent years, with the increasing maturity of genotypic rapid diagnostic technologies such as linear probe technology, Gene Xpert MTB/RIF technology, gene chip technology, and whole gene sequencing technology, their diagnostic value has gradually been widely validated and recognized due to their ease of operation, shorter positive reporting time, and lower biohazards [20, 21]. The results of drug sensitivity testing by molecular biology methods were put on the equally important position as traditional DST in Companion Handbook to the WHO Guidelines for the Programmatic Management of Drug-Resistant Tuberculosis published in 2014 from WHO because their testing methods were regard as same reference value, which gained valuable time to make an individualized and standardized treatment plan earlier for drug-resistant TB [15]. In January 2021, a categorical evaluation of nucleic acid amplification tests (NAATs) for TB/drug-resistant TB discovery conducted by WHO found that automated NAATs of varying complexity, such as the Abbott RealTime MTB and Abbott RealTime MTB RIF/INH (Abbott), Xpert MTB/XDR (Cepheid), and Genoscholar PZA-TB II (Nipro) were found to have high sensitivity and specificity for patient detection of TB/drug-resistant TB [22]. In addition, the Gene Xpert Omni®, a rapid molecular biology diagnostic for remote TB and rifampicin-resistant TB, was launched in

2015 by Cepheid and FIND in the USA as a battery-powered, portable, wireless device that is similar with Cepheid's other existing Gene Xpert systems. It is capable of running PCR kits with high quality and transmitting the result data in real time over a cellular data transmission network, but commercialization is still a way off [23]. Molecular assays such as Xpert MTB/RIF, Xpert MTB/RIF Ultra, Linear Probe, and TB-LAMP for TB/drug-resistant TB discovery have been approved by WHO at this stage. Safety and efficacy of eight molecular assays such as FluoroType MTBDR, BD Max MDR-TB, and Xpert XDR-TB test kits are evaluated by WHO. iCubate system, GeneChip, and other four molecular detection technologies are already applied in the market, but has not yet evaluated by WHO. Gendrive MTB/RIF ID, TruArray MDR-TB, and other eight molecular detection technologies are still under development [13]. Although the rapid diagnosis of drug-resistant tuberculosis represented by molecular biology can significantly shorten the diagnosis time, the cost of necessary equipment is much more than traditional testing methods, which limits its promotion and application [24].

Although imaging is not a confirmed diagnosis of tuberculosis or drug-resistant tuberculosis, it can provide clues and help in the early diagnosis of drug-resistant tuberculosis by summarizing the imaging manifestations and features. It was found that tree-in-bud sign and acinar nodule were the most frequent patterns of lung abnormality in primary multidrug-resistant TB [25], and the probability about involve lungs of lesion was close to 100%, with more than 50% of the lungs showing cavities, of which, more than 85% had more than one cavity [26]. Although there are many similarities in the CT imaging presentation of drug-resistant tuberculosis, the differences exhibited by extensively drug-resistant versus multidrug-resistant tuberculosis in terms of dendritic signs, pulmonary solidity, and cavity size are statistically significant [27, 28]. In the areas with high HIV prevalence, chest radiographic presentation of multidrug-resistant TB in children was not related to HIV infection, with solid lung changes (53.5%) being the most common presentation, followed by enlarged lymph nodes (35.6%), bronchiectasis (33.3%), and intrapulmonary cavities (31.1%) [29]. Thus, the expansion of intrapulmonary cavities in children with non-drug-resistant TB who are starting standardized treatment may indicate poor disease control, parenchymal lung damages and drug resistance increasing, and further medical disposal requiring.

It has been found that the mean age of patients with primary drug-resistant tuberculosis is lower than non-drug-resistant tuberculosis [30, 31] and the differences demonstrated by intrapulmonary nodules and bronchiectasis on CT imaging have statistically significant [30]. However, according to the researches that were done by Chung, M. J (2006) et al. [31], widely distributed bronchiectasis may be suggestive of non-tuberculous mycobacterial disease. In addition, the frequency of pulmonary cavitation was similarly higher in patients with primary drug-resistant tuberculosis than in non-drug-resistant tuberculosis, with the number of cavities mostly being 3 or more, and this was the only statistically significant factor [32–34].

1.3.2 Advances in the Treatment of Drug-Resistant Pulmonary Tuberculosis

Chemotherapy remains the mainstay of treatment for drug-resistant tuberculosis. As of 2019, there are 22 antituberculosis drugs in phase I, II, or III clinical trials worldwide, including 13 new antituberculosis drugs such as delpazolid (a new oxazolidinone antibiotic), pretomanid (a new nitroimidazole drug approved by the US FDA for the treatment of extensively drug-resistant tuberculosis in 2019), and 6 new uses of marketed drugs, such as clofazimine (a drug used to treat leprosy) and moxifloxacin for extensively drug-resistant/rifampicin-resistant treatment [13]. Although new antituberculosis drugs such as bedaquiline and delamanid have been introduced, chemotherapy for drug-resistant tuberculosis still requires prolonged injections and a combination of multiple oral antituberculosis drugs with high drug adverse effects, high treatment costs, and low cure rates [35].

As of August 2021, there were 25 drugs in phase I, II, or III clinical trials for the treatment of sensitive tuberculosis, MDR-TB, or tuberculosis infection, including 16 new chemical entities, 2 drugs that have received accelerated regulatory approval, 1 antibacterial and antifungal drugs that have recently approved by FDA under the limited stock pathway and 6 modified-use drugs. The treatment contains injectable drugs such as streptomycin for monoisoniazid-resistant tuberculosis was no longer recommended in WHO consolidated guidelines on drug-resistant tuberculosis treatment published in 2019, and a short course of chemotherapy regimen of 9–12 month may be used instead of a long course for multidrug/rifampicin-resistant TB that uses second-line antituberculosis drugs for less than a month or who are unable to use fluoroquinolones and second-line injectable drug regimens [36]. Previous studies have also shown that a 9-month short course of chemotherapy for multidrug-resistant pulmonary tuberculosis is cheaper and improved the cure rate considerably [37, 38].

In addition to conventional chemotherapy, timely surgical treatment can significantly improve the cure rate of multidrug-resistant TB meanwhile reduce the mortality and disease reversal rate [39].WHO guidelines on the treatment of drug-resistant TB also recommend the use of selective pneumonectomy as a complement to conventional chemotherapy regimens for multidrug/rifampicin-resistant TB [36]. For inoperable drug-resistant TB, adjunctive therapy based on conventional chemotherapy regimens, such as Chinese herbal therapy, immunotherapy, transbronchoscopic interventions, and nutritional support therapy, may be helpful for improving treatment outcomes [40].

References

1. Tang SHJ, Gao W. Clinical tuberculosis [M]. First2 edition. Beijing: People's Health Publishing House; 2019.
2. World Health Organization. Definitions and reporting framework for tuberculosis-2013 revision [R]. Geneva: World Health Organization; 2013. https://apps.who.int/iris/handle/10665/79199.
3. Meeting report of the WHO expert consultation on the definition of extensively drug-resistant tuberculosis, 27–29 Meeting report of the WHO expert consultation on the definition of extensively drug-resistant tuberculosis, 27–29 October 2020 [EB/OL]. Geneva: World Health Organization; 2021. https://apps.who.int/iris/handle/10665/338776.
4. World Health Organization. WHO treatment guidelines for isoniazid-resistant tuberculosis: supplement to the WHO treatment guidelines for drug-resistant tuberculosis [R]. Geneva: World Health Organization; 2018. https://apps.who.int/iris/handle/10665/260494.
5. World Health Organization. Guidelines for the programmatic management of drug-resistant tuberculosis: emergency update 2008 [R]. Geneva: World Health Organization; 2008. https://apps.who.int/iris/handle/10665/43965.
6. Piubello A, Aït-Khaled N, Caminero JA, et al. Field guide for the management of drug-resistant tuberculosis 2018[R]. Paris: International Union Against Tuberculosis and Lung Disease, 2018.
7. He GX, Wang LX. Evolution of tuberculosis control strategies [J]. Prevent Med Forum. 2008;14(6):481–4.
8. Shen X, Mei J, Gao Q. DOTS-Plus: a powerful weapon for controlling multidrug-resistant tuberculosis [J]. Shanghai J Prevent Med. 2006;18(5):225–6.
9. World Health Organization. Guidelines for the programmatic management of drug-resistant tuberculosis [R]. Geneva: World Health Organization; 2006. https://apps.who.int/iris/handle/10665/246249.
10. World Health Organization. The global plan to stop TB 2011–2015: transforming the fight towards elimination of tuberculosis [R]. Geneva: World Health Organization; 2010. https://apps.who.int/iris/handle/10665/44437.
11. World Health Organization. The end TB strategy [R]. Geneva: World Health Organization; 2014. https://apps.who.int/iris/handle/10665/331326.
12. World Health Organization. Global tuberculosis report 2021 [EB/OL]. [2021-10-14]. https://www.who.int/publications/digital/global-tuberculosis-report-2021.
13. World Health Organization. Global tuberculosis report 2020 [R]. Geneva: World Health Organization; 2020. https://apps.who.int/iris/handle/10665/336069.
14. Chunrong L, Hongxia F, Puxuan L, et al. The global tuberculosis report 2021: key data analysis for China and the global world [J/CD]. J Emerg Infect Dis. 2021;6(4):368–72.
15. World Health Organization. Companion handbook to the WHO guidelines for the programmatic management of drug-resistant tuberculosis [R]. Geneva: World Health Organization; 2014. https://apps.who.int/iris/handle/10665/130918.
16. World Health Organization. Guidelines for the programmatic management of drug-resistant tuberculosis, 2011 update [R]. Geneva: World Health Organization; 2011. https://apps.who.int/iris/handle/10665/44597.
17. World Health Organization. WHO treatment guidelines for drug-resistant tuberculosis, 2016 update [R]. Geneva: World Health Organization; 2016. https://apps.who.int/iris/handle/10665/250125.
18. World Health Organization. Rapid communication: key changes to treatment of multidrug- and rifampicin-resistant tuberculosis (MDR/RR-TB) [R]. Geneva: World Health Organization; 2018. https://apps.who.int/iris/handle/10665/275383.
19. Yan F. Evaluation of rapid diagnostic methods for drug-resistant tuberculosis and analysis of treatment effects [D]. Nanjing Medical University; 2014.
20. Wang L, Hu J, Guo Q. Diagnostic value of gene chip technology testing for drug resistance of Mycobacterium tuberculosis [J]. Chin J Pract Diagn Ther. 2018;32(4):393–4.
21. Lianshuang Z, Di D, Xin C, et al. Diagnostic value of gene microarray in mycobacterial strain identification and tuberculosis drug resistance gene detection [J]. Lab Med Clin. 2014;11(12):1595–8.
22. World Health Organization. Update on the use of nucleic acid amplification tests to detect TB and drug-resistant TB: rapid communication [R]. Geneva: World Health Organization; 2021. https://apps.who.int/iris/handle/10665/339611.
23. Accurate molecular diagnostics for remote locations—GeneXpert® Omni [EB/OL]. Cepheid. [2015-08-28]. https://www.rapidmicrobiology.com/news/accurate-molecular-diagnostics-for-remote-locations-genexpert-omni.
24. Yao WM, Chen CH, Zangya P, et al. Whole-gene sequencing analysis of methicillin-resistant Staphylococcus aureus linezolid resistance-associated variant loci [J]. Chin J Infect Control. 2017;16(1):1–5.
25. Kim W, Lee KS, Kim HS, et al. CT and microbiologic follow-up in primary multidrug-resistant pulmonary tuberculosis [J]. Acta Radiol. 2016;57(2):197–204.
26. Joshi AR, Mishra S, Sankhe AP, et al. HRCT spectrum of pulmonary multidrug-resistant tuberculosis in HIV negative patients: a study in Indian population [J]. Int J Sci Res. 2017;6(9):596–600.
27. Lee ES, Park CM, Goo JM, et al. Computed tomography features of extensively drug-resistant pulmonary tuberculosis in non-HIV-infected patients [J]. J Comput Assist Tomogr. 2010;34(4):559–63.
28. Cheon H. Comparison of CT findings of between MDR-TB and XDR-TB: a propensity score matching study [J]. Imaging Med. 2017;9(5):125–9.
29. Manikkam S, Archary M, Bobat R. Chest X-ray patterns of pulmonary multidrug-resistant tuberculosis in children in a high HIV-prevalence setting [J]. South Afr J Radiol. 2016;20(1):e1–6.
30. Li D, He W, Chen B, et al. Primary multidrug-resistant tuberculosis versus drug-sensitive tuberculosis in non-HIV-infected patients: comparisons of CT findings [J]. PLoS One. 2017;12(6):e176354.
31. Chung MJ, Lee KS, Koh W, et al. Drug-sensitive tuberculosis, multidrug-resistant tuberculosis, and nontuberculous mycobacterial pulmonary disease in non-AIDS adults: comparisons of thin-section CT findings [J]. Eur Radiol. 2006;16(9):1934–41.
32. Kim HC, Goo JM, Lee HJ, et al. Multidrug-resistant tuberculosis versus drug-sensitive tuberculosis in human immunodeficiency virus-negative patients: computed tomography features [J]. J Comput Assist Tomogr. 2004;28(3):366–71.
33. Wang Y-x, Chung MJ, Skrahin A, et al. Literature analysis of radiological signs related to multidrug-resistant tuberculosis [J]. Electron J Emerg Infect Dis. 2018;3(2):244–53.
34. Luyao M, Qiuting Z, Punxuan L, et al. Pulmonary multi-drug resistant tuberculosis: a radiological review [J]. Emerg Infect Dis. 2021;6(1):58–65.
35. Liu YH. The role of injectable antituberculosis drugs in the treatment of drug-resistant tuberculosis in China [J]. Chin J Tuberc Respir. 2019;42(6):401–4.

36. Would Health Organization. WHO consolidated guidelines on drug-resistant tuberculosis treatment [G]. Geneva: Would Health Organization; 2019. https://apps.who.int/iris/handle/10665/311389.
37. Moodley R, Godec TR. Short-course treatment for multidrug-resistant tuberculosis: the STREAM trials [J]. Eur Respir Rev. 2016;25(139):29–35.
38. Kurbatova EV, Dalton T, Ershova J, et al. Additional drug resistance of multidrug-resistant tuberculosis in patients in 9 countries [J]. Emerg Infect Dis. 2015;21(6):977–83.
39. Sikuan Y, Pan Z, Chuanli Y, et al. Clinical effect analysis of early surgical treatment of multidrug-resistant pulmonary tuberculosis [J]. J Third Milit Med Univ. 2013;35(7):685–7.
40. Shenjie T. Review and perspectives on the comprehensive treatment of drug-resistant tuberculosis [J]. J Tuberc Lung Health. 2014;3(3):141–7.

2 Detection of Drug-Resistant Pulmonary Tuberculosis and Its Epidemics

Fan Zhang, Yong-xiang Yi, Hong-zhou Lu, Qi An, Zhun Yu, and Pu-Xuan Lu

2.1 Detection of Drug-Resistant Tuberculosis

Timely detection of drug-resistant pulmonary is the vital step in controlling drug-resistant tuberculosis, and earlier detection of more patients with drug-resistant pulmonary tuberculosis is a powerful measure to reduce the spread of this disease. Moreover, earlier detection of drug-resistant pulmonary tuberculosis means lesser severity of pulmonary lesions with lesser pulmonary injuries. Lesser quantity and categories of drug-resistant tubercle bacillus are related to easier treatment with cheaper expenses. The earlier control and eradication of infectious source is performed, the lesser spreading of the drug-resistant bacteria among populations. The later the drug-resistant pulmonary tuberculosis is detected, the more prolonged course of disease will be, with progressing pulmonary lesions and greater pulmonary injuries. The increase in quantity and categories of drug-resistant tubercle bacillus in lungs means the decrease in susceptible drugs available with higher ratio of unresponsiveness to the treatment. The severe disease may develop into pulmonary destruction with a great impact on pulmonary function, leading to respiratory failure and endangering the life. Early detection and treatment for drug-resistant pulmonary tuberculosis, therefore, is of great benefits for both patients and the whole society [1].

2.1.1 Target Populations in Screening Drug-Resistant Pulmonary Tuberculosis

Drug susceptibility test should be carried out for all cases positive in sputum culture, and the screening of drug-resistant tuberculosis has become a commonly used strategy for controlling tuberculosis. This mass screening maximizes the successful detection of drug-resistant tuberculosis and facilitates us to achieve early detection, early diagnosis, early treatment or intervention of this disease as well as early control of infectious sources.

As for regions insufficient in expenses and capacities, surveillance should be performed with focuses at least on populations with high risks in drug-resistant tuberculosis, including: (1) close contacts of a patient with drug-resistant tuberculosis; (2) inhabitants in areas affected worst by the pandemic, where the newly found pulmonary tuberculosis patients should routinely receive the culture of tubercle bacillus and drug susceptibility test; (3) those with a family history of tuberculosis; (4) those exposed to an irregular anti-tuberculosis treatment for more than 1 month; (5) treatment-naive pulmonary tuberculosis patients still positive in sputum smear/culture after receiving the standard anti-tuberculosis for more than 2 or 3 months; (6) those unresponsive to the first-line treatment, i.e., persisting positiveness in sputum smear or culture until the end of month 5 or 6 of the treatment; (7) relapsing patients or those with chronic bacterial excretion. Treatment against drug-resistant tuberculosis can be launched directly in regions where drug susceptibility is

F. Zhang (✉)
Department of Tuberculosis Prevention and Control, Shenzhen Nanshan Center for Chronic Disease Control, Shenzhen, Guangdong, China

Y.-x. Yi
Hepatobiliary Surgery, Nanjing Drum Tower Hospital, Nanjing, China

H.-z. Lu
Infectious Disease, The Third People's Hospital of Shenzhen, Shenzhen, China
e-mail: luhongzhou@shphc.org.cn

Q. An
School of Architecture, Harbin Institute of Technology, Shenzhen, China

Z. Yu
Southern University of Science and Technology Hospital, Shenzhen, China

P.-X. Lu
Diagnostic Imaging, Shenzhen Center for Chronic Disease Control, Shenzhen, China

P.-x. Lu et al. (eds.), *Diagnostic Imaging of Drug Resistant Pulmonary Tuberculosis*,
https://doi.org/10.1007/978-981-99-8339-1_2

hard to carry out or regions with insufficient resources in patients including the following three groups [2]: (1) patients still unresponsive to a strictly standardized type-II therapeutic regimen, who often should be suspected as the sufferers with drug-resistant tuberculosis; (2) patients with active pulmonary tuberculosis who has the onset after close contact with any drug-resistant tuberculosis patient; (3) those unresponsive to type-I therapeutic regimen; given the great difference in pandemics of drug-resistant tuberculosis in this group of patients, a confirmation is necessary using a drug susceptibility test as far as possible.

2.1.2 Collection of Samples for Drug Susceptibility Test and Application of Rapid Drug-Resistance Test

The rapid diagnosis of drug resistance in Mycobacterium tuberculosis is the key in controlling drug-resistant pulmonary tuberculosis, based on which patients with drug-resistant pulmonary tuberculosis can be detected early, and effective quarantine and reasonable medication can be launched, thereby preventing from further transmission of drug-resistant pulmonary tuberculosis. Traditional drug susceptibility test (DST) is still the gold criteria for diagnosing drug-resistant tuberculosis, though its clinical application is limited by factors such as long reporting cycle and biological safety. Analytical techniques of molecular biology used widely in recent years may facilitate us to make the diagnosis for the drug resistance of Mycobacterium tuberculosis through detecting the target genes related to drug resistance, which overcomes the deficiency that the traditional phenotypic method depends on the growth of Mycobacterium tuberculosis and maximizes the efficiency in diagnosing drug-resistant patients. WHO recommends that the approved rapid DST in molecular biology be used as an initial method to detect rifampicin resistance in all tuberculosis patients (including treatment-naive and relapsing patients) before they begin to receive appropriate treatment [3].

Xpert MTB/RIF is an automatic integrated semi-nested real-time fluorescent quantitative PCR system, the unique one in the world, and characterized in simple operation, short time consumption, less cross pollution, safety to the environment and laboratory personnel, and quick detection of rifampicin resistance in early stage. Since its clinical application in 2010 as recommended by WHO, substantial evidences have been accumulated in the clinical practices, further confirming the value of Xpert MTB/RIF® to be a tool for the initial diagnosis of tuberculosis and rifampicin-resistant tuberculosis. Its sensibility and specificity, as shown by results of researches, are 96% and 98%, respectively, in detecting rifampicin resistance. Gene Xpert, however, is capable of detecting rifampicin resistance only. WHO provided the global estimate of the incidence of isoniazid resistance for the first time in 2019 that there were 1.4 million isoniazid-resistant TB cases, of which 1.1 million were susceptible to rifampicin. Most of these people had not been diagnosed as drug-resistant tuberculosis and had not received appropriate anti-TB treatment [4].

The second generation of Xpert MTB/RIF Ultra launched in 2017, as compared with its first generation (Xpert MTB/RIF), had enlarged chambers for kits detecting DNA amplification, with an augmentation of additional two molecular targets for detecting Mycobacterium tuberculosis. Its lower detection limit was equivalent to 1/8 of that of the first generation (i.e., <15 CFU/mL vs. 100 CFU/mL–120 CFU/mL), with its positiveness/negativeness reporting time shortened, respectively, to 77 and 66 min from the previous 110 min. Xpert MTB/RIF Ultra is applicable to the clinical scope for Gene Xpert recommended by WHO and to the detection of Mycobacterium tuberculosis in specific extra-pulmonary specimens (such as cerebrospinal fluid, lymph nodes, and biopsy specimens) [5]. As shown by meta-analysis, Xpert MTB/RIF Ultra has a sensitivity (a sensibility of 94% and a specificity of 99%) similar to that of Gene Xpert, in respect of the detection of rifampicin resistance.

Xpert MTB/XDR developed by Cepheid is capable of detecting the resistance to isoniazid, fluoroquinolones, ethylthioisonicotinamide, and the second-line injection drugs in sediment of original and concentrated sputum positive in Mycobacterium tuberculosis. This technique has shown a sensibility of 94–100% with a specificity of 100% in detecting the resistance to all drugs except for ethylthioisonicotinamide in 100 sputum specimens and 214 clinical isolation in comparison with results of sequencing, and its sensibility and specificity are in the same range when compared with phenotypic susceptibility test. It is anticipated to magnify the power of real-time detection of drug-resistant tuberculosis [6].

In patients with rifampicin-resistant tuberculosis, a timely detection of the additional resistance to isoniazid and fluoroquinolones should be performed at least to guide treatment decisions. Now WHO recommends using commercially available molecular linear probes for the initial detection of fluoroquinolones resistance in rifampicin-resistant patients. A linear probe, Geno-Type@MTBDRplus, is based on a hybridization between a specific probe fixed into a nitrocellulose membrane and amplified products carrying biotin post to multiplex-PCR using a primer modifying DNA of Mycobacterium tuberculosis, so as to determine drug resistance through an enzyme immunochromogenic reaction. Besides rifampicin resistance in MTB, it can also detect the resistance to isoniazid, fluoroquinolones, and the second-line injection drugs.

Crude et al. have reported [7] that the sensibility and specificity of this method are 94.3% and 96.0%, respectively, in detecting the simultaneous resistance to isoniazid and rifampicin. With a short detection cycle, linear probe can be completed within 24 h. Therefore, it is recommended by WHO as one of the main methods for the diagnosis of drug-resistant tuberculosis [8]. There is still a certain challenge, however, in popularizing the linear probe due to limitations on probes on the membrane making it impossible to detect all categories of drug-resistant tuberculosis, the high price of the kits, and the strict requirement on laboratory conditions and technicians.

The fundamental principle of DNA microarray (i.e., gene chip) is to hybridize the fluorescent labeled target nucleotide molecule (i.e., Mycobacterium tuberculosis DNA (MTB DNA)) with the probe on the chip, so as to obtain information about the number of molecules and the sequence of the tested sample by scanning. Microarray is mainly used to detect quickly the wild type and various mutations of three drug-resistant mutation genes including genes rpo, katG, and inhA related to the resistance to rifampicin and isoniazid. The coincidence rate between gene chip and traditional drug susceptibility tests for diagnosing isoniazid resistance, rifampicin resistance, and multidrug resistance is 98.8–100.0%, indicating that gene chip has high sensitivity and specificity. The commercialized gene chip limited by detection probes, however, detects only common mutant genes with the high price and necessitates specific laboratory equipment and professionals, so it is mostly used in scientific research now.

MTB DNA direct sequencing method, which is the most direct and reliable method in detecting the mutation of Mtb resistance gene, uses PCR to sequence directly the cloned DNA fragments, followed by a comparison with the sequence of the same DNA fragment from the standard susceptible strain, so as to identify mutated nucleotide sites. Characterized by high throughput, high automation, and automatic data processing, it has been applied successfully to the detection of mutations of multiple sites such as rpoB, ndh, KatG, rpsL, and rrs. However, this technology necessitates its operation in laboratory with a high operational requirement and a high cost and is mainly applied to scientific research now.

2.1.3 Detection of Pediatric Drug-Resistant Tuberculosis

It is a challenge to detect pediatric drug-resistant tuberculosis. Lower ratio of etiology diagnosis with more difficulties in drug susceptibility test can be seen in children than in adults due to the absence of specificity of clinical symptoms, difficulty in obtaining sputum, and low bacterial load in children.

Lack of monitoring data concerning the pediatric tuberculosis in the world and in China results in our uncertainty of drug resistance of tuberculosis in children. An analysis by Jiao et al. on drug resistance in Mycobacterium tuberculosis originating from China (including 100 strains in the cohort of children and 191 strains in that of adults) showed a general resistance rate of 55% and multi-resistance rate of 22% in pediatric tuberculosis, which seemed similar to data of adult patients with these two rates of 60.2% and 30.9%, respectively. Further researches showed that 52% of pediatric MDR-TB patients were treatment-naive, and further analysis is needed to evaluate the re-infection ratio in relapsing patients [9].

It is stipulated in WS288-2017 Pulmonary Tuberculosis Diagnosis China that positiveness at least in two specimens (smear, histology, or culture) is required for etiological diagnosis of pulmonary tuberculosis, and the etiological examination of gastric juice should be paid attention to in the diagnosis of pediatric tuberculosis [10]. It is difficult to obtain qualified sputum samples in children, and the positiveness rate in sputum smear is as low as 17.1–26.3% with negativeness in almost all other body fluid smears. Multiple sampling methods are recommended including continuous collection of biological samples, such as sputum, bronchoalveolar lavage fluid (BAL), nasopharyngeal aspirate, gastric aspirate (GA), lymph node aspirate, biopsy samples, cerebrospinal fluid, urine, etc., in order to improve the positiveness rate in bacteriological examination. Several studies support that gastric aspirate (GA) in combination with bronchoalveolar lavage fluid (BAL) may improve bacteriological detection rate for pediatric pulmonary tuberculosis. Therefore, composite reference criteria with a variety of non-pulmonary specimens are often adopted to evaluate the performance of new tools for diagnosing pediatric tuberculosis. Xpert MTB/RIF and Xpert Ultra are techniques available for disposing various types of the specimens such as sputum, stool, nasal/pharyngeal excretion, and gastric liquid, which facilitate the diagnosis of pediatric tuberculosis and rifampicin-resistant tuberculosis [5, 11].

All children exposed to infectious tuberculosis patients need to commonly undergo the tuberculosis screening. It is recommended, in particular, to closely follow up HIV-positive children and asymptomatic children exposed to family drug-resistant tuberculosis patients (once every 2–3 months in the first half year and once every 6 months within at least 2 years thereafter). If the latent infection progresses into tuberculosis, it is still necessary to sample sputum actively and find out the bacteriological evidence and drug-resistance type as far as possible, so as to guide the treatment based on the results of drug susceptibility test.

2.1.4 Detection of Patients Complicated with HIV

HIV infection is an important risk factor for drug susceptible or resistant tuberculosis. Patients with HIV-positive latent tuberculosis infection (LTBI) were 29 times (26–31 times) more likely to develop active pulmonary tuberculosis than those with HIV negative LTBIs [12]. Patients with HIV/TB double infection have atypical clinical manifestations of tuberculosis, with low positiveness rate in sputum smear and in acid fast bacilli culture, and they are prone to the complication with extra-pulmonary tuberculosis. Its imaging findings are atypical and easy to be confused with other pulmonary infections, which predisposes the diagnosis of AIDS/TB to difficulties, resulting in misdiagnosis and delay in diagnosis, and further leading to the wide spread of MDR/XDR-TB. Now bacterial culture is still the golden criteria for diagnosing MDR/XDR-TB, but even the newest method of liquid medium culture still needs at least 2 weeks, and this period of time is critical for MDR/XDR-TB patients complicated with HIV, who have a high mortality. Moreover, the failure to launch timely an anti-tuberculosis treatment will inevitably result in new cases of MDR/XDR-TB and their wide spreading. Therefore, Xpert Mtb/RIF should be used in the initial diagnosis for any HIV-positive patient suspected of MDR-TB, as that have been strongly recommended by WHO. In MDR/XDR-TB epidemic areas, TB patients with HIV infection are required to receive routine TB culture, drug susceptibility test, and other effective rapid diagnostic techniques. In addition to the first-line anti-TB drug susceptibility test, this test for the second-line injection and the fluoroquinolones should also be carried out to screen further XDR-TB. Data show that the mortality will increase significantly if HIV-positive patients have undetected drug resistance and use insufficient anti-tuberculosis treatment.

Although it is unrealistic to screen drug-resistant tuberculosis in all HIV-infected patients, especially in areas with high incidence of drug resistance, whereas drug susceptibility test should be carried out at least in high-risk groups of drug-resistant tuberculosis (such as those with unresponsiveness or close contacts of drug-resistant tuberculosis). Drug susceptibility test should also be performed in populations with low CD4+ T lymphocyte counts (e.g., lower than 200/mm^3), because these patients with drug-resistant tuberculosis will be confronted with a high mortality if undetected or not treated timely.

2.1.5 Application of Imaging Examination to the Detection of Patients with Drug-Resistant Tuberculosis

Although the diagnosis of drug-resistant pulmonary tuberculosis needs to be confirmed by microbiological examination and there is no significant difference in the chest imaging of drug-resistant pulmonary tuberculosis in comparison with the susceptible disease as reported by literature, many studies have found that the presence of multiple thick-walled cavities has the high specificity for diagnosing drug-resistant pulmonary tuberculosis, especially when the cavity number is ≥3 and the cavity diameter ≥30 mm, where the highest specificity is observed. However, there is no detailed index to quantify the cavities at present. Imaging examinations, therefore, may provide early warnings of suspected drug-resistant pulmonary tuberculosis.

Characteristic manifestations in image findings of single rifampicin-resistant pulmonary tuberculosis include: (1) Distributions of lesions: Lesions of pulmonary tuberculosis resistant to rifampicin are mainly distributed in the right middle lobe, the lingual segment of the left upper lobe, and the basal segment of the left lower lobe; (2) Morphological comparison of lesions: Multiple small lesions predominate, with more lesions with cavities, and their common diameter is <1.5 cm. (3) Extra-pulmonary lesions were mainly bilateral pleural effusion. Rifampicin resistance is suspected of in case of coexistence of these three characteristics in image findings, and a confirmation of this hypothesis can be made based on clinical responses.

The imaging features of multi-resistant pulmonary tuberculosis are complex and diverse, with their main features including: (1) Intrapulmonary lesions in MDR-TB patients mostly involve more than three lung fields, which is related to the prolonged course, repeated illness, and intrapulmonary spread of the lesions. (2) Three or more thick-walled cavities are commonly seen in the lungs with the incidence of lesions with cavitation of about 70%; multiple cavities are the prominent characteristics of acquired drug-resistant tuberculosis. Most of pulmonary cavities are fibrous thick-walled ones, due to their prolonged existence. The thicker the cavity wall is, the more difficult its close is. In addition, the blood vessels around the cavity wall are rare, hardened, or even closed, and it is difficult for anti-tuberculosis drugs to penetrate into the cavity, because of the barrier effect of tuberculosis cavity wall. Therefore, tuberculosis bacteria in the cavity are difficult to eradicate and prone to mutation resulting in drug resistance, and repeated and continuous bacterial excretion may lead to transmission. (3) Multi-resistant pulmonary tuberculosis is commonly complicated with mediastinal lymphadenopathy. CT and MRI enhanced scans often show circular enhancement of lymph nodes with a diameter larger than 1 cm. (4) It may be accompanied by lung nodular/mass, consolidation, mucus impaction, etc. [13, 14].

Imaging features of extensive drug-resistant (XDR) pulmonary tuberculosis. XDR pulmonary tuberculosis is the most serious type among all pulmonary tuberculosis, with its imaging features including extensive involvement by pulmonary lesions, disseminated pulmonary lesions, multiple cavities, and the complication with lung damage [13, 14].

1. XDR pulmonary tuberculosis spreads widely, often involves more than three lung fields complicated with unilateral lung damage, which is related to the prolonged

course of disease, poor response to the treatment, and repeated destruction of lung tissue in this cohort, making the disease extremely prone to intrapulmonary spread and resulting in extensive distribution of lung lesions. The percentage of patients with pulmonary infiltrating and spreading lesions in either XDR or MDR exceeds 50%, suggesting the significant activity in both cohorts. In addition, there are obviously more spreading lesions in XDR than in MDR, suggesting greater activity and extensiveness in the former.

2. Single cavity or multiple cavities are observed commonly in lungs. Studies showed that the number of cases with multiple cavities was significantly higher in XDR than in MDR, with a statistically significant difference ($P < 0.005$) [14].
3. During anti-tuberculosis treatment, pulmonary lesions in XDR pulmonary tuberculosis features are constant deterioration, with an increase in the number of spreading lesions and enlargement of the cavities, in contrast to a low ratio of shrinkage and closure of cavities, which reflect fully the continuous aggravation of pulmonary lesions with a poor responsiveness despite the active anti-tuberculosis treatment in XDR-TB patients.

2.2 Status and Characteristics of Epidemics of Drug-Resistant Pulmonary Tuberculosis

The spread and epidemics of drug-resistant pulmonary tuberculosis are the major challenge and dominant obstacle in the control of tuberculosis, especially that of MDR-TB and XDR-TB, which hinders seriously the progress of the control of tuberculosis and has become one of the serious issues of both public health and society.

2.2.1 Present Epidemic Status of Global Pulmonary Tuberculosis

Since directly observed treatment of short courses strategy (DOTS) launched by WHO in 1994, the progress of National Tuberculosis Program (NTP) in many countries has been boosted. The WHO global tuberculosis report showed that the estimated number of newly diagnosed tuberculosis worldwide in 2019 were 10 million, of which 58% were male, 32% were female, and 12% were children (<15 years old), and 8.2% of TB patients were complicated with HIV infection. Among all newly diagnosed patients with pulmonary tuberculosis, the number of those in the 30 countries with high tuberculosis burden accounted for 2/3, and those in 8 countries accounted for about 1/3 [3].

2.2.2 Present Epidemic Status of Global Drug-Resistant Pulmonary Tuberculosis

Since the launch of the Global Anti-TB Drug Resistance Monitoring Project in 1994, data of the drug resistance level of Mycobacterium tuberculosis have been collected and analyzed systematically in 169 countries accounting for 87% of 194 WHO member countries. The population and TB cases in these 169 countries, respectively, account for more than 99% of the global population and tuberculosis cases. These include 113 countries performing the continuous monitoring system of routine drug susceptibility test (DST) for all tuberculosis patients, and 59 carrying out epidemiological investigation relying on collected bacterial isolates. For those countries or regions deficient in laboratory capacity or resources and unable to conduct routine drug susceptibility tests on all tuberculosis patients, the approach most commonly used method is the national or regional drug resistance survey once every 5 years. Along with the present rapid development of fast molecular biology drug susceptibility tests, more and more countries are transferring from regular investigation to DST continuous monitoring system based on routine detections [3].

Among 30 countries with high tuberculosis burden and 30 countries with high burden of MDR tuberculosis (due to the overlap of these two groups, there are data on drug resistance levels in 40 countries), 37 countries have data on drug resistance levels, among which four countries (Brazil, Central African Republic, Democratic People's Republic of Korea, and Papua New Guinea) rely on the collection of local drug resistance monitoring data from various regions [3].

According to the WHO global tuberculosis report in 2021 [3], 132,222 cases of MDR-TB/RRTB and 25,681 cases of quasi extensive or extensive drug-resistant TB were detected worldwide in 2020, with a total number of 157,903, which was significantly lower than the total number of 201,997 cases in 2019 with a drop of 22%. Globally, a total of 150,359 MDR/rifampicin-resistant patients were registered for treatment in 2020, equivalent to 1/3 of annual MDR-TB/RRTB cases, showing a drop of 15% compared with the total number of 177,100 in 2019.

2.2.3 Present Epidemic Status of Drug-Resistant Tuberculosis in China

China is one of the countries with the severe epidemics of drug-resistant tuberculosis, one of the 22 countries with a high tuberculosis burden, and one of the 27 countries with the serious epidemics of MDR-TB around the world. As estimated by WHO Global TB Report in 2021 [3, 15], 83% of the newly diagnosed etiologically positive tuberculosis patients in 2020 in China received rifampicin resistance test, which was higher than the global average level of 71%. 16,343 cases of MDR/RRTB and 1185 cases of quasi-extensively or extensively drug-resistant tuberculosis were detected, with 17,528 cases in total, among whom 13,250 cases with MDR/RRTB had started their treatment. Since 1994, 13 provinces and cities in China (including Shandong Province, Zhejiang Province, Guangdong Province, Hubei Province, Liaoning Province, Henan Province, Inner Mongolia Autonomous Region, Hunan Province, Xinjiang Uygur Autonomous Region, Beijing City, Shanghai City, Chongqing city, and Heilongjiang Province) have successively participated in the Global Drug Resistance Monitoring Project of WHO/IUATLD and have carried out drug susceptible monitoring for INH, RFP, EMB, and SM in a row. The result available shows that the initial, acquired, and total drug-resistance rates in all provinces of China remain are at a high level. The drug-resistance level is extremely uneven, based on comparison among provinces, showing a higher epidemics of drug resistance in some provinces of China, such as Henan, Liaoning, Inner Mongolia Autonomous Region, etc.

China conducted five national epidemiological surveys (ES) of tuberculosis successively in 1979, 1984–1985, 1990, 2000, and 2010 [16–20]. The results of the former four showed that the initial drug-resistance rates were, respectively, 26.2%, 47.8%, 28.1%, and 18.6%, and the acquired drug-resistance rates were 68.1%, 64.1%, 41.1%, and 46.5%, respectively. However, only six anti-tuberculosis drugs were tested in these four epidemiological surveys, including four first-line drugs (i.e., isoniazid (INH), streptomycin (s), rifampicin (RFP), and ethambutol (EMB)), and two second-line drugs (i.e., sodium para-aminosalicylate (PAS) and thiourea (T)). In the fifth survey in 2010, 11 anti-tuberculosis drugs were tested, including 4 first-line drugs (h, R, s, e), and 7 second-line drugs (para-aminosalicylic acid (PAS), kanamycin (km), amikacin (AM), also known as BB-K8, capreomycin (CM), thioisonicotinamide (PTO), ofloxacin (ofx), and levofloxacin (LFX)). The overall resistance rate to any one of the 11 anti-tuberculosis drugs tested was 42.1% (95%CI: 36.3–48.2%), 42.7% for treatment-naive patients (95%ci: 36.4–49.2%), and 38.5% for relapsing patients (95%CI: 23.4–55.4%). The drug-resistance rate was 36.8% (95%CI:31.1–42.7%) and 24.6% (95%CI:19.7–30.1%), respectively, for the first-line and the second-line anti-tuberculosis drugs, with the total multi-resistance rate of 6.8% (95%CI:4.1–10.4%) and the extensive drug-resistance rate of 2.1% (95%CI:0.8–4.6%). At present, there are 339,000 cases of MDR-TB and 105,000 cases of XDR-TB in China, suggesting China has high MDR-TB incidence. The XDR-TB incidence previously reported by the national baseline survey report on drug-resistant tuberculosis were 68%, whereas the present data of XDR-TB incidence shows a rise. According to the China Tuberculosis Control Plan (2011–2015), with about 120,000 newly patients diagnosed with tuberculosis each year, the harm imposed by MDR-TB has become increasingly prominent during recent years, and epidemics of tuberculosis dominated by drug-resistant bacteria is anticipated possibly in the next few years.

2.2.4 Epidemic Features of Drug-Resistant Tuberculosis in China

Understanding whether the epidemics of drug-resistant tuberculosis in China or a certain region of China is caused by the treatment process using anti-TB drugs or by the direct transmission from drug-resistant TB patients may help us find more appropriate strategies for controlling drug-resistant tuberculosis. The team led by Professor Qian Gao, a Chinese expert in the control of tuberculosis, has found epidemic characteristics of drug-resistant pulmonary tuberculosis in China are as follows, through large-scale epidemiology surveys in combination with laboratory researches [21, 22]:

1. The percentage is significantly higher for treatment-naïve patients than in relapsing patients, among all drug-resistant tuberculosis patients

   The report of the fifth tuberculosis epidemiological survey in 2010 showed that 89 (86.4%) and 14 (13.6%) cases were, respectively, the treatment-naive and the relapsing among 103 tuberculosis patients resistant to the first-line drugs, compared with 62 (89.9%) and 7 (10.1%), respectively, among 69 patients resistant to the second-line drugs [20]. It was found by a study in Shanghai China that 1016 (72.5%) and 385 (27.4%) were treatment-naïve and relapsing patients, respectively, among 1401 first-line drug-resistant TB patients from 2000 to 2006, as compared to 199 (59.8%) and 134 (40.2%), respectively, among 333 TB patients resistant to second-line anti-TB drugs [23].

   It can be inferred that among drug-resistant TB patients, treatment-naïve patients far exceed the relapsing ones. Therefore, primary drug resistance is more common, and transmission is the culprit leading to primary drug resistance.

2. Recent advent transmission is the main reason for the emergence of drug-resistant tuberculosis

   Among the population with latent infection of Mycobacterium tuberculosis, 5% will show the onset of disease within 1–2 years post-infection, who is called pulmonary tuberculosis caused by recent transmission. In addition, 5% of patients with latent infection may have the onset during their lifetime or due to impaired body immunity, and these patients are called pulmonary tuberculosis caused by long-term transmission or endogenous resurgence.

Using the genotyping technology for Mycobacterium tuberculosis in five sites in China, researchers found that infection in 59 (43.7%) out of 135 patients with drug-resistant strains of Mycobacterium tuberculosis (MDR-Mtb) was caused by recent transmission, and further research found that MDR-Mtb was more likely to cause recent transmission than TB susceptible strains [21].

It can be inferred from the above that the main reason for the high incidence of drug-resistant tuberculosis in China is the direct spread of drug-resistant Mycobacterium tuberculosis. Correct treatment and control for the newly diagnosed tuberculosis can reduce significantly the advent of acquired drug-resistant tuberculosis, while the epidemics of drug-resistant tuberculosis cannot be curbed completely if early detection, diagnosis, and treatment cannot be achieved without the control of the spread of drug-resistant Mycobacterium tuberculosis. Efficient measures, therefore, comprise early detection and diagnosis of drug-resistant pulmonary tuberculosis and destruction of transmission routes, so as to control the high epidemics of drug-resistant tuberculosis, on the basis of standardized anti-tuberculosis treatment, strengthened tuberculosis management, and correct instruction for the medications of tuberculosis patients.

References

1. Zong Z-j, Jing W, Huo F-m, et al. Resistance analysis of extensively drug-resistant Mycobacterium tuberculosis isolates against linezolid [J/CD]. Electron J Emerg Infect Dis. 2017;2(3):160–3.
2. World Health Organization. Guidelines for the programmatic management of drug-resistant tuberculosis, 2011 update [EB/OL]. Geneva: World Health Organization; 2011. https://apps.who.int/iris/handle/10665/44597.
3. World Health Organization. Global tuberculosis report 2021 [EB/OL]. [2021-10-14]. https://www.who.int/publications/digital/global-tuberculosis-report-2021.
4. World Health Organization. Global tuberculosis report 2019 [EB/OL]. Geneva: World Health Organization; 2019. https://apps.who.int/iris/handle/10665/329368.
5. World Health Organization. WHO meeting report of a technical expert consultation: non-inferiority analysis of Xpert MTB/RIF ultra compared to Xpert MTB/RIF [EB/OL]. Geneva: World Health Organization; 2017. https://apps.who.int/iris/handle/10665/254792.
6. Cao Y, Parmar H, Gaur RL, et al. Xpert MTB/XDR: a 10-color reflex assay suitable for point-of-care settings to detect isoniazid, fluoroquinolone, and second-line-injectable-drug resistance directly from Mycobacterium tuberculosis-positive sputum [J]. J Clin Microbiol. 2021;59(3):e02314–20.
7. Crudu V, Stratan E, Romancenco E, et al. First evaluation of an improved assay for molecular genetic detection of tuberculosis as well as rifampin and isoniazid resistances [J]. J Clin Microbiol. 2012;50(4):1264–9.
8. Jian J, Yang X, Yang J, et al. Evaluation of the GenoType MTBDRplus and MTBDRsl for the detection of drug-resistant Mycobacterium tuberculosis on isolates from Beijing, China [J]. Infect Drug Resist, 2018, 11: 1627–1634.
9. Jiao WW, Liu ZG, Han R, et al. Prevalence of drug resistant Mycobacterium tuberculosis among children in China [J]. Tuberculosis (Edinb). 2015;95(3):315–20.
10. State Health Commission of the People's Republic of China, diagnostic criteria for pulmonary tuberculosis (WS 288-2017) [J/CD]. Electron J Emerg Infect Dis. 2018;3(1):59–61.
11. Lombardi G, Pellegrino MT, Denicolo A, et al. Quantiferon-TB performs better in children, including infants, than in adults with active tuberculosis: a multicenter study [J]. J Clin Microbiol. 2019;57(10):e01048–19.
12. World Health Organization. HIV-associated tuberculosis. 2014.
13. Wang, Yi-xiang, Myung Jin Chung, Aliaksandr Skrahin, et al. Literature analysis of radiological signs related to multidrug-resistant tuberculosis [J/CD] Electron J Emerg Infect Dis, 2018,3(2):244-253.
14. Yu W, Tan W-g, Lu P-x. Classification and imaging manifestations of drug-resistant pulmonary tuberculosis [J/CD]. Electron J Emerg Infect Dis. 2019;4(1):42–7.
15. Chunrong L, Hongxia F, Puxuan L, et al. The global tuberculosis report 2021: key data analysis for China and the global world [J/CD]. Electron J Emerg Infect Dis. 2021;6(4):368–72.
16. Ministry of Health of the People's Republic of China. Information compilation for sampling survey of national tuberculosis epidemiology 1979 [M]. 1981.
17. Ministry of Health of the People's Republic of China. Information compilation for sampling survey of national tuberculosis epidemiology 1984/1985 [M]. 1988.
18. Ministry of Health of the People's Republic of China. Information compilation for sampling survey of national tuberculosis epidemiology 1990 [M]. 1992.
19. Ministry of Health of the People's Republic of China. Information compilation for sampling survey of national tuberculosis epidemiology 2000 [M]. 2002.
20. Ministry of Health of the People's Republic of China. Information compilation for sampling survey of national tuberculosis epidemiology 2010 [M]. 2012.
21. Gao Q, Mei J. No reasons but transmission results in the high drug resistance rate of tuberculosis in China [J]. Chin J Antituberc. 2015;37(11):1091–6.
22. Gao Q, Yang C. Recent transmission of tuberculosis in China and its controlling strategies [J]. J Tuberc Lung Health. 2017;6(13):193–8.
23. Shen X, DeRiemer K, Yuan ZA, et al. Drug-resistant tuberculosis in drug-resistant pulmonary tuberculosis in Shanghai, China, 2000–2006: prevalence, trends and risk factors [J]. Int J Tuberc Lung Dis. 2009;13(2):253–9.

3 Laboratory Examination for Drug-Resistant Tubercle Bacillus

Yu-mei Zhu, Hou-ming Liu, Feng Wang, Wan-shui Shan, Qin Yin, and Kun-zhen Lu

The drug susceptibility test for Mycobacterium tuberculosis is an indispensable tool in controlling drug-resistant tuberculosis and plays a positive role in the diagnosis of drug-resistant tuberculosis, selection and modification of treatment regimens for this disease, the monitoring of drug resistances, and the control of patients with the drug resistances. The present drug susceptibility tests for tubercle bacillus can be categorized mainly into the phenotypic test and the genotype test. The phenotypic test can be divided into the test based on solid culture medium (the proportional method and the absolute concentration method), the test based on liquid culture medium (BACTEC, MGIT), and the rapid test with microdilution (microplate assays/MIC). Genotypic susceptibility tests can be categorized into (1) semi-nested automatic real-time fluorescent quantitative PCR; (2) melting curve; (3) membrane gene chips; (4) linear probe assay; (5) microarray chip; and (6) sequencing.

3.1 Pathogenic Detection of Drug-Resistant Tubercle Bacillus

Culture-isolation examination of Mycobacterium is the most reliable method for diagnosing tuberculosis, and the basis to obtain pure culture for strain identification, drug susceptibility test, and other biological researches. Now, the modified Lowenstein–Jensen medium is widely used in China to isolate and culture Mycobacterium tuberculosis. The sensitivity of the culture method is superior to that of smear microscopy, and generally a positiveness is shown in the culture when the microbial content in the sample reaches to 100 bacteria/mL. Due to the slow growth of Mycobacterium tuberculosis, the solid culture method takes more than 4 weeks, which affects the timeliness of diagnosis and treatment for tuberculosis patients. Many laboratories have begun to use liquid culture technology, and liquid rapid culture for Mycobacterium may shorten significantly instrument-positive time. Liquid culture is a method to detect the growth of Mycobacterium by measuring its growth and metabolism of bacteria using Mycobacterium rapid culture instrument (MIGT, BacT/Alert and ESP). Take BACTEC MGIT960 system as an example. The nutrients and oxygen in the tube will be consumed continuously, and the fluorescent agent in the MGIT culture tube will react and release fluorescence along with the change in oxygen concentration in the tube if Mycobacterium tuberculosis grows in the inoculated MGIT culture tube. The fluorescence intensity memory detector may measure continuously the fluorescence intensity in the culture tube once every 60 min, monitor and determine the growth of Mycobacterium in the tube. The liquid culture medium is rich in nutrients with a detector capable of monitoring continuously, thereby improving the sensitivity to the isolation and culture of Mycobacterium in the specimen and shortening the time needed for reporting the results [1–5]. In order to guarantee the reliability of the examination method, the present Mycobacterium rapid culture/examination system not only provides corresponding instruments and reagents, but also formulates examination procedures related to pre-treatment method of clinical samples, inoculation, detection and report of results based on the system, thereby achieving good repeatability and comparability. When a rapid culture and examination for Mycobacterium is performed, a decontamination should be carried out before inoculation of sample to reduce contamination rate. When the positiveness is reported by the system, the culture solution of corresponding sample must

Y.-m. Zhu (✉) · F. Wang
Department of Medical Laboratory, Shenzhen Center for Chronic Disease Control, Shenzhen, Guangdong, China

H.-m. Liu
Department of Clinical Laboratory, The Third People's Hospital of Shenzhen, Shenzhen, Guangdong, China

W.-s. Shan
Clinical Laboratory, The Third People's Hospital of Shenzhen, Shenzhen, Guangdong, China

Q. Yin · K.-z. Lu
Editorial Department of the Electronic Journal of Emerging Infectious Diseases, Shenzhen, Guangdong, China

P.-x. Lu et al. (eds.), *Diagnostic Imaging of Drug Resistant Pulmonary Tuberculosis*,
https://doi.org/10.1007/978-981-99-8339-1_3

first be subjected to microscopic examination of acid fast staining, and no positive report can be issued until the acid fast bacteria are found. Liquid isolation/culture of Mycobacterium tuberculosis has multiple advantages, including the advanced design, short time consumption for positiveness detection with its rate raised, the wide range of specimens applicable, and the fully automatic built-in quality control system, which reduces greatly the burden on the staff and helps improve the safety of the operation.

3.2 Phenotypic Drug Susceptibility Test for Drug-Resistant Tuberculosis

3.2.1 Solid Drug Susceptibility

The drug susceptibility test of solid Lowenstein–Jensen culture includes mainly the proportional method and the absolute concentration method, which were first proposed, respectively, by G. Canetti and J. Grossete from France and G. Meissner from Germany in the 1960s [6]. The proportional method is the one used in the current epidemiological surveillance and planning and management projects of poly-resistant tuberculosis in China. Drug susceptibility test can be categorized into the direct and the indirect. The direct method is defined as the drug susceptibility test that dilutes the clinical samples post to pre-treatment according to the amount of bacteria required by the smear microscopy, followed by a direct inoculation onto the control and culture medium containing drug. It is suitable for a sample with a large amount of bacteria verified by the microscope, and its advantages include the facts that the isolation, incubation, and drug susceptibility test can be carried out simultaneously, and that the results can be reported 3–4 weeks ahead of the indirect method. Its disadvantages are that the amount of inoculation is not easy to quantify and the pollution is difficult to control. The indirect method is to isolate and culture the clinical samples first and then conduct the drug sensitivity test after obtaining the pure bacterial culture visible to the naked eye. The indirect method reports the results more slowly than the direct method, but the operation based on the pure culture is easier to control the bacterial quantity, which has the advantages of a greater accuracy in its results and lower pollution rate. The basic operation of proportion method (indirect method) for drug susceptibility test is as follows: the inoculums containing 10^{-4} mg and 10^{-6} mg tested bacteria are cultured on the slope of the modified Lowenstein–Jensen (L-J) medium containing drug and on the control (without drug) for 4 weeks, and the drug resistance ratio is calculated and whether there is drug resistance is determined by comparing the difference in the number of colonies on the identically inoculated mediums with and without drug. Percentage of resistance = (number of colonies growing on the medium with drug)/(number of colonies growing on the control medium) × 100%. If the percentage of drug resistance is greater than 1%, the tested bacteria are considered to be resistant to the anti-tuberculosis drug. The basic operation of the absolute concentration method (indirect method) for drug susceptibility test is as follows: the bacteria to be tested with an inoculation amount of 10^{-3} mg are cultured on the slope of the control, modified Lowenstein–Jensen medium containing drugs in high and low concentration for 4 weeks, the culture medium is checked to observe the colony count, and the colony growth is recorded on the laboratory log. On the premise of good colony growth on the control medium, the number larger than 20 for colonies growing on the medium containing drug can be determined as drug resistance.

3.2.2 Liquid Drug Susceptibility

The traditional modified acid Lowenstein–Jensen culture is popularized in tuberculosis laboratories in China. As Mycobacterium tuberculosis is a bacterium growing slowly, however, it takes 4 weeks for a single bacterium growing on solid medium in the Lowenstein–Jensen tube to form a visible colony, which cannot meet the clinical needs for the diagnosis and treatment of tuberculosis. Liquid culture medium, the earliest in vitro culture medium used in microbiology, may provide bacteria with more sufficient nutrition and make it grow faster under good conditions, so it improves greatly the speed and rate of positiveness detection rate for Mycobacterium tuberculosis, in case of its combination with specific detection tools. Rapid liquid culture system for Mycobacterium, therefore, has been introduced gradually into clinical practice and has become one of the main detection methods in Tuberculosis Hospital, such as BD BACTEC™MGIT™960, ALERT 3D, and ESPII. The liquid susceptibility system, BD BACTEC™MGIT™960, will be introduced mainly in this Book.

BD BACTEC™MGIT™960 liquid drug susceptibility system is a rapid testing system based on the BD960 incubator, with its rational based on a successive detection with a fluorescent intensity memory detector in the incubator once every 60 min for fluorescent intensity released by fluorescent indicator activated by a specific light source, when the oxygen in the culture tube is used and the concentration of CO_2 increases. This system can detect the susceptibility of up to 14 anti-tuberculosis drugs, including four first-line drugs including rifampicin, isoniazid, ethambutol, and streptomycin, and five second-line drugs including amikacin, capreomycin, kanamycin, ofloxacin, and pyrazinamide. The test result is obtainable within 13 days, and for PZA drug sensitivity, within 21 days, which is conducive to the early diagnosis and treatment of patients. A proportional method is adopted by this liquid drug susceptibility system, with its criticality equaling 1% in determining drug susceptibility in Mycobacterium tuberculosis, and the MGIT incubation tube will be detected by the system when the GU value of the control tube not containing drug reaches to 400, with a result determined to be susceptible or resistant, respectively, in case of the GU in the drug tube less or larger than 100. BD BACTEC™MGIT™960 drug susceptible test has been launched in laboratories in China.

Aiming to compare the consistency between BACTEC-MGIT960 automatic Mycobacterium rapid drug susceptibility test and Lowenstein–Jensen proportional method, Yangshunli et al. [7] detected in parallel the susceptibility to rifampicin (RFP), isoniazid (INH), streptomycin (SM), and ethambutol (EMB) in 245 clinical isolates from inhospitalized patients and confirmed the capability of BACT-MGIT960 automatic Mycobacterium drug susceptibility test to obtain susceptibility to RFP, INH, SM, and EMB within 4–13 days, with the mean of 7.8 days. Its coincidence rate with Lowenstein–Jensen proportional susceptibility reaches 98.78%, 97.55%, 96.73%, and 96.73%, respectively, with a mean of 97.45%. Abe, Abe, Bergmann JS, Cambau et al. [8–10] evaluated the consistency between BACTEC-MGIT960 fully automatic Mycobacterium rapid susceptibility test and solid susceptibility test, and the results seemed also satisfactory. BACTEC-MGIT960 Mycobacterium liquid susceptibility system may obtain accurate susceptibility results and is especially suitable for fast susceptibility screening of clinical isolates. There is a certain difficulty, however, in generalizing this technique in rudimentary laboratories, due to the high price of reagents and apparatus required by the liquid susceptibility test, and its flux limited by the equipment.

3.2.3 Rapid Drug Susceptibility Test with Microdilution

Compared with the Lowenstein–Jensen culture, MIC assay has its manual operation time shortened greatly because only the addition of a certain amount of medium and bacterial suspension is required by the incubation due to the usage of the pre-prepared drug sensitive plates. The most important thing is that MIC assay can provide results within 7–21 days, which shortens greatly the reporting time of drug susceptibility results. In addition, the inclusive quantitative QC range may provide the test method with an immediate quality assurance. The result obtained by MIC assay, however, is the minimum inhibitory concentration, and it is necessary to determine whether a resistance exists, through utilizing the reference standards. Now the method of obtaining the minimum inhibitory concentration (MIC) of tubercle bacillus by microporous plate culture has been popularized in some hospitals in China. For example, Sensititre™ MIC drug susceptibility platform for Mycobacterium tuberculosis of Thermo and Zhuhai Yinke Medical Engineering Co., Ltd can realize comprehensive drug susceptibility test for Mycobacterium tuberculosis to a variety of first- and second-line anti-tuberculosis drugs. Jing Li et al. [11] used random number table to select 201 strains cultured by BACTEC MGIT 960 rapid incubation and identified as Mycobacterium tuberculosis isolates and used MicroDST™ microporous susceptibility method to test the susceptibility in isolates to the first- and second-line anti-tuberculosis drugs, including streptomycin (SM), isoniazid (INH), rifampicin (RFP), ethambutol (EMB), amikacin (AM), capreomycin (CM), levofloxacin (LFX), moxifloxacin (MFX), para-aminosalicylic acid (PAS), and propylthioisonicotinamide (PTO), with its result compared with that of Lowenstein–Jensen proportional method to evaluate the coincidence rate between them. Results showed that 7–14 days are required for determining drug susceptibility test results obtained by microporous susceptibility method in 201 Mycobacterium tuberculosis isolates, suggesting a sensitivity in this method not lower than 80% in comparison with Lowenstein–Jensen proportional susceptibility test, the golden standard, with a coincidence rate of 96.2%, 92.2%, 92.2%, 93.8%, 85.7%, 94.1%, 93.3%, 84.6%, 94.1%, and 100%, respectively, for streptomycin (SM), isoniazid (INH), ethambutol (EMB), rifampicin (RFP), levofloxacin (LFX), moxifloxacin (MFX), amikacin (AM), capreomycin (CM), para-aminosalicylic acid (PAS), and isonicotinamide propionate (PTO). This illustrates that microporous susceptibility method has a high consistency in its result of susceptibility to the first- and second-line anti-tuberculosis drugs compared with Lowenstein–Jensen proportional method and achieves a rapid test which is easily generalized and meeting present requirement in diagnosis of tuberculosis. Hao Wang et al. [12] performed drug susceptibility test on 124 clinical isolates from Mycobacterium tuberculosis complex using Sensititre tuberculosis susceptibility plate and L-J proportional method, respectively, on drugs including isoniazid, rifampicin, ethambutol, streptomycin, ofloxacin, moxifloxacin, amikacin, rifabutin, *p*-aminosalicylic acid, ethioisonicotinamide, cycloserine, and kanamycin, with a comparison on results between these two methods. Results showed that a coincidence ratio above 90.0% was achieved between Sensititre tuberculosis susceptibility plate and L-J proportional method in detecting susceptibility of 124 clinical isolates from Mycobacterium tuberculosis complex to each of the 12 drugs including isoniazid, rifampicin, ethambutol, streptomycin, ofloxacin, moxifloxacin, amikacin, rifabutin, *p*-aminosalicylic acid, ethioisonicotinamide, and cycloserine, illustrating Sensititre tuberculosis susceptibility plate had a high consistency in its results compared with traditional L-J proportional method, a shorter duration required by the detection, simpler manipulation, and the capability to obtain simultaneously the minimum inhibitory concentration of the anti-tuberculosis drugs.

3.3 Genotypic Susceptibility Test for Drug-Resistant Tuberculosis

With the soaring development of molecular biology in medicine, the molecular mechanism of bacterial drug resistance has been clarified gradually, and the relationship between phenotypes and genotypes for drug susceptibility in Mycobacterium tuberculosis has been recognized little by little and applied to clinical practice. The technologies for detecting drug-resistant mutant genes in Mycobacterium tuberculosis mainly fall into six categories as follows: (1) semi-nested fully automatic real-time fluorescent quantitative PCR; (2) probe melting curve; (3) membrane gene chip; (4) linear probe assay; (5) microarray chip; and (6) genetic sequencing. All these techniques are based on the analysis available for mutations (including insertion, deletion, and SNP) related to drug resistance in Mycobacterium tuberculosis, including rpoB/C mutation mediating rifampicin resistance, mutation of inhA, katG, and ahpC that mediate isoniazid resistance, embA/B/C/R mutation mediating ethambutol resistance, rrs and rpsl mutation mediating streptomycin resistance, gyrA and gyrB mutation mediating fluoroquinolones resistance, ethA/R and inhA mutation mediating ethionine isonicotinamide resistance, and mutation of pncA, rpsA, and panD that mediate pyrazinamide resistance. Because the discovery and confirmation of drug resistance genes are a continuously developing process, the gene mutations detected by the kit do not and cannot cover all the mutations related to phenotypic drug resistance. In addition, there are some complicated relationships between drug resistance phenotypes and genotypes, so there will be cases in which the drug resistance phenotypes are inconsistent or only partially consistent with gene mutations in clinical practice.

3.3.1 Semi-nested Automatic Real-Time Fluorescent Quantitative PCR

Cepheid U.S.A. developed a technology named Cepheid Gene Xpert System's MTB/RIF assay (abbreviated as XpertMTB/RIF) [13] based on a semi-nested fluorescent quantitative PCR in 2010, with a reagent capable of detecting simultaneously Mycobacterium tuberculosis and its rifampicin resistant mutation within 2 h. XpertMTB/RIF detection system mainly consists of two parts: (1) XpertMTB/RIF plastic detection box, which contains sample extraction reagent, PCR buffer, and lyophilized real-time fluorescent quantitative PCR reagent, and (2) Gene Xpert equipment: which controls the liquid contained in the plastic detection box and completes the post-PCR result analysis. Aiming to minimize the influence by cross amplification of non-tuberculosis mycobacterium (NTM) and detect better rifampicin resistance, amplification primers were designed in the rpoB region specifically chosen for Mycobacterium tuberculosis, and five molecular beacon probes (probes A–E) were designed, with their sequences covering the 81-bp rifampicin resistance determining region (RRDR) in rpoB, in respect of design of primers and probes for XpertMTB/RIF. In addition to the five probes for detecting rifampicin resistance, a quality control probe is contained in XpertMTB/RIF and has its design targeted at DNA of Bacillus globigii for monitoring extraction of samples and procedures of PCR amplification. The limit of detection (LOD) of XpertMTB/RIF is 4.5 genomes/reaction for detecting DNA of Mycobacterium tuberculosis, and 131 CFU/mL for detecting clinical sputum samples.

XpertMTB/RIF has multiple advantages in clinical application. First of all, its combination between reagents and equipment features the simplified and expedited operation. The integration and automation of sample extraction and PCR amplification are achievable in the fully closed state without too much requirement on manual operations, thereby reducing risks of sample pollution and post-PCR pollution. Meanwhile, it can realize a detection directly based on sputum samples to ensure that two vital clinical information can be obtained from the patient's sputum within 2 h—whether there is Mycobacterium and rifampicin resistance? Second, XpertMTB/RIF has the same sensitivity and specificity as culture, and its high sensitivity and high specificity have been verified by multi-site studies in various countries. Based on analysis by WHO, the sensitivity of XpertMTB/RIF is raised by 40% in comparison with acid fast microscopy. The data published in the New England Journal shows a sensitivity reaching to 98.2% with a specificity up to 99.2% in smear-positive patients, and a sensitivity reaching to 72.5–90.2% in culture-positive patients [14]. Recently, the First Affiliated Hospital of Chongqing Medical University conducted a meta-analysis on the efficacy of XpertMTB/RIF in diagnosing tuberculosis in HIV-infected people, which included 10 articles in total from samples consisting of 1878 patients, respectively, from 6 countries comprising South Africa, etc. Analytical results showed a comprehensive sensitivity of 69% for XpertMTB/RIF in diagnosing tuberculosis in HIV-infected patients with a comprehensive specificity of 97%, with its comprehensive sensitivity superior to that of acid fast staining smear (53%). Comprehensive sensitivity and specificity of Xpert for samples from respiratory tract, based on analyses for different types of samples, were 76% and 98%, respectively, and higher than 62% and 94%, respectively, for non-respiratory tract samples [15].

XpertMTB/RIF still has certain limitations in its application, although it has been recommended by WHO due to its technical advantages and has boosted the detection rate of multi-resistant tubercle bacillus by 3–8 times worldwide [16].

First of all, reagents of XpertMTB/RIF are more expensive in relative to those of traditional TB smear and culture with an expenditure up to several hundred Yuan for a single test and imposes a heavy economic burden on tuberculosis patients. In addition, XpertMTB/RIF provides information about the resistance to rifampicin alone, but not about isoniazid simultaneously. In countries with high tuberculosis burden, however, the accurate confirmation of MDR patients necessitates the clinical recognition of isoniazid resistance. Second, its sensibility is not so high for smear-negative sputum, sputum from patients co-infected with HIV and clinical extra-pulmonary specimens [17, 18]. Third, its potential is limited to detect mutated mixed samples and individual mutant site (C533G of gene rpoB) [19, 20].

Cepheid launched in 2017 a new generation of upgraded product, XpertMTB/RIF Ultra, aiming to solve these technical limitations of XpertMTB/RIF. The greatest technical difference between these two generations is the basis and methods for determining results. XpertMTB/RIF contains two procedures, i.e., DNA extraction and fluorescence quantitative PCR amplification, and determines rifampicin resistance mutation based on presence/absence of Ct value and its level for five rpoB drug resistance molecular beacon probes, as well as whether Ct difference (△Ct) among probes exceeds 3.5 cycles. XpertMTB/RIF Ultra, however, consists of three procedures including DNA extraction, fluorescent quantitative PCR amplification and post-PCR melting curve analysis, and detects rifampicin resistance through analyzing the variation of melting temperature (Tm) of melting curve peak of probes.

3.3.2 Multicolor Melting Curve Analysis

The concept of multicolor melting curve analysis (MMCA) was first proposed in 2011 by the investigation team led by Qingge Li of Xiamen University, China, and applied widely to researches on genetic mutation and/or genotyping in the field of microorganisms and genetic diseases [21–25]. The technical rationale of MMCA is to distinguish various target genes or mutations based on the difference of melting points resulted by stability differences among double-stranded hybrids formed by a hybridization between a self-quenching fluorescent probe with double end-labeling and target sequences, so as to realize detection and genotyping of multiple target sequences via a single PCR [26]. During the detection, in practical terms, the self-quenching fluorescent probe having double end-labeling will form a "probe-target sequence double-stranded hybrid" (hereinafter referred to as double-stranded hybrid) with the target sequence under detection. The stability of "double-stranded hybrid" can be reflected directly by melting temperatures. The fluorescence signal with the highest Tm (i.e., the melting temperature in case of complete matching) can be obtained during MMCA detection, if the target sequence under detection (wild type) is consistent with the probe sequence, suggesting the combination between them forms a 100% matched double-stranded hybrid. In case of non-complete consistency, on the contrary, between the target sequence under detection (the mutant) and the probe sequence, the double-stranded hybrid formed by their combination is not 100% matching, so the fluorescence signal of lower Tm (i.e., the melting temperature in case of non-complete matching) can be obtained. The stability of this double-stranded hybrid depends on the coincidence between the probe sequence and the target sequence to be tested. The higher the matching value is, the higher the stability will be, with higher melting point temperature obtained by the melting curve [27].

In the field of tuberculosis, a melting curve technology analysis platform with independent intellectual property rights was developed jointly by Xiamen University and Xiamen Zhishan Biotechnology Co., Ltd (http://www.zsandx.com/), and a set of one-stop overall scheme for rapid detection of both tuberculosis and drug-resistant tuberculosis "from sample DNA extraction to report of results." The technical services provided by their platform include nucleic acid extraction reagents, an automatic nucleic acid extraction instrument, automatic medical PCR analysis system, nucleic acid detection kit for complex group of Mycobacterium tuberculosis, a kit for detecting drug resistance mutation for 5 anti-tuberculosis drugs (rifampicin, isoniazid, ethambutol, streptomycin, and fluoroquinolones) and a strain identification kit for 19 common clinical Mycobacteria [28]. In the clinical test of resistance to anti-tuberculosis drugs, only the extracted sample DNA needs to be added into the pre-loaded PCR tube, mixed and spiked, followed by an immediate analysis of drug resistance mutation of PCR products post to PCR amplification. After the experiment, results of drug resistance test for the samples will be yielded directly based on the determination by result-interpretation software built in the instrument. This technology for detecting drug-resistant mutation not only has shorter manual operation time (only manual spiking is required) to complete all detection procedures within 3 h, but also makes it unnecessary to uncover PCR products and so eradicates the risk of cross contamination of PCR products induced by the uncovering. In summary, MMPC technology platform has the technical advantages of time saving, high efficiency, high automation, and reduction of cross contamination of PCR products in clinical application.

The details of kit in MeltProTB series for detecting mutations of resistance to five anti-tuberculosis drugs (rifampicin, isoniazid, ethambutol, streptomycin, and fluoroquinolones) are as follows: (1) rifampicin resistance mutation kit (MeltProTB/RIF), which detects mutations within 81-bp clip in rifampicin resistance determining region (RRDR) of ropB; an evaluation of clinical application of MeltProTB/RIF in 512 clinical isolates of Mycobacterium tuberculosis with the traditional proportional method as the golden criteria showed the sensitivity and the specificity of 97.4% and 96.2%, respectively, and positive predictive value, negative predictive value, and coincidence rate were 94.1%, 98.4%, and 96.7%, respectively. (2) Isoniazid resistance mutation kit (MeltProTB/INH) can be used to detect common mutation sites, such as katG315, inhA promoter region, ahpC promoter region, and inhA 94. A methodological evaluation was performed for the kit by using the standard strain of Mycobacterium tuberculosis (H37Rv) and Mycobacterium tuberculosis with known isoniazid resistance mutation site, and the minimum detection limit of MeltProTB/INH in detecting katG315 mutation site was 300 copies/reaction, which could distinguish simultaneously nine point mutations or deletions related to INH resistance. Thereafter 833 samples were used to evaluate the clinical application of the kit, with sequencing method as the golden standard, and 162 mutated samples were detected by MeltProTB/INH, which was consistent with the results of sequencing method. (3) The ethambutol resistance mutation Kit (MeltProTB/EMB) was used to detect four common mutated sites including embB 306, embB378-380, embB 406, and embB 497. A methodological evaluation was performed for the kit by using the standard strain of Mycobacterium tuberculosis (H37Rv) and 36 non-Mycobacterium tuberculosis strains. The minimum detection limit of MeltProTB/EMB was 3 copies/reaction, with a specificity of 100%. Thereafter 613 sputum samples were used to evaluate the clinical application of the kit with sequencing method as the golden standard, which showed that the results achieved by MeltProTB/EM were completely consistent with those by sequencing method. (4) Streptomycin resistance mutation kit (MeltProTB/STRr) was used to detect 15 drug resistance mutated sites including rpsL43, rpsL88, rrs513, rrs514, rrs517, rrs 905-908. A multi-site clinical study on streptomycin resistance in 1056 strains of Mycobacterium tuberculosis with the traditional proportional method as the golden standard showed the sensitivity and specificity of MeltProTB/STR were 88.8% and 95.8%, respectively, the minimum detection limit was 50 copies/reaction ~500 copies/reaction, and the Tm value of the melting curve had good repeatability, with a temperature fluctuation less than 1 °C. (5) Fluoroquinolones resistance mutation kit (MeltProTB/FQ) was used to detect the resistance mutant sites of gyrA and gyrB. The traditional proportional method was used as the golden standard when drug resistance was detected in 509 clinical isolates from Mycobacterium tuberculosis, showing sensitivity, specificity, positive predictive value, negative predictive value, and coincidence rate were, respectively, 97.01%, 99.55%, 97.01%, 99.55%, and 99.21%.

MeltProTB has five kits testing anti-tuberculosis drugs, covering the resistance detection for four first-line anti-tuberculosis drugs and fluoroquinolones, meeting requirement of clinical MDR test and pre-XDR test, and having irreplaceable application value in countries with high burden of tuberculosis.

3.3.3 Linear Probe Assay

Line probe assay (LPA), a technology integrating PCR amplification, reverse hybridization, and membrane strip color development, amplifies target DNA fragments using the primer, hybridizes the amplified products with the probe fixed on the membrane, and determines the result finally by rinsing and enzyme color development. Hain Lifescience Germany (https://www.hain-lifescience.de/en/) has developed kits detecting susceptibility to anti-tuberculosis drug, GenoType MTBDRplus and GenoType MTBDRsl, based on the linear probe assay. Among them, GenoType MTBDRplus kit, a molecular diagnostic technology recommended globally by WHO for controlling multi-resistant tuberculosis, is mainly used to detect mutation of resistance genes for rifampicin (rpoB) and isoniazid (KatG and InhA) in clinical sputum samples and positive cultures from patients with tuberculosis [29]. GenoType MTBDRsl kit is used to detect the resistance genes of fluoroquinolones, ethambutol, amikacin, kanamycin, and capreomycin. However, the kit has two models including VER 1.0 and VER 2.0, with a great difference between them in selecting and matching drug resistance genes. Mainly chosen resistance genes include gyrA, rrs, and emb for GenoType MTBDRslVER 1.0 [30, 31] and gyrA, gyrB, rrs and eis for GenoType MTBDRslVER2.0.

In order to guarantee the accuracy and reliability of the results, GenoType MTBDRplus has set up three quality control lines on the membrane strip to carry out quality control on the final results. The first is a conjugation quality control line to determine whether the conjugate and substrate are added to the reaction. The second is a quality control probe for Mycobacterium tuberculosis complex to confirm whether the bacteria detected is Mycobacterium tuberculosis complex. The third is a PCR amplification quality control probe comprising three probes: a general quality control probe, a katG positive quality control, and a rpoB positive quality control. Among them, the universal quality control probe is used to detect all Mycobacteria and Gram-positive bacteria with high GC% content, and its color development intensity is the key to determine the results of membrane strips. Only the probe with color development intensity identical to or stronger than the quality control probe can be determined to be as a valid result. Similarly, genotype MTBDRsl is also provided with three corresponding quality control probes.

The sensitivity and specificity were 80.00% and 84.62%, respectively, for sputum and 100.00% and 98.90%, respectively, for culture, as detected by GenoType MTBDRplus with the subjects including 145 cases of sputum specimen and 160 strains of clinical Mycobacterium tuberculosis with traditional drug susceptibility test as the standard. These findings suggest that GenoType MTBDRplus has high sensitivity and specificity, is capable of detecting quickly MDR Mycobacterium tuberculosis in smear-positive sputum specimens and cultured strains, and is conducive to the rapid screening and diagnosis of multi-resistant tuberculosis. The method per se, however, is cumbersome and has a high requirement on professional skills of operators and on detection environment of laboratories correspondingly due to the post-PCR uncovering detection as required, so it must be launched in strict accordance with the standards of the gene amplification laboratory [32].

A detection in subjects including 41 MDR strains, 8 XDR strains, and 3 non-MDR strains with sequencing method as the golden standard showed the sensitivity and the specificity of GenoType MTBDRsl of 87% and 96% for fluoroquinolones, 100% and 100% for amikacin, 77% and 100% for kanamycin, 80% and 98% for capreomycin, and 57% and 92%, respectively, for ethambutol. The results of GenoType MTBDRsl are not satisfactory, given our failure to grasp fully the molecular resistant mechanism of anti-tuberculosis drugs at present, and limited number of drug resistance genes detectable by the kit. Especially, 1/3 of ETB resistant strains remained undetectable in the study, because gyrB highly related to ethambutol (ETB) resistance was not included in the kit, and ETB resistance was of great significance for treating MDR patients. The insufficient sensitivity of the kit, however, made 2 out of 8 XDRs (25%) indistinguishable from MDR. Molecular drug resistance test is far from enough for patients with MDR or XDR, and traditional drug susceptibility tests must be supplemented to provide better and more accurate clinical services [32].

3.3.4 Membrane Gene Chip

PCR reverse dot blot is a DNA chip technology that integrates PCR amplification in vitro with reverse dot blot. This method may fix multiple oligonucleotide probes with specific sequences onto different sites of the solid-phase membrane, then hybridize the labeled PCR products with the solid-phase probes, and then complete the detection via enzymatic chemical color development to identify the nucleic acids with specific sequences. Based on a PCR reverse dot blot platform, Yaneng Bioscience (Shenzhen) Technology Co., Ltd (http://www.yanengbio.com/) developed a kit for detecting drug-resistant mutated genes of Mycobacterium tuberculosis, which could detect simultaneously 13 mutation types of 5 drug-resistant genes (rpoB, katG, InhA, rpsL, and embB) for 4 first-line anti-tuberculosis drugs (rifampicin, isoniazid, streptomycin, and ethambutol) within 8 h, with the minimum detection limit of 1.0×10^4copies/mL, and the specificity, accuracy, and repeatability, respectively, up to 98%, 95%, and 99%.

Chen et al. [33] carried out simultaneously sputum smear acid fast staining, simultaneous amplification testing (SAT) and BACTEC MGIT-960 rapid culture/drug susceptibility test on sputum samples collected from 225 patients suspected of pulmonary tuberculosis and 32 patients with other pulmonary diseases. Sputum samples from 53 patients with confirmed pulmonary tuberculosis were detected by PCR reverse dot blot and sequencing. PCR reverse dot blot has high sensitivity and high specificity in detecting the mutation sites of resistance genes for rifampicin, isoniazid, streptomycin, and ethambutol, with the coincidence rate of 92.5% and 98.1% compared, respectively, with culture method and sequencing method. Jincai He et al. [34] used PCR reverse dot blot to detect clinically isolated Mycobacterium tuberculosis strains or sputum samples positive in acid fast staining microscopy from 264 patients (including 141 treatment-naive patients and 123 relapsing patients). With DNA sequencing as the golden standard, the methodological performance of PCR reverse dot blot for detecting drug-resistant gene mutations in Mycobacterium tuberculosis was evaluated, showing the sensitivity, specificity, and accuracy of 94.74%, 100%, and 98 11%, respectively, with a kappa value of 0.9584 (95%CI: 0.8379–1.0789). The sensitivity, specificity, and accuracy of PCR reverse dot blot in detecting drug-resistant gene mutations in Mycobacterium tuberculosis meet the clinical requirements and is suitable for use in clinical laboratories.

3.3.5 Microarray Chip

TB drug resistance chip of Beijing Boao Jingdian Co., Ltd (https://www.capitalbiotech.com/) can diagnose within 6 h the resistance in Mycobacterium tuberculosis complex group carried by patients to rifampicin and isoniazid, the two first-line anti-tuberculosis drugs, which is conducive to targeted treatment and control of the disease as soon as possible. The kit is the product for rapidly diagnosing MDR tuberculosis first certified by CFDA in China and capable of completing quickly the assessment of drug resistance to two drugs (rifampicin and isoniazid), 3 genes, 8 loci, and 16 mutation types within 6 h (Fig. 3.1). Its coverage rate accounted for 96% of all genetic loci related to rifampicin resistance, con-

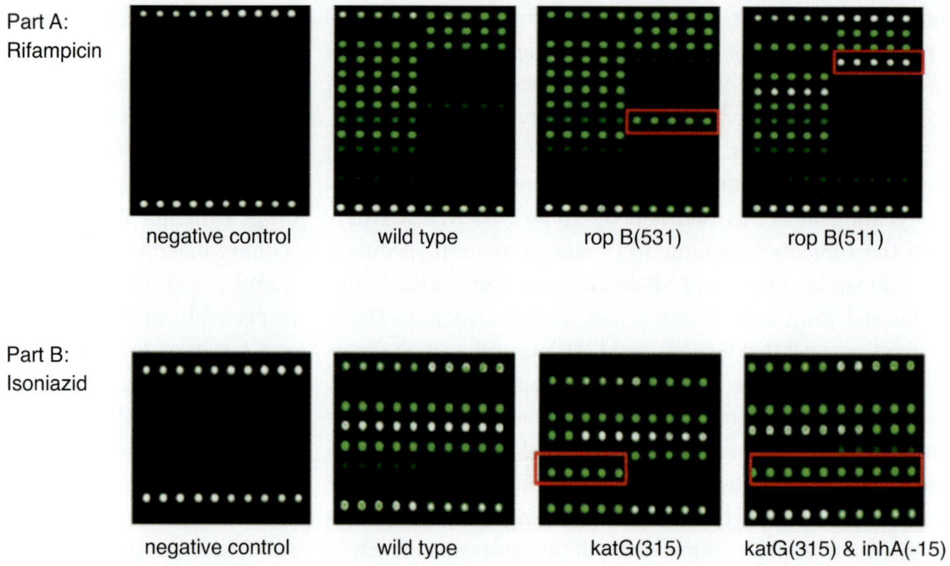

Fig. 3.1 Illustration of results in detecting drug-resistant genes in Mycobacterium tuberculosis

cerning the 6 most common loci related to drug resistance in rifampicin rpoB gene. Concerning two isoniazid genes including katG and inhA, the coverage rate accounted for 90% of all genetic loci related to isoniazid resistance. Jing Zhao et al. [35] used DNA microarray to detect the wild-type and various mutant types of the promoters of 3 resistance-related genes including genes rpoB, katG, and InhA for rifampicin (RFP) and isoniazid (INH). They also incubated Mycobacterium tuberculosis with BACTECTM MGIT 960 incubator. For a positive liquid culture, they switched back to modified Lowenstein–Jensen proportional method to perform drug susceptibility test. Results showed that there were 15 rpoB mutants in 174 sputum samples positive in Mycobacterium tuberculosis nucleic acid, with the highest mutation frequency observed at loci 531 and a mutation rate of 66.7%. 12 among 17 katG/inhA mutants were single mutations at locus katG, with a mutation rate of 70.6%. Compared with the drug susceptibility results of 68 cases by modified Lowenstein–Jensen proportional method, both coincidence rates for RFP and INH resistance detected by DNA microarray method were more than 90%. It is considered, therefore, that DNA microarray can detect quickly and accurately mutations of gene rpoB, katG, and inhA in clinical samples of the most of cases suspected of tuberculosis. It can be used to detect clinical drug resistance and guide clinical medication, with its generalization and application achievable during clinical diagnosis.

3.3.6 Sequencing

Compared with Sanger method, pyrophosphate sequencing technology has the advantages of high throughput, low cost, and shorter detection-report time [36]. Changtai Zhu et al. [37] used pyrophosphate sequencing technology to establish a poly-resistance detection method for Mycobacterium tuberculosis strains and compared it with BACTEC MGIT 960 drug susceptibility method. Pyrophosphate sequencing was used to detect resistance to rifampicin and isoniazid in 202 clinical isolates of poly-resistant Mycobacterium tuberculosis. Compared with drug resistance results obtained by BACTEC MGIT 960, the sensitivity and specificity of pyrophosphate sequencing in detecting clinical isolates of poly-resistant Mycobacterium tuberculosis were 72.8% [95% confidence interval (CI): 66.3–78.4%] and 90.0% (95% CI: 80.1–95.1%), respectively. It is considered that pyrophosphate sequencing can detect quickly the resistance in Mycobacterium tuberculosis to rifampicin and isoniazid, and it can be used as an effective tool to detect the drug susceptibility in poly-resistant Mycobacterium tuberculosis. Xiaoguang Chen et al. [38] used pyrophosphate sequencing to detect the embB306 gene of Mycobacterium tuberculosis, with the proportional drug susceptibility as the control, and evaluated the pyrophosphate sequencing in detecting poly-resistant strains. Results showed that the mutation rate of embB306 was 60.9% (14/23) for poly-resistant strains and 15.2% (7/46) for non poly-resistant strains, with a statistical significance between them ($\chi^2 = 15.09$, $P < 0.01$) (OR = 8.67, 95%CI: 2.38–33.27). Compared with proportional susceptibility test, pyrophosphate sequencing in detecting poly-resistant strains has its sensibility, specificity, and accuracy of 61%, 85%, and 77%, respectively. Direct DNA sequencing performed for Mycobacterium tuberculosis isolates that had obtained pyrophosphate sequencing showed a completely consistent result with a coincidence rate up to 100%. It is considered, therefore, that pyrophosphate sequencing as a tool for diagnosing poly-resistance in Mycobacterium tuberculosis has good clinical application value.

References

1. Kirihara JAL, Hillier SL, Coyle MB. Improved detection times of Mycobacterium avium complex and M. tuberculosis with the BACTEC radiometric system [J]. J Clin Microbiol. 1985;22(5):841–5.
2. Morgan MA, Horstmeier CD, DeYoung DR, et al. Comparison of a radiometric method (BACTEC) and conventional culture media for recovery of mycobacteria from smear-negative specimens [J]. J Clin Microbiol. 1983;18(2):384–8.
3. Roberts GD, Goodman NL, Heifets L, et al. Evaluation of the BACTEC radiometric method for recovery of mycobacteria and drug susceptibility testing of Mycobacterium tuberculosis from acid-fast smear-positive specimens [J]. J Clin Microbiol. 1983;18(3):689–96.
4. Siddiqi SH, Libonati JP, Middlebrook G. Evaluation of a rapid radiometric method for drug susceptibility testing of Mycobacterium tuberculosis [J]. J Clin Microbiol. 1981;13(5):908–12.
5. Zong Z-j, Jing W, Huo F-m, et al. Resistance analysis of extensively drug-resistant Mycobacterium tuberculosis isolates against linezolid [J]. Electron J Emerg Infect Dis. 2017;2(3):160–3.
6. Canetti G, Froman S, Grosset J, et al. Mycobacteria: laboratory methods for testing drug sensitivity and resistance [J]. Bull World Health Organ. 1963;29:565–78.
7. Yang S, Bu H, Fan M. A comparison between BACTEC-MGIT 960 rapid drug susceptibility test and Lowenstein-Jensen proportional susceptibility method [J]. Clin Med Pract. 2015;24(12):919–21.
8. Abe C, Aono A, Hirano K. Evaluation of the BACTEC MGIT 960 system for drug susceptibility testing of Mycobacterium tuberculosis isolates compared with the proportion method on solid media [J]. Kekkaku (Japanese). 2001;76(10):657–62.
9. Bergmann JS, Fish G, Woods GL. Evaluation of BBL MGIT (Mycobacteria Growth Indicator Tube) AST SIRE System for antimycobacterial susceptibility testing of Mycobacterium tuberculosis to 4 primary antituberculosis drugs [J]. Arch Pathol Lab Med. 2000;124(1):82–6.
10. Cambau E, Truffot-Pernot C, Boulahbal F, et al. Mycobacterial Growth Indicator Tube versus the proportion method on Lowenstein-Jensen medium for antibiotic susceptibility testing of Mycobacterium tuberculosis [J]. Eur J Clin Microbiol Infect Dis. 2000;19(12):938–42.
11. Li J, Wang Z, Bai G, et al. Clinical value of MicrioDST™ microporous plate in susceptibility test on the first- and second-line anti-tuberculosis drugs [J]. Chin J Lung Dis (Electrical Version). 2018;11(5):583–7.
12. Wang H, Zhao Q, Chen M. A methodological research on Sensititre tuberculosis susceptibility plate in detecting susceptibility of Mycobacterium tuberculosis [J]. Journal of Hebei Medical University. 2015;37(2):187–90.
13. Helb D, Jones M, Story E, et al. Rapid detection of Mycobacterium tuberculosis and rifampin resistance by use of on-demand, near-patient technology [J]. J Clin Microbiol. 2010;48(1):229–37.
14. Boehme CC, Nabeta P, Hillemann D, et al. Rapid molecular detection of tuberculosis and rifampin resistance [J]. N Engl J Med. 2010;363(11):1005–15.
15. Wu F, Li Y. A meta analysis of efficiency of GeneXpertMTB/RIF in diagnosing tuberculosis in population infected with HIV [J]. Chin J Antituberc. 2017;39(3):269–76.
16. Chakravorty S, Simmons AM, Rowneki M, et al. The new Xpert MTB/RIF Ultra: improving detection of Mycobacterium tuberculosis and resistance to rifampin in an assay suitable for point-of-care testing [J]. mBio. 2017;8(4):e00812–7.
17. Lawn SD, Brooks SV, Kranzer K, et al. Screening for HIV-Associated tuberculosis and rifampicin resistance before antiretroviral therapy using the Xpert MTB/RIF assay: a prospective study [J]. PLoS Med. 2011;8(7):e1001067.
18. Zeka AN, Tasbakan S, Cavusoglu C. Evaluation of the GeneXpert MTB/RIF assay for rapid diagnosis of tuberculosis and detection of rifampin resistance in pulmonary and extrapulmonary specimens [J]. J Clin Microbiol. 2011;49(12):4138–41.
19. Zetola NM, Shin SS, Tumedi KA, et al. Mixed Mycobacterium tuberculosis complex infections and false-negative results for rifampin resistance by GeneXpert MTB/RIF are associated with poor clinical outcomes [J]. J Clin Microbiol. 2014;52(7):2422–9.
20. Rufai SB, Kumar P, Singh A, et al. Comparison of Xpert MTB/RIF with line probe assay for detection of rifampin-monoresistant Mycobacterium tuberculosis [J]. J Clin Microbiol. 2014;52(6):1846–52.
21. Huang Q, Liu Z, Liao Y, et al. Multiplex fluorescence melting curve analysis for mutation detection with dual-labeled, self-quenched probes [J]. PLoS One. 2011;6(4):e19206.
22. Huang Q, Wang X, Tang N, et al. Rapid detection of non-deletional mutations causing α-thalassemia by multicolor melting curve analysis [J]. Clin Chem Lab Med. 2016;54(3):397–402.
23. Wang X, Hong Y, Cai P, et al. Rapid and reliable detection of non-syndromic hearing loss mutations by multicolor melting curve analysis [J]. Sci Rep. 2017;7:42894.
24. Liu N, Huang Q, Li Q, et al. Spectrum of PAH gene variants among a population of Han Chinese patients with phenylketonuria from northern China [J]. BMC Med Genet. 2017;18(1):108.
25. Liao Y, Li Q. Profile of MeltPro ® HPV test for human papillomavirus genotyping and cervical precancer screening [J]. Expert Rev Mol Diagn. 2019;19(10):857–62.
26. Li H, Wang S, Zhu Y, et al. A research on two methods detecting poly-resistant genes in Mycobacterium tuberculosis in diagnosing poly-resistant tuberculosis [J]. Chin J Health Lab Technol. 2015;25(15):2567–9.
27. Li Q, Huang Q. A method to detect mutations of nucleic acid sequence: China. CN102449167B [P]. 2014.
28. Xu Y, Liang B, Du C, et al. Rapid identification of clinically relevant Mycobacterium species by multicolor curve analysis [J]. J Clin Microbiol. 2019;57(1):e01096–18.
29. Makinen J, Marttila HJ, Marjamaki M, et al. Comparison of two commercially available DNA line probe assays for detection of multidrug-resistant Mycobacterium tuberculosis [J]. J Clin Microbiol. 2006;44(2):350–2.
30. Hillemann D, Rusch-Gerdes S, Richter E. Feasibility of the GenoType MTBDRsl assay for fluoroquinolone, amikacin-capreomycin, and ethambutol resistance testing of Mycobacterium tuberculosis strains and clinical specimens [J]. J Clin Microbiol. 2009;47(6):1767–72.
31. Zhu Y-m, Zhong Y-q, Li J-l, et al. Evaluation of GenoType Mycobacterium CMfor the rapid identification of non-tuberculous mycobacteria [J/CD]. Electron J Emerg Infect Dis. 2022;7(2):47–51.
32. Li H, Ma X, Shi J, et al. A research on linear probe assay MTBDRplus applied to detection of poly-resistance in smear-positive pulmonary tuberculosis [J]. Chin J Health Lab Technol. 2013;23(2):380–6.
33. Chen Y, Zhang L, Hong L, et al. Rapid diagnosis of pulmonary tuberculosis and detection of drug resistance by combined simultaneous amplification testing and reverse dot blot [J]. J Clin Pathol. 2018;71(6):498–503.
34. He J, Zhou D, Lao S, et al. The application of PCR-reverse dot blot to detection of drug-resistant genetic mutations in Mycobacterium tuberculosis [J]. Guangdong Med. 2013;34(3):395–7.
35. Zhao J, Wang F, Sun Q, et al. The role of DNA microarray in detecting resistance of Mycobacterium tuberculosis to rifampicin and isoniazid [J]. Med Bull Shanghai Jiaotong Univ. 2015;35(11):1651–4.
36. Nyren P. The history of pyrosequencing [J]. Methods Mol Biol. 2007;373(3):1–14.
37. Zhu C, Zheng R, Wang J, et al. The role of pyrophosphate sequencing technology in detecting poly-resistant Mycobacterium tuberculosis [J]. Exp Lab Med. 2012;30(6):528–30.
38. Chen X, Dong M, Teng X, et al. The role of pyrophosphate sequencing technology in detecting rapidly gene embB of poly-resistant Mycobacterium tuberculosis in Qingdao Region [J]. J Trop Med. 2018;18(3):354–61.

4 Pathogenic Mechanism of Drug-Resistant Pulmonary Tuberculosis and Its Diagnosis

Pu-Xuan Lu, Qiuting Zheng, Guofang Deng, Guang-ping Zheng, Yun Zhou, Fang-jun Wei, Gen-dong Yang, Ya-nan Hu, and Yu-xin Shi

Pulmonary tuberculosis is one of the main infectious respiratory diseases endangering human health. In comparison with drug-susceptible pulmonary tuberculosis once controlled in developed countries due to the active and effective measures taken by the government, drug-resistant tuberculosis is still one of the greatest challenges confronted by human being in striving to conquer tuberculosis [1–3].

Drug-resistant pulmonary tuberculosis is a disease caused by drug-resistant Mycobacteria tuberculosis resistant to drugs. There were 465,000 cases of rifampicin-resistant tuberculosis (RR-TB) around the world in 2019, and 78% of them were multidrug-resistant (MDR-TB). 3.3% of newly diagnosed tuberculosis and 17.7% of previously treated tuberculosis were MDR/RR-TB. The three countries with the largest burden around the world are India (27%), China (14%), and the Russian Federation (8%). Globally, the mean proportion of MDR-TB patients resistant to fluoroquinolones is 20.1%, based on the data reported by 105 countries and regions. More RR-TB patients have been identified during recent years, despite the persistent effort of nations in improving their capability in diagnosing drug-resistant pulmonary tuberculosis. Only 206,000 cases of patients were reported in 2019, however, accounting for 44% of the estimated number, which implied the severe insufficiency in the coverage rate for drug susceptibility tests. Most of MDR/RR-TB patients (86%) have been exposed to anti-tuberculosis treatment at their diagnosis [4].

P.-X. Lu (✉) · Q. Zheng
Diagnostic Imaging, Shenzhen Center for Chronic Disease Control, Shenzhen, China

G. Deng
Department of Tuberculosis, The Third People's Hospital of Shenzhen, Shenzhen, China

G.-p. Zheng · Y. Zhou · F.-j. Wei · G.-d. Yang
Department of Radiology, The Third People's Hospital of Shenzhen, Shenzhen, Guangdong, China

Y.-n. Hu
Department of General Practice, ZiWei Community Health Care Service Center of Longgang District People's Hospital, Shenzhen, Guangdong, China

Y.-x. Shi
Department of Radiology, Shanghai Public Health Clinical Center, Shanghai, China

The year of 2019 witnessed 65,000 cases of newly diagnosed MDR/RR-TB with an incidence of 4.5/100,000, and among them the ratio of patients previously exposed to anti-tuberculosis was 23/100,000 [4]. An analysis of data at baseline survey on drug resistance of tuberculosis in China carried out from 2007 to 2008 showed a drug resistance rate of 28.1% (853/3037) and a multidrug resistance rate of 5.8% (175/3037) in initial treatment of pulmonary tuberculosis patients, and the latter reached to 25.3% (226/892) in relapsing patients. An aggravation was observed for the epidemics of drug-resistant pulmonary tuberculosis in China, compared with the national epidemiological survey of tuberculosis in 2000 [5, 6]. In respect of the control of epidemics of drug-resistant pulmonary tuberculosis, therefore, it is still necessary to strengthen the discovery of drug-resistant/multidrug-resistant patients, the construction of control service systems, treatment management, and capital investment [7, 8].

According to WHO Global Tuberculosis Report 2021, 132,222 cases of MDR/RR-TB and 25,681 cases of pre-extensive or extensive drug-resistant tuberculosis were detected in 2020, with 157,903 cases in total, which was lower significantly than 201,997 cases observed in 2019, with a drop of 22% [4].

4.1 Definition and Categorization of Drug-Resistant Tuberculosis

1. Monoresistant tuberculosis (MR-TB): An Mtb infecting the tuberculosis patient is resistant to one anti-tuberculosis drug, as proven in vitro.
2. Poly-resistant tuberculosis (PDR-TB): An Mtb infecting the tuberculosis patient is resistant to more than one

P.-x. Lu et al. (eds.), *Diagnostic Imaging of Drug Resistant Pulmonary Tuberculosis*,
https://doi.org/10.1007/978-981-99-8339-1_4

anti-tuberculosis drug, as proven in vitro, but not including simultaneously isoniazid and rifampicin.

3. Multidrug-resistant tuberculosis (MDR-TB): An Mtb infecting the tuberculosis patient is resistant simultaneously to at least isoniazid and rifampicin, as proven in vitro.
4. Pre-extensive drug-resistant tuberculosis (Pre-XDR-TB) [9]: It is defined as a tuberculosis induced by a Mycobacteria tuberculosis strain, which meets the definition of MDR/RR-TB and is resistant to any fluoroquinolone.
5. Extensive drug-resistant tuberculosis (XDR-TB) [10]: It is defined as a tuberculosis induced by a Mycobacteria tuberculosis strain, which meets the definition of MDR/RR-TB and is resistant simultaneously to any fluoroquinolone and at least any other drug in Group A.
6. Rifampicin-resistant tuberculosis (RR-TB): It is defined as a tuberculosis proven resistant to rifampicin based on DST in vitro and includes any tuberculosis resistant to rifampicin, i.e., rifampicin monoresistant TB (RMD-TB), rifampicin multiresistant TB (RPR-TB), MDR-TB, and XDR-TB.

The diagnosis of drug-resistant pulmonary tuberculosis is mainly based on drug-resistant Mycobacteria tuberculosis identified by laboratory tests and confirmed by drug susceptibility tests. Laboratory tests include mainly sputum smear staining, isolation and culture of Mycobacterium tuberculosis, detection of nucleic acid of Mycobacterium tuberculosis (TB-PCR) in sputum samples, identification of Mycobacterium tuberculosis species, drug susceptibility test of Mycobacterium tuberculosis, detection of drug-resistant mutant gene of Mycobacterium tuberculosis, and immunological detection of mycobacteria. The WHO-recommended rapid detection technology now available for tubercle bacillus and for rifampicin resistance includes GeneXpert MTB/RIF. By the end of 2017, this WHO-recommended test has been used as the initial method for screening suspected cases of tuberculosis by 32 out of the 48 countries with high burden of tuberculosis [11].

Correct clinical classification of drug-resistant pulmonary tuberculosis is helpful to guide clinical diagnosis, treatment, and evaluation of responses. Drug-resistant tuberculosis, based on the Report of Global Project of Monitoring Resistance to Anti-Tuberculosis Drugs (version 3) issued by World Health Organization/International Union Against Tuberculosis and Lung Diseases (WHO/IUATLD), can be divided into new drug-resistant tuberculosis and relapsing drug-resistant tuberculosis, corresponding to the absence/presence of exposure to any anti-tuberculosis drug [12, 13].

New drug-resistant tuberculosis (NDR-TB), also known as primary drug-resistant tuberculosis, happens in an initial treatment patient or a patient exposed to any anti-tuberculosis drug for less than 1 month. NDR-TB includes the infection with a Mycobacteria tuberculosis strain with a preexisting resistance and a resistance induced by a genetic mutation in vivo in a Mycobacteria tuberculosis infecting people (i.e., a natural resistance).

(Remark: New drug-resistant tuberculosis is induced by the transmission from another person infected by a drug-resistant strain.)

Relapsing drug-resistant tuberculosis (RDR-TB) is defined as a resistance in a patient with a previous exposure to anti-tuberculosis treatment or on an anti-tuberculosis treatment for at least 1 month. This resistance forms in most cases because a few flora with drug-resistant mutants becomes dominant due to the eradication of originally drug-susceptible flora by improper treatment or other factors. (Remark: They include generally patients with treatment failure or recurrence, or those on treatment and lost to follow-up. The possibility is that resistance has been generated in the tuberculosis during the treatment for these patients, or their diseases are transmitted from any person with drug-resistant Mycobacteria tuberculosis in vivo.)

Relapsing drug-resistant tuberculosis can be caused by three conditions as follows: (1) Re-infection. A relapsing tuberculosis patient is infected again with another new strain of drug-resistant Mycobacteria tuberculosis during or after anti-tuberculosis treatment, and this is a primary resistance; (2) Mixed infection, also known as multiple infections. A tuberculosis patient on re-treatment is infected with two or more Mycobacterium tuberculosis strains, including drug-susceptible one and drug-resistant one. The susceptible strain is eradicated during anti-tuberculosis treatment, while the replication of drug-resistant bacteria increases, so this resistance during re-treatment is also caused by the initially infected drug-resistant bacteria and belongs also to primary drug resistance. (3) Relapsing drug-resistant tuberculosis, i.e., a resistance formed by a flora with resistant mutation which is screened due to the use of anti-tuberculosis drugs during the former treatment in a relapsing tuberculosis patient. Because there is no way to discriminate different floras based on phenotypes of bacteria (i.e., colonial morphology), not all drug resistances occurring during an anti-tuberculosis treatment for more than 1 month can be regarded for granted as the relapsing drug-resistant tuberculosis.

4.2 Mechanism of Drug Resistance in Tuberculosis and Its Risk Factors

4.2.1 Mechanism of Drug Resistance in Tuberculosis

The mechanisms vary for drug resistance of Mycobacterium tuberculosis, which are currently considered related to the mutation of targeting genes of Mycobacterium tuberculosis, bacterial adaptability, and the genetic background of the bacteria themselves.

Clinically, the main mechanism for drug resistance in Mycobacterium tuberculosis is genetic mutation, which mostly occurs in drug target genes and genes related to drug activating enzymes. Genetic mutation of Mycobacterium tuberculosis may change drug targets, so that some precursor drugs (such as isoniazid and pyrazinamide) cannot be activated in the cells of Mycobacterium tuberculosis and even result in over expression of drug targets, thereby causing resistance to drug [14]. Meanwhile, mutations of the drug-efflux system and of genes related to cell wall synthesis of Mycobacterium tuberculosis may enhance the inherent drug resistance and raise further drug resistance of Mycobacterium tuberculosis.

Adaptability is an important indicator for evaluating the ability of growth and reproduction of bacteria living in a specific environment. The decreased viability of bacteria is called fitness cost, and strains with stronger adaptability may spread more easily. The present whole-genome sequencing of MDR-TB reveals multiple mutations, some of which are compensatory mutations [14]. Though not inducing drug resistance by themselves, these mutations may compensate for the harmful effects caused by mutations and restore the initial growing capacity of the strain, thereby improving the adaptability of drug-resistant tuberculosis strains [15, 16].

Drug resistance of Mycobacterium tuberculosis correlates closely to its genetic background, and the strain Lineage 2 has always been considered more toxic and a greater tendency to form drug resistance [17].

The joint action of genetic mutation, compensatory mutation, and gene background endows Mycobacterium tuberculosis with stronger adaptability and higher drug resistance. The research on the mechanism of drug resistance in Mycobacterium tuberculosis is helpful to understand further the evolutionary process of its drug resistance, so as to provide a theoretical basis for rapid diagnosis of drug-resistant tuberculosis and development of a new generation of anti-tuberculosis drugs.

4.2.2 Causes of Drug Resistance in Tuberculosis and Its Risk Factors

4.2.2.1 Causes of Drug Resistance Tuberculosis

The occurrence of drug-resistant tuberculosis results from a joint action of multiple factors, including mainly three groups as follows: (1) Individual factors: First, improper treatments performed without the guidance by the principle of tuberculosis treatment, such as the absence of combined treatment, insufficient dosage below effectiveness, inadequate treatment, and intermittent dosing due to poor compliance in the patient. These are the most important factors for inducing acquired drug-resistant tuberculosis, which act via a mechanism of inducing chromosomal mutation of MTB allowing the selective growth of drug-resistant MTB strains, thereby inducing drug-resistant tuberculosis. Second, opportunities and intensity of individual contact with and exposure to pathogens and even hereditary susceptibility may also affect the probability for an individual to get drug-resistant tuberculosis [18]. (2) Social factors, including the shortage of anti-tuberculosis drugs, poor quality of drugs, the failure of relevant social departments in implementing effective supervision and management, the lack of publicity, education and popularization of relevant knowledge in populations of patients, and the lack of control of tuberculosis infection due to floating population and loose management of anti-tuberculosis drugs, may lead to the spread of drug-resistant tuberculosis, and its spread and epidemics may result in the occurrence of drug-resistant tuberculosis among initial treatment patients [19]. (3) Bacterial factors. The occurrence of resistance, based on a molecular consideration, is mostly caused by the change of bacterial cellular wall, mutations of enzyme genes related to specific drug resistance and of target genes, and the genesis of a drug-efflux mechanism, which result in the lowered permeability of cellular wall to anti-tuberculosis drugs, the difficulty for drugs to enter the bacteria effectively and their accelerated discharge under the effect of efflux mechanism, so that no effective drug concentration can be achieved and no anti-tuberculosis effect can be exerted [14, 20]. In summary, many reasons account for drug resistance, including drug insufficiency, poor quality of drugs, improper treatment, poor compliance in patients or termination of treatment and social monitoring strength, all of which may not only result in the emergence of drug-resistant tuberculosis but also lead to the gradual increase in drug resistance spectrum of Mycobacterium tuberculosis during anti-tuberculosis treatment. Direct transmission of drug-resistant tubercle bacilli between humans is an important way to causing the prevalence of drug-resistant TB.

4.2.2.2 Risk Factors of Drug-Resistant Tuberculosis

Risk factors of drug-resistant tuberculosis include [21]: (1) history of exposure to anti-tuberculosis drugs; (2) persistently positive in smear or culture after 3-month anti-tuberculosis treatment; (3) history of contact with any patient with drug-resistant tuberculosis; (4) coming from an area with high incidence of drug-resistant tuberculosis; and (5) poor response to persistent 2-week treatment using the first-line anti-tuberculosis drugs, where in the failure of anti-tuberculosis drug treatment is an independent prognostic indicator of extensively drug-resistant tuberculosis (XDR-TB).

4.3 Diagnosis of Drug-Resistant Pulmonary Tuberculosis

WHO categorizes drug-resistant tuberculosis into five groups, including the isoniazid-resistant, the rifampicin resistant, and the multidrug resistant, as well as the pre-extensively resistant and the extensively resistant. Pre-extensively drug-resistant tuberculosis is defined as a tuberculosis resistant to rifampicin and any of fluoroquinolones. Extensively drug-resistant tuberculosis is defined as a tuberculosis resistant to rifampicin and any of fluoroquinolones, as well as at least one of the following two drugs: bedaquiline and linezolid.

The proportion of multidrug-resistant or rifampicin-resistant tuberculosis has remained around 3–4% (the best estimate) among all patients diagnosed with tuberculosis for the first time during more than recent 10 years, and around 18–21% among those having received anti-tuberculosis treatment. The burden of multidrug-resistant tuberculosis or rifampicin-resistant tuberculosis is relatively stable.

4.3.1 Present Condition of Diagnosis of Drug-Resistant Pulmonary Tuberculosis

With complex and diverse clinical manifestations, drug-resistant tuberculosis has multiple factors intervening with the evaluation of responses. Methods for clinical diagnosis of drug-resistant tuberculosis have both advantages and disadvantages, so clinical diagnosis is very important. The emergence of drug-resistant tuberculosis is highly suspected of, if the patient shows no amelioration of tuberculosis-related symptoms such as cough, expectoration, fever, and night sweat but deterioration instead after more than 3 months of standardized anti-tuberculosis treatment by a specialist or after two times of unstandardized treatment, with an increased number and enlarged infiltrating scope of lesions compared with their pre-treatment condition, as confirmed by imaging examinations such as chest X-ray and CT scans [22, 23]. Clinical manifestations of drug-resistant tuberculosis, however, are often atypical and show milder symptoms, even without obvious changes in image findings compared with the status prior to the emergence of the resistance, which brings a great challenge to the clinical diagnosis.

Culture of Mycobacterium tuberculosis, identification of strains, and drug susceptibility test are reliable methods for determining drug-susceptible/resistant pulmonary tuberculosis. The diagnosis of drug-resistant pulmonary tuberculosis mainly depends upon laboratory tests, including bacteriological and molecular ones (such as GeneXpert MTB/RIF, GeneXpert MTB/RIF Ultra, probe melting curve, gene chip, and linear probe assay). Molecular biological methods may realize rapid and precise diagnosis of pulmonary tuberculosis and the detection of drug resistance. The rapid detection technologies recommended by the World Health Organization for tuberculosis and rifampicin resistance include GeneXpert MTB/RIF and GeneXpert MTB/RIF Ultra. The present gold standard for the cultivation and detection of drug-resistant tubercle bacillus is still bacterial culture and drug sensitivity test, which are time-consuming. Moreover, the detection of resistance to the first- and the second-line anti-tuberculosis drugs is usually not performed until the disease shows no response to conventional empirical treatment given to an initial treatment patient, so as to make a large number of drug-resistant tuberculosis patients miss the best timepoint for treatment [24–27].

Early diagnosis and timely modification of treatment regimen are the keys to control the progression of drug-resistant pulmonary tuberculosis. Imaging examination, an important adjuvant method, may provide not only a hint of a possible drug-resistant tuberculosis in a patient based on imaging signs but also the necessity of timely detection of drug-resistant Mycobacteria tuberculosis so as to offer diagnostic evidence. In addition, image examination has also great significance in clinical imaging diagnosis, differential diagnosis, and evaluation of responses and prognosis.

4.3.2 Laboratory Tests and Diagnosis of Drug-Resistant Pulmonary Tuberculosis

4.3.2.1 Traditional Laboratory Tests for Drug-Resistant Pulmonary Tuberculosis

Phenotypic drug sensitivity test (pDST) is the gold standard for determining the resistance to anti-tuberculosis drugs, but it is time-consuming and requires professionals and good laboratory infrastructure to minimize biosafety risks. pDST still has a certain value in detecting newly identified resistance to drugs, the resistance to new anti-tuberculosis drugs and to drugs with uncertainty shown by molecular biological detection.

4.3.2.2 Molecular Technologies for Detecting Susceptibility of Drugs

WHO recommends to use GeneXpert MTB/RIF and GeneXpert MTB/RIF Ultra for rapid diagnosis of pulmonary tuberculosis and extra-pulmonary tuberculosis in adults and children as well as rifampicin resistance. As for tuberculosis patients, WHO [28] recommends to use commercially available line probe assays (LPAs) as the initial susceptibility test for anti-tuberculosis drugs, but not the susceptibility test based on phenotype culture, in detecting rapidly the presence of genetic mutation inducing rifampicin and isoniazid resistance in positive sputum smear (direct detection) or

Mycobacterium tuberculosis complex culture (indirect detection). The consistency is more than 90% between rifampicin resistance and rpoB mutation in Mycobacterium tuberculosis, but more than 70% between isoniazid resistance and its mutations of inhA and KatG. Therefore, it is still necessary to perform the classical drug sensitivity test (DST) to prevent from the missed detection of isoniazid resistance, even if it is not detected by LPAs.

In addition to detecting mutations for resistance to rifampicin and isoniazid, LPAs can also detect genetic mutations related to the resistance to fluoroquinolones and the second-line anti-tuberculosis injections.

As for the second-line anti-tuberculosis drugs, WHO still recommends to use LPAs as the initial screening test to detect the resistance to fluoroquinolones and the second-line injections in patients with RR-TB or MDR-TB. WHO recommends to use LPAs to detect isolates from sputum specimen (direct detection) and extra-pulmonary Mycobacterium tuberculosis complex (indirect detection). Mutations inducing the resistance to the second-line injections, as detected by LPAs, are highly correlated to results of phenotype DST based on cultures. A similar high correlation is also observed for the resistance to fluoroquinolones between these two detections. LPAs are applicable to patients confirmed eligible for receiving any short-term regimen against multidrug-resistant tuberculosis.

Other molecular diagnostic techniques: Detection of Mycobacterium tuberculosis by loop-mediated isothermal amplification (TB-LAMP), which can be used as an alternative test or a subsequent test of sputum smear microscopy for diagnosing adult pulmonary tuberculosis in patients with symptoms and signs consistent with this disease. These recommendations are applicable to any environment permitting routine sputum smear microscopy. TB-LAMP should not replace rapid molecular test, which is used to detect tuberculosis and rifampicin resistance, especially in the population with risks of multidrug-resistant tuberculosis. Another molecular detection technique is polymerase chain reaction single strand conformation polymorphism (PCR-SSCP), and it is of the great importance in understanding the resistance to isoniazid and rifampicin in Mycobacterium tuberculosis through using PCR-SSCP to detect its genetic mutation related to drug resistance. The PCR-SSCP technology is characterized in simple operation, short duration required by the detection, no special requirements on equipment and reagents, no radioactive pollution, mature technical conditions, relatively high detection rate, and extensive use. It is affected, however, by length of DAN fragments under detection, concentration of polyacrylamide, ionic strength of buffer solution, and temperature during electrophoresis. PCR-SSCP cannot provide specific loci of mutations and their nature, so it can be applied to only screening of genetic mutation, which limits its practical clinical application. Centralized platform, including Abbott RealTime MTB and MTB-RIF/INH detection, Roche Cobas® MTB and MTB-RIF/INH test, Hain FluoroType® MTBDR method, and BDMAX™MDR-TB method, has value in detecting the resistance in rifampicin and isoniazid resistance determining genotype regions. Genoscholar®PZA-TB II Detection (Nipro, Ōsaka of Japan) is the only one method commercially available for detecting the mutation within pnaA gene (including the region of promoter) potentially inducing the resistance to pyrazinamide.

4.3.2.3 Gene Sequencing

Next generation gene sequencing (NGS), also known as high throughput sequencing, is a method recommended by WHO for the rapid detection of tuberculosis and capable of diagnosing drug-resistant tuberculosis on the basis of reducing the delay in treatment due to drug resistance. NGS available now can neither distinguish completely mutations for low resistance from those for high resistance, nor can it distinguish some mutations irrelevant to drug resistance. In comparison with such a disadvantage of NGS for clinical isolates that it necessitates the culture of Mycobacterium tuberculosis to yield sufficient quantity of bacteria, targeted NGS can realize directly both the sequencing for clinical isolates and the rapid detection of multidrug resistance through analyzing sputum specimen of the patient. Therefore, NGS may provide profound and complete data for all mutations related to clinical resistance and replace diagnostic methods of either the phenotype diagnosis or molecular drug susceptibility test, which are available now for diagnosing multidrug resistance. Characterized in advantages including high throughput, short time consumed by the detection, high precision, and abundance of information, NGS is applied widely to detection of drug-resistant tuberculosis, especially multidrug-resistant tuberculosis.

4.3.3 Imaging Diagnosis of Drug-Resistant Pulmonary Tuberculosis

4.3.3.1 Basic Imaging Findings of Drug-Resistant Pulmonary Tuberculosis

Predilection sites of drug-resistant pulmonary tuberculosis: Sites for intrapulmonary lesions of drug-resistant pulmonary tuberculosis are extensive, including the middle lobe of the right lung, the lingual segment of the left upper lobe, and basal segments of both lower lobes. Compared with the population with drug-susceptible pulmonary tuberculosis, the population with drug-resistant disease has significantly more sufferers with lesions affecting more than three pulmonary lobes. 87.07% of this population manifest a simultaneous involvement of non-predilection sites of tuberculosis, such as the anterior segment of the upper lobe and the basal segment of the lower lobe. The difference concerning distribution of lesions in pulmonary fields and occurrence sites seems unobvious among groups differing in types of drug resistance [22, 23].

Drug-resistant pulmonary tuberculosis, having the same imaging features as those of drug-susceptible secondary pulmonary tuberculosis [23], manifests the main signs including pulmonary consolidation, nodules (including centrilobular and acinar nodules), cavity sign, tree-in-bud sign, thickening of bronchial wall, bronchiectasis, pleural thickening and/or calcification, pneumothorax and/or pleural effusion, mediastinal and/or hilar lymph lymphadenectasis.

1. Nodule and cavity: Drug-resistant pulmonary tuberculosis is more prone to pulmonary nodules and cavities, in comparison with drug-susceptible pulmonary tuberculosis. Multiple nodules measuring often 6–30 mm (Fig. 4.1) can be observed in a patient with a history less than 1 month of drug-resistant pulmonary tuberculosis. For patients with a much shorter history (less than 1 month), as revealed by some authors, the prevalence of pulmonary nodules showed a significant difference between drug-susceptible pulmonary tuberculosis and drug-resistant one (36.84% vs. 73.68%, $P = 0.049$), illustrating a higher prevalence for the latter [29]. Pulmonary cavitation, as shown by researches, is a characteristic manifestation of drug-resistant pulmonary tuberculosis, and its incidence and number are higher if compared with patients suffering from drug-susceptible one, with statistical significance [23]. Patients with drug-resistant pulmonary tuberculosis manifest cavities distributed more extensively and occurring at more foci, and the ratio with lesions involving at least three lobes is significantly higher than that in drug-susceptible pulmonary tuberculosis (Fig. 4.2). The occurrence of cavities, including their number as well as lobes and segments that they involve, is related to the length of medical history of the patient. Among all patients with a history longer than 1 month, those with drug-resistant pulmonary tuberculosis have much more cavities, when compared with those with drug-susceptible one (7.18 vs. 2.36, $P = 0.003$) [29]. Pulmonary nodules and cavities may coexist in some of drug-resistant pulmonary tuberculosis cases, and the incidence of intrapulmonary nodule (mass) and intra-consolidation cavitation is also higher in drug-resistant pulmonary tuberculosis than in drug-susceptible one.
2. Tree-in-bud sign: It is a characteristic manifestation of bronchial dissemination of tubercle bacillus and correlates to bacteriologically positive pulmonary tuberculosis [22]. Tree-in-bud sign, therefore, is one of the typical manifestations in imaging diagnosis of active pulmonary tuberculosis, despite its lack of value in differential diagnosis among various types of drug-resistant pulmonary tuberculosis and drug-susceptible one (Fig. 4.3).
3. Consolidation: Pathologically, the pulmonary consolidations shown by image findings are mainly exudative or proliferative changes of pulmonary tuberculosis and one of the main signs suggesting the presence of active pulmonary tuberculosis. The consolidation can be complicated with cavitation and has no specificity in either drug-resistant or drug-susceptible tuberculosis. Multiple consolidations observed at non-predilection sites for secondary pulmonary tuberculosis in multiple lobes and segments and complicated with intra-cavity nodules and/or tree-in-bud sign help to prompt the diagnosis of drug-resistant pulmonary tuberculosis [22] (Fig. 4.4).
4. Thickening of bronchial wall and bronchiectasis: Extensive thickening of bronchial wall and bronchiecta-

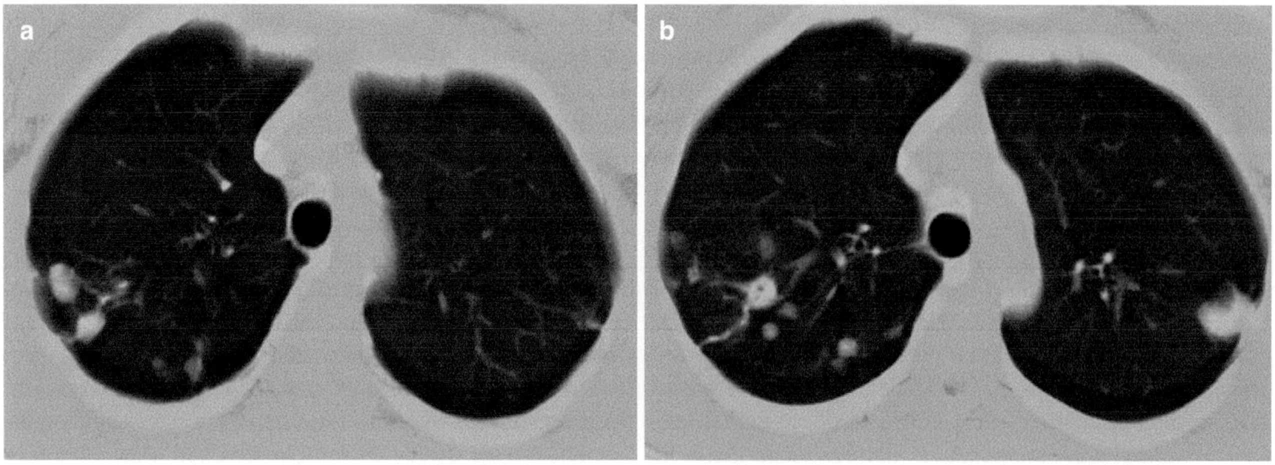

Fig. 4.1 (**a**, **b**) A 23-year-old female, with a chief complaint of cough for more than 20 days, showing resistance to H, R, Ofx, and S. Multidrug-resistant pulmonary tuberculosis with nodules. (**a**, **b**) Multiple nodules complicated with cavities in the right upper lobe are shown by lung window of CT scans. A consolidation is seen in the left upper lobe, showing adhesion with pleura

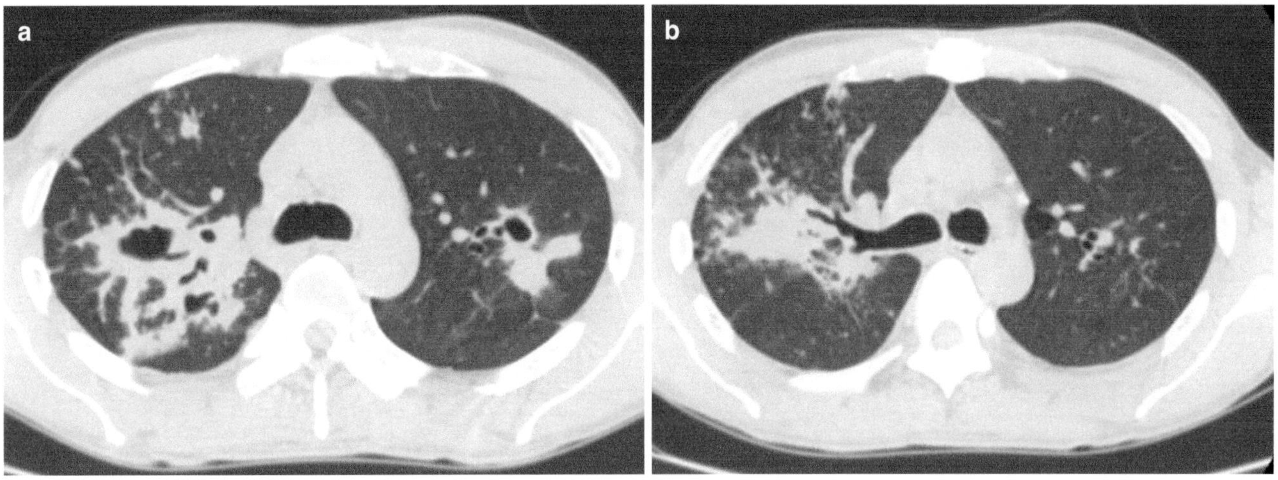

Fig. 4.2 (**a**, **b**) A male aged 38 years, with single drug-resistant pulmonary tuberculosis with cavitation. (**a**, **b**) Cavities are shown in upper lobes of both lungs by the lung window. A segmental consolidation and small nodules are observed in the right upper and middle lobes, with thickening of bronchial wall and stenosis of its lumen in the anterior segment of the right upper lobe

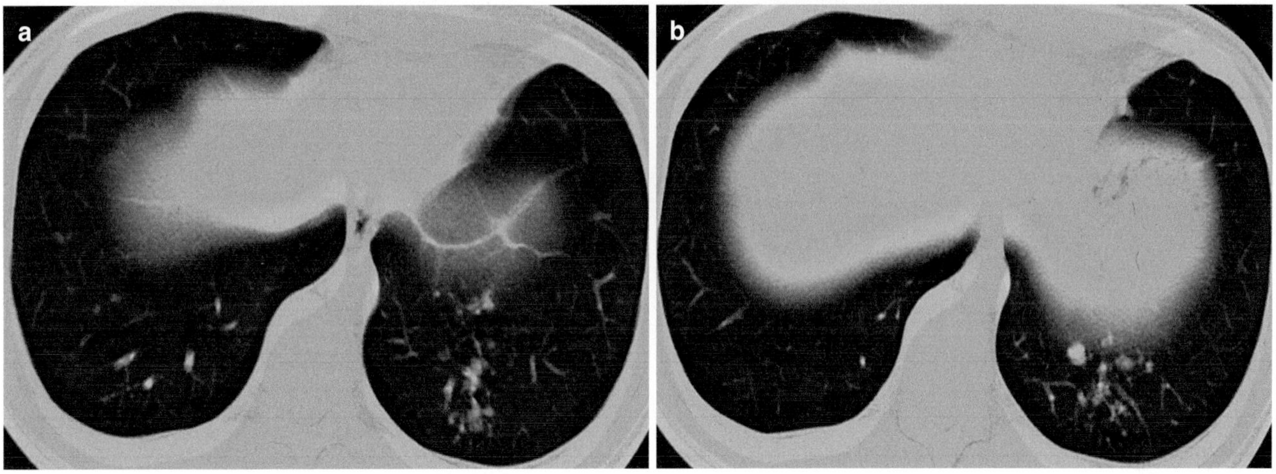

Fig. 4.3 (**a**, **b**) A male aged 25 years, with resistance to H, Cm, and Pto. Image findings show a drug-resistant pulmonary tuberculosis with tree-in-bud sign as the main manifestation. (**a**, **b**) Lung window of CT scans shows mucus impaction in the left lower lobular central bronchus and in its distal airway, and the combination of images in different sections appears similar to the sign of "sprouting in spring," which is called tree-in-bud sign

sis can be induced by drug-resistant pulmonary tuberculosis [23], which involves often smaller bronchial branches in lungs and manifests as thickening of the walls of multiple adjacent bronchioles complicated often with bronchiolectasis (Fig. 4.5), in contrast to bronchial tuberculosis as the complication of drug-susceptible pulmonary tuberculosis, which involves mainly large bronchi.

5. Pleural thickening and calcification, pleural effusion, and pneumothorax: Drug-resistant tuberculosis can cause exudative pleurisy and pleural effusion at the early stage. After penetrating visceral pleura, intrapulmonary tuberculosis lesions may cause pneumothorax, tuberculosis empyema, or pyopneumothorax. Along with the protracted course of the disease, the affected pleura continues to proliferate, followed by the occurrence of irreversible pleural thickening and adhesion, which forms encapsulated pyothorax or pyopneumothorax and induces strip calcification. Therefore, extensive pleural hypertrophy, calcification, and adhesions complicated with encapsulated pyothorax or pyopneumothorax help to prompt the diagnosis of drug-resistant pulmonary tuberculosis.
6. Destroyed lung: Drug-resistant pulmonary tuberculosis with protracted course is more prone to destroyed lung, in comparison with drug-susceptible tuberculosis. Tuberculosis destroyed lung manifests as extensive lesions in a lobe or in unilateral lung, which are mainly pulmonary collapse and atelectasis induced by extensive caseous lesions and fibrosis and are complicated

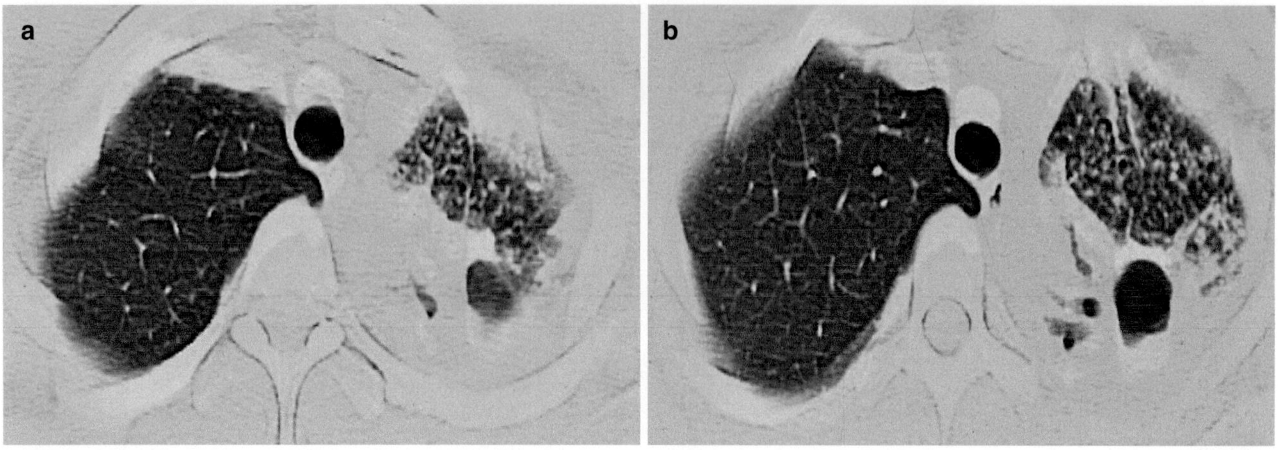

Fig. 4.4 (**a**, **b**) A 23-year-old female, with resistance to H, R, and S. Drug-resistant pulmonary tuberculosis with consolidations and cavities. (**a**, **b**) A large consolidation with a thick-wall cavitation was observed in the upper lobe of the left lung, as shown by lung window of CT scans, and miliary nodules are seen in the left upper lobe with local pleural thickening

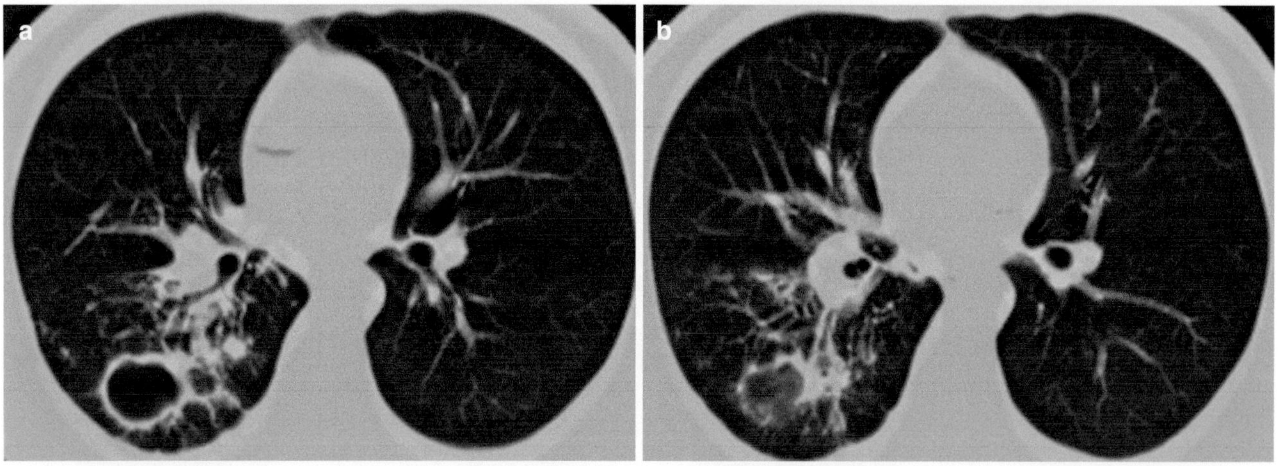

Fig. 4.5 (**a**, **b**) A male aged 29 years, with resistance to H, R, Ofx, and S. Thickening of bronchial wall in drug-resistant pulmonary tuberculosis, complicated with bronchiectasis. (**a**, **b**) A cavity with smooth interior wall is observed in the right lower lobe in lung window of CT scans, and the wall of drainage bronchi is thickened, and complicated with bronchiectasis

with solitary or multiple tuberculous fibrous cavities and bronchiectasis and/or bronchoconstriction, severe destruction of pulmonary tissues, structural distortion, and general loss of pulmonary functions. Unilateral chest collapse may occur, with mediastinal shift toward the affected side and complications including severe pleural hypertrophy, adhesion, and calcification (Fig. 4.6).

4.3.3.2 Characteristic Image Findings Shown by CT Scans for Drug-Resistant Pulmonary

Drug-resistant pulmonary tuberculosis has extensively distributed intrapulmonary lesions, among which exudative lesions are commonly observed and complicated often with intrapulmonary disseminated lesions and multiple cavities. This disease has multiple complications and is characterized in morphological diversity of its lesions.

1. Extensive distribution of lesions: Chest image findings of drug-resistant tuberculosis are complex and diverse, with extensive lesions involving often at least three lobes.
2. Morphological diversity: Co-existence of diverse image findings of pulmonary tuberculosis can be observed, such as pulmonary nodules, cavities, consolidations, pleural thickening, emphysema, bronchial disseminating lesions, atelectasis, and destroyed lung.
3. Multiple cavities: Cavitation, its main image finding, manifests as multiple cavities in most cases, which can be thin/thick-walled cavities and fibrotic ones. The mean number of cavities is often more than 2 in patients with drug-resistant pulmonary tuberculosis, and multiple small cavities concentrated in a single lobe is the characteristic image finding of drug-resistant pulmonary tuberculosis patients, especially those who are initial treatment. A few patients manifest a solitary thick-walled cavity

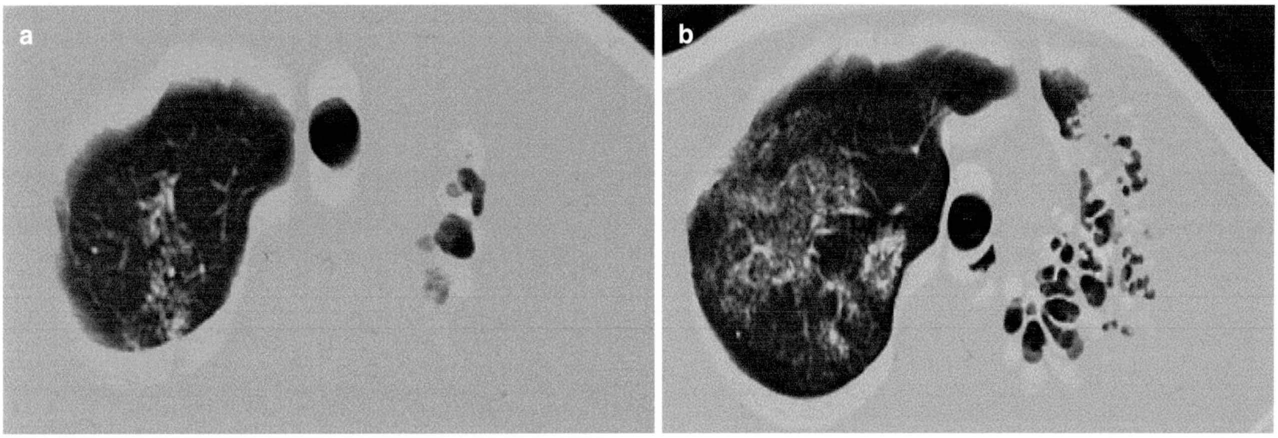

Fig. 4.6 (**a**, **b**) A female aged 30 years, with resistance to H, R, and S. Drug-resistant pulmonary tuberculosis with destroyed lung. (**a**, **b**) The destroyed left lung is shown by lung window of CT scans, with extensive multiple caseous fibrotic cavities, severe destructions of pulmonary tissues, the collapse of the left thorax and the left mediastinal shift. In addition, diffusive bronchial disseminating lesions are seen in the right upper lobe

complicated with multiple segmental and lobar acinar and nodular dissemination, and the cavity may remain unchanged for a long time post to treatment.

4. Multiple consolidations and destroyed lung: Patients with drug-resistant pulmonary tuberculosis have a high incidence of pulmonary parenchyma damage with multiple tortuous and dilated intrapulmonary bronchi and cavities. Destroyed lung is commonly observed, especially in those with extensive drug-resistant pulmonary tuberculosis, most of which have lesions involving at least three lung fields and are commonly complicated with unilateral destroyed lung, with an obvious increase in disseminating lesions and the complications of multiple cavities.
5. High incidence is observed for multiple intrapulmonary nodules, intrapulmonary disseminating lesions, and atelectasis [23].
6. Bronchiectasis, pleural thickening, emphysema, and fibrotic changes. Multi or extensive drug-resistant pulmonary tuberculosis shows extensive scope of lesions, prolonged course, multiple bronchoconstrictions and bronchiectasis, and the potential to cause obstructive emphysema. Extensive pulmonary fibrosis may lead to constrictive ventilatory disorder, and emphysema occurs when the pleura is pulled by the fibers. The unilateral destroyed lung is often accompanied by the contralateral symmetrical emphysema.
7. The patient is prone to extra-pulmonary lesions. Lymph nodes in enhanced scans often manifest as annular enhancement, if the patient is complicated with bilateral pleural effusion, mediastinal or superficial lymphadenectasis.

References

1. Corbett EL, Marston B, Churchyard GJ. Tuberculosis in sub-Saharan Africa :opportunities, challenges, and change in the era of antiretroviral treatment [J]. Lancet. 2006;367(9514):926–37.
2. Professional Committee of Infectious Diseases and Radiology of Radiation Branch under Chinese Medical Association. Experts' consensus on grading diagnosis and imaging diagnosis of pulmonary tuberculosis [J/CD]. Electron J Emerg Infect Dis. 2018;3(2):118–27.
3. Tang S, Xu S, Li L. Drug-resistant phthisiology [M]. Beijing: People's Medical Publishing House; 2014.
4. World Health Organization. Global tuberculosis report 2021 [EB/OL]. https://www.who.int/publications/i/item/9789240037021.
5. Global tuberculosis report 2017 [EB/OL]. Geneva: World Health Organization; 2017. https://apps.who.int/iris/handle/10665/259366.
6. Sheng F, Zhao B, Song Y, et al. Risk factors of drug-resistant tuberculosis in China: an analysis on baseline data of national drug-resistant tuberculosis 2007 [J]. Chin J Antituberc. 2013;35(4):221–6.
7. Technical Guiding Group for National Tuberculosis Epidemiological Sampling Survey. A sample survey report of national tuberculosis epidemiology 2000 [J]. Chin J Antituberc. 2002;24(2):65–108.
8. Cheng S. Current situation and suggestions on control of multidrug-resistant tuberculosis in China [J]. China Trop Med. 2017;17(3):213–5.
9. Yu W, Tan W-g, Lu P-x. Classification and imaging manifestations of drug-resistant pulmonary tuberculosis [J]. Electron J Emerg Infect Dis. 2019;4(1):42–7.
10. Meeting report of the WHO expert consultation on the definition of extensively drug-resistant tuberculosis, 27–29 October 2020 [EB/OL]. Geneva: World Health Organization; 2021. https://apps.who.int/iris/handle/10665/338776.
11. Yu W-y, Tan W-g, Luo Y-t, et al. 2018 WHO Tuberculosis Report: key data analysis for global and China [J]. Electron J Emerg Infect Dis. 2018;3(4):229–34.
12. International Union Against Tuberculosis and Lung Disease. Field guide for the management of drug-resistant tuberculosis [M]. Paris, France; September 2018. ISBN: 979-10-91287-20-3.

13. World Health Organization. Global tuberculosis report 2014 [R]. Geneva: World Health Organization; 2014.
14. Dookie N, Rambaran S, Padayatehi N, et al. Evolution of drug resistance in Mycobacterium tuberculosis: a review on the molecular determinants of resistance and implications for personalized-care [J]. J Antimicrob Chemother. 2018;73(5):1138–51.
15. Gagneux S. Ecology and evolution of Mycobacterium tuberculosis [J]. Nat Rev Microbiol. 2018;16(4):202–13.
16. Dheda K, Gumbo T, Maartens G, et al. The epidemiology, pathogenesis, transmission, diagnosis, and management of multidrug-resistant, extensively drug-resistant, and incurable tuberculosis [J]. Lancet Respir Med. 2017;5(4):291–360.
17. Al-Saeedi M, Al-Hajoj S. Diversity and evolution of drug resistance mechanisms in Mycobacterium tuberculosis [J]. Infect Drug Resist. 2017;10:333–42.
18. Mathema B, Andrews JR, Cohen T, et al. Drivers of tuberculosis transmission [J]. J Infect Dis. 2017;216(6):S644–53.
19. Nguyen QH, Contamin L, Nguyen TVA, et al. Insights into the processes that drive the evolution of drug resistance in Mycobacterium tuberculosis [J]. Evol Appl. 2018;11(9):1498–511.
20. Hameed HMA, Islam MM, Chhotaray C, et al. Molecular targets related drug resistance mechanisms in MDR-, XDR-, and TDR-Mycobacterium tuberculosis strains [J]. Front Cell Infect Microbiol. 2018;8(10):114.
21. Jagielski T, Minias A, van Ingen J, et al. Methodological and clinical aspects of the molecular epidemiology of Mycobacterium tuberculosis and other mycobacteria [J]. Clin Microbiol Rev. 2016;29(2):239–90.
22. Chen G, Cheng G-x, Zhu S-q, et al. CT scanning of mono-resistant pulmonary tuberculosis during initial treatment [J/CD]. Electron J Emerg Infect Dis. 2018;3(2):111–4.
23. Wang, Yi-xiang, Myung Jin Chung, Aliaksandr Skrahin, et al. Literature analysis of radiological signs related to multidrug-resistant tuberculosis [J/CD]. Electron J Emerg Infect Dis, 2018,3(2):244-253.
24. Rasool G, Khan AM, Mohy-Ud-Din R, et al. Detection of Mycobacterium tuberculosis in AFB smear-negative sputum specimens through MTB culture and GeneXpert® MTB/RIF assay [J]. Int J Immunopathol Pharmacol. 2019;33:1–6.
25. Cohen KA, Manson AL, Desjardins CA, et al. Deciphering drug resistance in Mycobacterium tuberculosis using whole-genome sequencing: progress, promise, and challenges [J]. Genome Med. 2019;11(1):45.
26. Zignol M, Cabibbe AM, Dean AS, et al. Genetic sequencing for surveillance of drug resistance in tuberculosis in highly endemic countries: a multi-country population-based surveillance study [J]. Lancet Infect Dis. 2018;18(6):675–83.
27. Nguyen TNA, Anton-Le Berre V, Bañuls AL, et al. Molecular diagnosis of drug-resistant tuberculosis: a literature review [J]. Front Microbiol. 2019;10:794.
28. Compendium of WHO guidelines and associated standards: ensuring optimum delivery of the cascade of care for patients with tuberculosis, second edition [EB/OL]. Geneva: World Health Organization; 2018. https://apps.who.int/iris/handle/10665/272644.
29. Song Q-S, Zheng C-J, Wang K-P, et al. Differences in pulmonary nodular consolidation and pulmonary cavity among drug-sensitive, rifampicin-resistant and multi-drug resistant tuberculosis patients: a computerized tomography study with history length matched cases [J]. J Thorac Dis. 2022;14(7):2522–31.

Mono-Drug Resistant Pulmonary Tuberculosis

5

Gen-Ming Chen, Hua Huang, Xin-nian Wen, Xiao-li Gu, Jie-qi Luo, Xin-jiang Liu, and Jing-zhe Liu

5.1 Summary of Mono-Drug Resistant Pulmonary Tuberculosis

The pandemic and the spread of drug-resistant tuberculosis have introduced new challenges to efforts aimed at preventing and controlling tuberculosis. Mono-drug resistant pulmonary tuberculosis (MR-TB) is defined as a disease with the mycobacterium tuberculosis identified in vitro resistant to any of the first-line anti-tuberculosis drugs [1]. Results of the China's Fifth Tuberculosis Epidemiological Sampling Survey in 2010 showed the mono-resistance rate for China's first-line anti-TB drugs was 16.8%, much higher than multidrug resistant rate (6.8%) [2]. Drug resistance rate, as shown by Baseline Survey of TB Resistance in China (2007–2008), was 18.96%, 9.63%, 6.52%, and 28.93%, respectively, for rifampin (RFP), isoniazid (INH), ethambutol (EMB), and streptomycin (SM) in TB patients in China [3]. The majority of mono-drug resistant pulmonary tuberculosis is the primary drug resistance in an initial infection of the drug-resistant mycobacterium tuberculosis, and timely cure of mono-drug resistant tuberculosis is an effective way to eliminate infectious source of drug resistance and control its spread. Emphasis should be laid upon prevention and control of mono-resistant tuberculosis, so as to terminate tuberculosis epidemic by the year 2030.

An effective way to improve the efficacy in treating mono-resistant pulmonary tuberculosis is to raise the diagnostic capability of drug sensitivity test (DST) for mycobacterium tuberculosis. DST can be divided into phenotype DST and genotype DST, based on different detection principles. Phenotypic DST, a method based on the positiveness in drug-resistant bacteria culture with its result determined according to the growth and metabolism of drug-resistant bacteria, is time consuming and often lags behind clinical requirement. With the development of molecular biology, however, genotype DST has become capable of detecting directly nucleic acids of pathogens in the specimens, thereby improve significantly the diagnostic efficiency of tuberculosis. It is one of the diagnostic methods for diagnosing tuberculosis, as recommended by *WS 288–2017 Tuberculosis Diagnosis* formulated by National Health Commission of People's Republic of China [4], wherein hypersensitive mycobacterium tuberculosis and rifampin-resistant gene detection (GeneXpert MTB/RIF) shows a high sensitivity in diagnosing pulmonary tuberculosis and provides early clinical diagnostic quickly and sensitively. GeneXpert MTB/RIF is one of the fast detection methods recommended by WHO and capable of achieving simultaneous identification of both Mycobacterium tuberculosis and rifampicin resistance within 2 h. The relevant kit developed at the end of 2019, which shows further improved efficacy in detecting the sensitivity to isoniazid, fluoroquinolones, and the second-line injections, is characterized in easy operation, less time consumption, high sensitivity and specificity, and low pollution rate and has been widely applied to the diagnosis of tuberculosis and detection of drug resistance. Semi-automatic gene detection, including the first-line and the second-line linear probe analysis, enables relatively rapid diagnosis of tubercu-

G.-M. Chen (✉)
Department of Radiology, Baoan Central Hospital of Shenzhen, Shenzhen, Guangdong, China

H. Huang · J.-q. Luo
Department of Radiology, The Third People's Hospital of Shenzhen, Shenzhen, Guangdong, China

X.-n. Wen
Department of Medical Imaging, Chest Hospital of Guangxi Zhuang Autonomous Region, Liuzhou, Guangxi, China

X.-l. Gu
Department of Radiology, Luohu Hospital of Traditional Chinese Medicine, Shenzhen, Guangdong, China

X.-j. Liu
Department of Radiology, Fudan University Pudong Medical Center, Shanghai, China

J.-z. Liu
Department of Medical Imaging, The First Hospital of Tsinghua University, Beijing, China

P.-x. Lu et al. (eds.), *Diagnostic Imaging of Drug Resistant Pulmonary Tuberculosis*, https://doi.org/10.1007/978-981-99-8339-1_5

losis. However, during the DNA extraction process, false negatives can occur easily when there is a low quantity of Mycobacterium tuberculosis present in sputum or the presence of DNA inhibitors. In addition, high-throughput sequencing can also be used for diagnosis. Fast diagnosis of drug-resistant pulmonary tuberculosis has been made possible by these molecular biological detections, which have opened up a new path for the early diagnosis and early treatment of mono-resistant pulmonary tuberculosis. Recommendation by WHO [1] for pulmonary tuberculosis diagnosis is the fast DST detection, if permitted by laboratory conditions, for isoniazid/rifampin or rifampin alone performed simultaneously with the diagnosis of tuberculosis, which helps to find more mono-resistant TB patients. A fast diagnosis through drug resistance gene detections should be carried out as soon as possible for patients at high risk of drug resistance (including chronic excretors) and/or patients unresponsive to re-treatment, smear-positive pulmonary TB patients in close contact with multidrug resistant tuberculosis patients, patients unresponsive to the initial treatment, recurrent patients or patients in return visit, and patients positive in initial sputum smear whose positiveness persists up to the end of month 3), so as to know about drug resistance and formulate individualized therapeutic regimens timely, thereby improving curative ratio and reducing the risk of recurrence.

The mechanism of resistance in mono-drug resistant pulmonary tuberculosis is complex, and the main molecular mechanism predisposing mycobacterium tuberculosis to drug resistance is the mutation of chromosomal gene encoding targets of drugs against mycobacterium tuberculosis or related metabolic enzymes. Possible factors resulting in drug resistance include drug shortage, poor quality of drugs, improper treatment, and poor compliance in patients. Voluntary discontinuation or termination of treatment by patients can also lead to the emergence of drug resistance and the gradual increase in drug resistance spectrum of mycobacterium tuberculosis during anti-tuberculosis treatment. Drug-resistant mycobacterium tuberculosis spreads primarily through direct interpersonal transmission [5]. To control the epidemics of drug-resistant tuberculosis, timely detection, proper treatment, cure of patients with mono-resistant pulmonary tuberculosis, and elimination of infectious sources are effective approaches. Drug-resistant tuberculosis can be categorized into the newly diagnosed resistance and re-treatment resistance, depending on whether there has been previous treatment with anti-tuberculosis drugs, as recommended by Monitoring Project Report of Global Anti-Tuberculosis Drug Resistance implemented by World Health Organization (WHO)/International Union Against Tuberculosis and Lung Disease (IUATLD) [6]. Mono-resistant pulmonary tuberculosis (MR-TB) can also be grouped based on this categorization into newly diagnosed MR-TB and re-treatment MR-TB. Newly diagnosed MR-TB, defined as a disease occurring in an anti-tuberculosis-naive patient or a patient with an exposure to anti-tuberculosis drug for less than 1 month, which includes infection with drug-resistant mycobacterium tuberculosis or the resistance induced by a genetic mutation in a sensitive mycobacterium tuberculosis at the time of infection (i.e., natural resistance) (N.B. these patients have been infected by people with drug-resistant strain infection). Re-treatment MR-TB is defined as a disease occurring in a patient having been exposed to anti-tuberculosis treatment or anti-tuberculosis drug for at least 1 month. MR-TB mostly occurs because of the dominance by a few strains appearing post to the eradication of previously sensitive dominant strains due to factors such as improper treatment, and it includes generally unresponsiveness to treatment, recurrence or lost to follow-up of patients undergoing treatment. Drug-resistant mycobacterium has developed in these patients during their treatment, or they have been infected by a drug-resistant mycobacterium through interpersonal transmission. Epidemiological Characteristics of Pulmonary Tuberculosis in Hebei Province, China 2008–2014 [7] showed a smear-positive drug resistance rate of 8.2% for initial treatment patients and 8.9% for those undergoing re-treatment, suggesting that the situation of mono-resistant pulmonary tuberculosis should not be underestimated for those pulmonary tuberculosis patients receiving re-treatment.

Rifampin mono-resistant tuberculosis (RMR-TB), a common mono-resistant tuberculosis, is defined as a disease infected with the Mycobacterium tuberculosis strain resistant only to rifampin, as proved by drug sensitivity test in vitro [1]. Global tuberculosis report 2020 showed that there were 465,000 cases of rifampin-resistant tuberculosis (RR-TB) around the world in 2019, of which 22% were mono-resistant tuberculosis. The incidence is low with a dropping tendency for rifampin mono-resistant tuberculosis in developed countries in Europe and America. For example, a retrospective study on tuberculosis in California during the year from 1993 to 2008 years showed that the ratio of rifampin mono-resistant tuberculosis in all rifampin-resistant tuberculosis decreased from 31% to 11% [8]. However, the incidence of rifampin mono-resistant tuberculosis shows an increasing trend in high-burden TB countries such as African countries [9]. The fifth tuberculosis epidemiological survey in China in 2010 showed a ratio of 1.4% for rifampin mono-resistant tuberculosis, occupying 1.2% in treatment-naive tuberculosis patients and 2.6% in re-treatment tuberculosis patients [2]. The ratio of rifampin mono-resistant tuberculosis, as reported by the research [10], was 0.6% for strains from newly diagnosed initial treatment tuberculosis patients in Burundi in Africa, compared with 12% for strains from re-treatment tuberculosis. From the year 2007–2009, the ratio of rifampin mono-resistant tuberculosis in South Africa increased from 7.3% to 10.0% [11]. Greater increase in ratio of rifampin mono-resistant tuberculosis was observed in males than in females, and in patients aged over 50 years than in those aged between 25 and 29 years. Another study [12] in South Africa showed an over two-time growth for rifampin mono-resistant tuberculosis in Western Cape from the year 2004–2008, witnessing an increase from 31 patients in 2004 to 98 patients in 2008, with a doubling time of 1.63 years (95% CI:1.18–2.66). Moreover, South African is a country with serious rifampin mono-resistant tuberculosis in children, because of the untypical symptoms in children predisposing them to delay in treatment, facilitating the widespread of rifampin-resistant tuberculosis. It can be inferred that rifampin mono-resistant tuberculosis occurs frequently in re-treatment patients and cannot be underestimated. Patients with rifampin mono-resistant TB patients should be identified timely, followed by proper treatment as soon as possible.

The latest data show that the treatment success rate is 85% for drug-sensitive TB, compared with only 57% for drug-resistant TB [13]. The clinical treatment seems not so difficult for mono-resistant pulmonary tuberculosis, except for rifampin mono-resistant patients [14]. As for rifampin mono-resistant tuberculosis, however, poor responses were achieved by WHO standard 6-month chemotherapy regimen (2HREZ/4HR) for initial treatment patients and 8-month treatment plan (2SHREZ/1HREZ/5HRE) for re-treatment patients [14, 15]. Clinical treatment of rifampin mono-resistant pulmonary tuberculosis has a certain difficulty, in that satisfactory clinical response are hardly achieved by 12-month anti-tuberculosis treatment [16]. Rifamycin, one of the major first-line anti-tuberculosis drugs, triggers genetic mutation very easily resulting in drug resistance, in case of improper treatment or abnormal metabolism of liver enzymes. It has been revealed by studies [17] that rifampin-resistant pulmonary TB patients have an obviously lower treatment completion rate and an obviously higher mortality compared with TB patients resistant to the second-line medication. That is because the prognosis of rifampin mono-resistant pulmonary tuberculosis is poor, and rifampin-resistant Mycobacterium tuberculosis strain exposed to rifampin may reduce the efficacy of the second-line treatment regimen containing ofloxacin. Moreover, the risks of treatment failure and acquired drug resistance may increase and even multidrug-resistant tuberculosis (MDR-TB) possibly occurs, if mono-resistant tuberculosis cannot be identified and medications/individualized treatment cannot be modified in time. Therefore, timely diagnosis and cure of initial treatment mono-resistant tuberculosis constitute the effective approach to eradicate the infectious source of drug resistance tuberculosis and control its spread. Both WHO and China recommend a chemotherapy with a total course no less than 12 months for rifampin-resistant pulmonary tuberculosis, while 3SHLfxZE/9HLfxZE or 3SHLfxZE/15HLfxZE is recommended by Chinese Guideline for Chemotherapy of Drug-Resistant Tuberculosis 2015 [18]. Recent years, some scholars have witnessed certain responses about immune agents in tuberculosis patients of adjuvant therapy, and immune preparations developed maturely include mainly cytokine preparations and Mycobacterium vaccine, which though are not recommended generally to patients with mono-resistant pulmonary tuberculosis or those in good condition due to prices of these preparations [18]. In respect of new therapeutic drugs, 25 drugs for treating sensitive TB, MDR-TB, or tuberculosis infections had been in phase I, II, or III clinical trials by August 2021, including 16 new chemical entities, 2 drugs with accelerated approval by regulatory authorities, 1 antibacterial and antifungal agent recently approved based on limited-species model by US food and Drug Administration, and 6 drugs with changed indications [13]. Given the absence of definite randomized or controlled trials to determine the best therapeutic regimens against various drug resistances, we still lack sufficient evidences from randomized clinical trials to rationalize the best regimen against mono-resistant pulmonary tuberculosis [14, 19]. The design of regimens in treating mono-resistant tuberculosis can be based on experiences of clinicians. For patients with drug-resistant tuberculosis, an individualized treatment regimen is typically designed and needs to be routinely reviewed by an expert panel. This review may include factors such as the patient's treatment history, results of drug sensitivity testing, and the possibility of newly acquired drug resistance in Mycobacterium tuberculosis.

5.2 Image Findings of Newly Diagnosed and Re-Treatment Mono-Resistant Tuberculosis

Imaging examination plays a vital role in diagnosis and treatment of drug-resistant pulmonary tuberculosis. Imaging methods recommended by the latest version of Imaging Diagnostic Criteria for Pulmonary Tuberculosis (guideline) include X-ray and CT scans [20]. Chest X-ray can be used as a method for screening pulmonary tuberculosis and evaluating effect post the treatment for this disease. It is the simplest imaging method to detect pulmonary tuberculosis lesion. Due to its advantages of high-density resolution and thin-layer reconstruction, CT imaging can not only show the subtle changes of the lesions on the level of tissue structure of pulmonary lobules but also display the pathophysiological characteristics of the lesions in respect of blood supply and metabolism with the help of enhanced scanning. At present, multi-slice spiral CT plays an important role in the diagnosis, differential diagnosis, evaluation of response, and prognosis of pulmonary tuberculosis. The tangibility and display of features of pulmonary tuberculosis as well as improvement and application of CT imaging are the key factors determining not only the imaging diagnostic level for pulmonary tuberculosis but also the progression and improvement in imaging diagnosis technology. In recent years, CT scans plays an important role increasingly in the diagnosis of drug-resistant pulmonary tuberculosis, and it is of great significance in the clinical diagnosis, differential diagnosis, evaluation of response, and prognosis for drug-resistant pulmonary tuberculosis. Drug-resistant pulmonary tuberculosis is the most serious type of all tuberculosis and has the specific feature in the imaging findings. Treatment and control of pulmonary tuberculosis will benefit from the raised awareness and familiarity with imaging findings of drug-resistant pulmonary tuberculosis.

CT scans for pulmonary tuberculosis may have various imaging findings [21–23]. Drug-resistant pulmonary tuberculosis has a long and protracted course with an inclination of deterioration and progression, due to its poor response to conventional anti-tuberculosis treatment. Drug-resistant pulmonary tuberculosis not only has imaging features of non-resistant pulmonary tuberculosis but also is characterized in extensive distribution and diversified shapes of lesions, obvious exudation, common cavitation, and frequent complications such as pulmonary emphysema and pleural thickening [5]. Common features of drug-resistant tuberculosis include cavitation and involvement of bilateral lungs, and both indicate the presence of a higher risk inducing drug-resistant tuberculosis. Therefore, suspected pulmonary TB patients with either sign in their imaging findings should undergo drug sensitivity test as soon as possible, based on which a reasonable chemotherapy regimen is formulated.

There are fewer reports on the characteristic imaging findings of mono-resistant pulmonary tuberculosis, and only a few literature summaries are available now [5, 24]. It has been revealed through multivariate logistic regression analysis in a study [24] on imaging findings in treatment-naive mono-resistant pulmonary tuberculosis that main risk factors inducing MR pulmonary tuberculosis include large lobar or segmental consolidation, mouth-eaten cavity, bronchial thickening and stenosis, and absence of calcification of hilar/mediastinal lymph node; Besides common features in CT scans for smear-positive pulmonary tuberculosis, as shown by results of this study, treatment-naive mono-resistant pulmonary tuberculosis has still following features: acute onset and high severity (the reason may be that lobar or segmental consolidation and mouth-eaten cavity both represent that the disease is in the acute state, when a large amount of exudate is rapidly produced at the infected site to fill the alveoli and spread around, forming lobar or segmental consolidation within a short time, while the mouth-eaten cavity is formed by liquefaction necrosis and discharge on the basis of consolidation); Bronchi are easily invaded and damaged, and the occurrence rate of bronchial wall thickening and stenosis is correlated positively with the amount of Mycobacterium tuberculosis. The more bacteria number, the easier it damages the airway. The highest bacteria number are observed in pulmonary tuberculosis patients with the mouth-eaten cavity. Calcification of hilar and mediastinal lymph nodes unlikely occurs, because of possible difficulty of calcium deposit due to rapid progression and hypersensitivity state of treatment-naïve mono-resistant pulmonary tuberculosis. All these findings suggest that the possibility of treatment-naive mono-resistant pulmonary tuberculosis should be suspected in case of widely distributed lesions with CT scans featuring dominantly active tuberculosis, as well as the coexistence of consolidation of large pulmonary lobes or segments, mouth-eaten cavities, thickening and stenosis of bronchi, and absence of calcified hilar/mediastinal lymph nodes in an initial treatment mono-resistant pulmonary tuberculosis patient. For re-treatment drug-resistant pulmonary tuberculosis, it is believed generally that the focus is prone to occurrence in the upper lobe of the lungs and easy cavitation, usually without lymphadenopathy. Early imaging findings include often consolidations with poorly defined border, accompanied by grid or nodular opacities. Cavitation is a characteristic manifestation of re-treatment pulmonary tuberculosis, featuring usually an irregular thick-walled cavity within the consolidation. Intra-bronchial dissemination induced by cavitation can appear further a typical tree-in-bud sign. Pleural thickening is also common in re-treatment pulmonary tuberculosis. Re-treatment drug-resistant pulmonary tuberculosis with obscure symptoms often results in delayed diagnosis and is prone to fibrous foci, bronchial stenosis, or bronchiectasis, which is one of the common complications of re-treatment drug-resistant pulmonary tuberculosis and secondary to the destruction and fibrosis of pulmonary tissues. There is still no relevant literature, however, concerning whether re-treatment mono-resistant pulmonary tuberculosis has characteristic imaging findings.

Rifamycin is one of the main first-line anti-tuberculosis drug, and it is of great significance to understand the imaging findings of rifampin mono-resistant pulmonary tuberculosis so as to guide clinical medication. CT imaging findings of rifampin mono-resistant pulmonary tuberculosis has certain characteristics [25]. First, lesions are mainly located in apicoposterior segment of the upper lobe and the dorsal segment of the lower lobe in typical tuberculosis, and the middle lobe, the lingual segment of the upper lobe, and the basal segment of the lower lobe in rifamycin mono-resistant pulmonary tuberculosis. In respect of lesion morphology, rifamycin mono-resistant pulmonary tuberculosis is more prone to pulmonary cavitation, and cavities with the diameter <1.5 cm are common. The major extra-pulmonary manifestation is bilateral pleural effusion. The coexistence of all these imaging findings implies the probable presence of rifamycin mono-resistant pulmonary tuberculosis.

In respect of differential diagnosis, the imaging findings are characterized in extended distribution, morphological diversity, and severity of pulmonary lesions in mono-resistant pulmonary tuberculosis, which should be differentiated from diabetes, pneumoconiosis, and pulmonary tuberculosis accompanied by immunocompromised patients such as HIV/AIDS. However, the amelioration of these underlying diseases often precedes the control of pulmonary tuberculosis, which can be used to distinguish them from mono-resistant pulmonary tuberculosis.

5.3 Introduction of Typical Cases of Mono-Resistant Pulmonary Tuberculosis

Case 1. Newly Diagnosed Isoniazid Mono-Resistant Pulmonary Tuberculosis

Summary of medical history

The patient was 18-year-old male, admitted on June 1, 2016, with the chief complaint of "repeated cough and expectoration for 2 months, with chest pain, chest tightness, and low fever for 7 days." The patient initially experienced cough, expectoration, chest tightness, chest pain, night sweats, and fever without obvious cause 2 months prior and sought medical advice from a social health medical center. He received symptomatic treatment to relieve cough and reduce sputum, but the specific medication is unknown. The initial diagnosis was acute bronchitis, and the symptoms improved. Nevertheless, he experienced recurrent cough and expectoration and used over-the-counter medication with an unknown name and long duration. Subsequently, he went to a comprehensive hospital on May 25, 2016, for chest pain, chest tightness, and low fever. A chest X-ray revealed patchy high-density opacities in both lungs and consolidation with lucid areas inside the lower left lung, which was secondary pulmonary tuberculosis of both lungs with a cavitation in the left lower lung. According to relevant provisions of the centralized control of tuberculosis, he was referred to a district-level chronic disease prevention and treatment hospital for further treatment. Fatigue, poor spirits, loss of appetite and sleep, and a weight loss of approximately 3 kg were present since the onset of illness, but the patient's urination and defecation were normal. Past history: The patient reports no prior episodes of infectious diseases, including hepatitis and tuberculosis. He has no history of diabetes, hypertension, bronchiectasis, or bronchial asthma.

Personal history: He was born and raised in the domicile of origin, he left there 4 months ago to work as an assembly line worker. He denies the history of TB contact, family history of any hereditary disease, and history of infection. He has irregular word/rest schedules and likes playing games in internet cafe. He smokes about 10 cigarettes per day, but is not addicted to wine.

Physical examination: T 38.8 °C, P89/min, R 20/min, and BP 119/79 mmHg. Development below the average, malnutritious, consciousness, poor mentality, and cooperative in physical examination. Symmetrical thorax, with trachea in the middle; respiratory harshness in both lungs, vocal fremitus in the left lung is enhanced with partial flatness in percussion; moist crackles are heard in the left lung. The heart rate is 90 beats/min, regular rhythm, and no murmur is heard in each auscultatory valve area. The abdomen seems flat and touches soft, without tenderness or rebound tenderness; the liver and spleen are not touchable in the infracostal margin. No edema in both lower extremities.

Preliminary diagnosis: Infiltrating pulmonary tuberculosis of both lungs with a cavitation in the lower left lung.

Diagnosis and treatment process

The patient sought medical service at Department of Pulmonary Diseases on June 1, 2016, and laboratory tests and imaging examinations were completed on that. Laboratory examination included blood routine, eight items of liver function, five items of renal function, tuberculosis antibody, ESR, sputum tuberculosis smear, sputum culture, drug sensitivity test, and PPD test. Normal blood routine and renal function. Albumin (ALB) 30 g/L, positive tuberculosis antibody, erythrocyte sedimentation rate (ESR) 26 mm/h, positive sputum tuberculosis smear (2+): 5 strips/100 fields under oil immersion lens; a mean diameter of 12 mm for scleroma in PPD test, suggesting moderate positiveness. Chest plain CT scans (Fig. 5.1) showed in both lungs nodular, patchy and large blocky opacities with increased density as well as consolidations, with clear or blurred borders; a thick-walled cavity was observed in the apical segment of upper right lobe and a mouth-eaten cavity within the consolidation in the lower left lobe; there was a small amount of pleural effusion in the left thoracic cavity with thickness and adhesion of pleura. The definite diagnosis of active pulmonary tuberculosis was established, based on comprehensive considerations of clinical information, laboratory tests, and chest CT scans. He received anti-tuberculosis treatment with the regimen FDC-2HRZE/4HR, together with liver protection using Compound Yiganling. Sputum culture on June 25, 2016, was positive (3+), and phenotypic drug sensitivity test on July 17, 2016, showed sensitivity to all first-line drugs. His cough and expectoration were not relieved yet by August 8, 2016, when he underwent the re-examination, and positiveness still remained for sputum smear (2+) that he underwent again together with sputum culture and drug sensitivity test. Re-examination of chest plain CT scans (Fig. 5.2) showed enlarged lesions with blurred boundary in both lungs; enlarged consolidation with the cavity unobservable inside it in the lower left lobe; the persistence of the

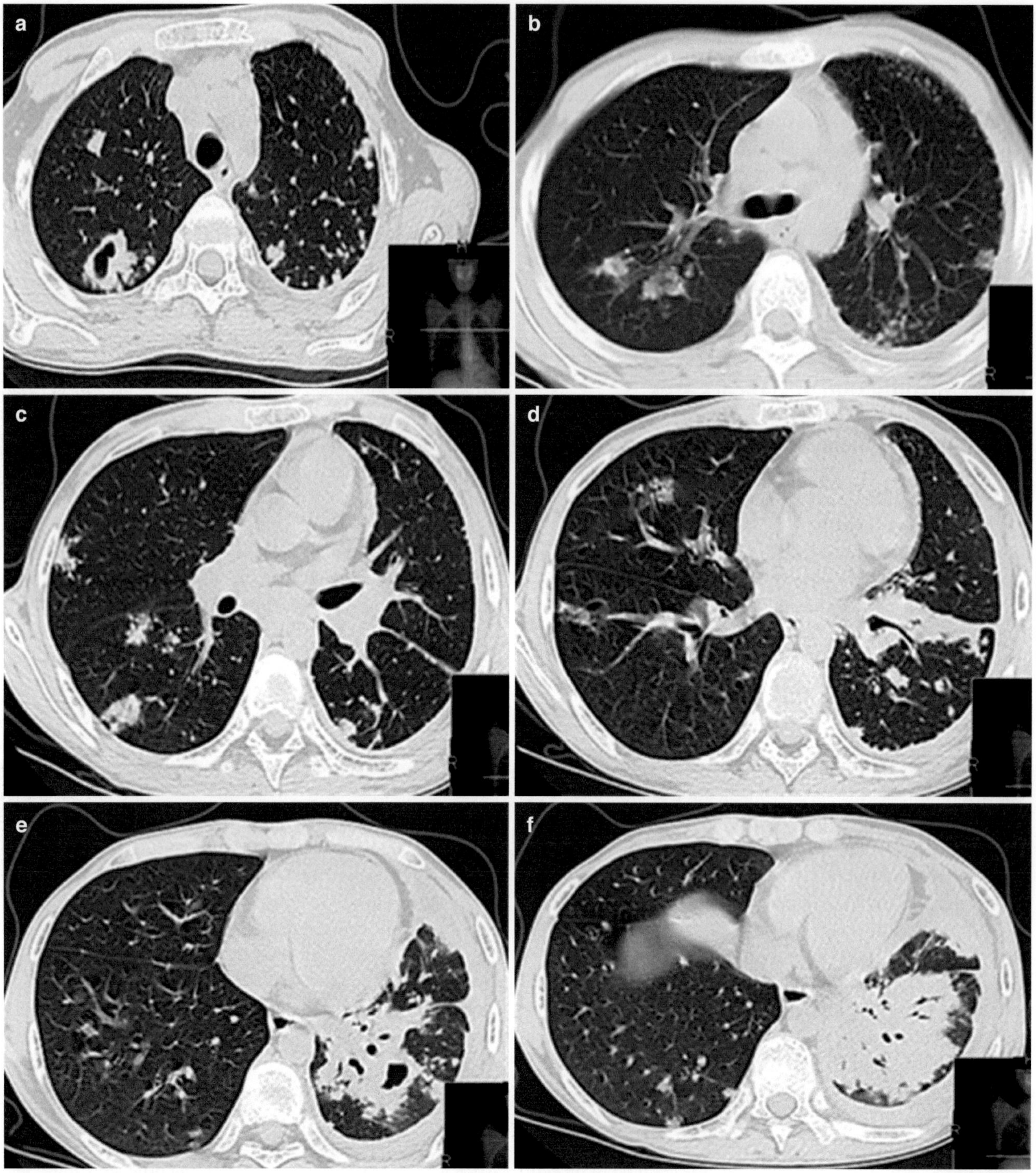

Fig. 5.1 (**a**–**f**) Chest plain CT scans on June 1, 2016. Lung window: nodular and patchy high-density opacities are observed in all lobes of both lungs, with clear or blurred boundaries; a thick-walled cavity with smooth interior wall and clear edge of the exterior wall exists in the apical segment of the upper right lobe; large blocky consolidations are seen in the lower left lobe, which have blurred boundaries and smooth interior wall, as well as inflatable bronchi and mouth-eaten cavities inside; there is a small amount of pleural effusion with thickening and adhesion of pleura

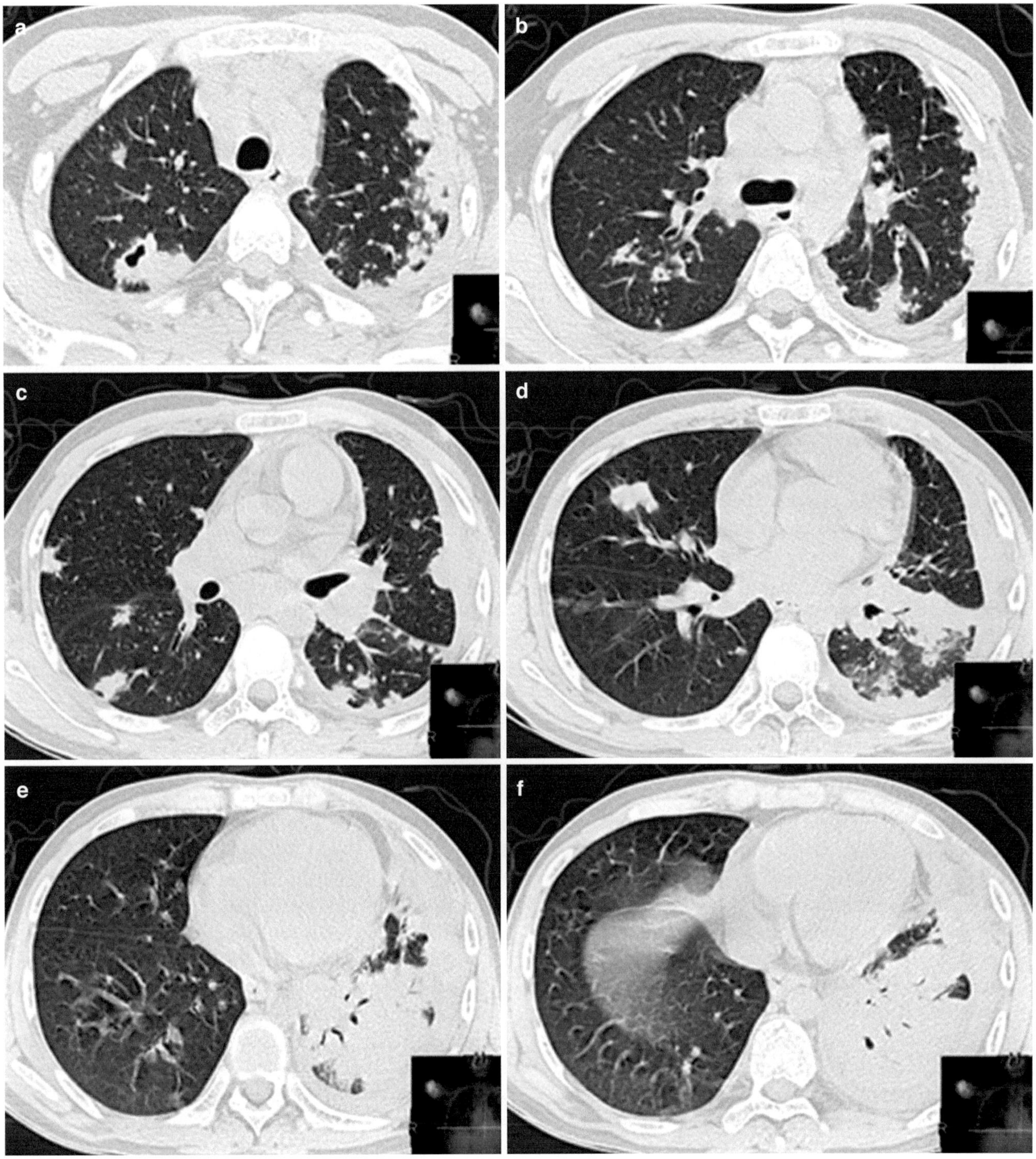

Fig. 5.2 (**a**–**f**) Re-examination of chest plain CT scans on August 8, 2016. Compared with chest plain CT scans on June 1, 2016, an enlargement of lesions on both lungs is observable with more blurred boundaries; an increase in the consolidation in the left lower lobe is seen, with the disappearance of the cavity inside the consolidation; the thick-walled cavity in the upper right lobe still exists with its wall thickened and its exterior wall more blurred compared to its previous imaging; and slight increase in the left pleural effusion than before

thick-walled cavity in the upper right lobe with the wall thickened and the exterior wall blurred than before; and the increase in the left pleural effusion, which suggested the poor response to the anti-tuberculosis treatment. He underwent Xpert Mtb/RIF test on August 9, 2016, showing mycobacterium tuberculosis complex sensitive to rifampin, which was suspected clinically to be Herxheimer-like reaction, and the original regimen was continued. The result of sputum culture on August 23, 2016, was positive (3+), and phenotype drug sensitivity test on September 15, 2016, showed the sensitivity to rifampin, ethambutol, and chloramphenicol and resistance to isoniazid. The anti-tuberculosis medication, therefore, was modified together with the therapeutic course, and the regimen 6RZELfx was used to continue his anti-tuberculosis treatment. Negativeness was detected on December 16, 2016, and re-examination of chest plain CT scans (Fig. 5.3) showed the obvious absorption of lesions in both lungs with disappearance of the cavity, an appreciable absorption of the left pleural effusion succeeded by the dominance by pleural thickening and adhesion, and a disease evolving toward amelioration and healing. Re-examination of chest X-ray (Fig. 5.4) on March 20, 2017, showed a small amount of strip high-density opacities with dominant fibrotic lesions; a slightly thickening of the left pleura was observed, which suggested the stabilization of the lesions, and the sputum smear was negative. Therefore, the medication was discontinued, and the patient was instructed to re-visit timely in case of any discomfort.

Final diagnosis: newly diagnosed isoniazid mono-resistant pulmonary tuberculosis.

Discussion

In contrast to reports on multidrug resistance flooding the imaging study of drug-resistant pulmonary tuberculosis, fewer reports are available on the mono-resistant pulmonary TB. It can be inferred from findings of chest CT scans in this patient that CT findings are of a great value in diagnosis, differential diagnosis, and dynamic changes of lesions under treatment for the newly diagnosed mono-resistant pulmonary tuberculosis. Also, newly diagnosed mono-resistant pulmonary TB has a CT manifestation identical to that of newly diagnosed drug-sensitive pulmonary TB, and between them there is only a difference of incidence of manifestations of lesions. It is reported in the literature [24] that compared with newly diagnosed drug-sensitive pulmonary TB, newly diagnosed mono-resistant pulmonary TB has CT findings characterized in extensive distribution of lesions, acute onset and high severity, the inclination to form lobar or segmental consolidation and mouth-eaten cavity, the inclination to invade and harm bronchi, and the difficulties in calcification of hilar and mediastinal lymph nodes. Therefore, the characteristics of CT finding are conducive to the diagnosis of newly diagnosed mono-resistant pulmonary TB.

Newly diagnosed mono-resistant pulmonary TB patients, with the first-line resistance unknown, may ameliorate within a short period with relief or disappearance of clinical symptoms, improved results of bacteriological examination and absorption/decrease of lesions shown by imaging finding, after undergoing a treatment with normalized and standardized chemotherapy regimens. However, continuous absorption and decrease may happen subsequently in some of lesions, in comparison to the other showing increase in sizes or numbers or emergence of new lesions, indicating progression and deterioration. This often needs to be differentiated from the Herxheimer-like reaction in treatment-naive pulmonary tuberculosis patients, the authentic exacerbation of pulmonary tuberculosis caused by low or deficient immunity. It is considered by related literature [27] that Herxheimer-like reaction is a transient reversible so-called deterioration, i.e., the increase in size and number of lesions in contrast to minor or absent symptoms with negativeness in sputum smear or culture, showing a paradox. CT imaging findings often show the increase in original lesions with blurred boundaries, and newly emerging lesions characterized in consolidation or exudative lesions of ground glass opacities for Herxheimer-like reaction, differing from drug-resistant pulmonary TB, which manifests often the enlargement of original lesions accompanied with expansion of the original cavities or new cavitation. New lesions are dominantly nodular ones, characterized in aggravation of clinical symptoms, positiveness in sputum smear and sputum culture, and large bacterial load. These two diseases, therefore, can be differentiated based on clinical symptoms, laboratory tests, and imaging findings. Low or deficient immunity often exists in pulmonary tuberculosis patients complicated with underlying diseases such as diabetes, HIV, or malnutrition, predisposing their pulmonary lesions to exacerbation despite regular anti-tuberculosis treatment if blood glucose is controlled poorly or the decrease in CD4+ lymphocytes cannot be corrected.

Of course, some newly diagnosed treatment-naive patients with mono-resistant pulmonary tuberculosis keep showing poor response to regular treatment using standardized chemotherapeutic regimen, with no relief of symptoms and no absorption of lesions, but deterioration instead. This patient was one of these cases, who showed a poor response suggested by an aggravating tendency and positiveness (++) in sputum smear without any alleviation of cough or expectoration at re-examination post to 2-month regular anti-tuberculosis treatment for the treatment-naive smear-positive pulmonary TB patients. Despite the disappearance of the cavity in the lower left lobe and the seemingly vanishing lesion shown by chest plain CT scans, the original lesion showed a significant enlargement, the increase in the left pleural effusion, and the persistent presence of the thick-walled cavity in the upper right lobe with increased thickness

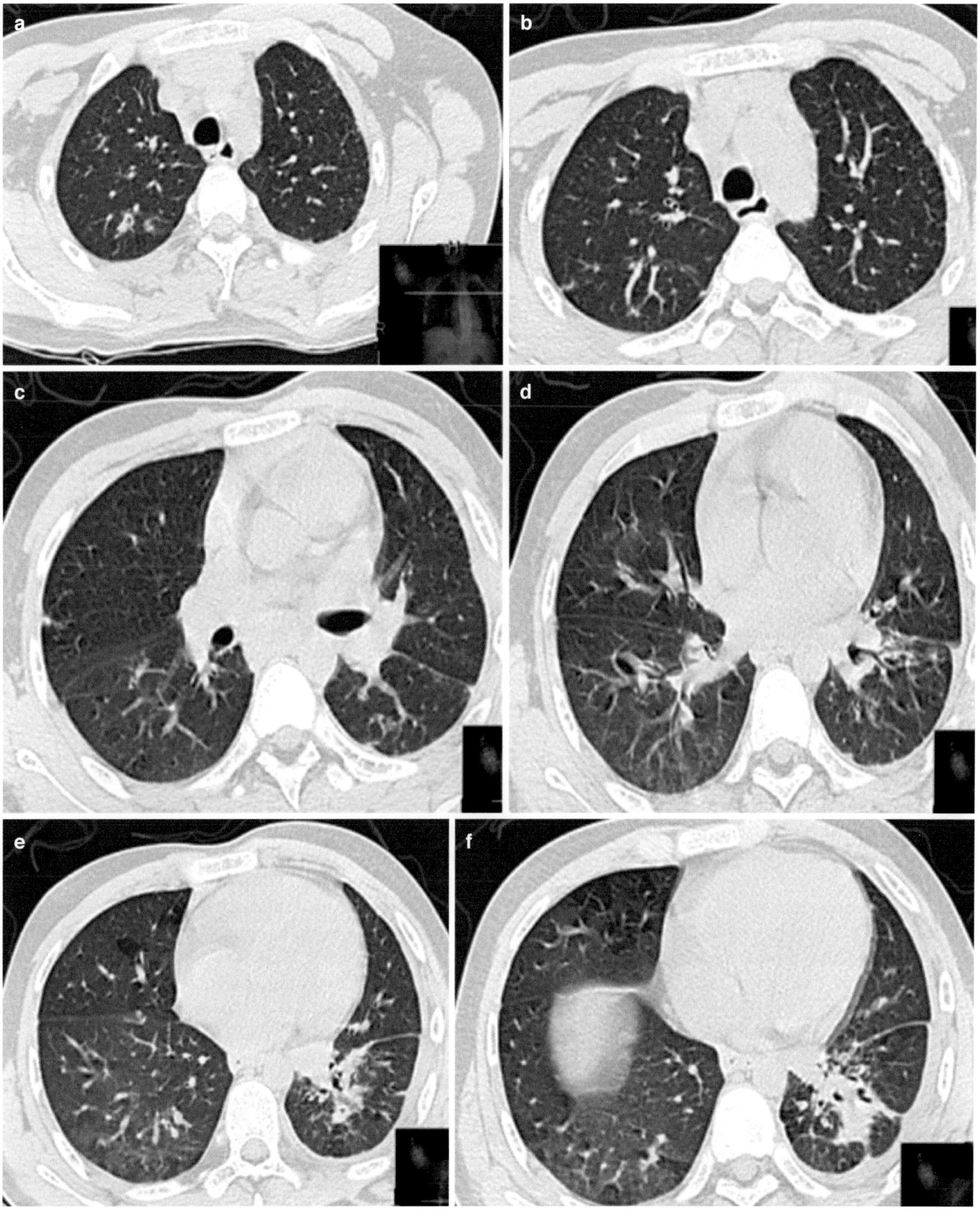

Fig. 5.3 (**a**–**f**) Re-examination of chest plain CT scans on December 16, 2016. Compared with chest plain CT scans on August 8, 2016, an obvious absorption and decrease in nodular opacities and consolidations in both lungs are observed, with their boundaries becoming clearer than before; disappearance of the cavity in the upper right lobe; significant decrease and absorption of the left pleural effusion are noticed, and now the dominant imaging is thickening and adhesion of pleura

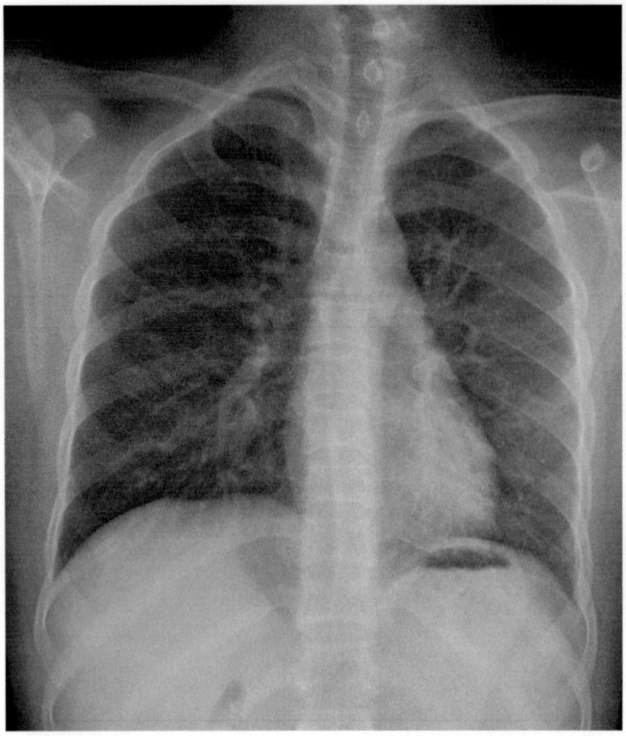

Fig. 5.4 Re-examination of chest X-ray on March 20, 2017, showing a small amount of strip-like high-density opacities, and the feature of lesions is dominantly fibrosis, with a slight thickening of the left pleura

of its wall compared with its previous size. This dynamic change of the lesion cannot be distinguished temporarily from Herxheimer-like reaction, and it is difficult to distinguish the true and false deterioration. In this case, it is necessary to perform a rapid drug sensitivity test under conditions allowed. If not allowed, a traditional drug sensitivity test should be carried out to find out the potential resistance to isoniazid and rifampin, because it is of great significance for choosing subsequent treatment regimens. The author considers, therefore, that genetic test should be done timely for all patients with poor response to the treatment, including those persistently positive in sputum Mycobacterium tuberculosis and those with progressive disease, which is of positive realistic significance in the timely diagnosis, improvement of effectiveness/price ratio of the treatment, and the control of the spread of drug-resistant pulmonary tuberculosis in populations.

Isoniazid exhibits a very strong bactericidal action on Mycobacterium tuberculosis either in the reproductive period and stationary period with low risks of side effects. It is one of the two preferred options with the highest safety and efficacy among anti-tuberculosis drugs for treating active and latent pulmonary tuberculosis. Despite the great severity and extensiveness of lesions in this case, the patient responded well after an individualized regimen was launched with the modified anti-tuberculosis drugs, and lesions were absorbed almost completely at the end of treatment. Isoniazid-resistant tuberculosis, therefore, is more amenable to treatment when compared with multidrug-resistant and rifampin-resistant tuberculosis. It was revealed by WHO report in 2018 [28], however, that isoniazid-resistance rate was 7.1% in rifampin-susceptible strains in newly diagnosed tuberculosis patients, which was significantly higher than that of multidrug resistance/rifampin resistance (3.5%). Compared with drug-sensitive TB patients, isoniazid-resistant TB patients showed the higher rates for treatment failure, relapse, and acquired resistance [29]. Therefore, the puzzles in isoniazid resistance and its countermeasures can never be underestimated. We must take it seriously and never let our guard down. In line with this commitment, the WHO in 2018 provided supplementary guidelines for the treatment of isoniazid drug-resistant tuberculosis, building upon the 2016 edition of the treatment guidelines for drug-resistant TB. This effort aimed to develop a more suitable regimen and offer recommendations for the treatment course specific to isoniazid drugresistant TB.

Case 2. Newly Diagnosed Isoniazid Mono-Resistant Pulmonary Tuberculosis

Summary of medical history

The patient is a 46-year-old male who presented with a persistent cough with expectoration for over 1 month, which was worse at night and companied by white viscous sputum. He had also experienced unexplained shivering and fever 9 days prior with a temperature of 38.6 °C and the fever often happens during night with night sweats and afternoon tidal fever. He did not report chest pain, stuffy/runny nose, shortness of breath, or hemoptysis. The patient attempted self-treatment using unknown medicines that he bought in a pharmacy, but no amelioration was noticed and his cough exacerbated. He was admitted to a district hospital where he received intravenous Piperacillin-Sulbactam for anti-infection treatment and showed improvement, with a diagnosis of "probable secondary pulmonary tuberculosis of both lungs with cavitation in both upper lobes" based on chest X-ray. He was subsequently referred to the outpatient department of pulmonary diseases at a district chronic disease prevention and treatment hospital.

Past history: He has a history of diabetes for 3 years, treated regularly using hypoglycemic drugs such as Metformin with his blood glucose level controlled well, which was monitored routinely. He denies the history of infectious diseases such as tuberculosis, viral hepatitis, paragonimiasis, and schistosomiasis and denies the history of chronic diseases such as chronic bronchitis, hypertension, coronary heart disease, and kidney diseases.

Personal history: no unhealthy habits; no smoking or drinking.

Physical examination: T: 36.8, P: 110 beats/min, R: 20/min, Bp: 128/89 mmHg. Consciousness, mental state generally well. The neck touches soft, no palpable swollen lymph nodes; the trachea is situated in the middle; harshness in the breathing sound of both lungs, no wheezes or moist crackles. The heart rate is 110 beats/min; regular rhythm, without murmurs at each auscultatory valve area. The abdomen seems flat and touches soft, without tenderness or rebound tenderness; liver and spleen not palpable in the infracostal margin; no percussion pain in liver area; negative shifting dullness; no edema in lower extremities.

Preliminary diagnosis: (1) Invasive pulmonary tuberculosis; (2) type-2 diabetes mellitus.

Diagnosis and treatment process

Adjuvant examinations on the day of his hospital visit: white blood cell count: 9.66×10^9/L, neutrophils%: 82.6%; lymphocyte%: 7.5%; eosinophils%: 0.1%; fasting blood glucose: 7.0 mmol/L; C-creative protein: 77.09 mm/L; erythrocyte sedimentation rate (ESR): 47.00 mm/L; normal hepatic function. Antibodies against Mycobacterium tuberculosis: IgG positive and IgM negative. Plain and enhanced CT scans of the chest (Fig. 5.5) showed multiple spotty and nodular high-density opacities, patchy ground glass opacities, as well as patchy consolidations, multiple thick-walled cavities, small cavities, and mouth-eaten cavities, with right hilar lymphadenopathy; no obvious enhancement was noticed in pulmonary lesions by enhanced CT scans, but annular enhancements were observed on the exterior wall of large cavities and on hilar lymph nodes. Anti-infection treatment was continued, using intravenous Piperacillin and Sulbactam for 5 days. On February 6, 2017, when the re-examination was performed, his cough kept ameliorating, but the expectoration was not relieved obviously. His sputum samples were smeared, cultured, and tested for drug sensitivity. Sputum smear on February 6, 2017, showed 4+ for acid-fast bacilli, and the result of sputum culture on February 27, 2017, was 4+. An anti-tuberculosis was launched on February 6, 2017, using FDC-2HRZE/4HR regimen, together with a therapy of liver protection. His cough and expectoration were ameliorated significantly with 2+ for sputum smear on March 6, 2017, when the re-examination was carried out, and the anti-tuberculosis treatment was continued with the previous regimen. On April 27, 2017, sensitivity tests on traditional drugs showed the resistance to isoniazid and the sensitivity to rifampin, ethambutol, and chloramphenicol, so the chemotherapy was modified to use 6RZELfx for the continuous anti-tuberculosis treatment. Chest plain CT scans (Fig. 5.6) on re-examination on August 5, 2017, showed obvious absorption and decrease in active lesion in both lungs, an increase in strip-like opacities, paracicatricial emphysema, and formation of bronchiectasis. Negativeness was observed for sputum smear at re-examination on August 5, September 6, and October 6, 2017. Chest X-ray on October 6, 2017 (Fig. 5.7) suggested the lesions were dominantly non-active ones, showing a tendency prone to stabilization. The final diagnosis was newly isoniazid mono-resistant pulmonary tuberculosis.

Discussion

With rapid generalization and application of DST technology, more and more newly diagnosed treatment-naive mono-resistant pulmonary tuberculosis have been diagnosed in time, and individualized treatment regimens have been given based on the drug resistances, thereby reducing risks of treatment failure and re-treatment. In case of limited laboratory capacity, however, imaging examination seems extremely important, especially the important value of CT signs of lesions for diagnosis and differential diagnosis of drug-sensitive pulmonary tuberculosis.

Despite the similarity of CT findings on both morphology and characteristics of lesions (i.e., coexistence of multiple forms and properties dominated by activity signs) between the mono-resistant patients and the drug-sensitive ones among all those with newly diagnosed pulmonary tuberculosis patients, the former differs from the latter in CT findings as shown by related researches [24, 25], mainly in respect of: (1) extensive distribution of lesions involving several pulmonary lobes and segments and involving easily sites not vulnerable to tuberculosis, including the middle of right lobe, the lingual segment of the upper left lobe and basal segments of both lower lobes. The reason might be further decrease in systemic cellular immunity with severer damage and impaired capability in eradicating Mycobacterium tuberculosis in patients suffering from drug-resistant tuberculosis compared with those with drug-sensitive tuberculosis, and therefore Mycobacterium tuberculosis grows and proliferates actively with larger bacterial load and greater risks in spreading randomly to pulmonary lobes and segments through bronchi. (2) Cavities are common. The research [25] has reported that the diameter of cavities is lower than 15 mm, and nodules with multiple small cavities are frequently observed, which tend to distribute in clusters. It has been reported that mouth-eaten cavities more likely occur within large lobular or segmental consolidations. All these results are related to immunity compromised and the infection with drug-resistant stains. (3) It is likely to invade and damage bronchi, leading to thickening bronchial wall. (4) Large lobular consolidation is more likely to occur, because CD4 + T lymphocytes tend to be fewer in patients with drug-resistant tuberculosis compared with those with non-resistant TB [29], thereby predisposing the former to poor immunity and facilitating the entry of a great amount of Mycobacterium tuberculosis into pulmonary tissue via bronchi to cause rapidly caseous pneumonia, which manifests a segmental or large lobular consolidation with blurred boundaries. Therefore, a diagnosis of a newly mono-resistant pulmonary tuberculosis is suggested in a TB patient by coexistence of various CT findings including extensive lesions, great lobular or segmental consolidations, multiple small cavities and

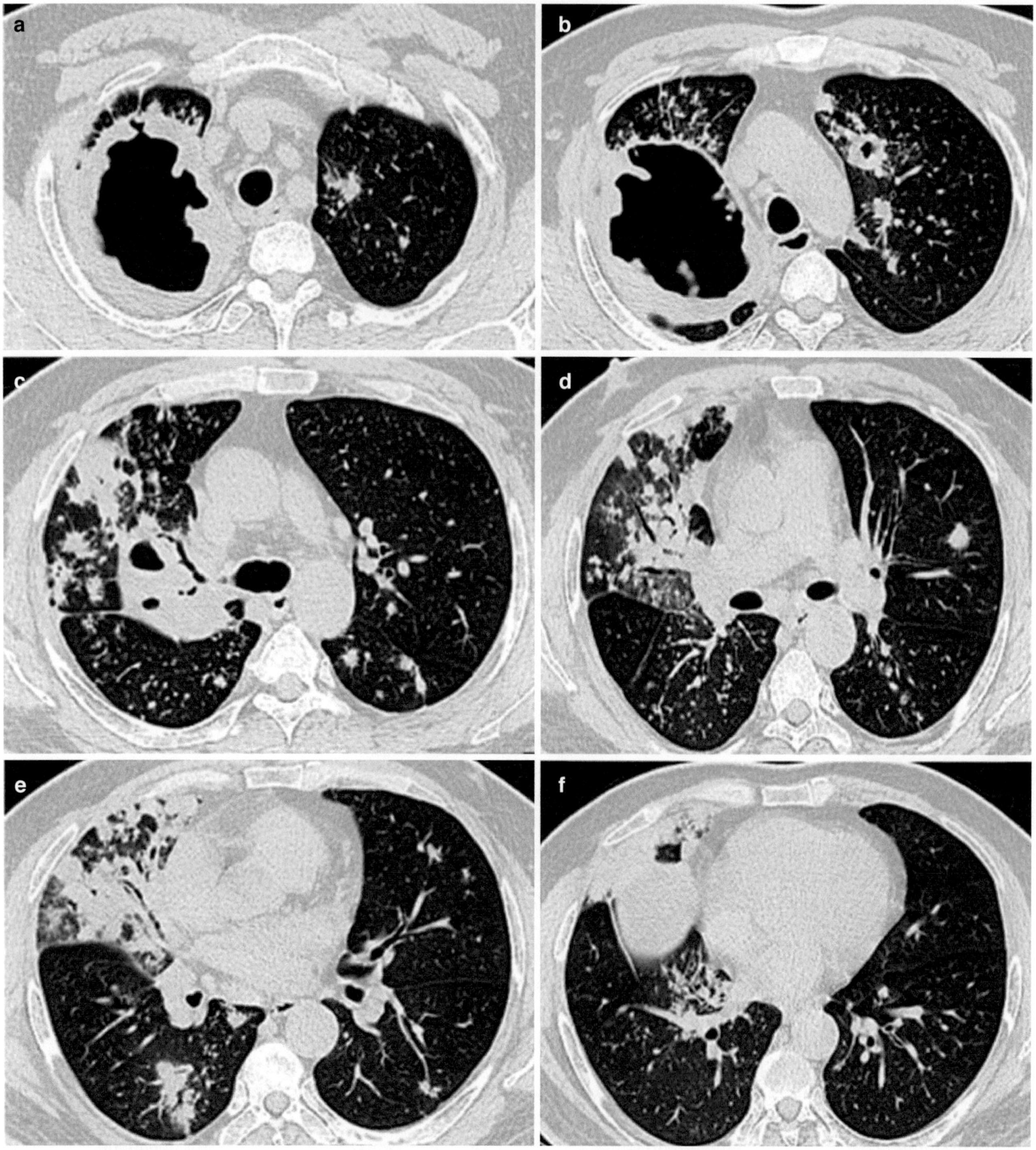

Fig. 5.5 (**a**–**j**) Plain and enhanced CT scans of the chest on January 31, 2017. Lung windows (**a**–**f**) showed multiple spotted and nodular high-density opacities in both lungs, as well as lobular and segmental consolidations, and patchy ground glass opacities; a giant thick-walled cavity was observed in the posterior apical segment of the upper right lobe, with the rugged interior wall and multiple mural nodules; a small mouth-eaten cavity is seen in the consolidation in the upper right lobe, and a thick-walled cavity in the posterior apical segment of the upper left lobe. Mediastinal window (**g**–**j**) shows a circular enhancement (i.e., a mild enhancement during the arterial phase and an obvious enhancement during the venous phase) in the tuberculous granulation tissue within the exterior wall of the giant thick-walled cavity in the upper right lobe, compared with the absence of enhancement in the caseous necrotic tissue within the interior wall. Some liquid is observed in the cavity. No obvious enhancement is found in other pulmonary lesions. Right hilar lymphadenopathy is observed, showing a circular enhancement

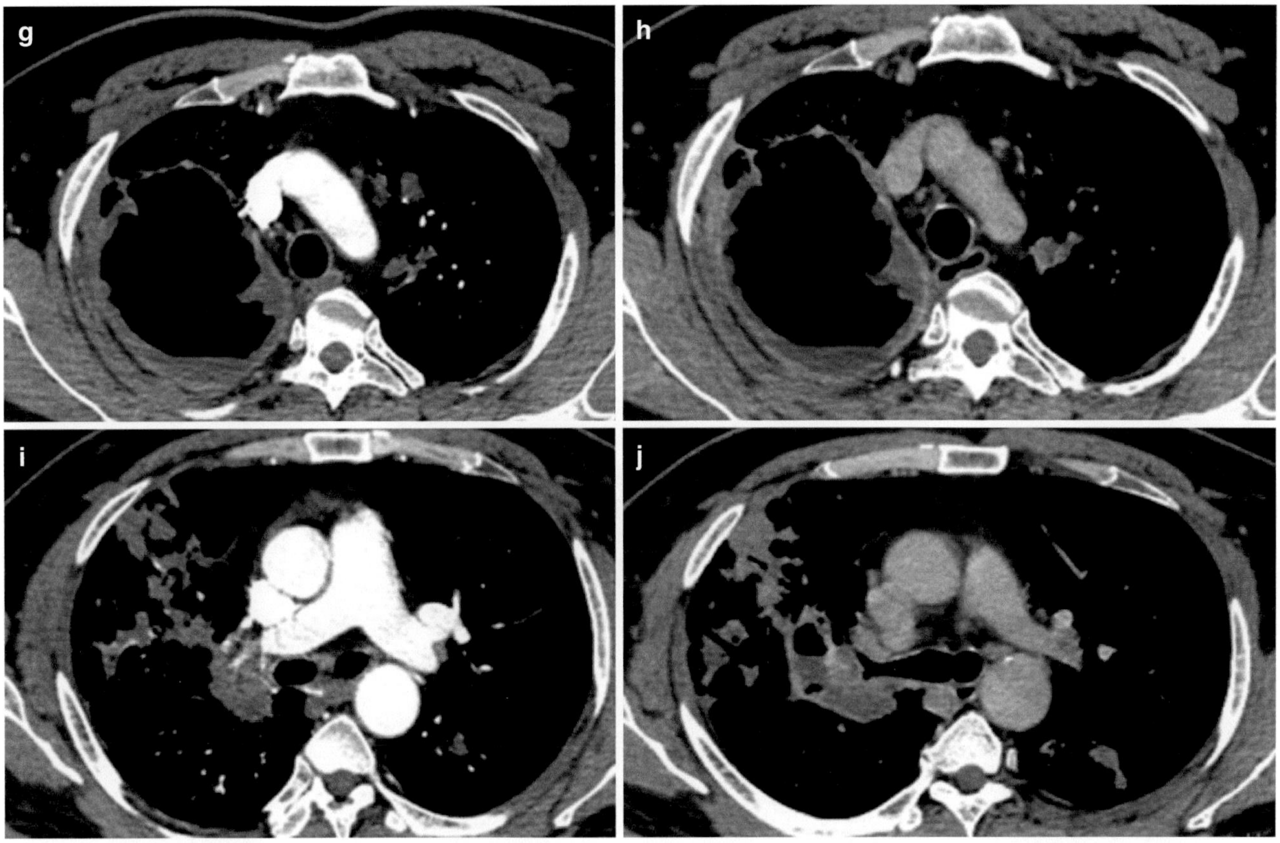

Fig. 5.5 (continued)

mouth-eaten cavities, and thickening of bronchial wall. The confirmation of the diagnosis, however, still requires the comprehensive consideration of both clinical information and results of drug sensitivity test in vitro. The preliminary diagnosis for this patient was active pulmonary tuberculosis, based on a comprehensive consideration of clinical symptoms and results of laboratory test. The possibility of drug-resistant pulmonary TB, however, should be considered, according to CT findings characterized in the distribution of lesions in five lobes bilaterally, infrequent sites of TB, lesions of bronchial distribution, segmental consolidation, multiple active lesions such as thick-walled or mouth-eaten cavities.

The patient had concomitantly type-2 diabetes, which is underlying disease predisposing the patient to increased risk of drug-resistant tuberculosis, for there is a correlation between diabetes and drug-resistant tuberculosis [30]. A study [31] revealed that diabetes induced a 2-time increased of risk of rifampin resistance in TB patients and raised the probability of drug-resistant pulmonary TB. The reason is that the high serum glucose environment in diabetes patients is conducive to the growth and proliferation of Mycobacterium tuberculosis, and high bacterial loads in a patient with low immunity induce immune escape of Mycobacterium tuberculosis. Drug-resistant pulmonary tuberculosis, as reported by the literature, has similar features of imaging findings such as cavitation, bronchial dissemination, and extra-pulmonary manifestations, irrespective of the presence or absence of concomitant underlying diseases, except for older age, more cases with sputum positiveness, and greater bacterial loads for those complicated with diabetes. The occurrence of severe disease with untypical manifestations, including the giant cavity in the upper right lobe, multiple thick-wall nodules with amount caseous necrotic tissue, circular enhancement manifested by granulation tissue in the exterior wall of the cavity shown by enhanced CT scans, the absence of obvious enhancement of caseous necrotic tissue in the interior cavity wall, seemed to be the outcome of a joint effect by dual factors including diabetes and drug resistance. Rapid DST detection for rifampin- and Isoniazid-resistance, if allowable by laboratory conditions, should be done prior to anti-tuberculosis treatment for a patient complicated with an underlying disease (such as diabetes and HIV/AIDS) predisposing him/her to high risk of emerging drug-resistant tuberculosis, who manifests imaging findings including extensive distribution of lesions, and coexistence of multiple cavities, consolidations, and thickening of bronchial wall, so as to launch individualized therapeutic regimens as soon as possible, minimize the risk of treatment

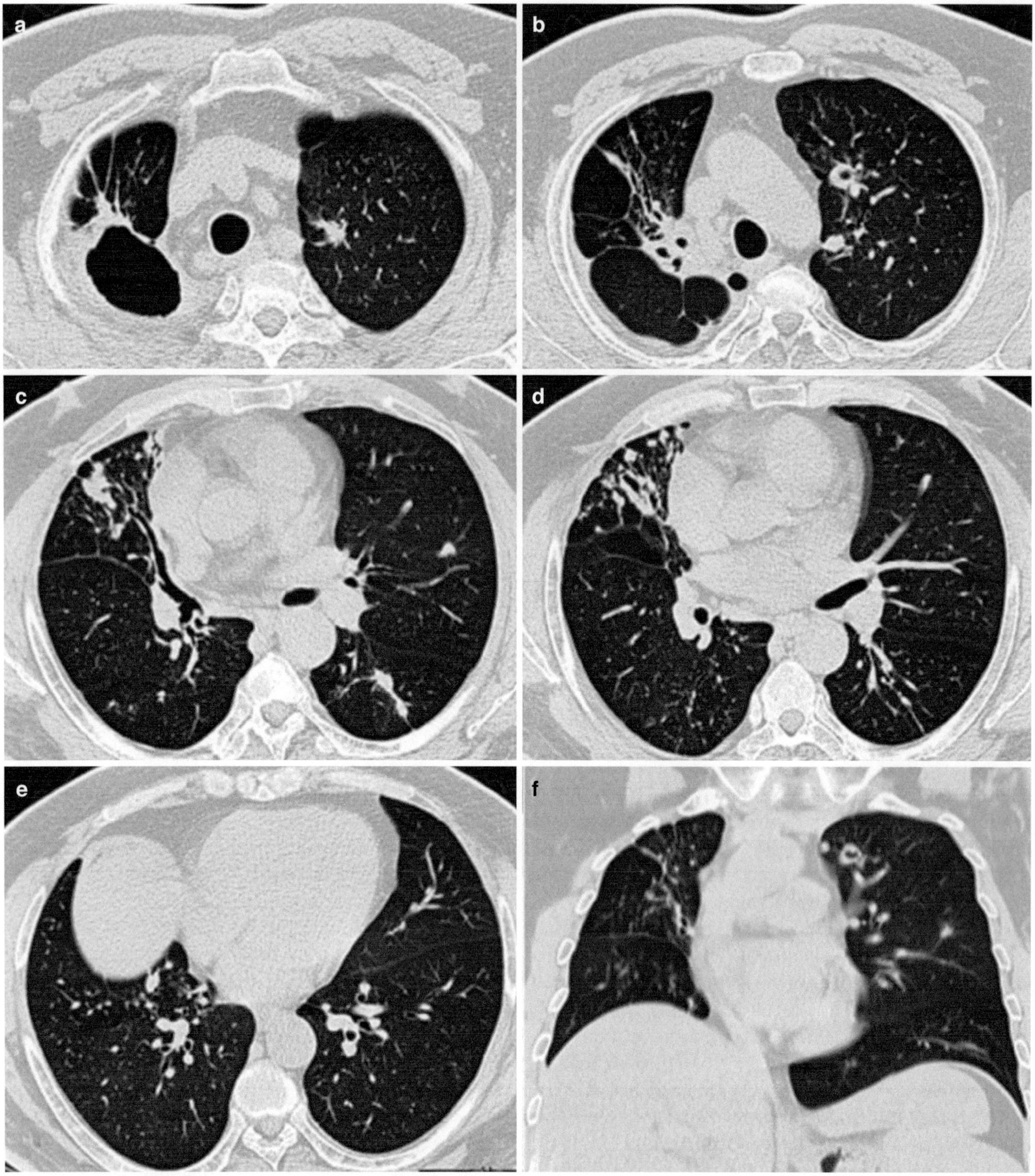

Fig. 5.6 (**a**–**f**) Re-examination of chest CT (August 5, 2017). Compared with CT findings in January 31, 2017, lung lesions decrease significantly with clear boundaries; the giant cavity in the right upper lobe shrinks with the smooth interior wall; mural nodules and liquid in the cavity disappear, with surrounding strip-like high-density opacities with clear boundaries, thickening and adhesion of adjacent pleura; multiple paracicatricial emphysema appear in the upper and middle right lobes; bronchiectasis is seen for the right middle lobe with thickened bronchial walls; the small thick-walled cavity in the left upper lobe still exists, but the wall becomes thinner than before and the exterior wall becomes smoother

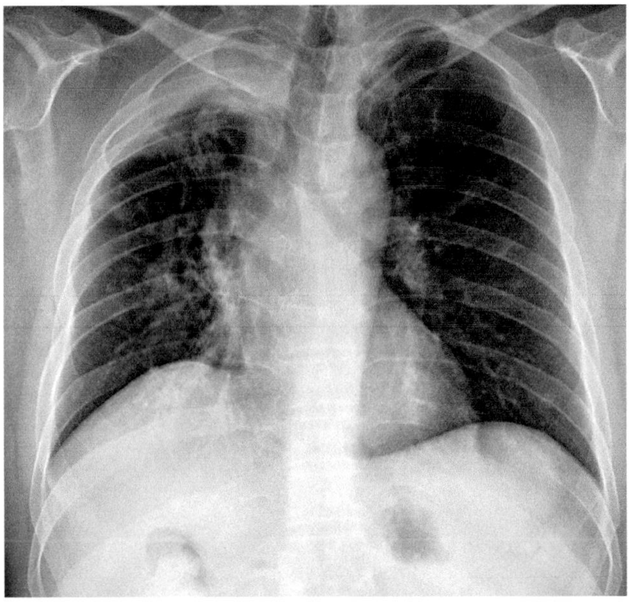

Fig. 5.7 Re-examination of chest X-ray on October 6, 2017. Nodular and strip-like high-density opacities in both lungs, with shrunk size of the right upper lobe; obviously thickening and adhesion are observed for the right pleura, with slight collapse of the right thorax; slight right shifting of the trachea; elevation of the right diaphragm

failure, and avoid the progression from mono-resistance to multiple resistance TB.

Case 3. Re-Treatment Rifampin Mono-Resistance Pulmonary Tuberculosis

Abstract of disease history

The patient was a 34-year-old female, who was admitted on June 3, 2016, with a recurring cough and expectoration for 1 month. She had previously sought medical service in a local hospital 1 month prior, complaining of worsened cough and expectoration that lasted for 7 days, but it was relieved with antibiotics and expectorants (details unknown). She experienced hemoptysis several times with 2 mL per episode prior to admission. Upon re-examination of X-ray in the local hospital, a patchy high-density opacity with blurred boundaries was observed in her right lung, indicating pulmonary tuberculosis. Consequently, the patient was referred to the outpatient department of lung diseases in a chronic disease control hospital for further treatment. Since the onset of the disease, she has reported poor mental state, loss of appetite and sleep, fatigue, and weight loss of about 4 kg. Urination and defecation have been normal.

Past history: The patient denies the history of hepatitis or tuberculosis; the history of hypertension, coronary heart disease, or diabetes.

Physical examination: T: 36.5 °C, Bp: 120/75 mmHg, R: 18/min, P: 75 beats/min. Consciousness, poor mentality, and cooperative in physical examination. No jaundice or bleeding spots on skin or mucous membrane of the whole body; superficial lymph nodes not palpable or swollen, no congestion of the pharynx; no swelling of bilateral tonsils; the neck touches soft, with trachea positioned in the middle; harshness in the breathing sound of both lungs, no wheezes or moist crackles; no pleural friction sound is heard; no bulge in precordial region; the heart rate is 75 beats/min; regular rhythm, without pathological murmurs; the abdomen seems flat and touches soft, without tenderness or rebound tenderness; liver and spleen not palpable in the infracostal margin; negative shifting dullness; normal bowel sounds.

Preliminary diagnosis: invasive pulmonary tuberculosis.

Diagnosis and treatment process

Blood routine: Leukocyte count 7.21 × 10^9/L, neutrophils percentage: 62.5%, lymphocytes percentage: 29.7%, eosinophils percentage: 0.1%; 8 items of liver function: direct bilirubin 3.9 μmol/L, total bilirubin 8.1 μmol/L, total protein 70 g/L, albumin 38 g/L, alkaline phosphatase 104 μ/L, γ-glutamyltransferase 18.5 μ/L, aspartate aminotransferase 16.2 μ/L, and glucose 5.1 mmol/L; items of renal function: urea nitrogen 7.22 mmol/L, creatinine 72 μmol/L, bicarbonate 27.3 mmol/L, uric acid 246.3 μmmol/L, cystatin C 0.64 mg/L; erythrocyte sedimentation rate (ESR) 21 mm/h; negative in tuberculosis antibody IgG and IgM; negative in acid-fast stain of sputum smear. Chest CT scans (Fig. 5.8): patchy, nodular, and tree-in-bud patterns and ground glass opacities; multiple and small thick-walled cavities; bronchiectasia, with a small amount of strip-like and spotty opacities in the middle lobe (Fig. 5.8e). Clinical diagnosis based on clinical symptoms and CT findings: (1) invasive pulmonary tuberculosis; (2) right middle lobe bronchiectasis complicated with infection; (3) the probable diagnose: alveolar hematocele (apical segment of the upper lobe of the right lung).

Lemahui Capsule and Adrenaline Hydrazone Tablet were given to stop bleeding; Moxifloxacin hydrochloride tablets were given for 2 weeks; Anti-tuberculosis treatment for 2 months was used, consisting of oral Isoniazid tablet 0.3 g, oral Rifampin capsule 0.45 g, and oral Ethambutol 0.75, once a day. Compound glycyrrhizin capsule 20 mg three times a day was given to protect the liver, and the symptoms of cough and expectoration were relieved gradually and disappeared. Revisit on July 4, and August 5, 2016, showed that the blood routine, liver function, kidney function, and urine routine were normal, with negative result of sputum smear. Anti-tuberculosis treatment was continued for another 4 months, using oral isoniazid tablet 0.3 g and oral rifampin capsule 0.45 g once a day. Given the absence of symptoms and adverse reaction, the patient received the medication intermittently without regular, sufficient, and whole-course therapy, and multiple sputum smears showed negative results during the treatment. The patient complained of cough and expectoration again 3 months after the end of the treatment, and then

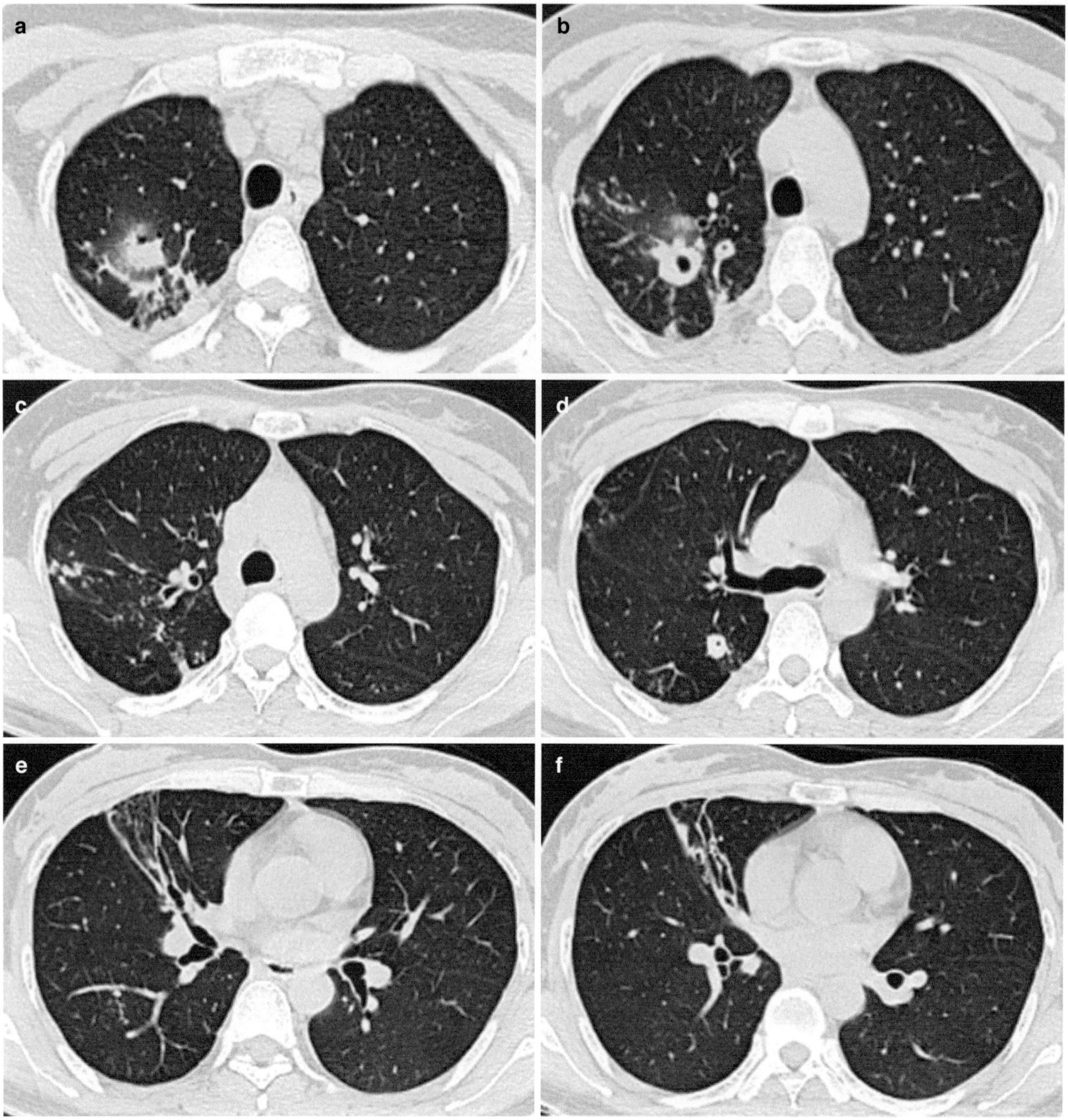

Fig. 5.8 (**a–f**) Chest CT on June 3, 2016, for this newly diagnosed patient prior to treatment. (**a–d**). Lung window showed patchy, nodular, and tree-in-bud in the upper lobe and the dorsal segment of the right lung, a small amount of ground glass opacities in the apical segment of upper lobe of the right lung, with multiple small cavities within nodules and thickening and adhesion pleura adjacent to lesions. (**e**, **f**). Lung window showed multiple bronchiectasis of the middle lobe of the right lung with thickening of bronchial wall and strip-like and dotty high-density opacities, as well as tree-in-bud high-density opacities in the dorsal segment of the lower right lobe

he re-visited our hospital on April 5, 2017. Chest CT scans (Fig. 5.9) showed the obvious increase in the number of nodules and consolidation in the right lung, with the enlargement of multiple thick-walled cavities; bronchiectasis in the anterior segment of the upper lobe and the middle lobe of the right lung; and formation of non-active lesions including strip-like opacities, calcification and thickening and adhesion of pleura. The result of acid-fast staining test of sputum smear was 4+, and Xpert Mtb/RIF of sputum showed a result of mycobacterium tuberculosis complex, which was resistant to rifampin.

Final diagnosis: Re-treatment rifampin mono-resistant pulmonary tuberculosis.

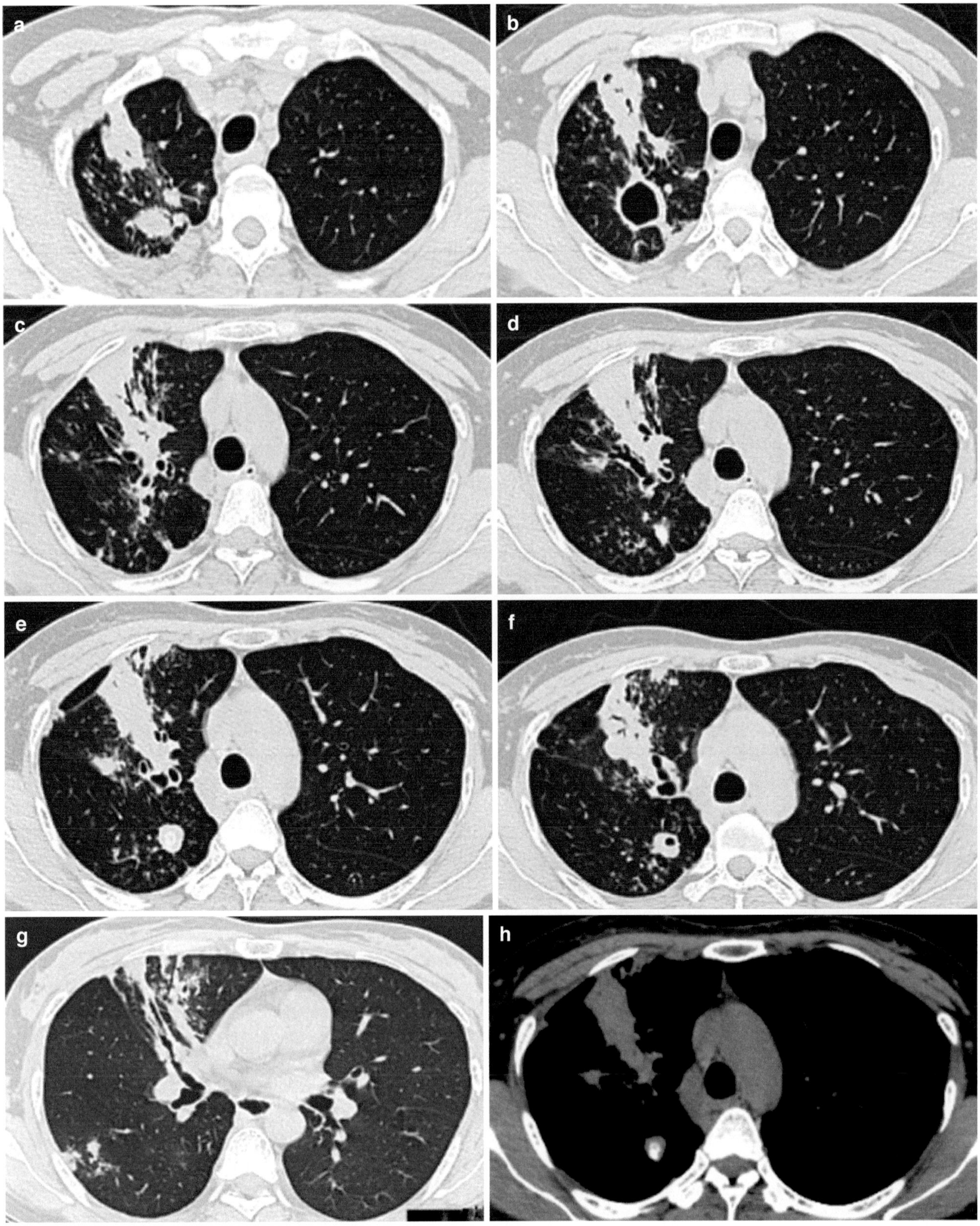

Fig. 5.9 (**a**–**h**) Re-examination of chest CT on April 5, 2017. (**a**–**h**) Compared with chest CT on June 3, 2016, lung window and mediastinal window showed the lesions increase (number and size) in upper lobe, middle lobe and lower lobe of the right lung. The lesions are mainly consolidations and nodules, with air-bronchogram observed within the consolidation; the increase in the size was noticed for the thick-walled cavities in the apical segment of upper lobe and the dorsal segment of the lower lobe of the right lung. The bronchus in anterior segment of the upper right lobe seems tortuous and dilated, with coexistence of bronchial stenosis and bronchiectasis in the middle right lobe. Strip-like opacities in the apical segment of the upper right lobe, with nodular calcification observed in the lesions in the dorsal segment of the lower right lobe, and thickening and adhesion of the right pleura

Discussion

Re-treatment tuberculosis patients, including those receiving unreasonable or nonstandard anti-tuberculosis medication for at least 1 month and those with recurrent disease unresponsive to the initial treatment, have multiple factors predisposing them to drug resistance [1], including medical factors, factors of patients themselves, and the factor of anti-tuberculosis drugs, wherein the nonstandard anti-tuberculosis treatment and irregular medication accepted by the patients are the mainly triggers. As reported in the literature [32], another reason for the development of drug resistance in pulmonary tuberculosis is the poor blood circulation in the lesions, which leads to prolonged exposure of Mycobacterium tuberculosis to antibiotics at low concentration. These factors can cause incomplete absorption of pulmonary lesions during anti-tuberculosis treatment, leading to oscillating between amelioration and deterioration while repeatedly transforming among exudation, proliferation, and caseous necrosis. The outcome at the end of the therapeutic cycle can be not only non-active lesions including fibrosis, calcification, purified cavity, and thickening/adhesion of pleura but also active manifestations prone to deterioration including enlargement of lesions, increase in both number and size of cavities, and increased number of lesions spreading via bronchi. This patient had the characteristics concerning factors triggering drug resistance and inducing the outcome, in that the patients showed a poor compliance, as well as intermittence and irregularity in his medication. Re-examination of CT scans at the end of treatment showed the phenomenon of the active diseases, including the increase but not the reduction of lesions, greater extension of their sizes, presence of cavities, enlargement of the nodules and segmental consolidations compared with the previous imagines. There was a response in a certain degree observed for previous lesions with presence of some non-active lesions including a small amount of fibrotic change, calcification within nodules, thickening and adhesion of pleura and tortuous bronchiectasis, because of chemotherapy. It can be inferred, therefore, that poor response or no response during anti-tuberculosis treatment or recurrence post to the cure may suggest the mixed lesions before the re-treatment is launched and the coexistence of active and non-active lesions. Some researchers [33] gathered a group of patients with drug-resistant pulmonary tuberculosis, and most of them were receiving re-treatment. The comparison of CT findings for patients with various drug resistance and drug-sensitive TB showed that more extensive lesion was observed in the former, who manifested more pulmonary nodules, thickening of bronchi wall and cavities compared with the latter. No statistic difference of lesion distribution or CT findings was revealed between different categories of drug resistances, suggesting the similarity of CT findings between re-treatment mono-resistant pulmonary tuberculosis and other drug-resistant pulmonary tuberculosis, concerning the extensive lesions, tendency to form nodules and cavities with thickening of bronchi wall. Despite the golden criteria discerning drug resistance emerged in re-treatment pulmonary tuberculosis is still drug sensitivity test, CT imaging remains to be the ideal method to observe these lesions directly and intuitively. Chest CT, therefore, is recommended as one of the routine clinical procedures for pulmonary tuberculosis patients requiring re-examination, so as to evaluate scope better, nature, and severity of lesions and suggest the drug resistance to help clarify the differentiation diagnosis.

Re-treatment tuberculosis patients are the populations with a high risk of drug resistance, showing high ratio of general drug resistance and the highest incidence of mono-resistance. The efficient approach, therefore, consists of the timely detection of re-treatment mono-resistant pulmonary tuberculosis and individualized chemotherapeutic regimens launched as soon as possible to avoid the development of multi-resistant tuberculosis and further spreading of drug-resistant Mycobacterium tuberculosis. WHO [1] has suggested, therefore, that Xpert Mtb/RIF, the molecular biological diagnostic tool, should be preferred for patient belonging to the population with high risk of drug-resistant tuberculosis, because of the long time required by phenotype drug-resistant test to obtain its results. Xpert Mtb/RIF, capable of identifying directly DNA of bacteria strains and detecting genetic mutations related to rifampin resistance, shows a similar sensitivity, specificity, and accuracy with the traditional solid culture and is of advantages of short time consumption, high level of biological safety and low cost, which is in favor of early diagnosis and treatment in clinical practice.

Since the patient in this case had mono-resistant rifampin pulmonary tuberculosis, it was essential to exercise great prudence when formulating therapeutic regimens. Rifampin is a sterilizing agent and one of the most important core drugs, and its resistance is not easily recoverable. Once resistance to rifampin occurs, it predisposes isoniazid, another core drugs, to a reduction of efficacy and makes treatment challenging, which is almost equivalent to MDR-TB. According to literature reports [34], 80% of strains resistant to rifampin are also resistant to isoniazid. Tuberculosis with rifampin resistance shows a poorer response and prognosis compared to tuberculosis not resistant to rifampin, so regimens for rifampin mono-resistant tuberculosis must be formulated and controlled according to regimens for multi-resistance disease.

References

1. World Health Organization. Companion handbook to the WHO guidelines for the programmatic management of drug-resistant tuberculosis. WHO/HTM/TB/2014.11. Geneva: World Health Organization; 2014.
2. Technical Guidance Group for the Fifth National Epidemiological Sampling Survey of Tuberculosis, Office for the Fifth National Epidemiological Sampling Survey of tuberculosis, and tuberculosis control Center of China Disease Control Center. Report on the fifth national epidemiological sampling survey of tuberculosis in 2010 [J]. Chin J Antituberc. 2012;34(8):485–508.
3. Ministry of Public Health of the Peoples Republic of China. A report on baseline survey of tuberculosis in China (2007–2008) [M]. Beijing: People's Medical Publishing House; 2010. p. 49–51.
4. State health and family planning Commission of the People's Republic of China. Diagnostic criteria for pulmonary tuberculosis (WS 288-2017) [J/CD]. Electr J Emerg Infect Dis. 2018;3(1):59–61.
5. Yu W, Tan W-G, Lu P-X. Classification and imaging manifestations of drug-resistant pulmonary tuberculosis [J/CD]. Electr J Emerg Infect Dis. 2019;4(1):42–7.
6. World Health Organization. Anti-tuberculosis drug resistant in the world: report NO4.WHO/HTM/TB/2008.394. Geneva: World Health Organization; 2008.
7. Zhang H, Xu H, Fan L, et al. An analysis on epidemiological features of pulmonary tuberculosis in Hebei Province 2008-2014 [J]. J Med Pest Control. 2016;32(09):977–80, 983.
8. Prach LM, Pascopella L, Barry PM, et al. Rifampin mono-resistant tuberculosis and HIV comorbidity in California, 1993-2008: a retrospective cohort study [J]. AIDS. 2013;27(16):2615–22.
9. Mukinda FK, Theron D, van der Spuy GD, et al. Rise in rifampin-monoresistant tuberculosis in Western Cape, South Africa [J]. Int J Tuberc Lung Dis. 2012;16(2):196–202.
10. Sanders M, Van Deun A, Ntakirutimana D, et al. Rifampicin mono-resistant mycobacterium tuberculosis in Bujumbura, Burundi: results of a drug resistance survey [J]. Int J Tuberc Lung Dis. 2006;10(2):178–83.
11. Coovadia YM, Mahomed S, Pillay M, et al. Rifampicin mono-resistance in mycobacterium tuberculosis in KwaZulu-Natal, South Africa: a significant phenomenon in a high prevalence TB-HIV region [J]. PLoS One. 2013;8(11):e77712.
12. Dramowski A, Morsheimer MM, Jordaan AM, et al. Rifampin-monoresistant mycobacterium tuberculosis disease among children in Cape Town, South Africa [J]. Int J Tuberc Lung Dis. 2012;16(1):76–81.
13. World Health Organization. Global tuberculosis report 2021[EB/OL]. [2021-10-14]. https://www.who.int/publications/digital/global-tuberculosis-report-2021.
14. WHO treatment guidelines for drug-resistant tuberculosis, 2016 update. WHO/HTM/TB/2016.04. Geneva: World Health Organization; 2016.
15. Gu J, Tang S. Thoughts on the diagnosis and treatment of rifampin-resistant tuberculosis [J]. Chin J Antituberc. 2015;37(11):1097–101.
16. Tuberculosis clinical professional Committee of China Anti Tuberculosis Association. Annual report on the progress of clinical diagnosis and treatment of tuberculosis (2014) (part II: clinical treatment of tuberculosis) [J]. Chin J Antituberc. 2015;37(7):673–721.
17. Althomsons SP, Cegielski JP. Impact of second-line drug resistance on tuberculosis treatment outcomes in the United States: MDR-TB is bad enough [J]. Int J Tuberc Lung Dis. 2012;16(10):1331–4.
18. Tang S, Xu S, Li L. Drug resistant tuberculosis [M]. Beijing: People's Medical Publishing House; 2014. p. 126–287.
19. Chinese Association of Antituberculosis. Guideline on chemotherapy for drug-resistant tuberculosis (2015) [J]. Chin J Antituberc. 2015;37(5):421–69.
20. Imaging Committee on infections, Chinese Society of Radiology; Committee on Infectious Disease; Radiology Committee, Chinese Medical Doctor Association, et al. Imaging diagnostic criteria of pulmonary tuberculosis [J/CD]. Electr J Emerg Infect Dis. 2021;6(1):1–6.
21. Bomanji JB, Gupta N, Gulati P, et al. Imaging in tuberculosis [J]. Cold Spring Harb Perspect Med. 2015;5(6):a017814.
22. Curvo-Semedo L, Teixeira L, Caseiro-Alves F. Tuberculosis of the chest [J]. Eur J Radiol. 2005;55(2):158–72.
23. Van Dyck P, Vanhoenacker FM, Van den Brande P, et al. Imaging of pulmonary tuberculosis [J]. Eur Radiol. 2003;13(8):1771–85.
24. Chen G, Cheng G-x, Zhu S-q, et al. CT scanning of mono-resistant pulmonary tuberculosis during initial treatment [J]. Electr J Emerg Infect Dis. 2018;3(2):111–4.
25. Zhang Z, Ren G, Tan Y, et al. CT findings of rifampin mono-resistant pulmonary tuberculosis [J]. Guide China Med. 2015;13(25):65–6.
26. Akira M, Sakatani M, Ishikawa H. Transient radiographic progression during initial treatment of pulmonary tuberculosis: CT findings [J]. J Comput Assist Tomogr. 2000;24(3):426–31.
27. Gegia M, Winters N, Benedetti A, et al. Treatment of isoniazid-resistant tuberculosis with first-line drugs: a systematic review and meta-analysis [J]. Lancet Infect Dis. 2017;17(2):223–34.
28. World Health Organization. WHO treatment guidelines for isoniazid-resistant tuberculosis: supplement to the WHO treatment guidelines for drug-resistant tuberculosis [R]. Geneva: WHO; 2018. p. 1–31.
29. Hu Y, Zhang H, Liu J, et al. An analysis on drug sensitivity in correlation to count of blood CD4 cells and separation/identification of sputum bacteria in patients with multi-resistant pulmonary tuberculosis [J]. Chin J Antituberc. 2015;37(4):360–5.
30. Chang JT, Dou HY, Yen CL, et al. Effect of type 2 diabetes mellitus on the clinical severity and treatment outcome in patients with pulmonary tuberculosis: a potential role in the emergence of multidrug-resistance [J]. J Formos Med Assoc. 2011;110(6):372–81.
31. Mehta S, Yu EA, Ahamed SF, et al. Rifampin resistance and diabetes mellitus in a cross-sectional study of adult patients in rural South India [J]. BMC Infect Dis. 2015;15(1):451.
32. Li L, Wang D, Liu Q, et al. The observation of characteristics of focal perfusion in re-treatment smear-positive pulmonary tuberculosis patients by 32-slice CT double inlet perfusion technique [J]. Chin J Antituberc. 2016;66(7):1417–30.
33. Li C, Zhou X, Lu Y, et al. An analysis of CT findings in patients of different categories of drug-resistant tuberculosis and those with drug-sensitive tuberculosis [J]. Chin J Antituberc. 2018;40(7):707–12.
34. World Health Organization. Anti-tuberculosis drug resistance in the world, WHO Report No. 3[R]. Geneva: World Health Organization; 2004.

Multidrug-Resistant Tuberculosis

6

Chun-hua Li, Jie Zhou, Xian-rong Long, Sheng-xiu Lv, Dong Yu, Wei-Jun Luo, and Jin-ping Wu

6.1 Summary of Multidrug-Resistant Tuberculosis

Multidrug-resistant tuberculosis (MDR-TB) is defined as a tuberculosis induced by Mycobacterium tuberculosis resistant at least simultaneously to isoniazid and rifampin, as confirmed by drug susceptibility testing (DST) in vitro [1]. Based on the presence/absence of previous exposure to anti-tuberculosis treatment, MDR-TB can be categorized into the new multidrug-resistant tuberculosis (nMDR-TB) and the relapsing multidrug-resistant tuberculosis (rMDR-TB) [2]. The nMDR-TB are the MDR-TB patients who have not received anti-TB therapy or have taken anti-TB drugs for less than 1 month, and the latter defined as MDR-TB occurring in patients with such a previous exposure or in those undergoing anti-tuberculosis treatment lasting more than 1 month.

In 2019, there were about ten million persons suffering from tuberculosis, equaling 130 every 100,000 in average。 As indicated by WHO Report of Global Tuberculosis 2020, there were 465,000 patients with rifampicin-resistant tuberculosis (RR-TB) worldwide in 2019, and 78% of them were MDR-TB. Among three nations with the greatest burden of drug-resistant tuberculosis in the world, as shown by the report, China ranked the second only after India and witnessed about 833,000 newly diagnosed TB patients and about 65,000 newly emerging MDR/rifampicin-resistant TB(MDR/RR-TB) cases in China [1]. The latest data about outcome in treatment for MDR/RR-TB patients in 2019 showed a global successful ratio of 57%. Moreover, the population having received treatment occupied only 38% in estimated MDR-TB patients in 2019. In order to control MDR-TB, it is an important measure to improve the diagnostic rate of tuberculosis, expand coverage of drug resistance tests for patients with bacteriologically confirmed tuberculosis, and ensure all patients diagnosed with MDR-TB can be treated.

According to the 2021 WHO Global Tuberculosis Report, 132,222 cases of MDR/RR-TB and 25,681 cases of extensively drug-resistant TB(XDR-TB) or pre-extensively drug-resistant TB (pre-XDR-TB) were detected in 2020, equaling 157,903 cases in total, which was lower significantly than 201,997 in 2019, with a decrease of 22%. During the past 10 years, the ratio of MDR/RR-TB has remained at about 3–4% for treatment-naive patients, and 18–21% (the best estimate) for relapsing tuberculosis patients, with a stabilized burden imposed by MDR/RR-TB. The year 2020 witnessed 150,359 cases of MDR/RR-TB registered for treatment around the world, which accounted only for 1/3 of annual MDR/RR-TB number and showed a drop for 15% compared with 177,100 cases in 2019 [3].

When MDR-TB is diagnosed, sputum culture identification and DST are the main methods for diagnosing MDR-TB. The culture of Mycobacterium tuberculosis, however, requires generally several weeks, which is greatly detrimental to early diagnosis, treatment, and control of the spread of MDR-TB. Imaging examination (especially CT scans), on the contrary, is of great important method in diagnosis and treatment of tuberculosis.

Compared with drug-sensitive tuberculosis (DS-TB), MDR-TB is characterized in CT findings more complex with

C.-h. Li (✉) · S.-x. Lv
Department of Medical Imaging, Chongqing Public Health Medical Center, Chongqing, China

J. Zhou
Department of Tuberculosis, Foshan Hospital of Traditional Chinese Medicine, Foshan, Guangdong, China

X.-r. Long
Department of Medical Imaging, Foshan Fourth People's Hospital, Foshan, Guangdong, China

D. Yu
Department of Prehospital Care, Shenzhen Center for Prehospital Care, Shenzhen, Guangdong, China

W-J. Luo

Department of Medical Imaging, Shenzhen Center for Chronic Disease Control, Shenzhen, Guangdong, China

J.-p. Wu
Department of Radiology, Third People's Hospital of Changzhou City, Changzhou, Jiangsu, China

P.-x. Lu et al. (eds.), *Diagnostic Imaging of Drug Resistant Pulmonary Tuberculosis*,
https://doi.org/10.1007/978-981-99-8339-1_6

greater multiformity distributed more extensively and more prone to involvement of multiple lobes and segments [4]. Its ratio is up to 86.1% for the involvement of at least 3 lobes, and 61.3% for that of whole lungs. This is related probably to the inherent attribute in most MDR-TB as the acquired drug resistance with a prolonged course, multiple recurrences, and intrapulmonary dissemination. Another feature of MDR is multiple cavities, which is reported to appear in nearly 70% of rMDR-TB patients, compared with about only 20% in DS-TB patients. Presence of lesions in no less than 2 lung fields, as proposed by some researchers, correlates to MDR-TB, and the number of cavities no less than 3 suggests a high probability of MDR-TB [5]. Besides involvement of both lungs, manifestations including multiple bronchial disseminating lesions, bronchiectasis, and destroyed lungs are more often observed in MDR-TB, which is probably related to the prolonged course of this disease, and repeated infiltration and destruction of pulmonary tissues by Mycobacterium tuberculosis.

Despite the certain feature in chest CT findings for MDR-TB, its overall image finding has no substantial difference with DS-TB [4, 6], both of which may manifest extensive distribution, bronchial disseminating lesions, multiple cavities, destroyed lungs, pleura thickening and bronchiectasis, with the exception of the higher incidence observed in MDR-TB patients.

6.2 Introduction of Typical Cases of Multidrug-Resistant Tuberculosis

Case 1

The patient, a 48-year-old female, was admitted with the chief complaint of "cough with intermittent fever for 6 months, with an exacerbation for 20 days." She had the onset of cough without obvious inducement 6 months before, which was mainly dry cough complicated with fever dominantly in the morning, with the highest temperature up to 38.5 °C. She was diagnosed with "pulmonary infection" for several times at the local hospital, and her symptoms ameliorated to some extent post to the treatment with cefixime and levofloxacin, though she had intermittent cough and expectoration. She felt an exacerbation of her cough and expectoration, and CT scans in the local county hospital suggested tuberculosis in both lungs, with positiveness (2+) in sputum smear. Detection on sputum drug-resistant gene showed Mycobacterium tuberculosis with R resistance. On July 14, 2020, she underwent anti-tuberculosis treatment with a combination regimen (HERZ) in the local Tuberculosis Prevention and Control Institute. Her cough ameliorated slightly, but abdominal distension and nausea appeared and aggravated gradually. Fever occurred 1 day before with the temperature of 38.5 °C, and she was admitted for further treatment. Chest CT scans on August 31, 2020 (Fig. 6.1) showed small patchy consolidations with a small cavity and bronchiectasis in the middle and lower lobes of the right lung.

DST showed the resistance to H on September 30, 2020, and an anti-tuberculosis treatment with H-R-E-Clr regimen in normal dosage was given. On December 29, 2020, positiveness was indicated by a rapid culture of sputum Mycobacterium tuberculosis. Given the persistent positiveness post to more than 5 months of anti-tuberculosis treatment, a potential of multidrug resistance was considered. Re-examination of chest CT (Fig. 6.2) suggested absorption and amelioration of lesions with local fusion and consolidation, and an anti-tuberculosis treatment was planned, using regimen of "Lfx-Lzd-Cfx-Cs-E-Z," but the patient denied it on the ground of the partial absorption of pulmonary lesions and the low-income of the family and accepted "H-R-E-Z-Lfx" regimen instead.

Roche DST on March 23, 2021, with the sputum specimen sampled on December 29, 2020, suggested Mycobacterium tuberculosis resistant to H, R, Sm, RFT, Pa, and Mfx. Re-examination of chest CT scans (Fig. 6.3) showed the increase in lesions in both lungs. She underwent an anti-tuberculosis treatment using "Lfx-Lzd-Cfx-Cs-E-Z" regimen on March 30, 2021.

Roche DST on May 21, 2021, showed resistance to H, R, Sm, RFT, and Mfx, and re-examination of CT scans (Fig. 6.4) showed obvious absorption of intra-pulmonary lesions and the closure of the cavity, suggesting the response to the treatment, based on which the anti-tuberculosis with "Lfx-Lzd-Cfx-Cs-E-Z" regimen was continued.

Discussion

This case was a middle-aged woman diagnosed with "pulmonary infection" on many occasions in the local primary hospital due to cough and intermittent fever for 6 months and was given anti-infection treatment for many times, including levofloxacin, which is a broad-spectrum antibiotic, is not only effective against bacterial pneumonia, but also one of the important drugs in anti-tuberculosis treatment. The previous misdiagnosis of pneumonia, however, made her exposed repeatedly to anti-infection treatment using levofloxacin alone. The combined medication is the focus in treating tuberculosis, and any anti-tuberculosis drug used alone will inevitably increase the risk of drug resistance. With the protracted course, she did not visit the local county hospital, until the disease aggravated after 6 months. Pulmonary tuberculosis was considered based on chest CT scans, with positiveness (2+) in acid-fast stains of sputum smear. Results of DST suggested the presence of Mycobacterium tuberculosis with R resistance. Due to the positiveness in sputum tuberculosis bacteria, she began to receive anti-tuberculosis treatment with combined drugs in the blister pack (HREZ) at the local Tuberculosis Prevention and Control Institute. The severe gastrointestinal reaction

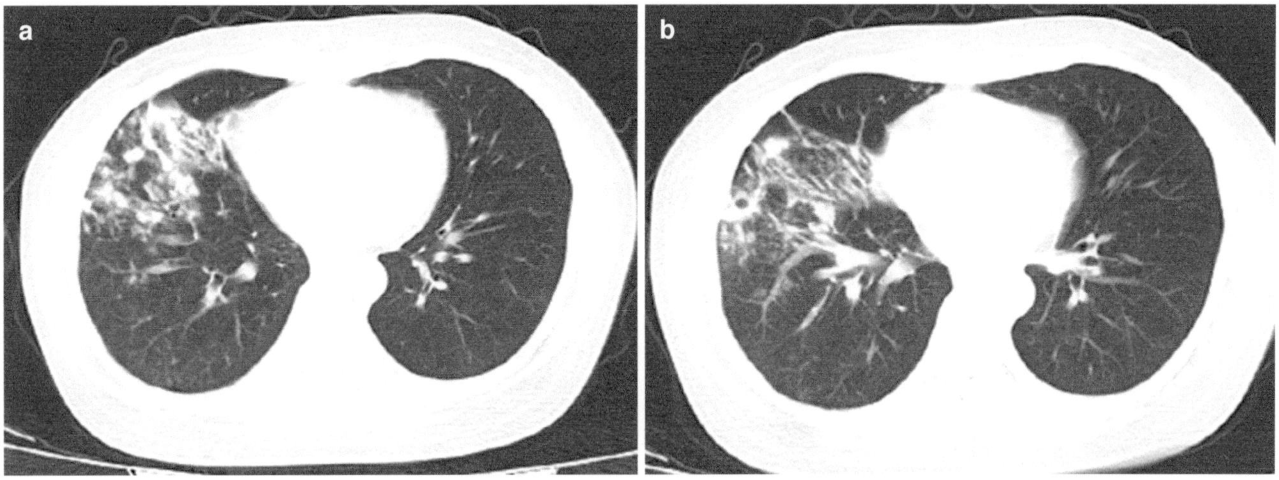

Fig. 6.1 (**a**, **b**) Chest CT scans on August 31, 2020, showed acinar nodular opacities, small patchy and segmental consolidations in the middle and lower lobes of the right lung, with bronchiectasis and thickening bronchial wall observed in the right middle lobe

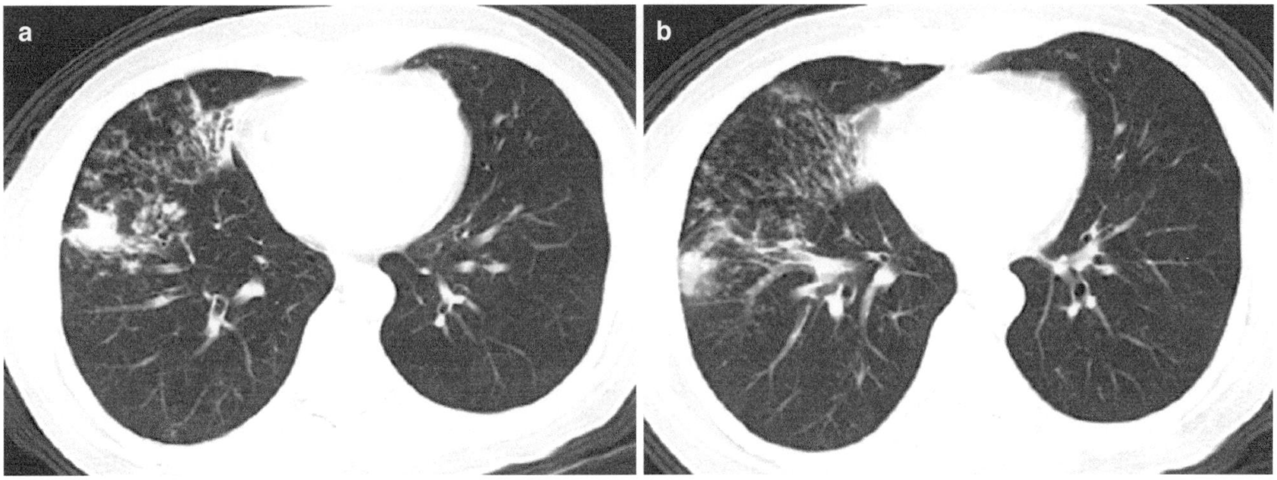

Fig. 6.2 (**a**, **b**) Chest CT scans on December 29, 2020, show partial absorption of the lesion in the middle lobe of the right lung, and amelioration of consolidation and bronchiectasis showing dominantly tree-in-bud sign and centrilobular nodules, fusion of lesions in anterior basal segment manifesting patchy consolidations, and absence of the small cavity, as compared with CT scans on August 31, 2020

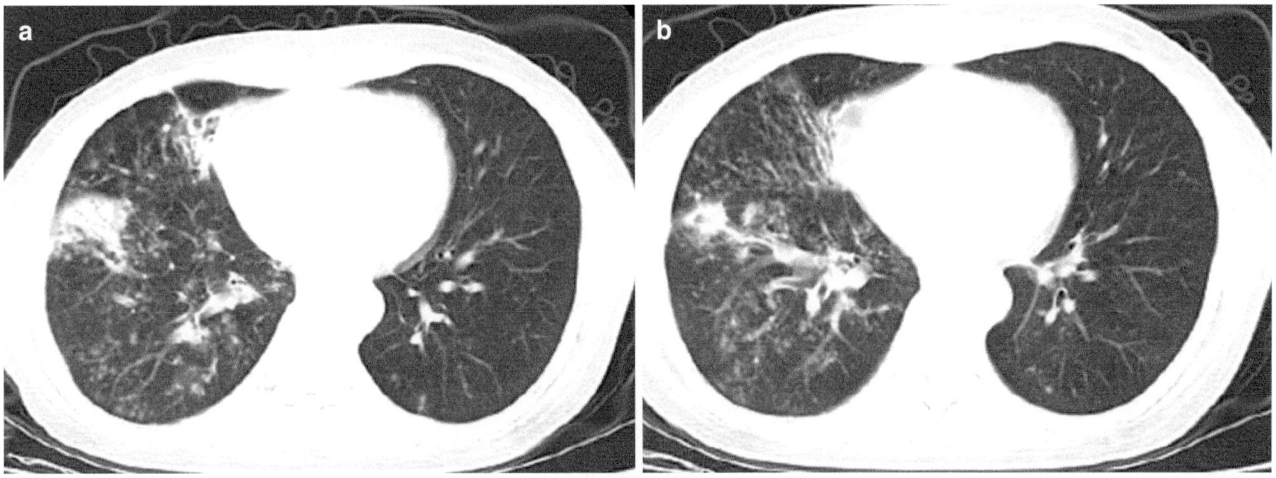

Fig. 6.3 (**a**, **b**) Chest CT scans on March 30, 2021, show the increase in the consolidation in the right lower lobe and re-emergence of a small cavity inside the consolidation, as compared with findings in chest CT scans on December 29, 2020. New emergence of bronchial disseminating lesions is observed in basal segments in both lower lobes, with slight decrease in number of bronchial disseminating lesions in the lateral segment of right middle lobe

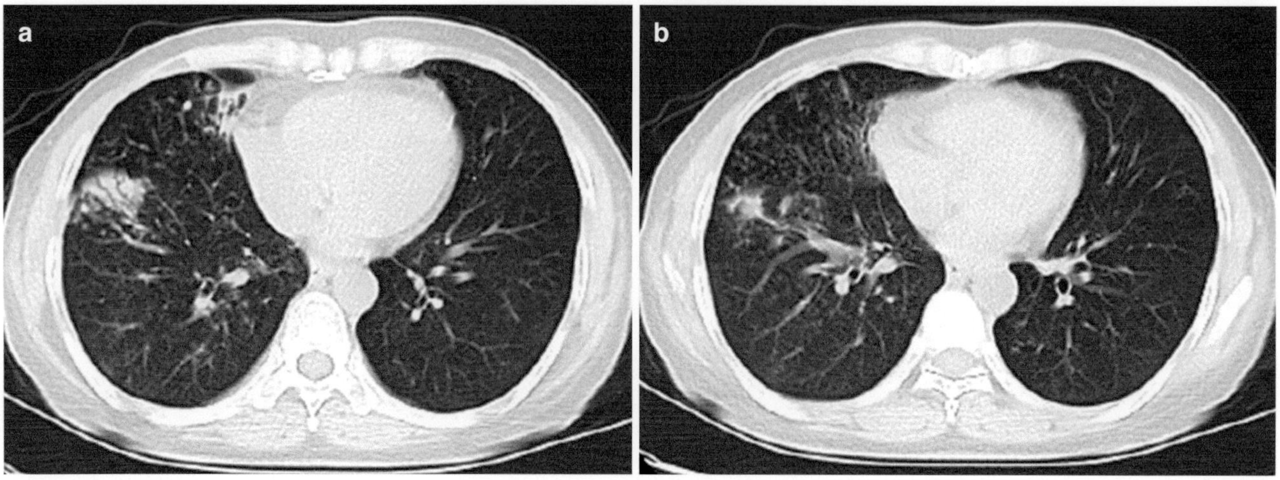

Fig. 6.4 (**a**, **b**) Chest CT scans on May 6, 2021, show the obvious absorption of bronchial disseminating lesions in the right middle and lower lobes, and the decrease in scope of consolidation, with closure of the small cavity inside, as compared with CT scans on March 30, 2021

post to medication, however, lowered her compliance and increased again the risk of drug resistance. Chest CT scans on August 31, 2020, revealed lesions differing in attributes, including multiple patches, nodules, cavity and bronchiectasis, in right middle and lower lobes, which were dominantly hyperplasia and consolidation, implying the disease had evolved for a certain period with a conversion from exudation to hyperplasia and degenerescence. Based on CT findings, however, the lesion involved two adjacent lobes. Though a cavity appeared, it was small size without multifocality, which was not a typical manifestation of CT findings for MDR-TB concerning both the scope of lesions and the appearance of the cavity.

Resistance to H was revealed by DST on September 30, 2020, and an anti-tuberculosis treatment was given using H-R-E-Clr in routine dosage. We had reason to believe that this patient had a great chance of MDR-TB, due to the persistent positiveness post to the anti-tuberculosis treatment for more than 5 months as confirmed by positiveness in the rapid culture of sputum tuberculosis on December 29, 2020, considering her previous rifampin resistance together with the ratio of 78% of MDR-TB in RR-TB patients, her non-standardized medication, and the re-examination of chest CT showing some lesions absorbed and some enlarged and fused. The "Lfx-Lzd-Cfx-Cs-E-Z" regimen, therefore, was planned for her anti-tuberculosis treatment, though it was denied by her on the ground of the partial absorption of pulmonary lesions and financial reasons, and finally substituted for "H-R-E-Z-Lfx." This regimen, though obviously unreasonable for treating MDR-TB, was continued until March 30, 2021, when the latest DST confirmed the multidrug resistance to H, R, Sm, RFT, Pa, and Mfx in the tuberculosis of this patient. Then the re-examination of chest CT scans (Fig. 6.3) showed the reappearance of the small cavity in the right lower lobe, new emergence of bronchial disseminating lesions in the basal segments of both lower lobes, and absorption of only a small amount of lesions in the right middle lobe. Considering comprehensively previous CT scans showing lesions waxing and waning with obvious increase in number observed at the last examination without complete absorption, which implied the poor response, the regimen was changed at last and "Lfx-Lzd-Cfx-Cs-E-Z" regimen was used for anti-tuberculosis treatment. Roche DST on May 21, 2021, showed that the strain was resistant to H, R, Sm, RFT, and Mfx, almost identical to results 2 months before. Re-examination of chest CT scans showed the obvious absorption of bronchial disseminating lesions in right middle and lower lobes, the consolidation shrunk, and closure of the small cavity in the consolidation, which implied the treatment was effective, so the regimen was continued.

It could be inferred from the history of her visits and medication that the initial "anti-tuberculosis treatment" for 5 months followed by the blister pack for "combined" treatment caused the development from R resistance gradually to H resistance and then to multidrug resistance, implying this case was most likely a relapsing MDR-TB induced by improper medication. CT findings in this case, however, manifested acinar nodular shadows, small patches, bronchiectasia, and smaller number of cavity, which were not typical features of CT findings in MDR-TB. It can be inferred, therefore, that it is hard to determine accurately MDR-TB based on chest CT findings alone, and early DST is necessitated especially by treatment-naive MDR-TB patients. A regimen for anti-tuberculosis treatment should be formulated reasonably and actively based on the results of the DST, which is an important approach to control the development of MDR-TB and block its disseminating. MDR-TB induced by improper medication should be avoided clinically as far as possible.

Case 2

The patient, a female aged 43 years, complained repeated cough and gasp for 5 years with the recurrence 10 days before. She had cough and expectoration with a small amount of white sticky sputum without obvious inducement 5 years before (in January 2016), with chest pain characterized in a pain referred to the left chest and an exacerbation when she coughed and inhaled. She was diagnosed with pulmonary tuberculosis at the Tuberculosis Prevention and Control Institute and received an anti-tuberculosis treatment using "combined reagents (HREZ)" for 3 months. She manifested shortness of breath with fever in April 2016 and was admitted on April 5, 2016. Direct sputum smear microscopy (DSSM) for acid-fast bacilli (AFB) showed a positive result, and drug-resistant gene for tuberculosis detected in sputum showed Mycobacterium tuberculosis with the DST suggesting resistance to H, R, and Sm. An anti-tuberculosis regimen containing "Pa-Z-Pto-Am-Lfx-PAS" was given and she was discharged after her disease ameliorated. Then this regimen was continued. In December 2016 the anti-tuberculosis regimen of "Pa-Z-Pto-Lfx" was launched, which was discontinued in June 2017. She complained about the recurrent cough and chest pain (dominantly the right chest pain) in November 2017, which was considered to be recurrent pulmonary tuberculosis by the local hospital. Roche DST in March 2018 showed Mycobacterium tuberculosis resistant to H, R, Sm, and Rft. She underwent an anti-tuberculosis treatment containing "Lfx-Cm-Pto-Cs-Z-Pa" in routine dosage, but discontinued Capreomycin by herself 2 months later. She withdrew all anti-tuberculosis medications voluntarily in May 2019. After that, she received repeated anti-infection treatment locally due to cough and expectoration. She was admitted for the fourth time in July 2019 due to cough, expectoration, fever, and shortness of breath, with positiveness (4+) in DSSM for AFB and DST showing Mycobacterium tuberculosis resistant to H, R, Sm, and Rft. An anti-tuberculosis treatment containing "Mfx-Cm-Cs-Lzd-Cfz-PAS" was given, together with anti-infection and liver protection, and after that her symptoms including cough and expectoration ameliorated obviously. Rapid DST of sputum tuberculosis on August 10, 2019, showed Mycobacterium tuberculosis resistant to H, R, Sm, E, and Rft, and a treatment containing "Mfx-Cm-Lzd-Cfz-PAS-Z" was given. On May 20, 2020, the same result was shown in the same test, and again, she received the same treatment. Her cough and expectoration exacerbated significantly on February 15, 2021, when her fluorescent staining of sputum tuberculosis was positive (4+) with positiveness (3+) in detection of acid-fast bacilli by Sandwich Cup Collecting Bacteria and Smear Method. Rapid DST of sputum tuberculosis showed Mycobacterium tuberculosis resistant to H, R, Sm, Rft, Rft, PAS, and Pa and the treatment containing "Mfx-Cm-Lzd-Cfz-PAS-Z" was started and continued up to August 2021. The patient underwent multiple chest CT scans during the course of the disease, which showed that both lung injuries and number of cavities progressed with prolonged duration of the illness, with more significant clustering of cavities (Figs. 6.5, 6.6, 6.7, 6.8, 6.9, 6.10, 6.11, 6.12 and 6.13).

Discussion

The patient was diagnosed with pulmonary tuberculosis at the onset of disease 5 years before and given with anti-tuberculosis treatment. Despite 3-month anti-tuberculosis treatment with "combined reagents (HREZ)" initiated by Tuberculosis Prevention and Control Institute, a diagnosis of MDR-TB was established, as confirmed by DST performed vigorously. An active standardized treatment was launched with proper anti-tuberculosis medication optioned based on results of DST and discontinued post to the completion of cycles. She suffered again from cough and chest pain 5 months post to the discontinuation, which was considered as recurrent pulmonary tuberculosis by the hospital, and she received an anti-tuberculosis treatment containing "Lfx-Cm-Pto-Cs-Z-Pa." However, she discontinued the medication or

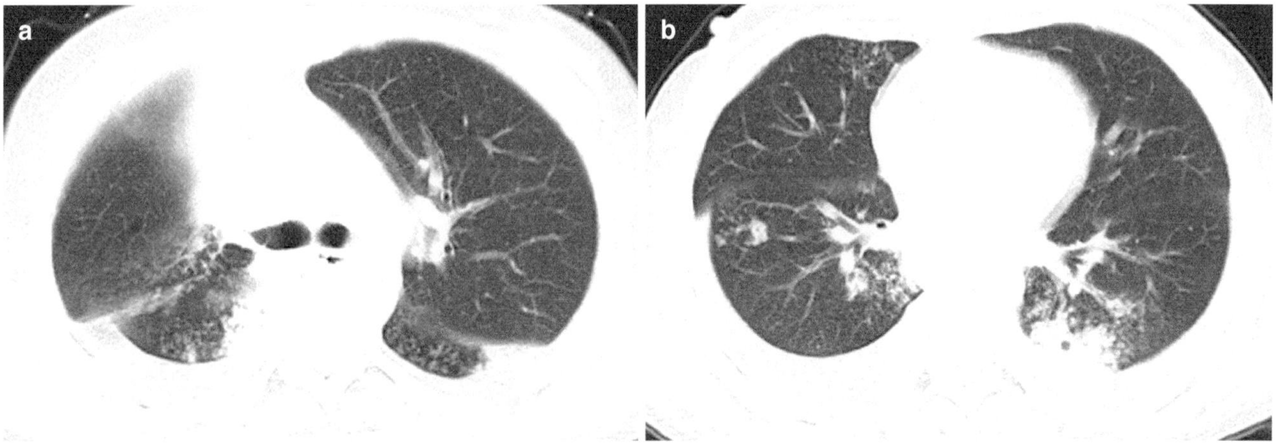

Fig. 6.5 (**a**, **b**) Chest CT scans on April 13, 2016, shows centrilobular nodules and tree-in-bud sign in the posterior segment of the upper lobe of the right lung, the right middle lobe, and both lower lobes, with small size cavities in consolidations in both lower lobes and a small amount of bilateral pleural effusion

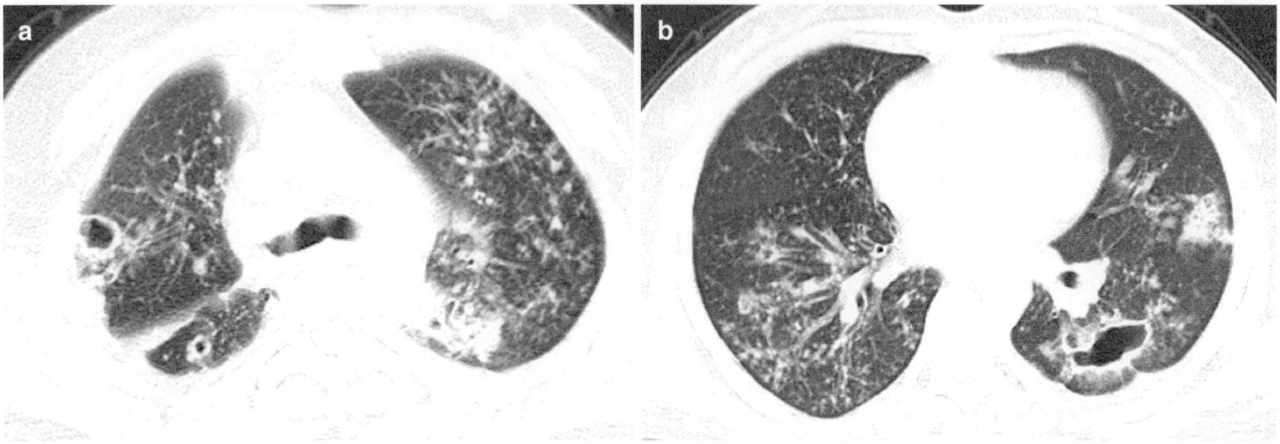

Fig. 6.6 (**a**, **b**) Chest CT scans on January 18, 2018, show the increase in lesions in both lungs, thickening of bronchial wall and tram-track sign, with emergence of new cavities in the right upper and lower lobes, enlargement of the cavity in the left lower lobe, and the decrease in both pleural effusion

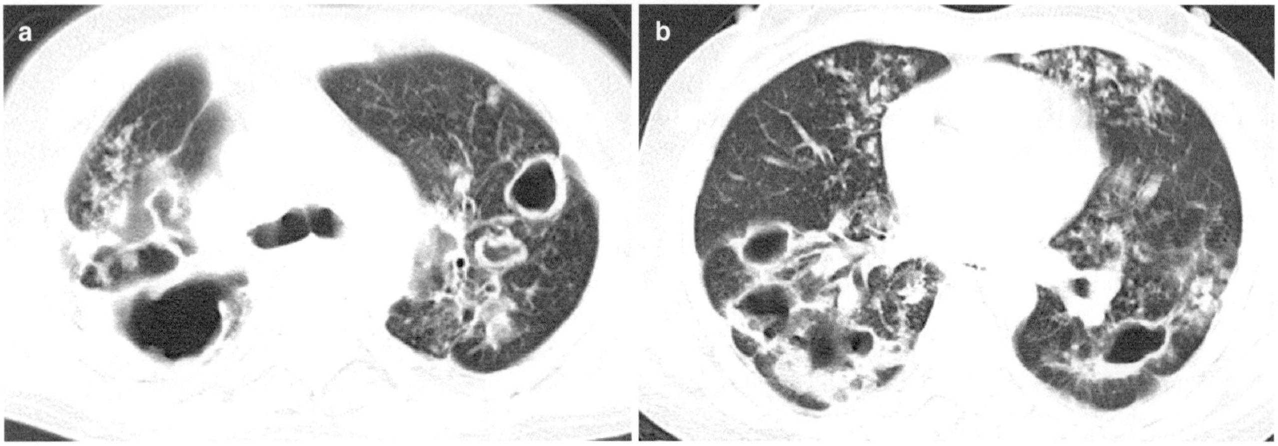

Fig. 6.7 (**a**, **b**) Chest CT scans on September 3, 2019, show the increase in lesions in the right middle lobe and the left lingual segment, compared with CT findings on January 18, 2018. There is an increase for cavities in the left upper lobe, and for those with fusion in the posterior segment in the right upper lobe and the right lower lobes. Absorption with amelioration is observed for some of lesions in the left upper lobe

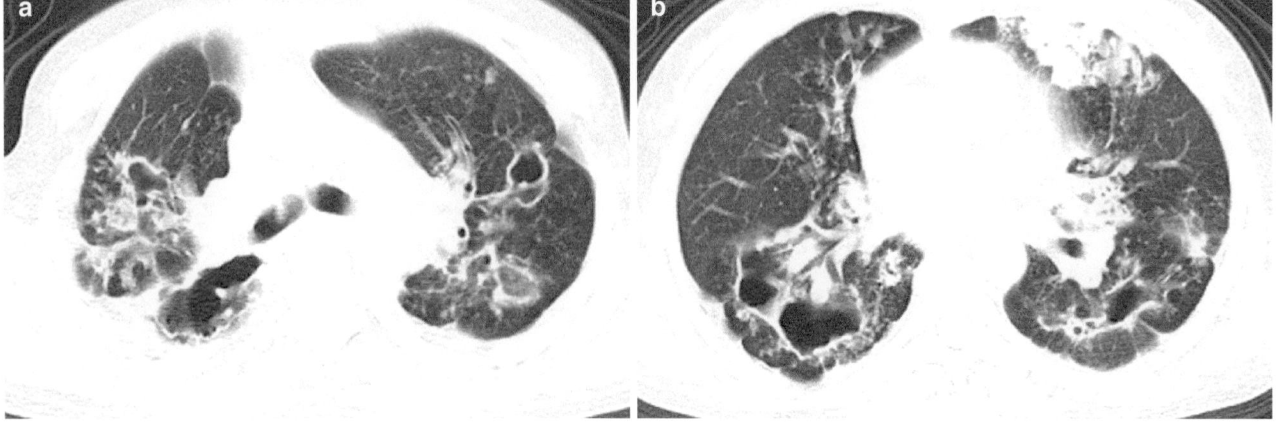

Fig. 6.8 (**a**, **b**) Chest CT scans on December 9, 2019, show a slight shrinkage for cavities in both lungs with thinning of cavities wall, absorption and decrease in some of lesions, and significant fusion and consolidation in the left upper lobe, as compared with July 3, 2019

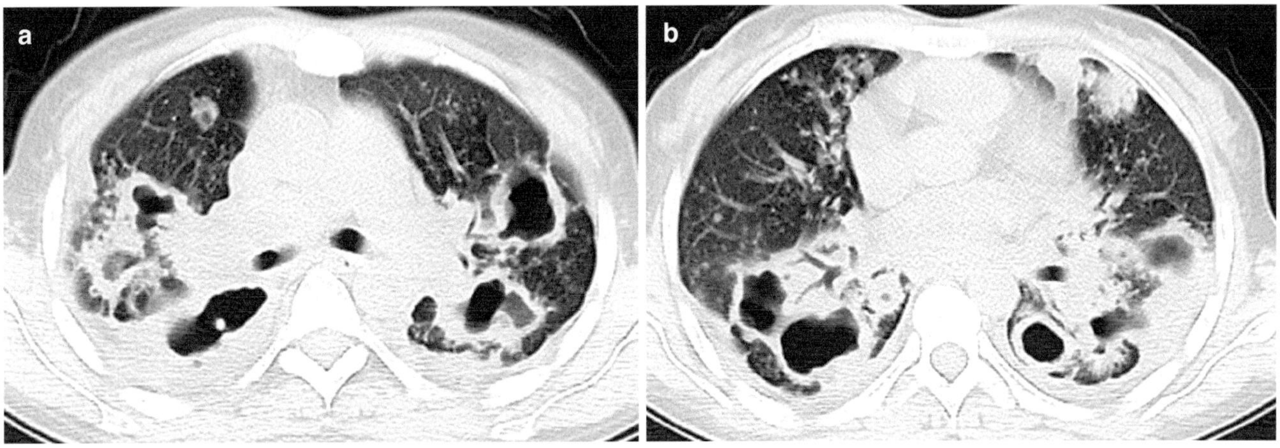

Fig. 6.9 (**a**, **b**) Chest CT scans on May 9, 2020, show enlargement of cavities in both lungs, with significant thickening cavities wall and in bilateral pleura, as compared with chest CT scans on December 9, 2019. New bronchial disseminating lesions and consolidations are observed in the right upper and middle lobes and both lower lobes

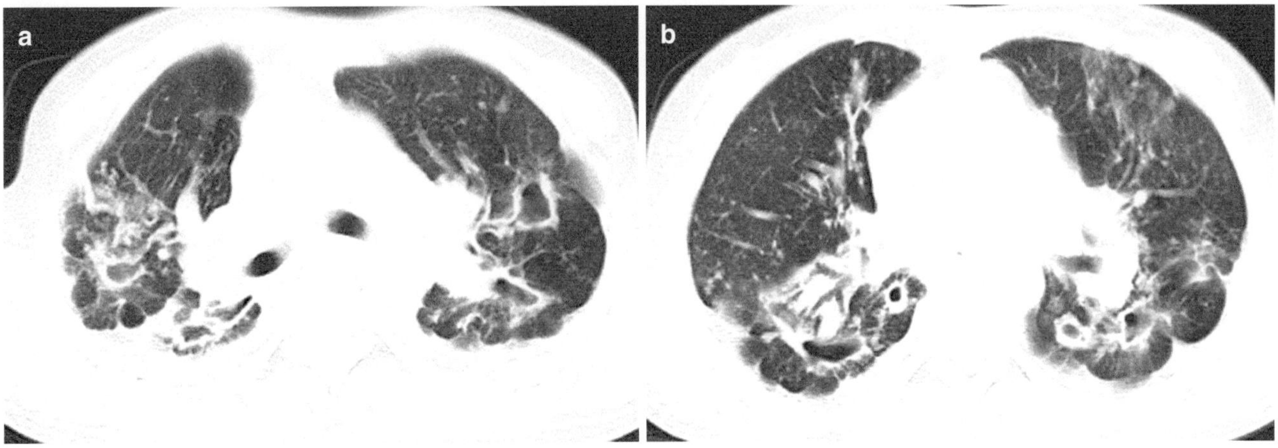

Fig. 6.10 (**a**, **b**) Chest CT scans on September 7, 2020, show the absorption and decrease in lesions in both lungs, and the shrinkage of cavities in both lungs with the thinning of their wall, as compared with chest CT scans on May 9, 2020

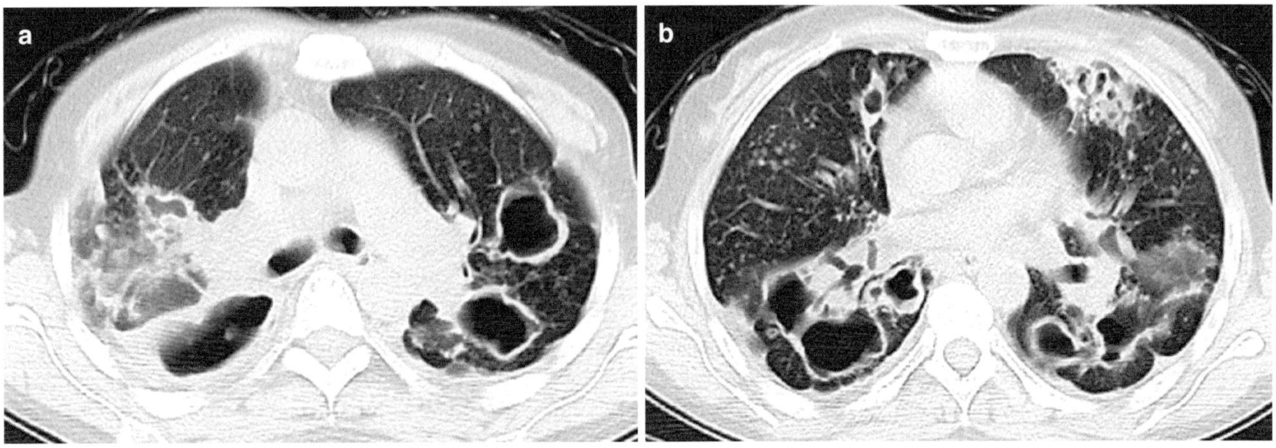

Fig. 6.11 (**a**, **b**) Chest CT scans on January 23, 2021, cavities wall thickening in both lungs, as compared with chest CT scans on September seventh 2020. In addition, the increase is observed for cavities in the lingual segment of left lung, and bronchial disseminating lesions in both upper lobes

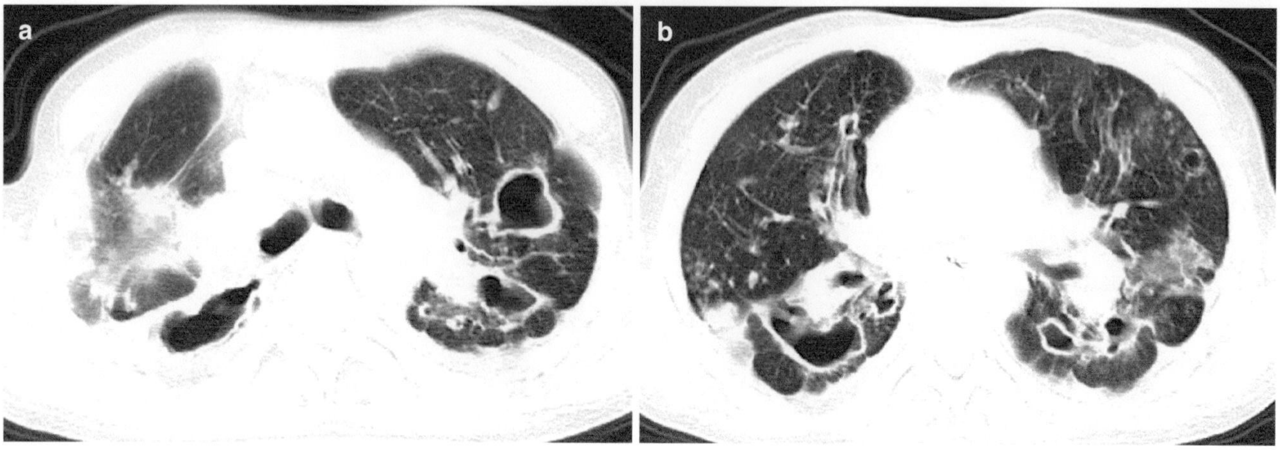

Fig. 6.12 (**a**, **b**) Chest CT scans on March 9, 2021, show the decreased size of cavities in both lungs, with wall thinned in some of them, and decrease in intra-pulmonary bronchial disseminating lesions, as compared with chest CT scans on January 23, 2021

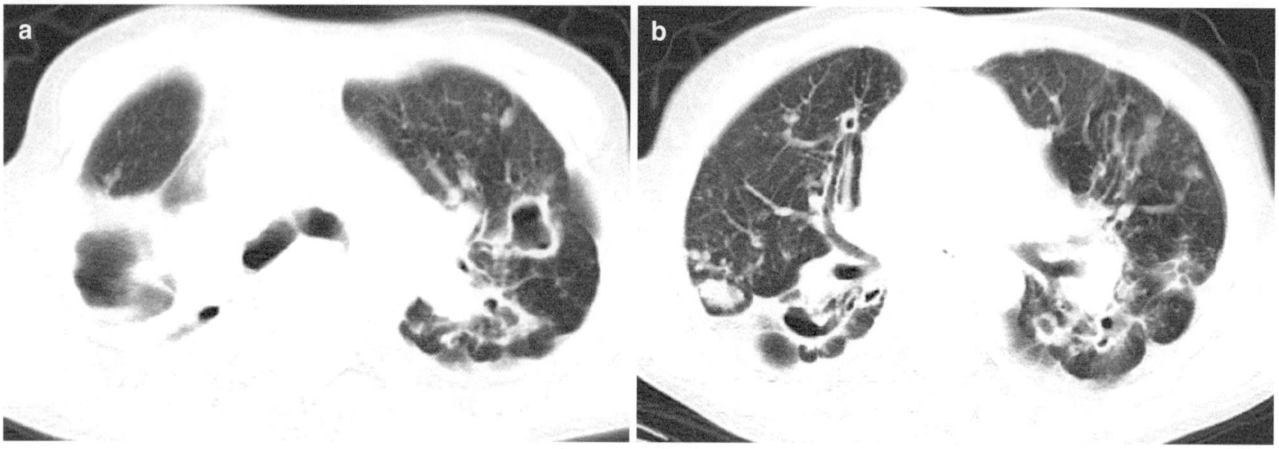

Fig. 6.13 (**a**, **b**) Chest CT scans on June 8, 2021, show shrinkage of cavities in both lungs with absorption and amelioration of intra-pulmonary lesions, as compared with chest CT scans on March 9, 2021

took the medication irregularly later during the treatment and was admitted repeatedly due to cough, expectoration, fever, and short of breath. Persistent positiveness was shown by sputum smear and sputum culture, with all DSTs suggesting MDR-TB, which developed from the initial resistance to "H, R, Sm" to the resistance to "H, R, Sm, E, and Rft" or "H, R, Sm, and Rf" confirmed by multiple DSTs during 2 years, and finally to the resistance to "H, R, Sm, Rft, PAS, and Pa." Early findings in CT scans included centrilobular nodules and tree-in-bud sign in both lungs and consolidations in both lower lobes with minor cavities inside. CT findings post to treatment manifested gradual increase in intra-pulmonary lesions, especially the gradual increase in number and size of cavities with thickening of their walls. Despite the amelioration of disease during the treatment with shrinkage of the cavities, their closure seemed hard at last. Symptoms of the patient had no complete amelioration, though the anti-tuberculosis treatment was modified for several times based on DSTs and chest CT findings. The 5-year intermittent anti-tuberculosis treatment imposed a great burden on the patient both physically and psychologically, with her compliance dropping significantly, and factors such as her voluntary withdrawal of medication predisposed to her poor response and increased risk of resistance. However, this also implied the inconsistency between result of DST in vitro and actual response, i.e., factors such as poor compliance might cause poor or even no response to the drug, even if the strains were supposed to be susceptible as shown by the test in vitro.

Besides voluntary withdrawal of medication by the patient, common reasons for poor responses in MDR-TB patients to medication include also multiple cavities and thick-walled cavities. The small amounts of consolidations in both lungs and the small cavity in the left lower lobe, as shown by CT scans in this patient, progressed into multiple cavities in both lungs in July 2019, which manifested dominantly an aggregation in clusters with the gradual increase in size. The size of cavities varied frequently post to the treatment with repeated thickening or thinning of their walls, implying the high tuberculosis burden and insufficient potential of anti-tuberculosis drugs in eradicating tubercle bacillus inside cavities predisposed pulmonary tissues to repeated destruction by tuberculosis [6]. The formation of cavities is related to immune reaction in the host to Mycobacterium tuberculosis [7]. Cavities are also an inducement of MDR-TB, due to poor blood supply around the cavities, the concentration of anti tuberculosis drugs entering the cavities is low, which cannot effectively kill the MTB inside the cavity, low concentrations of anti tuberculosis drugs stimulate the MTB in the cavities by prolonged, increasing the risk of developing drug resistance [8, 9], therefore, pulmonary tuberculosis patients with cavities are more prone to development of drug resistance. Meanwhile, cavities are also the result of the development of drug-resistant tuberculosis. The development into multiple cavities in this patient took a long time, nearly 2 years. Due to prolonged positiveness in sputum strains in the patient exposed to the prolonged treatment, the probability is greater for cavities and lung injuries post to destruction of pulmonary tissues. It has been revealed by researches [10] that severe hypoxia existing in pulmonary consolidations and peripheries of cavities correlates positively to lung injuries and cavitation [11, 12]. There is a reciprocal causation, therefore, between pulmonary consolidation and cavities promoting each other in MDR-TB patients responding poorly to medication. In this patient who responded poorly to medication, both lung injuries and number of cavities progressed with prolonged duration of the illness, with more significant clustering of cavities. The great deal of tubercle bacillus in cavities in MDR-TB patients caused easily their intra-pulmonary dissemination, which was one of the reasons for poor responses in MDR-TB patients.

Case 3

The patient, a female aged 28 years, visited the hospital on June 17, 2018, with a chief complaint of cough with expectoration of a great deal of yellow sputum, complicated with fever, chest tightness, night sweat, and body weight loss of 2–3 kg for 2 weeks. Chest X-ray examination in primary chronic disease control institution showed spotty and patchy shadows with uneven density and unclear border in the left upper lobe, which suggested "infection in the left lung, with possibility not excludable for pulmonary tuberculosis" (Fig. 6.14).

Laboratory test on June 19, 2018, showed positiveness in IgG antibody against Mycobacterium tuberculosis. PPD (June 20, 2018) showed a size of 15 mm × 16 mm.

Positiveness (+) for Mycobacterium tuberculosis was reported on June 30, 2018, for the specimen submitted on June 20, 2018.

Regimen FDC-2HRZE/4HR was launched on June 20, 2018, which persisted for nearly 2 months until August 15, 2018, when the patient reported remission of her symptoms to some extent.

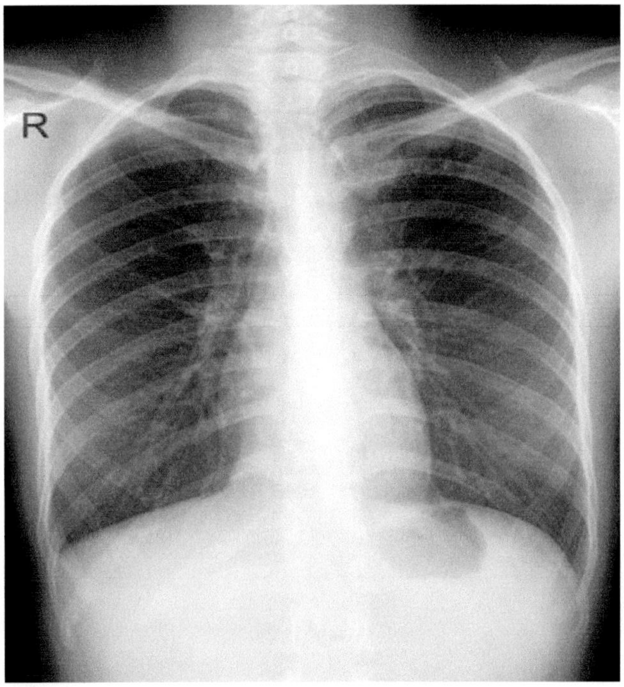

Fig. 6.14 Chest X-ray on June 17, 2018. A high-density patchy opacity is observed at the overlap between the left apex and the first anterior rib, with small patchy high-density opacities seen in outer zone of the second to the third anterior intercostal space in the left upper lung field. The right costophrenic angle seems blunt

Mutation of inhA gene and rpoB gene was detected of Mycobacterium tuberculosis on August 16, 2018.

Resistance to H, R, Km, Am, S, and Rb was reported on October 10, 2018, by susceptibility test on a specimen sampled on August 19, 2018. A regimen "R-E-Z-Am-Ofx-Pto" against the MDR-TB was launched on August 20, 2018. Chest CT scans on August 29, 2018, showed multiple patchy, spotted, and nodule in posterior apical segment of left upper lung, with spotty opacities in the right middle lobe and localized thickening of posteromedial pleura in the right lower lobe (Fig. 6.15).

Re-examination of chest CT on November 20, 2018, post to 5.5-month anti-tuberculosis treatment comprising the 3-month treatment against MDR-TB showed absorption with amelioration of lesions in both lungs (Fig. 6.16).

The regimen was modified into "E-Z-Pto" for the anti-tuberculosis treatment due to abnormal hepatic function on January 24, 2019, with compound glycyrrhizin tablets and ornithine aspartate granules for liver protection. This regimen was continued until May 26, 2019, when re-examination of CT scans revealed an obvious absorption with amelioration of lesions in both the left upper lobe and the local thickening of the right posterior pleura (Fig. 6.17).

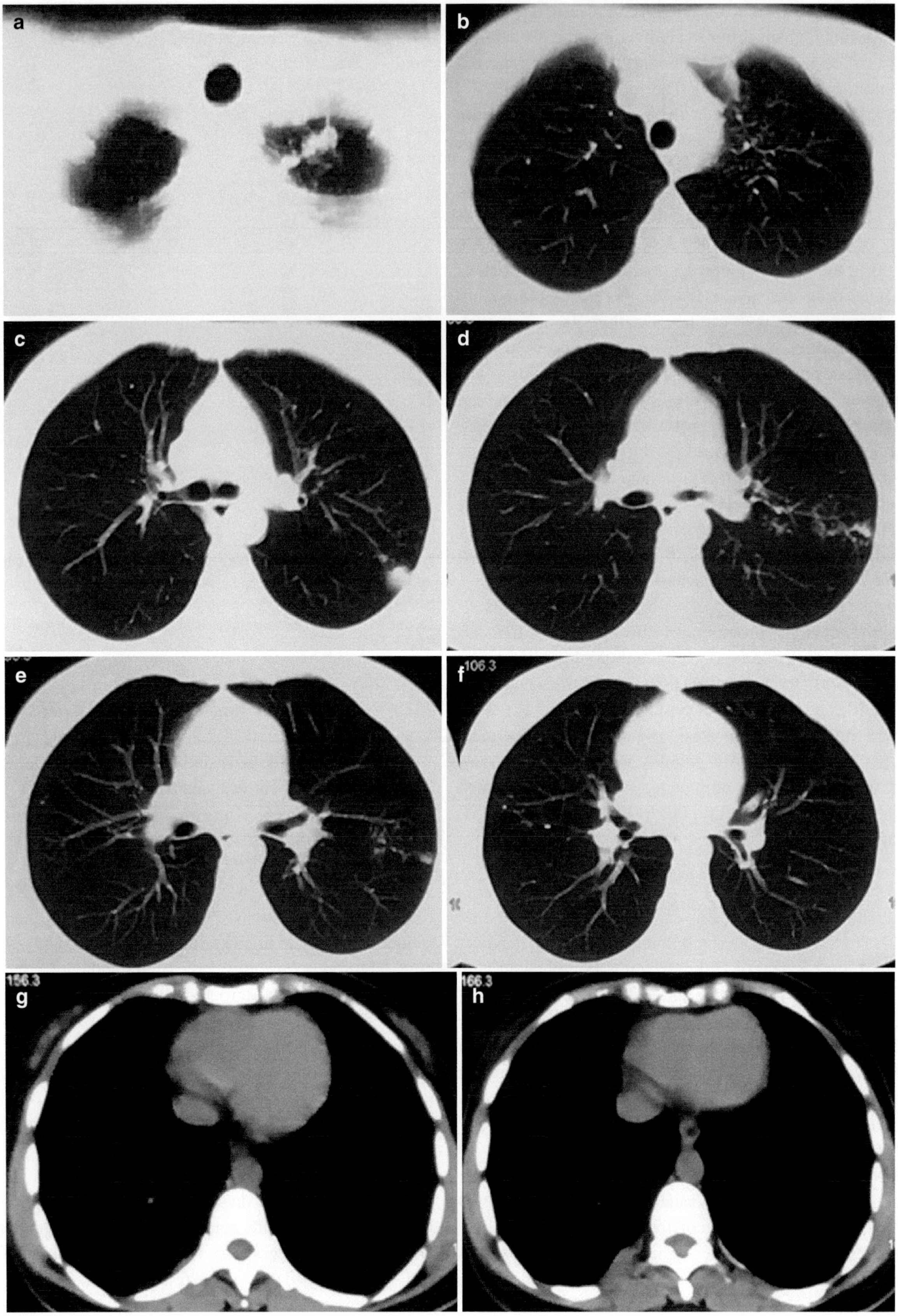

Fig. 6.15 (**a**–**h**) Chest CT scans on August 29, 2018. (**a**–**e**) (lung window) shows multiple irregular patchy, spotted, and nodule in the apex and posterior segment of the left lung. (**f**) (lung window) shows a small amount of spotty high-density opacities in the right middle lobe. (**g**, **h**) (mediastinum window) shows a localized thickening of posteromedial pleura in the right lower lobe

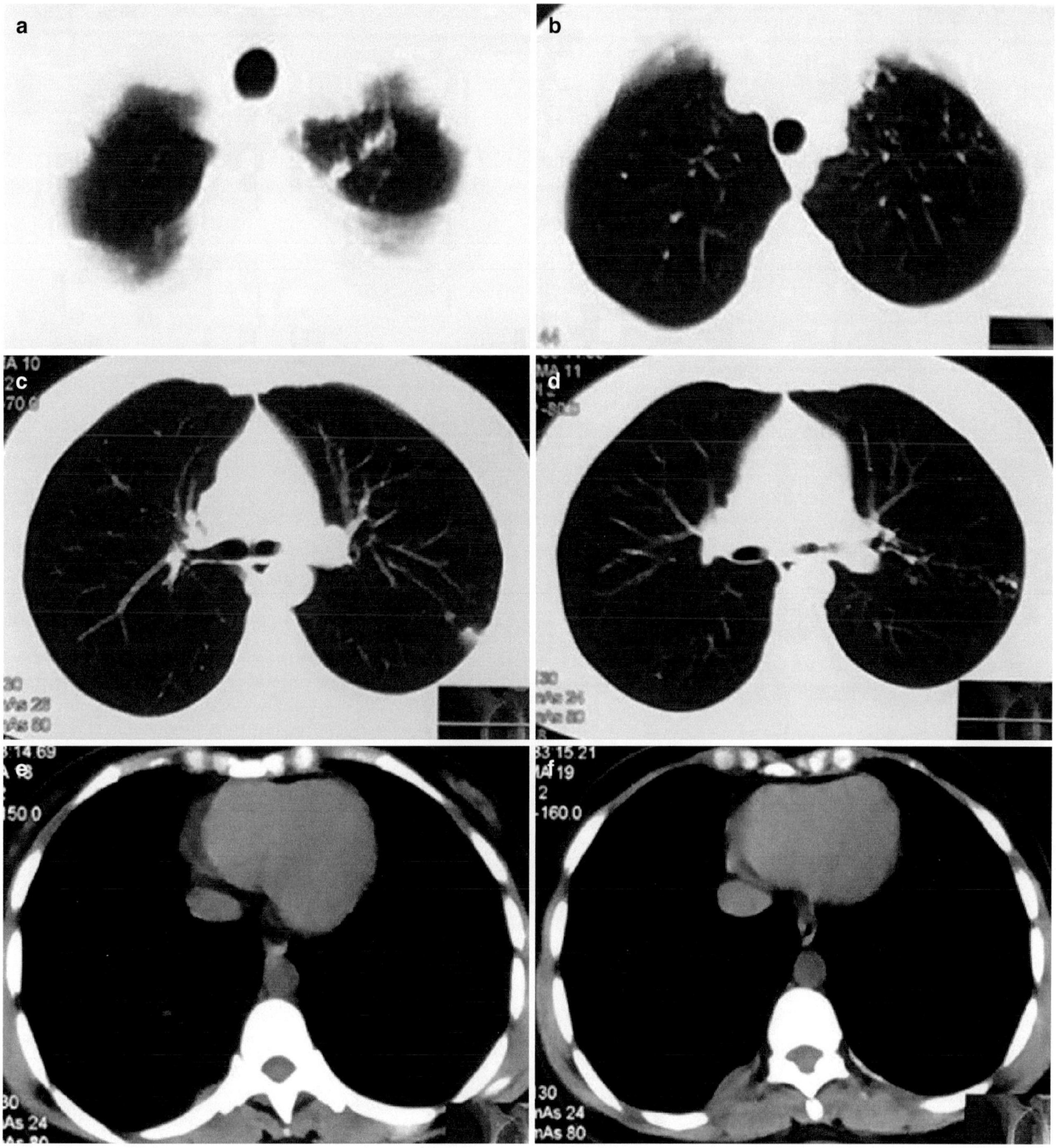

Fig. 6.16 (**a**–**f**) Chest CT scans on November 20, 2018. (**a**–**d**) (lung window) shows spotty, patchy, and small nodule high-density opacities in the left upper lobe, manifesting absorption and amelioration compared with CT findings on August 29, 2018. (**e**, **f**) (mediastinum window) shows no significant change about pleura thickening in the right lower lobe compared with its previous imaging

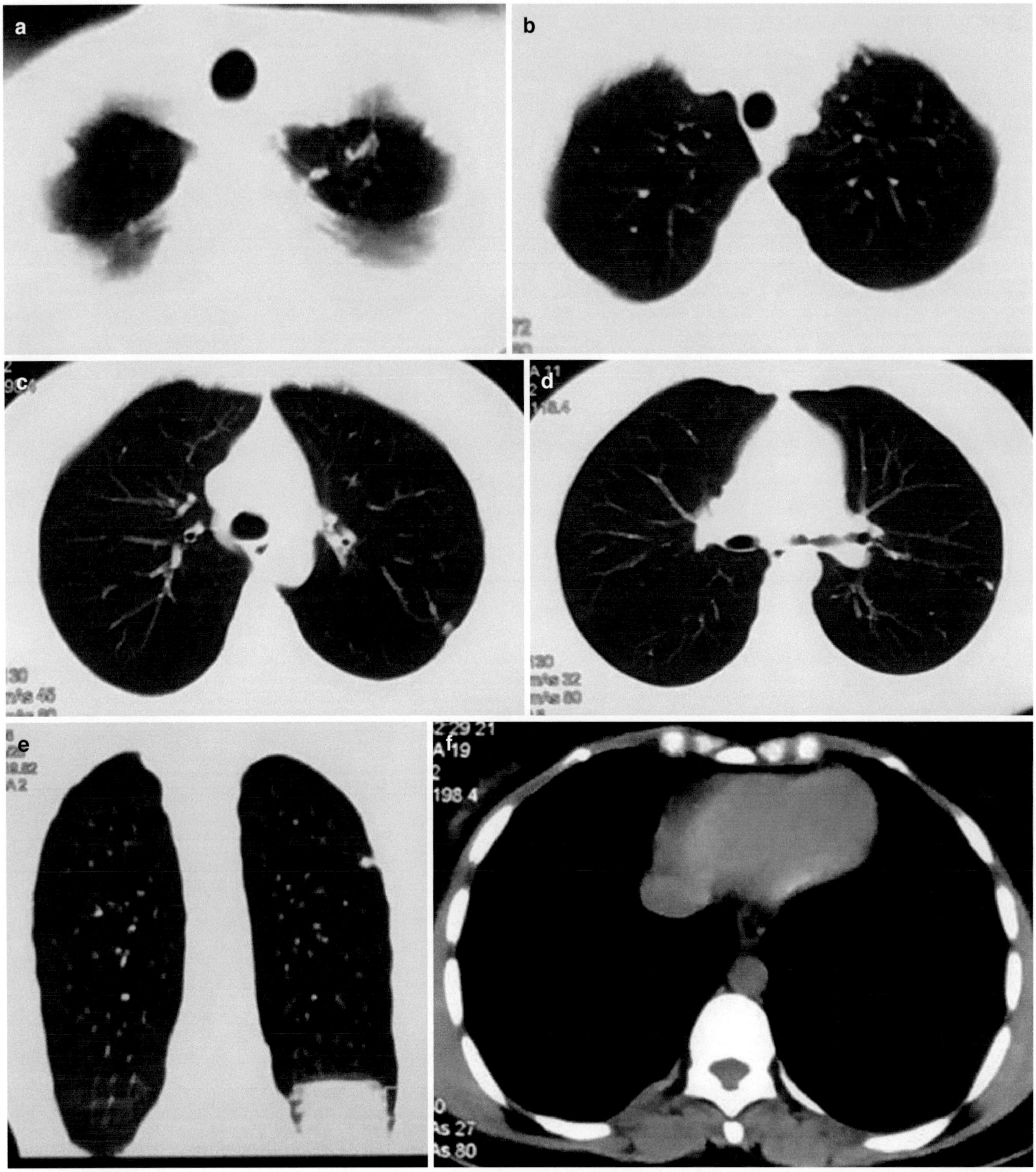

Fig. 6.17 (**a**–**f**) Re-examination of chest CT scans on May 26, 2019. (**a**–**e**) (lung window) shows a small nodule with clear boundary in the left upper lobe. (**f**) CT scans in mediastinal window show a slight thickening of posteromedial pleura in the right lower lobe. Compared with chest CT scans on November 20, 2018, both the lesion in the upper left lobe and the local hypertrophy in the right pleura show absorption and amelioration

Discussion

This case could be categorized into the rMDR-TB, based on the latest classification criteria for drug-resistant pulmonary tuberculosis [2, 13]. This patient was a young female with typical clinical symptoms of tuberculosis, characterized by significant cough, expectoration, fever, night sweat, and body weight loss of 2–3 kg. Chest X-ray examination at the primary hospital which she visited showed a small patchy high-density opacity in the left upper lobe, findings not so severe without obvious caseous pneumonia or cavity, seeming not so consistent with her clinical symptoms or signs. Pulmonary tuberculosis, however, was highly suspected by the clinician, based on clinical symptoms, signs and findings in chest X-ray. She underwent instantly PPD test, test on IgG antibody against Mycobacterium tuberculosis and sputum smear, showing the results of 15 mm × 16 mm for PPD. Positiveness in both IgG antibody against Mycobacterium tuberculosis, and positiveness (+) in Mycobacterium tuberculosis in sputum smear 2 weeks later, and she was diagnosed as active pulmonary tuberculosis.

Mutation was detected for inhA gene and rpoB gene of Mycobacterium tuberculosis post to 2-month standardized anti-tuberculosis treatment. A modification for the former therapeutic regimen was made, so as to perform a well-directed effective treatment. Three re-examinations of chest CT scans were done during 10 months post to anti-MDR-TB treatment, with image findings showing a gradual absorption and amelioration of pulmonary lesions.

Pulmonary lesions seem severer in a larger number with significantly higher incidence of tuberculosis cavitation, as observed by researchers, in drug-resistant tuberculosis, especially those with MDR-TB, than in DS-TB [5]. However, the number of pulmonary lesions and the severity are not correlated necessarily to the presence of MDR-TB, as observed in this case. Despite minor manifestations of pulmonary lesions, lower severity in pulmonary exudative lesions and absence of cavity, as high as 6 drug-resistant tuberculosis strains were identified, approximating an extensive resistance. Despite this patient seemed to be an rMDR-TB considering timepoints during the treatment, there are reasons to believe that her original disease was MDR-TB but not that a genetic mutation of Mycobacterium tuberculosis, which seemed improbable to be induced during 2-month anti-tuberculosis treatment, resulted in a simultaneous resistance to six anti-tuberculosis drugs, based on pulmonary lesions not so extensive and the resistance to 6 drugs detected within so short period. The patient responded satisfactorily to the treatment, due to timely scientific modification of regimen against DR-TB based on guidance by DST and mutation detection. Another characteristic of this case, in addition to irregular patchy and dotty lesions in the upper left lobe, was the localized hypertrophic protrusion in posteromedial pleura in the right lower lobe, with a length about 6.0 cm and a protrusion of about 1.2 cm into pleural cavity, but without effusion. A significant absorption noticed for pleural thickening post to 10-month anti-tuberculosis treatment indicated that MDR-TB might manifest localized pleural thickening persisting for a prolonged duration, but the lesion may be absorbed after positive treatment.

References

1. WHO. Global Tuberculosis Report 2020 [DB/OL]. https://www.who.int/teams/global-tuberculosis-programme/tb-reports.
2. Yu W, Tan W-g, Lu P-x. Classification and imaging manifestations of drug-resistant pulmonary tuberculosis [J/CD]. Electr J Emerg Infect Dis. 2019;4(1):42–7.
3. World Health Organization. Global tuberculosis report 2021 [EB/OL]. [2021-10-14]. https://www.who.int/publications/digital/global-tuberculosis-report-2021.
4. Li C, Lu S, Wang H, et al. CT scan findings of multi-drug resistant pulmonary tuberculosis patients and its correlation to CD4 cells [J]. Chin J Antituberc. 2017;39(6):597–603.
5. Chuchottaworn C, Thanachartwet V, Sangsayunh P, et al. Risk factors for multidrug-resistant tuberculosis among patients with pulmonary tuberculosis at the central chest Institute of Thailand [J]. PLoS One. 2015;10(10):e0139986.
6. Wang Y-x, Chung MJ, Skrahin A, et al. Literature analysis of radiological signs related to multidrug-resistant tuberculosis [J/CD]. Electr J Emerg Infect Dis. 2018;3(2):244–53.
7. Yang J, Lu S, Tang G, et al. An analysis of CT scan findings of treatment-naive and relapsing multidrug resistant pulmonary tuberculosis [J]. Chin J Antituberc. 2020;42(1):38–43.
8. Ong CW, Elkington PT, Friedland JS. Tuberculosis, pulmonary cavitation, and matrix metalloproteinases [J]. Am J Respir Crit Care Med. 2014;190(1):9–18.
9. Li C, Zhou X, Lu Y, et al. An analysis of CT scan findings of pulmonary tuberculosis differing in the category of drug-resistance and drug-susceptible pulmonary tuberculosis [J]. Chin J Antituberc. 2018;40(7):707–12.
10. Wáng YXJ, Chung MJ, Skrahin A, et al. Radiological signs associated with pulmonary multi-drug resistant tuberculosis: an analysis of published evidences [J]. Quant Imaging Med Surg. 2018;8(2):161–73.
11. Belton M, Brilha S, Manavaki R, et al. Hypoxia and tissue destruction in pulmonary TB [J]. Thorax. 2016;71(12):1145–53.
12. Volkman HE, Pozos TC, Zheng J, et al. Tuberculous granuloma induction via interaction of a bacterial secreted protein with host epithelium [J]. Science. 2010;327(5964):466–9.
13. Elkington P, Shiomi T, Breen R, et al. MMP-1 drives immunopathology in human tuberculosis and transgenic mice [J]. J Clin Invest. 2011;121(5):1827–33.

7 Poly-Resistant Tuberculosis (PDR-TB)

Min Song, Wei-jun Fang, Yuan-yuan Han,
Qian-qian Zhang, Hong-jun Li, and Luo-lin Wang

7.1 Summary of Poly-Resistant Tuberculosis (PDR-TB)

7.1.1 Definition

Poly-resistant tuberculosis (PDR-TB) is defined as the Mycobacterium tuberculosis infecting a pulmonary tuberculosis patient and confirmed by drug susceptibility testing (DST) in vitro to be resistant to more than one anti-tuberculosis drug, but not simultaneously including isoniazid (INH) and rifampicin (RFP).

7.1.2 Epidemiology and Incidence of Drug Resistance

As indicated by WHO Report of Global Tuberculosis 2022 [1], there were 450,000 patients with rifampicin-resistant tuberculosis (RR-TB) worldwide in 2021, up 3.1% from 437,000 in 2020. In recent years, the incidence of drug-resistant tuberculosis in China has declined, but the epidemic situation is still not optimistic. It was estimated that there were about 33,000 MDR/RR-TB patients in China with an incidence of 2.3/100,000 population. Ratio for MDR/RR-TB was estimated to be 3.4% among newly diagnosed tuberculosis patients, and 19% among those with relapsing tuberculosis. Resistance rate in tuberculosis patients in China differed greatly in different areas in China. The multi-resistance rate was high in treatment-naive smear-positive pulmonary tuberculosis patients in middle and eastern China with developed economy [2, 3]. In Western China with underdeveloped economy, however, mono-resistance rate was high in relapsing smear-positive pulmonary tuberculosis patients [4]. In some regions of China, the poly-resistance rate was 2.9–7.2% [5, 6].

Drug resistance tuberculosis can be categorized into five groups, based on WHO Global Tuberculosis Report, including isoniazid-resistant tuberculosis (Hr-TB), rifampicin-resistant tuberculosis (RR-TB), multidrug-resistant tuberculosis (MDR-TB), pre-extensively drug-resistant tuberculosis (Pre-XDR-TB), and extensively drug-resistant tuberculosis (XDR-TB). Pre-XDR-TB is a tuberculosis resistant to rifampicin and any of fluoroquinolones, and XDR-TB is a tuberculosis resistant to rifampicin, any of fluoroquinolones and at least one of the two drugs including bedaquiline and linezolid [6]. Incidence of poly-resistance tuberculosis (PDR-TB) was not mentioned by WHO Global Tuberculosis Report in 2021 and in 2022 [1, 7]. The number of cases of PDR-TB should be summarized into the category of MDR-TBs. It can be inferred from the concept of poly-resistant pulmonary tuberculosis that this is a disease with the Mycobacterium tuberculosis resistant to more than one anti-tuberculosis drugs not including simultaneously isoniazid and rifampicin, these two first-line anti-tuberculosis drugs. More detailed classification is helpful to guide clinical treatment more accurately!

7.2 Image Findings of Poly-Resistance Tuberculosis

The image findings of poly-resistant pulmonary tuberculosis are complex and diverse, which are closely related to its pathological changes. Given the absence of report on image findings of poly-resistant pulmonary tuberculosis, all follow-

M. Song (✉) · W.-j. Fang · Y.-y. Han
Department of Radiology, Guangzhou Chest Hospital, Guangzhou, Guangdong, China

Q.-q. Zhang
Magnetic Resonance Room, Zhoukou Central Hospital, Zhoukou, Henan Province, China

H.-j. Li
Department of Radiology, Beijing You'an Hospital, Capital Medical University, Beijing, China

L.-l. Wang
Department of Gastroenterology, Shenzhen People's Hospital, Shenzhen, Guangdong, China

P.-x. Lu et al. (eds.), *Diagnostic Imaging of Drug Resistant Pulmonary Tuberculosis*,
https://doi.org/10.1007/978-981-99-8339-1_7

ing data of this disease are from Guangzhou Chest Hospital in China, except for cases with special remarks. Onset age was 44.3 years old on average and concentrated in the age group of 18–40 years old, accounting for about 40.9%. Patients were mainly middle-aged and young people. It might be related to the living habits of middle-aged and young patients and the great burden on their working and educations. The ratio of men to women was about 7:3. The proportion of treatment-naive patients was about 30%, and that of patients with relapsing diseases was about 70%. Patients with diabetes accounted for 36.8%.

Diagnosis was confirmed in all patients, based on positiveness in sputum culture and sputum smear as well as drug susceptibility test. Their image findings showed some characteristics.

1. Poly-resistance tuberculosis (PDR-TB) has the common characteristics of smear-positive pulmonary tuberculosis, including manifestations of active tuberculosis such as centrilobular nodules, tree-in-bud sign, single or multiple cavitation(s), and thickening of bronchial wall with stenosis and/or expansion, similar to active drug sensitive pulmonary tuberculosis (DS-TB) [8]. It has much fewer calcified lesions in active PDR-TB than that in DS-TB, but similar to MDR-TB in previous researches [9, 10]. About 60% of patients in this cohort manifested consolidation and exudation (Figs. 7.1, 7.2, 7.3, 7.4 and 7.5). Many studies have shown that consolidation and consolidation with cavities in patients with tuberculosis, especially consolidation in or above multiple pulmonary segments with mouth-eaten cavities and bronchial damage, suggest the possibility of multidrug resistance [11, 12]. Chest high-resolution and enhanced CT scans in poly-resistance pulmonary tuberculosis patients also show pulmonary mass, mucoid impaction, and mediastinal lymphadenectasis, and most of the lesions show peripheral enhancement in enhanced CT scans (Figs. 7.6 and 7.7).
2. Distribution in lung lobes: The ratio of PDR-TB patients with lesions involving three lobes was 70.5% (Figs. 7.5, 7.8, and 7.9). Patients with drug-resistant tuberculosis all showed positiveness in sputum smear, and pulmonary tuberculosis with this positiveness formed easily extensive bronchial dissemination [13]. Compared with the cohort of drug susceptible pulmonary tuberculosis, MDR-TB has its intra-pulmonary lesions reported by corresponding literature to involve commonly more than 3 lobes [14, 15], showing statistical significance ($P < 0.005$), which is related to the protracted course, recurrent attack, and intra-pulmonary dissemination of MDR-TB.
3. Predilection sites: Predilection sites are similar for the cohort of PDR-TB patients without diabetes and for those with drug susceptible tuberculosis, including dominantly posterior apical segment of the upper lobes and dorsal segment of the lower lobes, but rarely involve pulmonary lobes. Pulmonary tuberculosis lesions in most of PDR-TB cases in Guangzhou Chest Hospital, China were widely distributed in both lung fields. Consolidations were common and more extensively in these cases, and some consolidations were with mouth-eaten cavities (Fig. 7.10). Song et al. [12] analyzed, limited drug penetration into the consolidation in or above multiple pulmonary segments with multiple mouth-eaten cavities and bronchial damage that harbor large numbers of mycobacteria, together with the immunodeficiency caused by the poor glucose levels control, might contribute to the drug resistance.
4. Cavities: Ratio of patients with cavitation in PDR-TB cases in Guangzhou Chest Hospital was 72.1%, similar to the incidence of cavitation (70%) in MDR-TB patients, and higher than that (30–40%) in DS-TB patients, according to the statistical data in the relevant literature [16]. About 50.8% of the patients have multiple cavities in lungs (Figs. 7.1 and 7.9). Among all PDR-TB cases with cavities, ratios for patients with thick-walled cavities (Fig. 7.4), patients with non-walled cavities, patients with coexisting thick- and thin-walled cavities, and patients with thin-walled cavities were 70.5%, 18.2%, 6.8%, and 4.5%, respectively. The tuberculous cavity wall is composed of collagen outside the cavity, cheese like material inside the cavity and granulation tissue in the middle, which are lacking blood supply. Anti-tuberculosis drugs are not easy to penetrate the cavity wall, predisposing cavity wall to an exposure to a low blood drug concentration, so that a large number of hidden Mycobacterium tuberculosis can survive in the cavity and eventually result in the formation of drug resistance. Statistics of several studies [17–20] show that, the existence of cavity, especially multiple cavities, is a risk factor for multidrug-resistant tuberculosis, and cavities in multiple drug resistance tuberculosis are more common than that in drug sensitive tuberculosis. But some scholars' research shows that the incidence of cavitation of drug sensitive pulmonary tuberculosis is higher than that of drug-resistant pulmonary tuberculosis [10]. However, most researchers demonstrated that thick-walled cavities, especially multiple thick-walled cavities, are a significant feature of acquired drug-resistant pulmonary tuberculosis [9, 16]. The thicker cavity wall often shows a higher concentration of bacteria in the sputum [21]. A large number of mycobacteria in the cavity and limited drug penetration may lead to drug-resistant tuberculosis [22]. Thus, scholars have concluded that severe drug-resistant pulmonary tuberculosis, including XDR-TB and

MRR-TB, may overall appear even more aggressive than DS-TB, with more number of cavities, larger cavities, and cavities of thicker wall [16, 23]. In addition, data from Guangzhou Chest Hospital in China suggested about 20% of patients had consolidations with mouth-eaten cavities (Figs. 7.1, 7.7 and 7.9), and most of these patients were complicated with diabetes. Enhanced CT scans showed low-density liquefaction

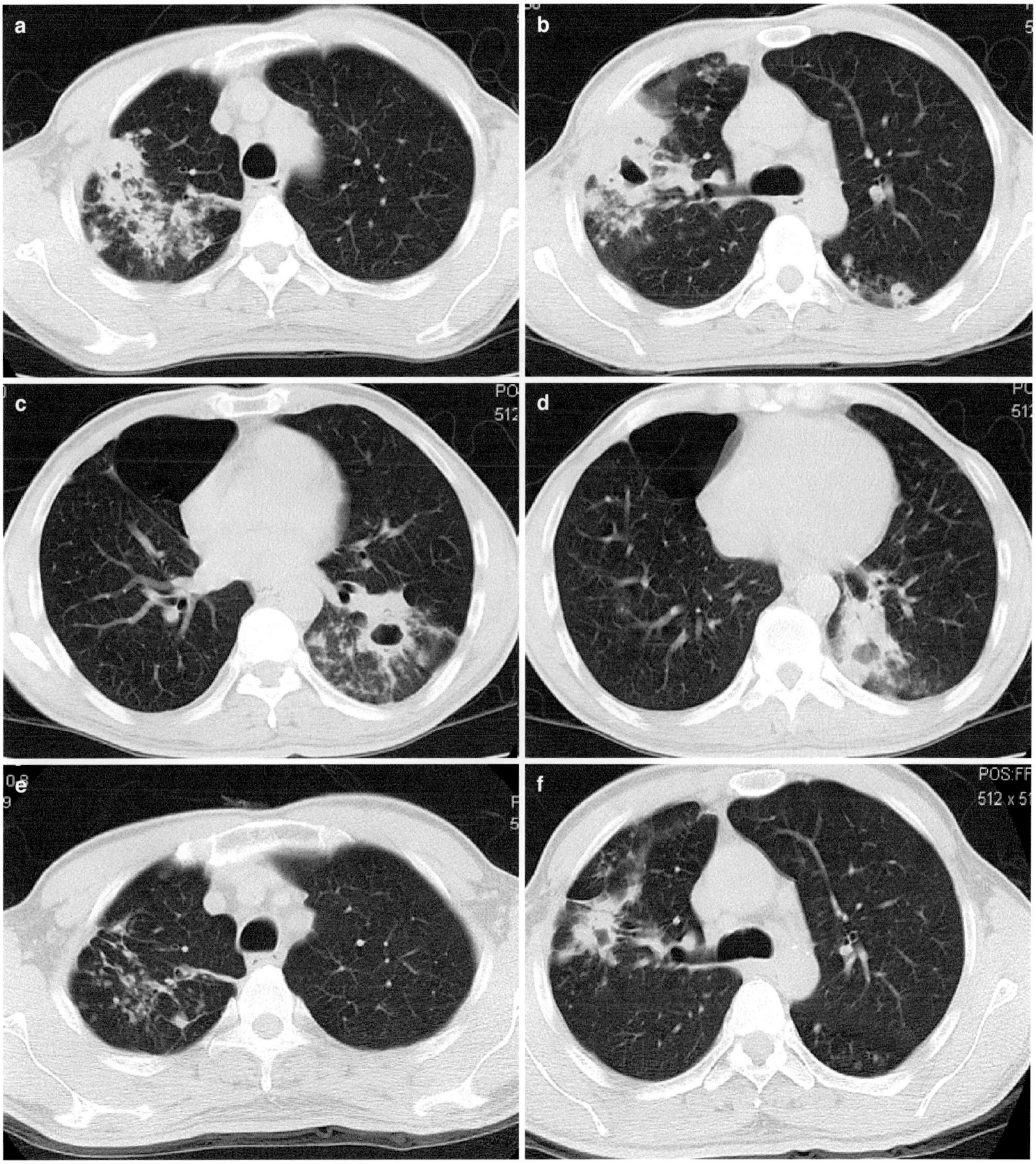

Fig. 7.1 (**a–h**) Primary poly-resistant TB in a 55-year-old man, with resistance to isoniazid and streptomycin. Chief complaint of cough and expectoration with white mucus sputum or foam-like sputum for 2 months. (**a–d**) Chest CT scans showed patchy, nodular, linear opacities, and consolidations with mouth-eaten cavities in the right upper and lower lobes, and the left lower lobe. (**e–h**) Image findings in re-examination of chest CT scans on October 8, 2019, post to 15-month anti-tuberculosis treatment, showing the obvious absorption of pulmonary lesions and decreased size of cavities, with the thin-walled appearance

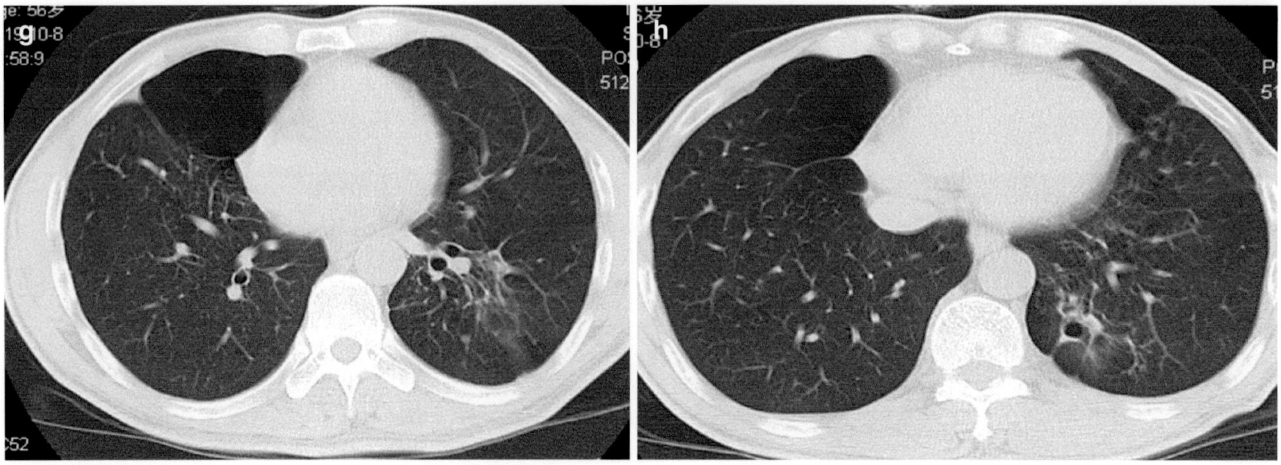

Fig. 7.1 (continued)

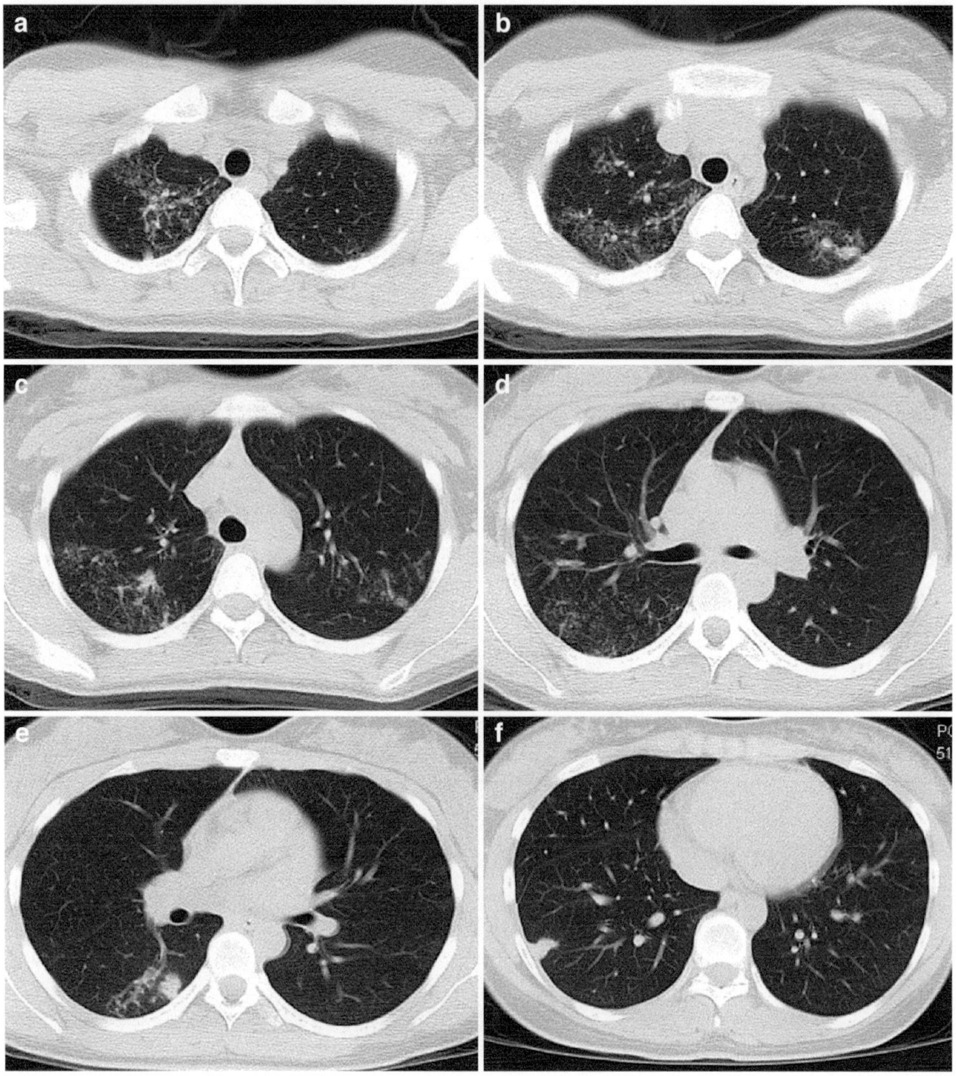

Fig. 7.2 (**a**–**l**) Primary poly-resistant TB in a 17-year-old woman, with resistance to rifampicin, streptomycin, ethambutol. Chief complaint of bilateral anterior chest pain without obvious inducement for 2 weeks. (**a**–**f**) Chest CT scans on October 16, 2018, showed multiple centrilobular nodules, tree-in-bud signs, consolidations and patchy opacities in both lungs. (**g**–**l**) Chest CT scans on March 13, 2020, post to 17-month anti-tuberculosis treatment showed the obvious absorption of pulmonary lesions, with residue of small amount of sclerotic foci in linear and small nodular appearance

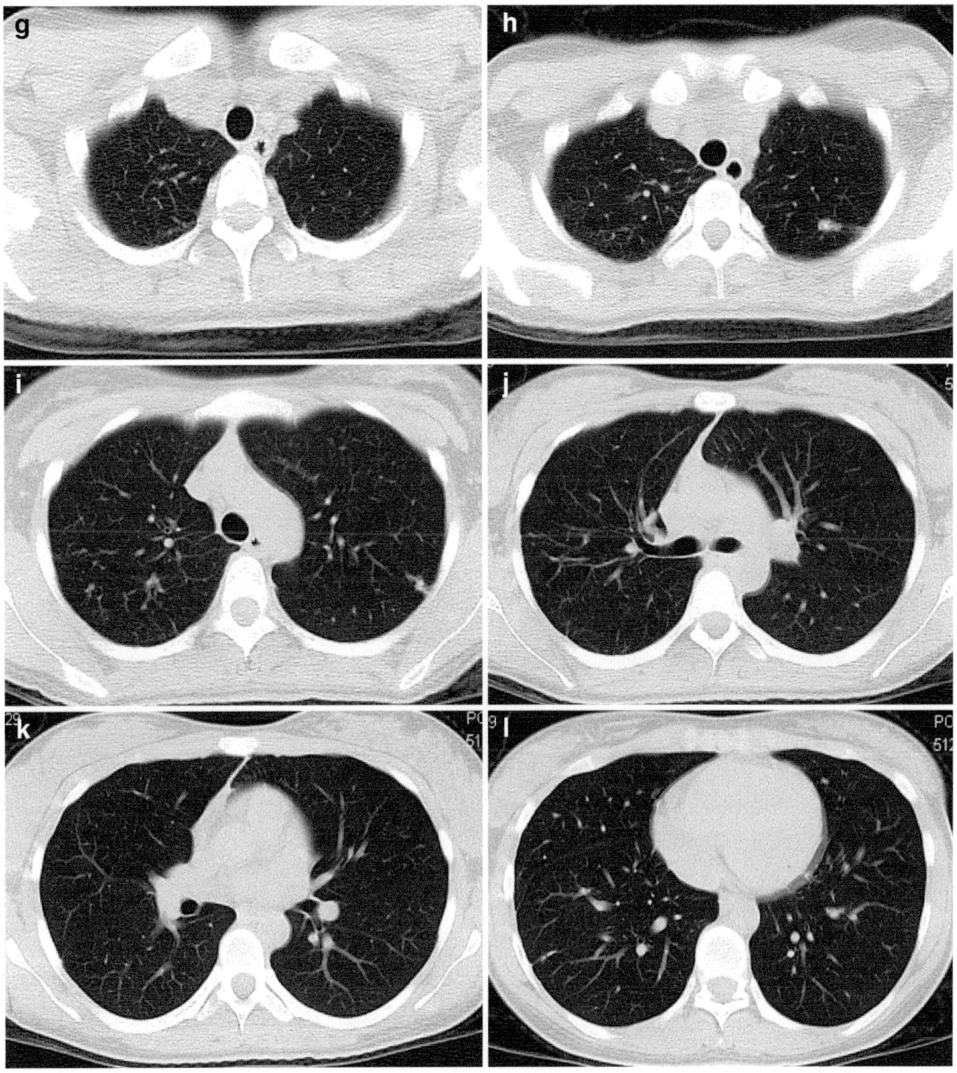

Fig. 7.2 (continued)

area with inhomogeneous enhancement of segmental or lobular consolidation around it. Biopsy showed that the low-density area was caseous substance and the surrounding was granulation tissue. This imaging manifestation may be related to the cellular immune response in patients with drug-resistant pulmonary tuberculosis. The number of CD4 + CD25 + Foxp3 + T lymphocytes and levels detected for transforming growth factor β1 (TGF-β1) and interleukin-10 (IL-10), as found in some studies [24], were much higher in drug-resistant pulmonary tuberculosis patients than in those with nondrug-resistant disease. As a result, the cellular immunity of the body was weakened, and the invasiveness of DR-TB patients against drug-resistant tuberculosis bacteria was suppressed, which predisposed the lesions to the formation of lobar or segmental consolidation, liquefaction necrosis, and mouth-eaten cavities. It was found that consolidations with cavities were significantly correlated with MDB-TB [11, 12].

5. Bronchial tuberculosis and bronchiectasis: About 75% of patients in PDR-TB group were complicated with bronchial tuberculosis (Figs. 7.5, 7.6 and 7.10; Case 2), and 40% complicated with bronchiectasis (Fig. 7.9). Patients with drug-resistant tuberculosis all showed positiveness in sputum bacteria, which easily invade bronchi. Invasion of large segmental bronchi presented as typical signs of bronchial tuberculosis, while invasion of small bronchi leads to airway obstruction and would cause consolidation or consolidation with cavities. Most bronchiectasis was associated with chronic infection. PDR-TB patients often have a long history of anti-tuberculosis treatment, so bronchiectasis and fibrous lesions were common in these patients.
6. Hilar and mediastinal lymph nodes, pleural effusion and pleura: Hilar and mediastinal lymphadenopathy in PDR-TB was rarely observed. Only 25% of patients had mild lymphadenopathy, and lymph nodes with a transverse diameter greater than 1.3 cm were rare. No calcified

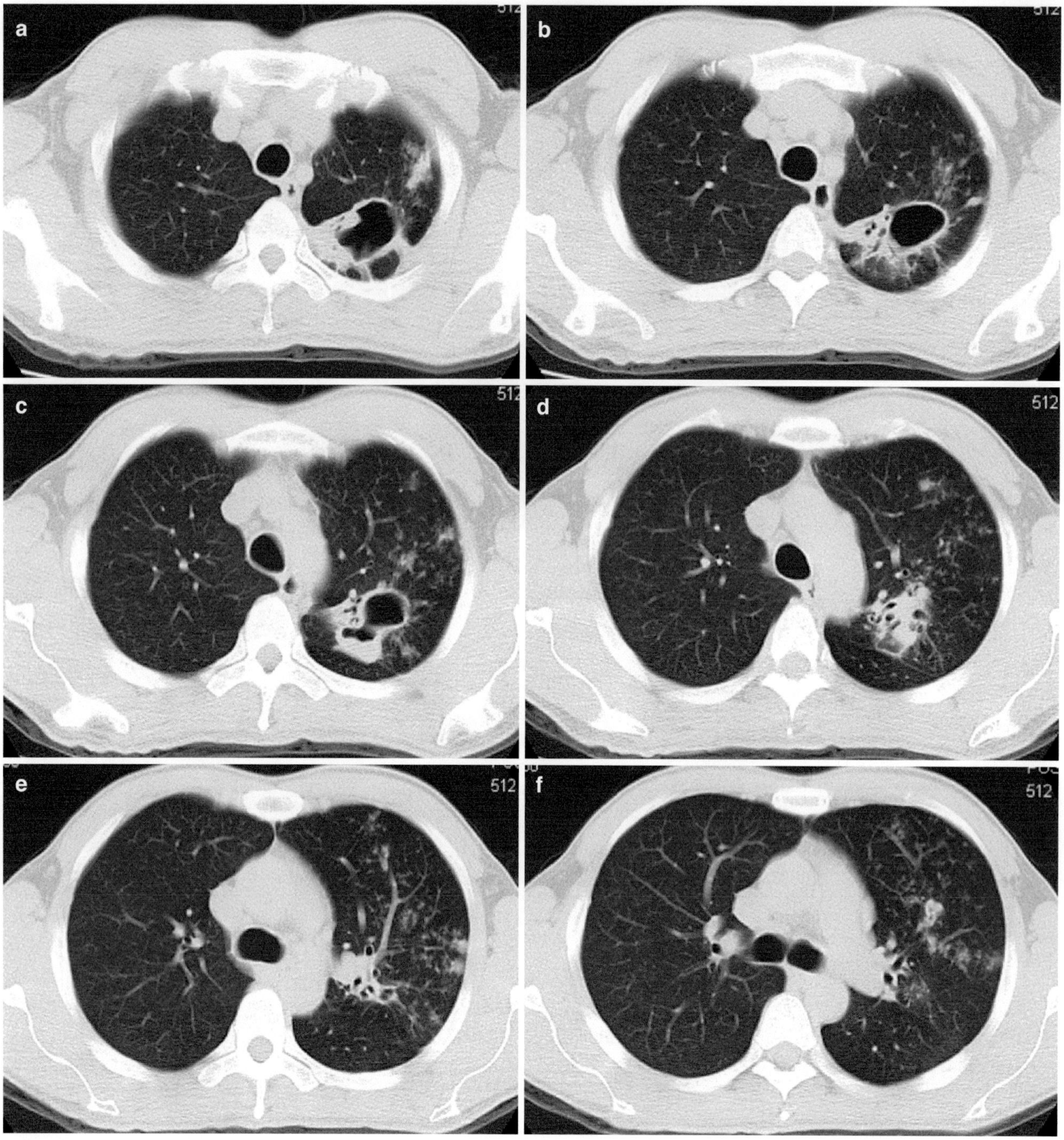

Fig. 7.3 (**a**–**r**) Primary poly-resistant TB in a 35-year-old man, with resistance to rifampicin, moxifloxacin, and rifabutin. Chief complaint of cough, expectoration, and fever without an obvious inducement for 2 days. Fibrobronchoscope showed the changes of left upper bronchitis. He had diabetes for 3 years. (**a**–**j**) Chest CT scans on June 8, 2020, showed multiple centrilobular nodules, tree-in-bud signs, patchy opacities in the left lung, with thick-walled cavity in apicoposterior segment of upper lobe of left lung. (**k**–**r**) Chest CT scans on August 9, 2020, showed the decreased size of the cavity with increased area of consolidation around the cavity, lesions in anterior segment of the left upper lobe were more than before, with a certain absorption of the rest of lesions, as compared with CT scans on June 8, 2020

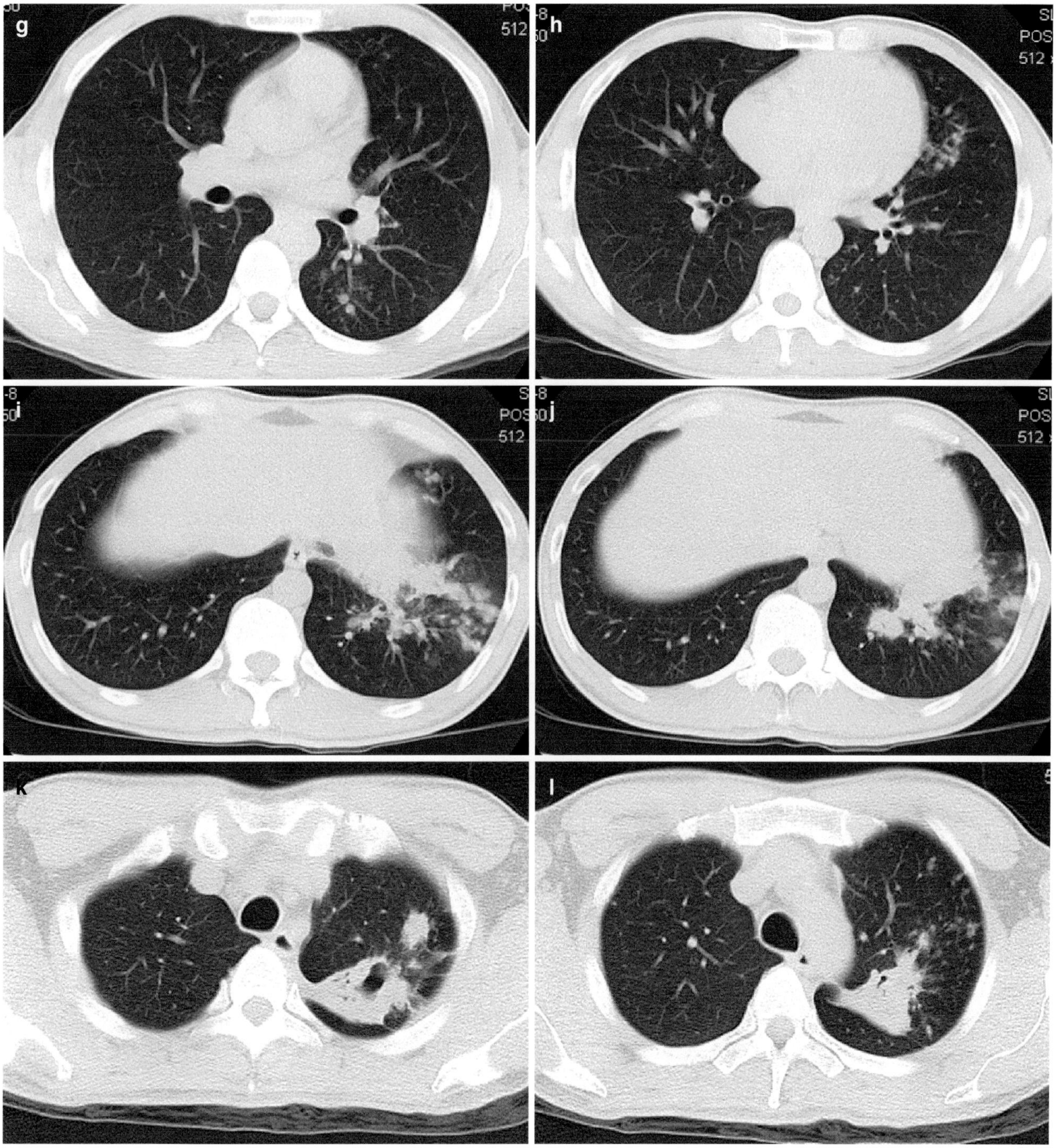

Fig. 7.3 (continued)

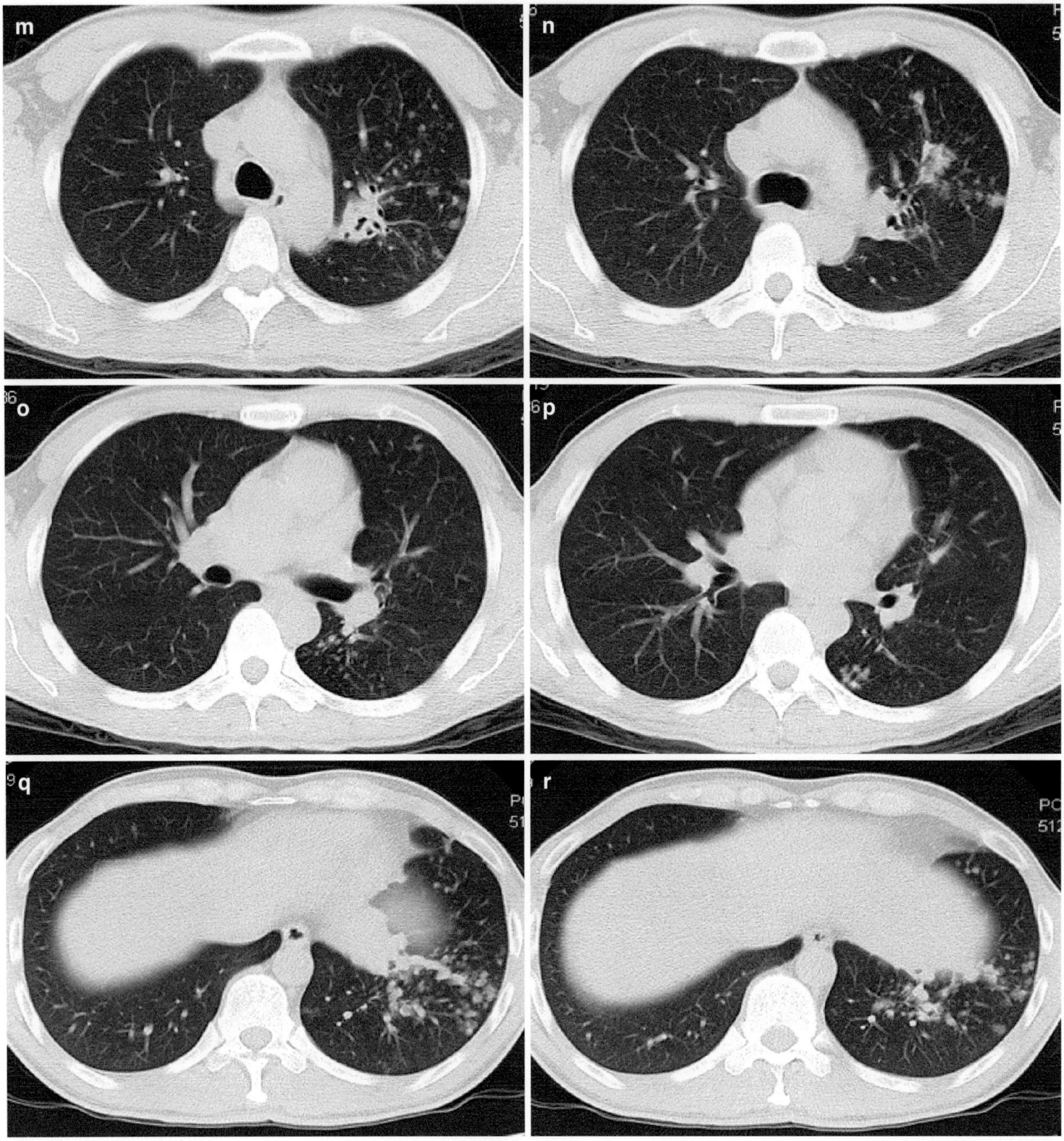

Fig. 7.3 (continued)

lymph nodes were observed in hilum and mediastinum in PDR-TB, which were similar to the rare calcification foci in the lungs. The reason is unclearly, which might be related to the pathogenicity of drug-resistant bacteria and the big proportion of diabetic patients in the study group. A previous study reported that the incidence of calcification foci in MDR-TB patients with diabetes mellitus was very low [12]. No calcified lymph node lesions were found, and the possible reason was that lesions in PDR pulmonary tuberculosis progressed rapidly in a hypersensitive state, which made it hard for calcium to deposit. Unilateral or bilateral pleural effusion occurred in about 11.4% of these patients, and those with pleural thickening were seldom seen.

7. Follow-up showed that waxing and waning were easily observed for lesion in patients exposed to irregular treatment (Fig. 7.4; case 1). PDR-TB patients with diabetes mellitus would show a rapid progression of pulmonary

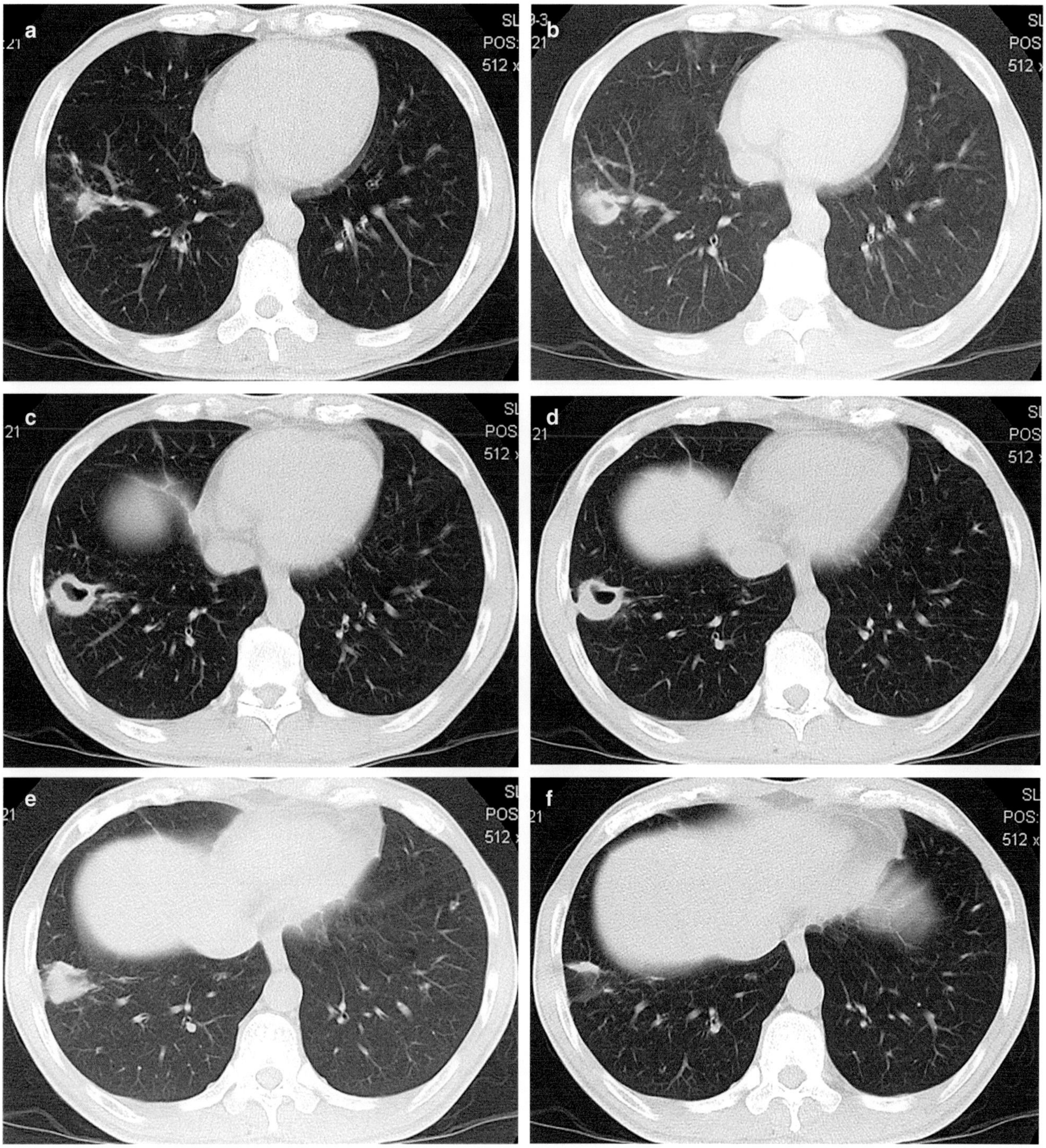

Fig. 7.4 (**a**–**l**) Primary poly-resistant TB in a 46-year-old man, with resistance to isoniazid, ofloxacin, moxifloxacin, and ethioisonicotinamide. Chief complaint of cough with an expectoration of a small amount of blood-streaked sputum for 3 months. (**a**–**f**) Chest CT scans on September 30, 2018, showed thick-walled cavity was observed in the lateral basal segment of the right lower lobe, with spotty, nodular, and patchy opacities around it, and some nodular and patchy opacities were observed in other lung fields. (**g**–**l**) Re-examination of chest CT scans on September 26, 2019, showed lesions around the cavity in the right lower lobe increased but the wall of the cavity became thinner, as compared with CT scans on September 30, 2018

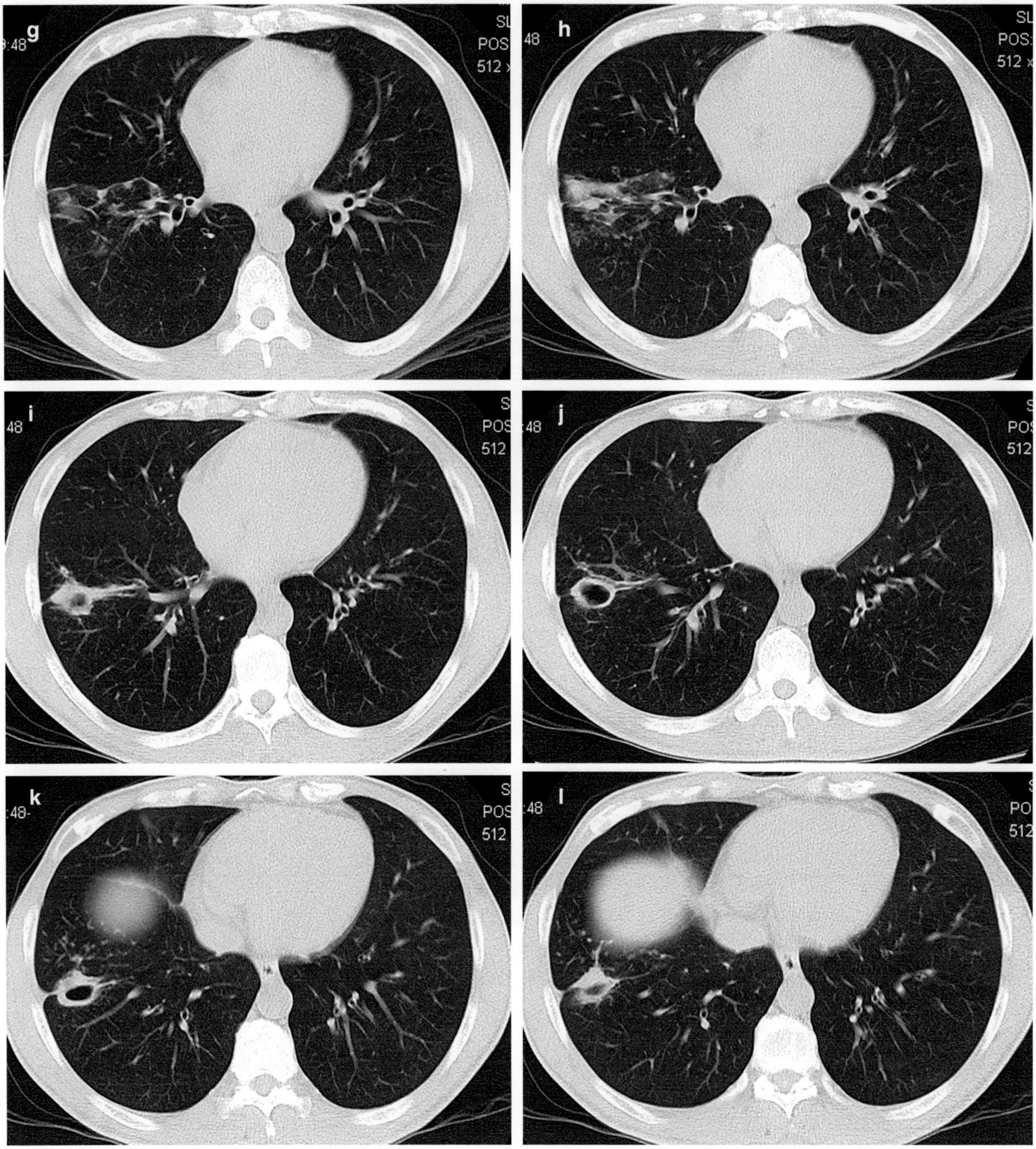

Fig. 7.4 (continued)

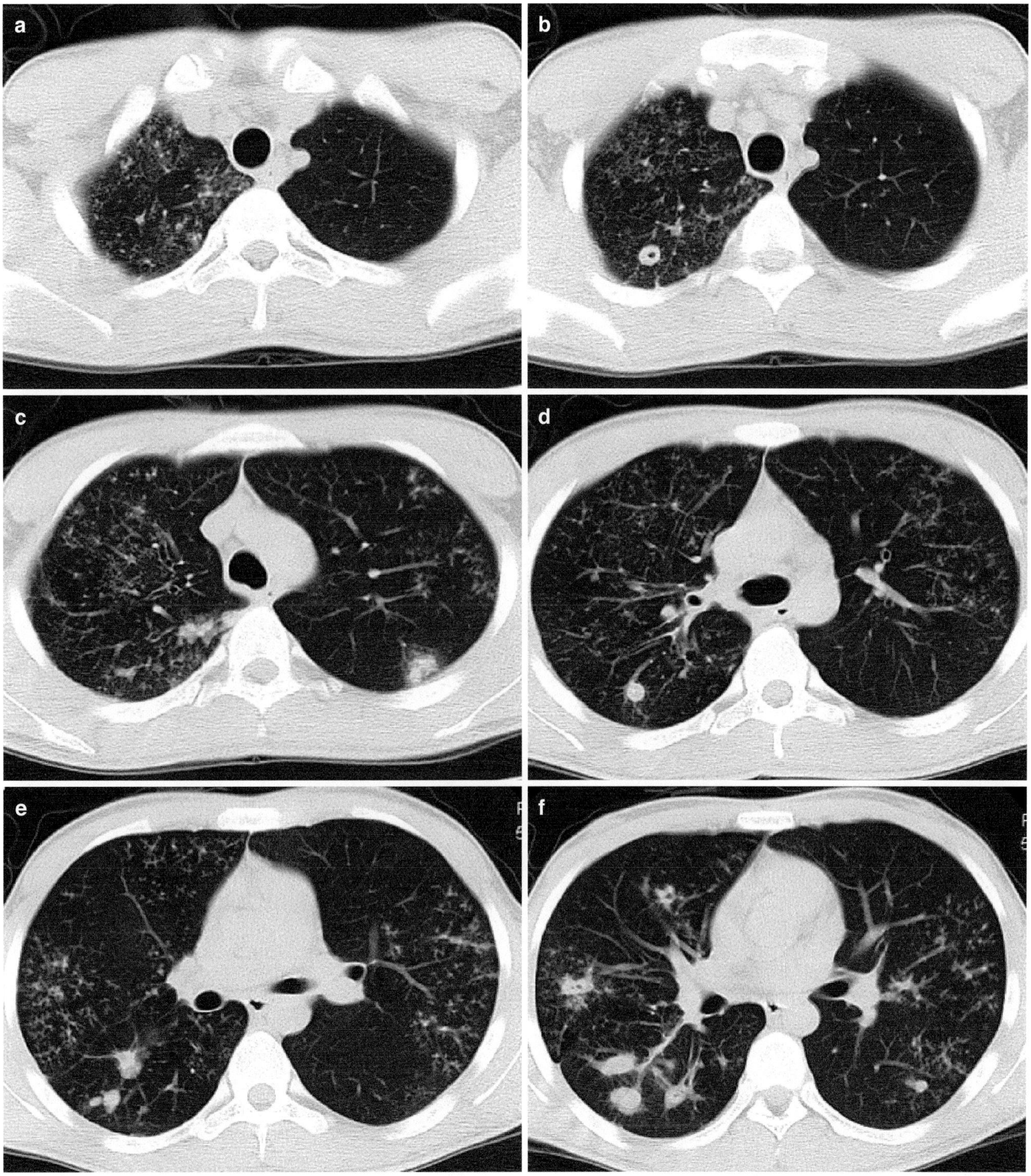

Fig. 7.5 (**a**–**r**) Primary poly-resistant TB in a 17-year-old man, with resistance to rifampicin, pyrazinamide, and rifabutin. Chief complaint of recurrent cough with expectoration without an obvious inducement for 2 years, and he had an onset of fresh hemoptysis in a volume of about 10 mL per day without an obvious inducement in May 2019. (**a**–**h**) chest CT scans on August 16, 2019, showed multiple tree-in-bud signs, centrilobular nodules, patchy opacities with unclear boundary in lobes of both lungs, with multiple cavities in the right lung; the wall of the lower part of the trachea and the starting part of the right main bronchus was thick and less smooth locally, with blunt protuberances observable. (**o**–**r**) Bronchoscope on August 29, 2019: tuberculosis of trachea and the right main bronchus (ulcerative necrotic type). (**i**–**n**) chest CT scans on May 23, 2020, post to 9-month anti-tuberculosis treatment formulated based on results of drug susceptible test showed the obvious absorption of lesions and the closure of the cavity in both lungs, as compared with CT scans on August 16, 2019

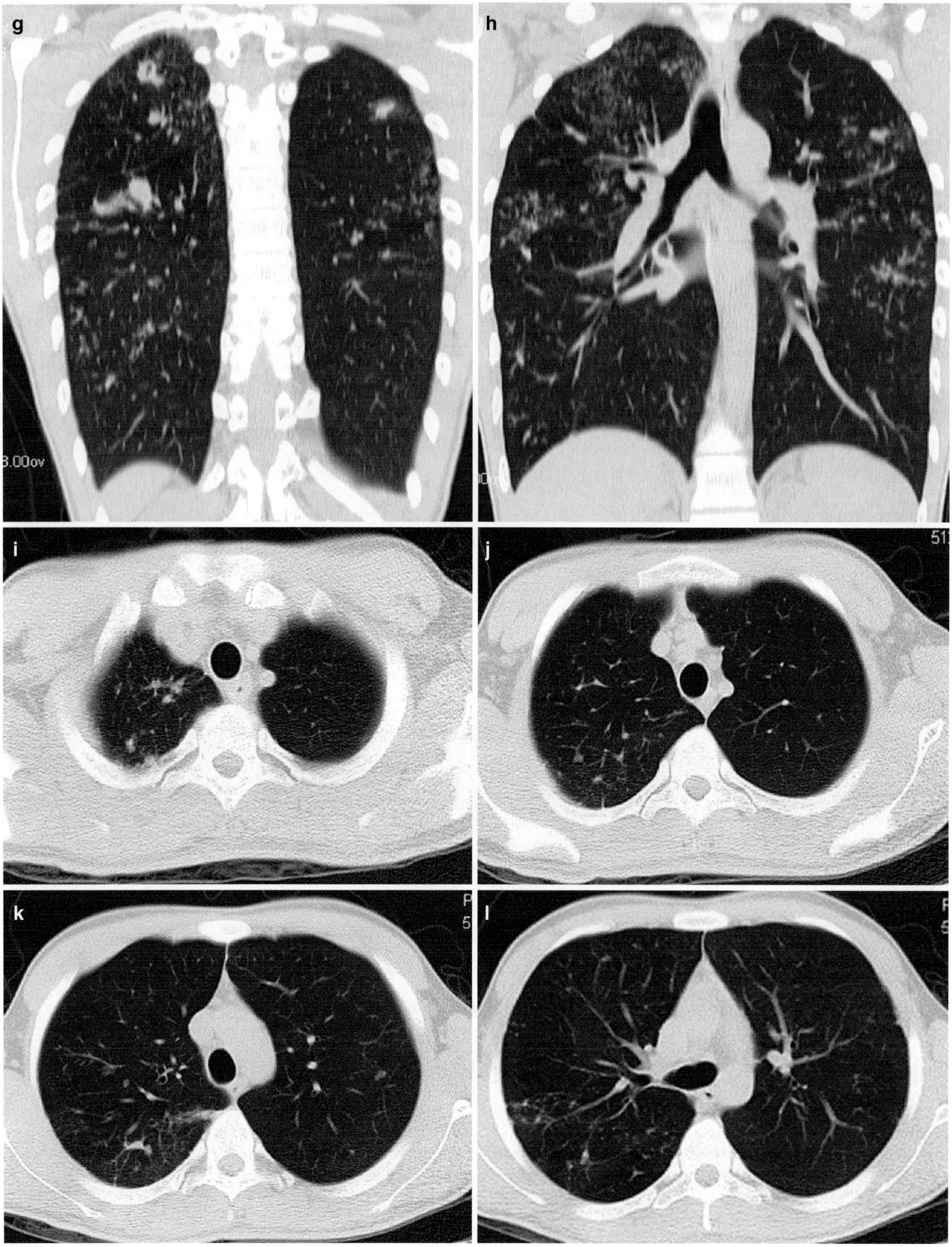

Fig. 7.5 (continued)

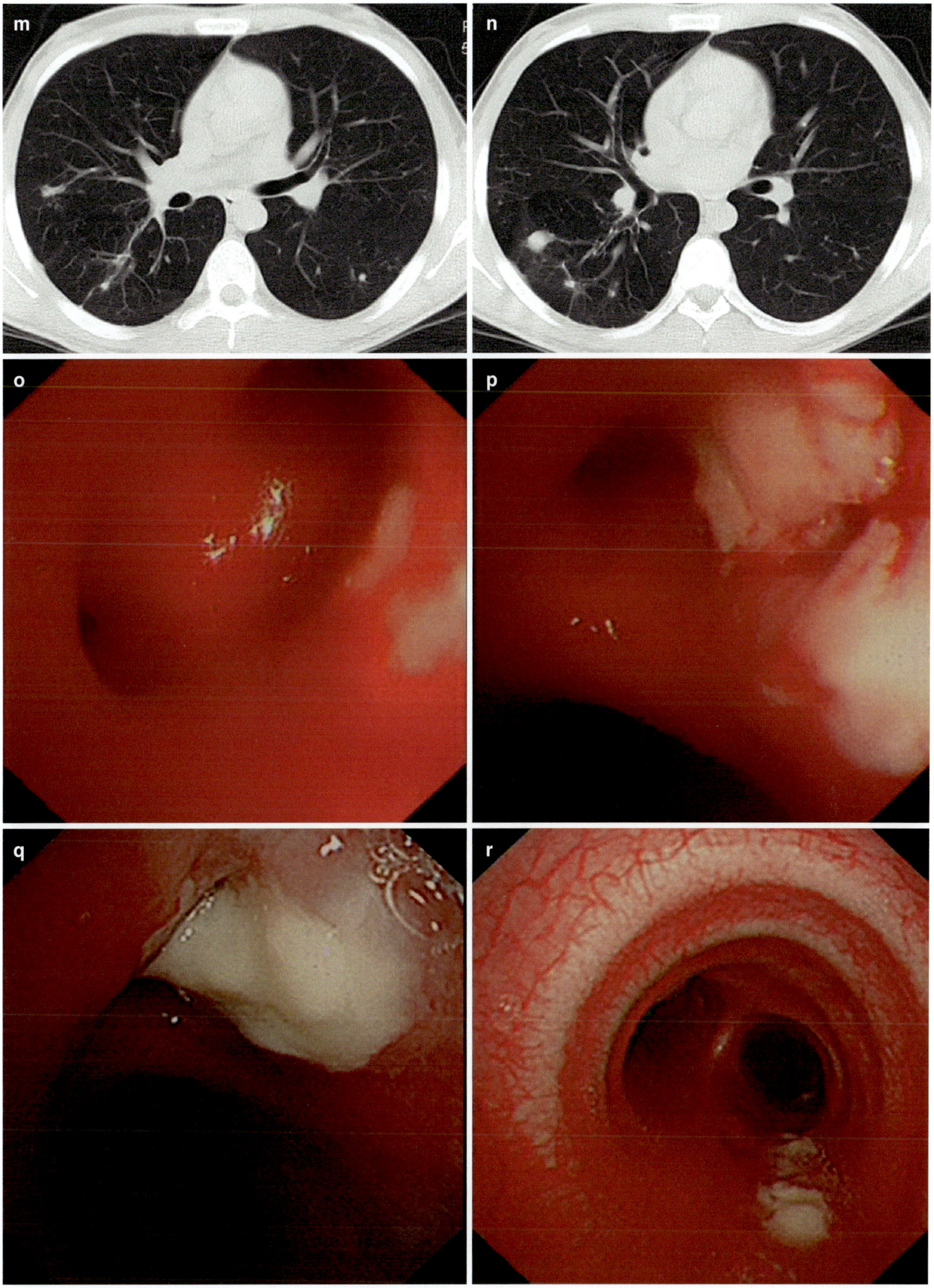

Fig. 7.5 (continued)

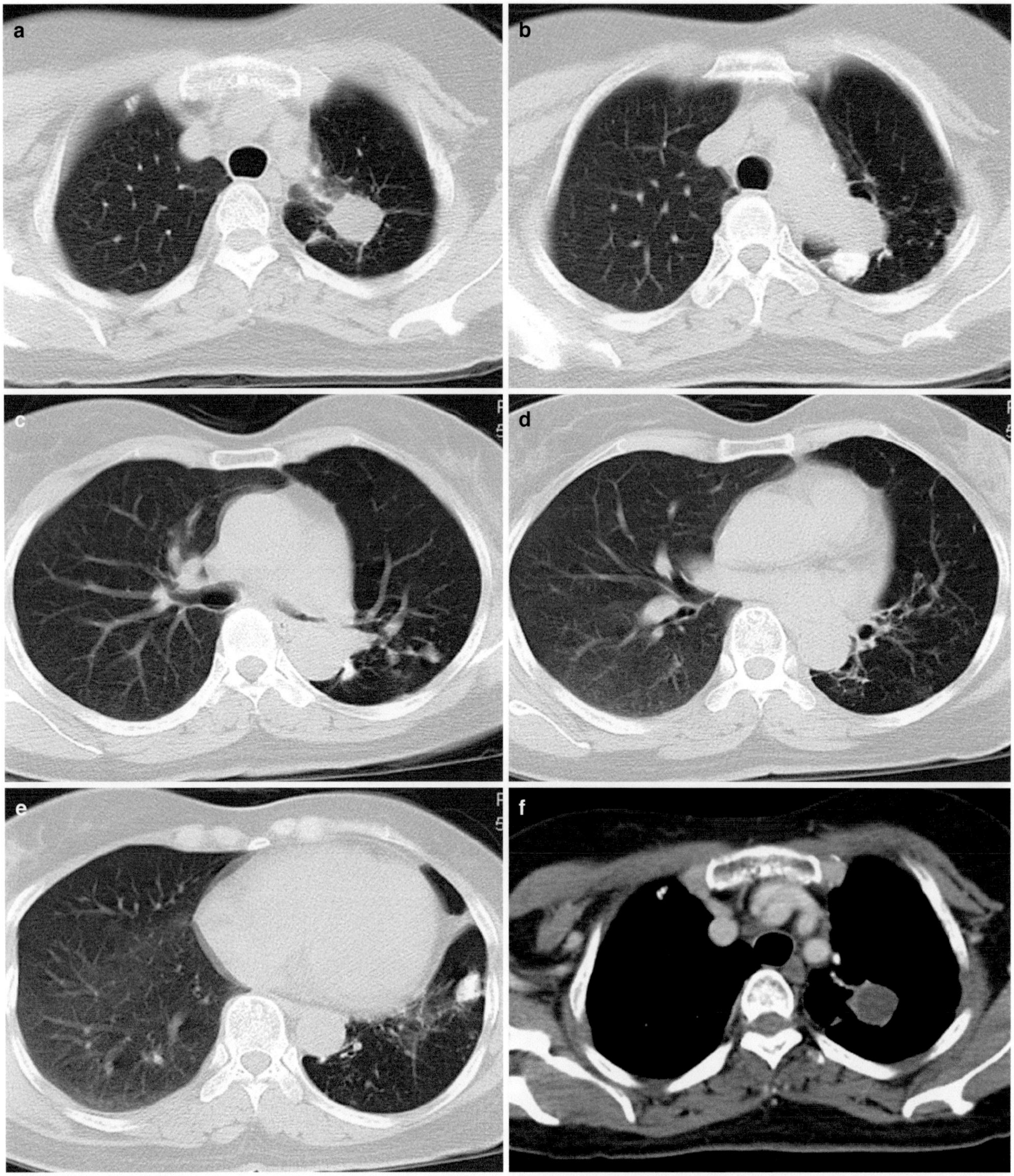

Fig. 7.6 (**a**–**h**) Relapsing poly-resistant TB in a 42-year-old woman, with resistance to rifampicin, pyrazinamide, and streptomycin. Chief complaint of cough with expectoration for 1 month, with chest tightness and short of breath after physical exertions. Chest CT scans showed multiple nodules and linear shadows in the left lung, with obvious stenosis of the left main bronchus; multiple calcified nodules were also observed in the left lung; enhanced CT scans showed peripheral enhancement of the biggest nodule in the left upper lobe

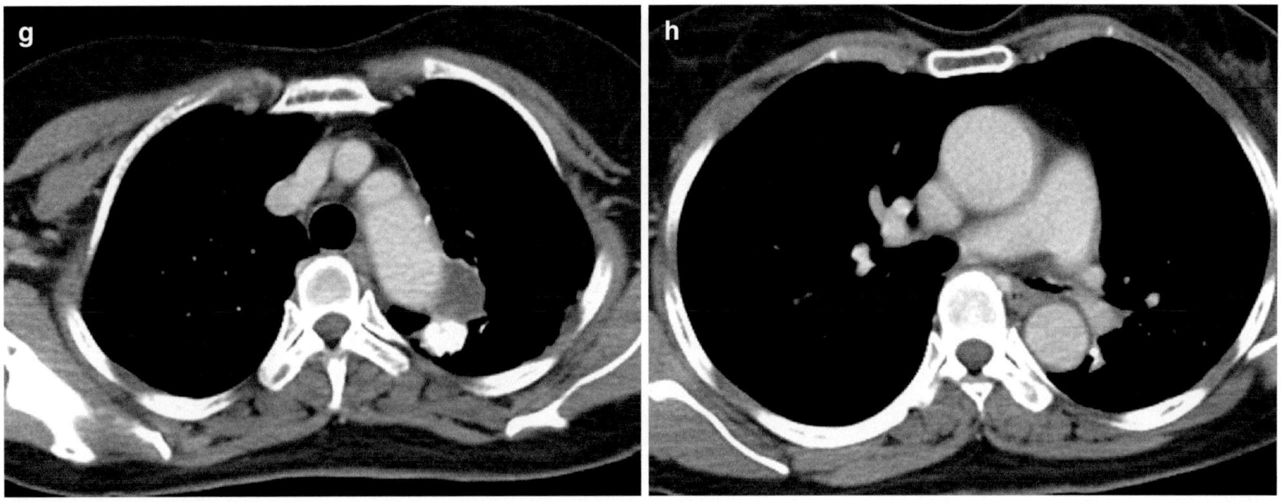

Fig. 7.6 (continued)

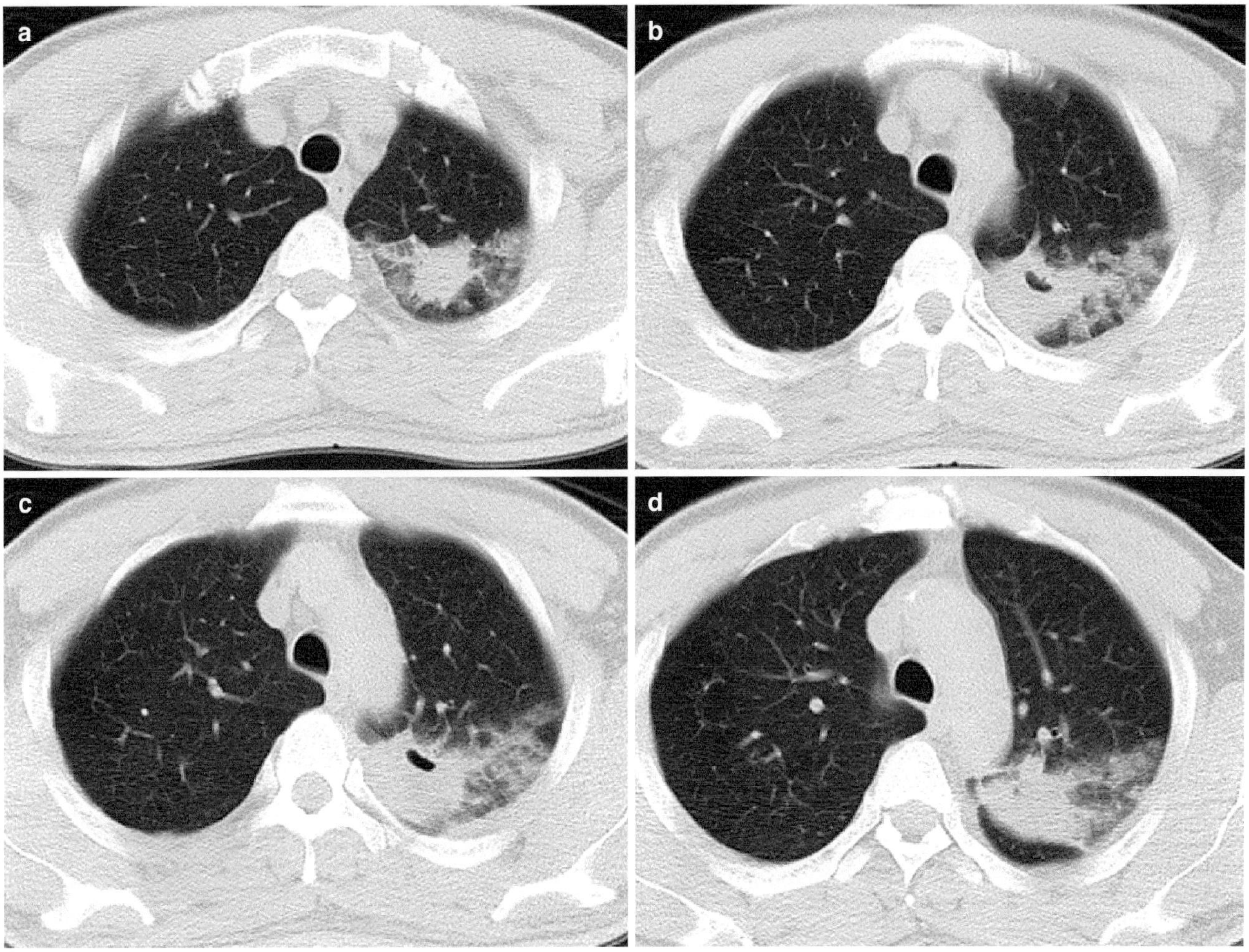

Fig. 7.7 (**a**–**j**) Primary poly-resistant TB in a 47-year-old man, with resistance to isoniazid and *p*-aminosalicylic acid. Chief complaint of recurrent chest tightness without an obvious inducement for 1 year. He had an episodic fever with temperature of 38.0 °C, and the symptoms were relievable post to symptomatic treatment. The patient had a history of diabetes for 20 years. Chest CT scans showed patchy opacities and consolidations with cavity in the apical posterior segment of the left upper lobe with unclear border along the circumference of the lesion; enhanced CT scans showed low-density liquefaction area in consolidations with cavity, with peripheral enhancement

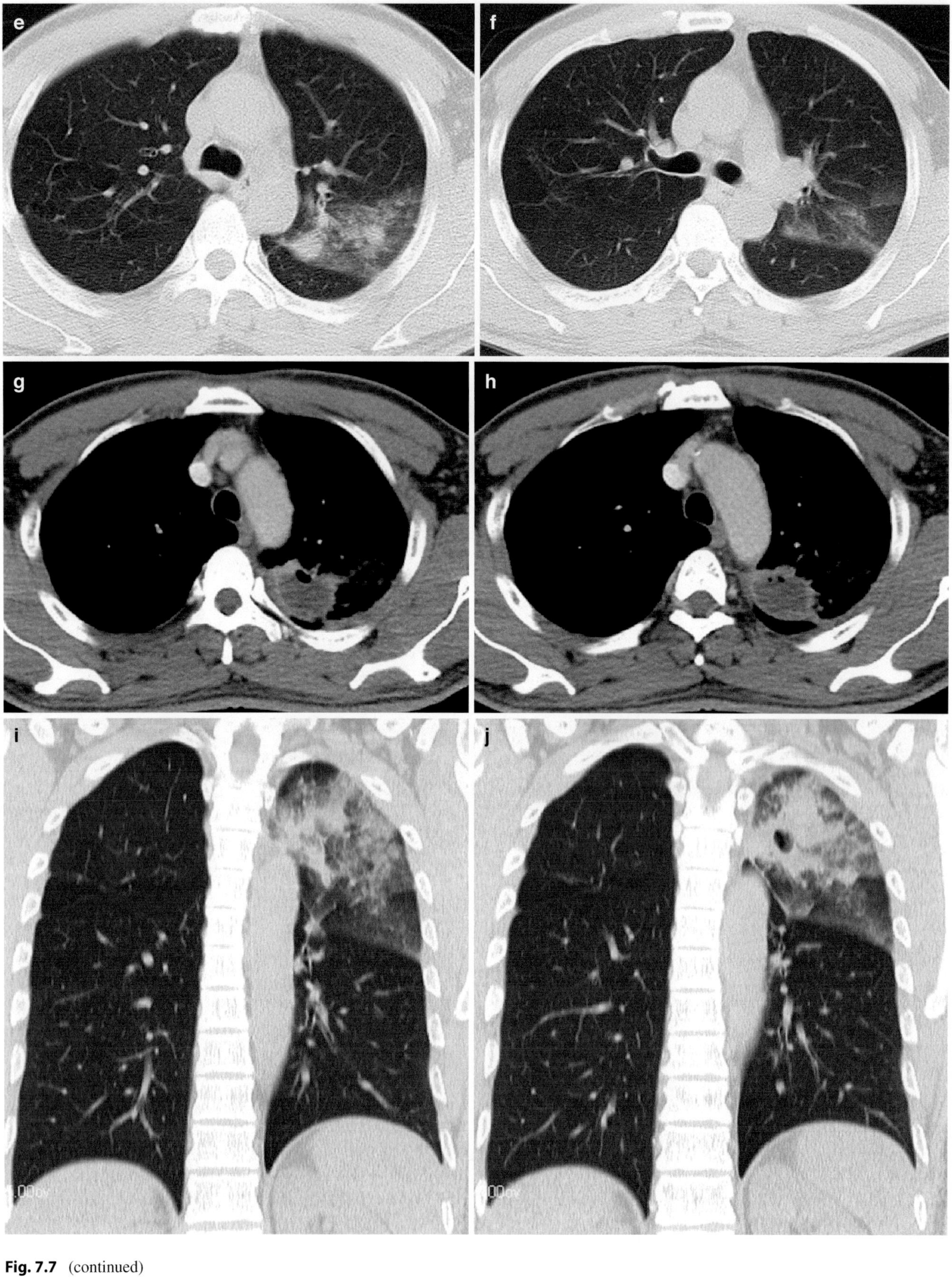

Fig. 7.7 (continued)

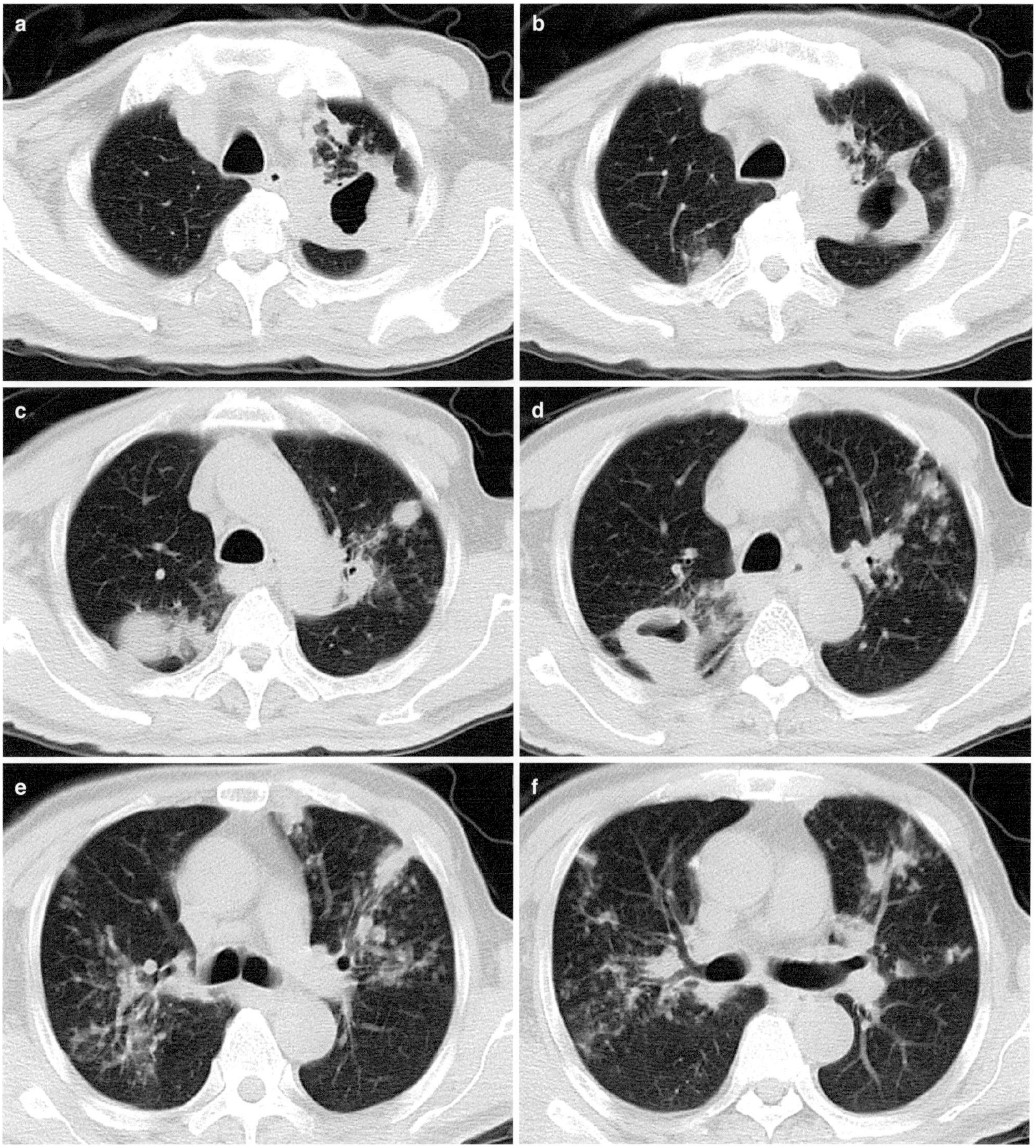

Fig. 7.8 (**a–n**) Primary poly-resistant TB in a 72-year-old man, with resistance to rifampicin and fluoroquinolones. Chief complaint of "recurrent cough with expectoration for one year, with fatigue and anorexia." (**a–h**) Chest CT scans on December 17, 2019, showed multiple centrilobular nodules and patchy high-density opacities, with thick-walled cavities in lesions in both upper lobes. Formation of mucus emboli was observed in multiple slightly enlarged bronchi in both upper lungs. (**i–n**) Chest CT scans on September 9, 2020, showed the obvious absorption of lesions with cavities shrank in both upper lungs, the intrabronchial mucus emboli disappeared, as compared with CT scans on December 17, 2019

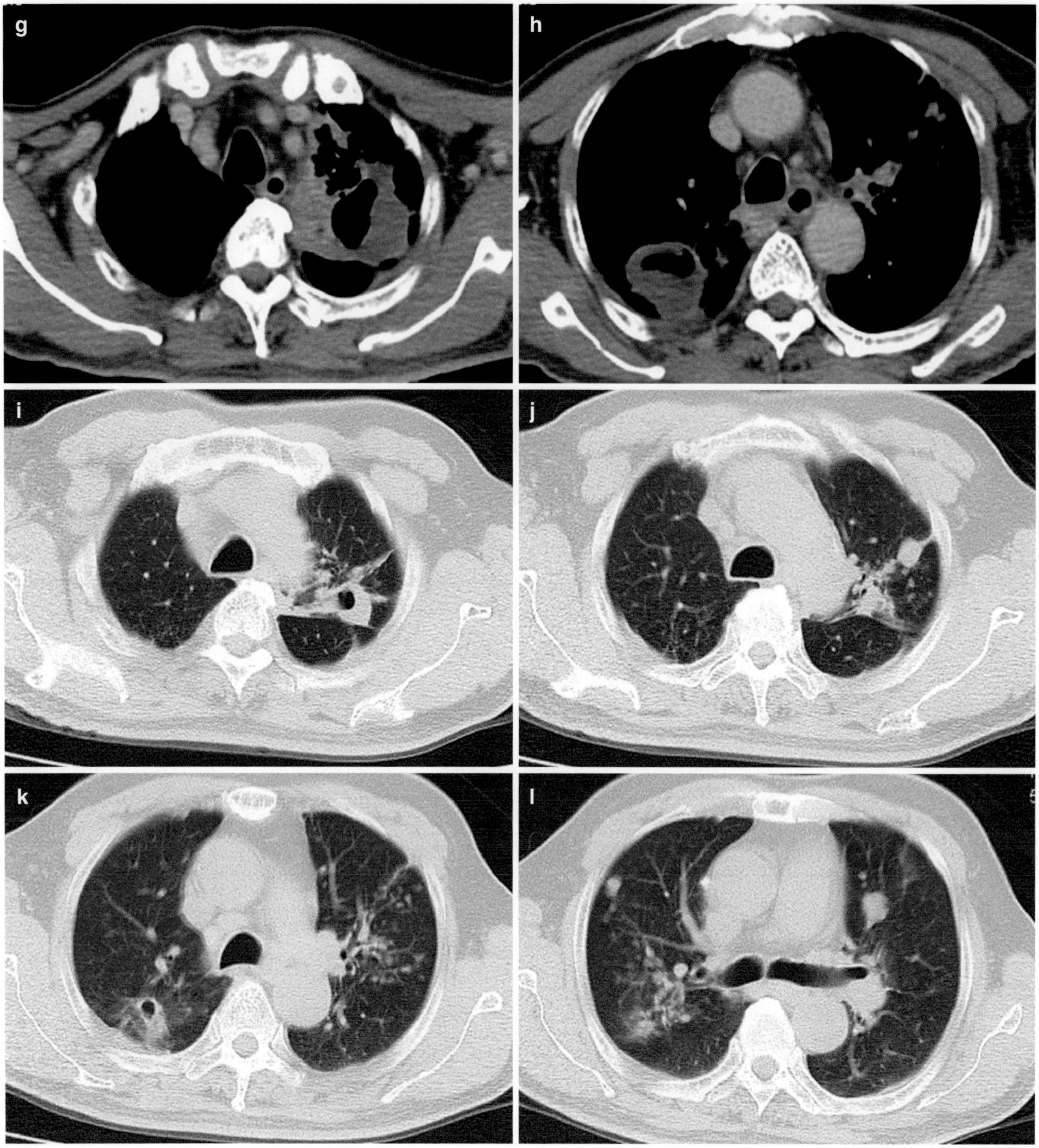

Fig. 7.8 (continued)

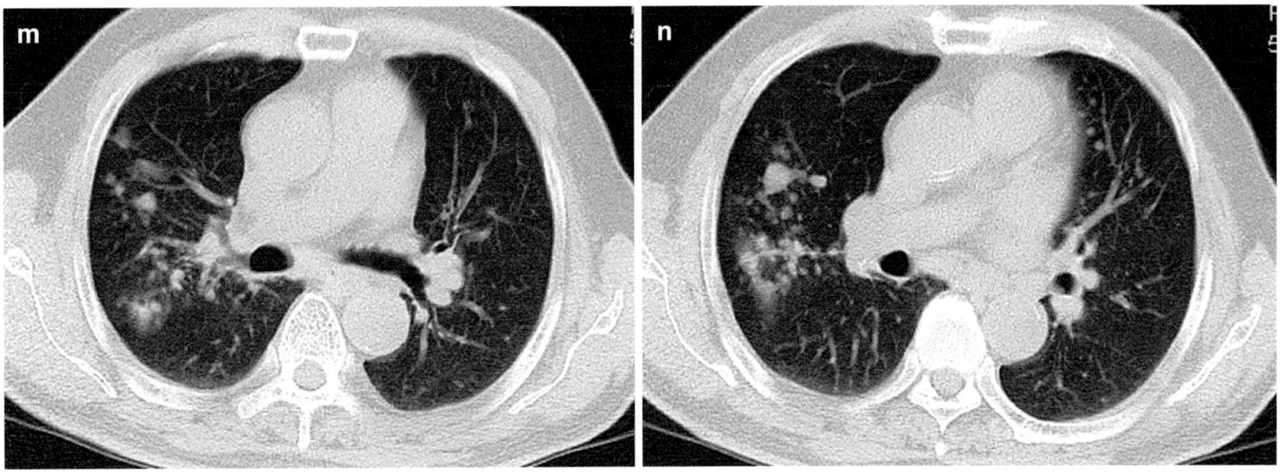

Fig. 7.8 (continued)

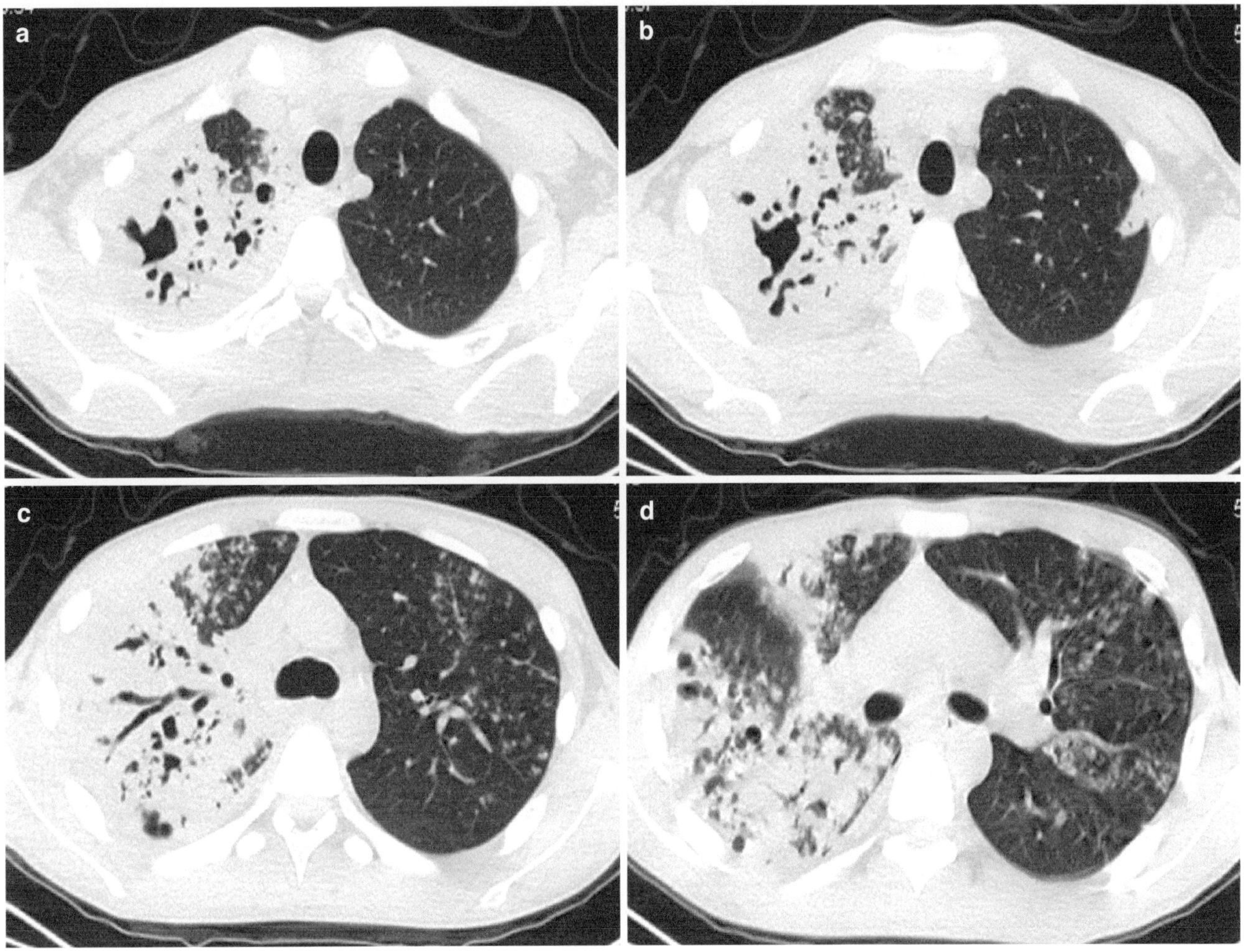

Fig. 7.9 (**a**–**n**) Primary poly-resistant TB in a 30-year-old man, with resistance to isoniazid, streptomycin, and ofloxacin. Chief complaint of cough with an expectoration of a small amount of white sputum for 3 months, complicated with fever for 1 week and a temperature up to 40 °C. (**a**–**h**) Chest CT scans on March 24, 2008, showed multiple centrilobular nodules, tree-in-bud signs, consolidation, and ground glass opacities in both lungs, with multiple mouth-eaten cavities inside the consolidation in the right upper and lower lobes, and the right pleural effusion. (**i**–**n**) Chest CT scans on September 29, 2009, in comparison with CT scans on March 24, 2008, showed that there was an emergence of new consolidation in apical posterior segment in the left upper lobe and the left pleural effusion, with absorption of the rest of pulmonary lesions and the right pleural effusion, a cavity appeared in the previous pulmonary nodule of the left upper lobe. Bronchiectasis was observed in the right upper and lower lobes

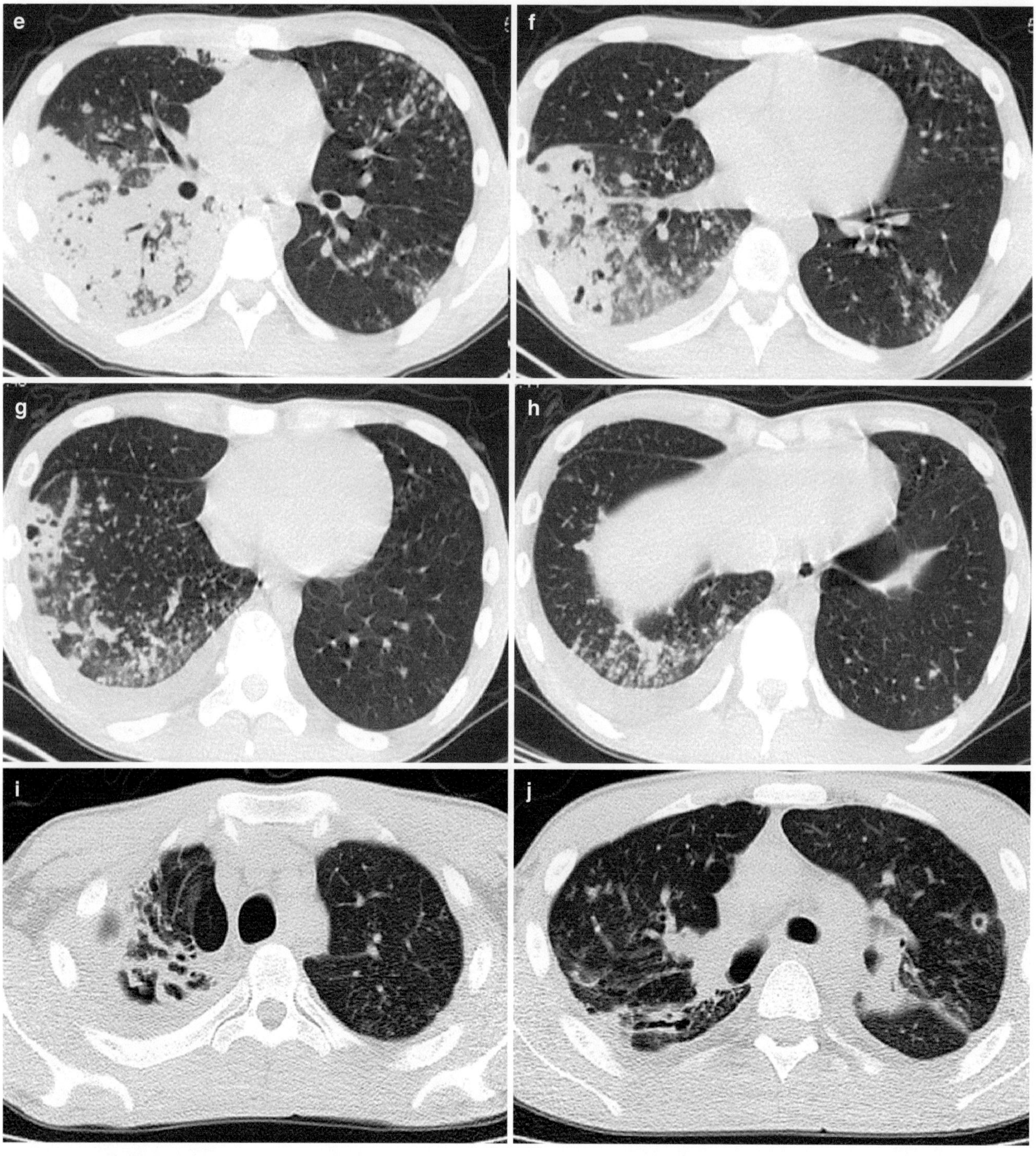

Fig. 7.9 (continued)

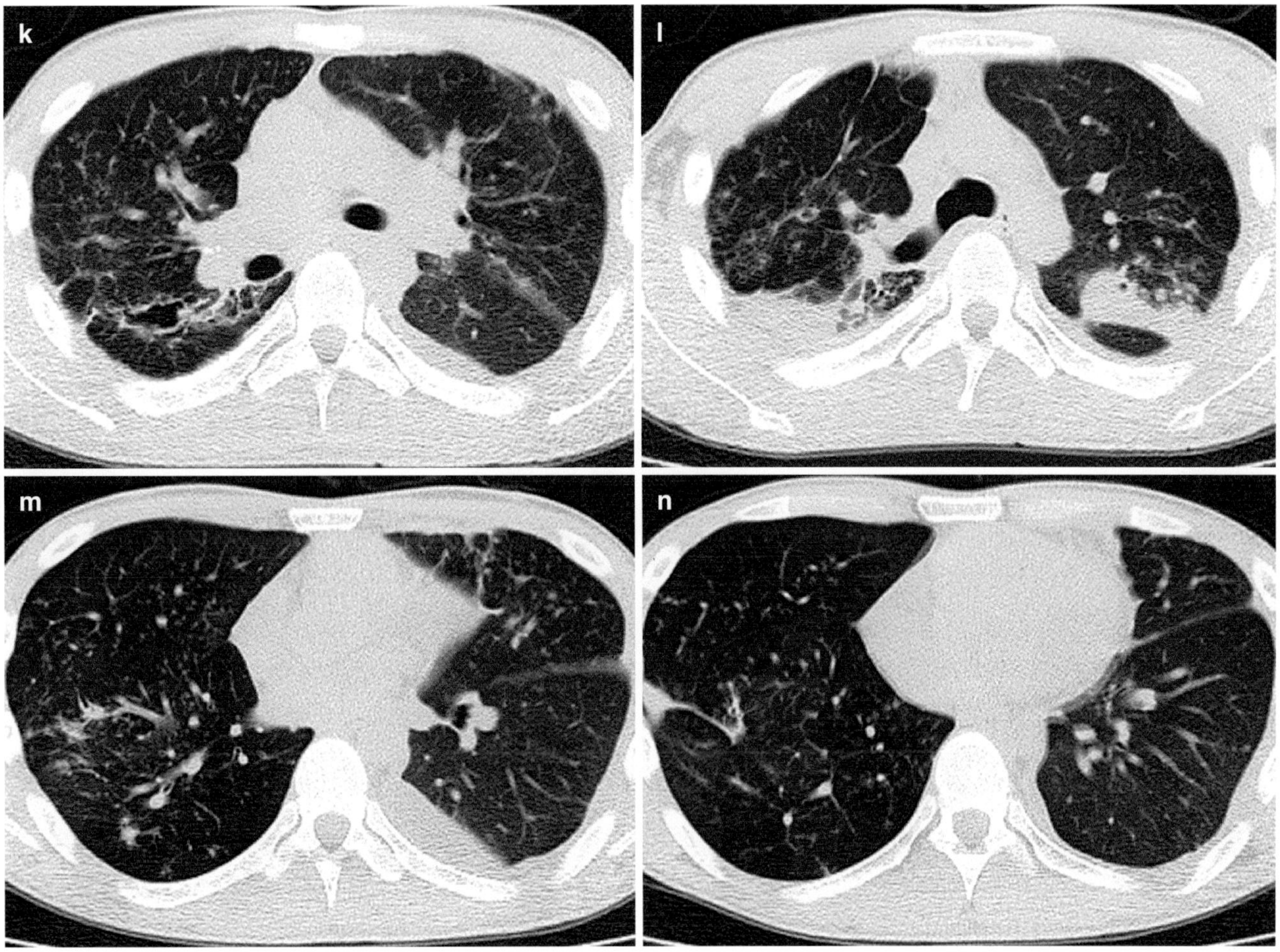

Fig. 7.9 (continued)

lesions in the absence of timely treatment or irregular treatment (Figs. 7.3 and 7.10, case 1 and 2).

In conclusion, drug-resistant pulmonary tuberculosis is one of the most difficult problems in the diagnosis and treatment of tuberculosis. The potential presence of drug resistance in a patient should be evaluated by clinicians based on a comprehensive analysis of image characteristic, and laboratory test should be performed timely for a patient suspected of drug-resistant tuberculosis to clarify drug susceptibility results, which will facilitate early diagnosis and early effective treatment for those with drug-resistant tuberculosis and help to achieve lower incidence and mortality.

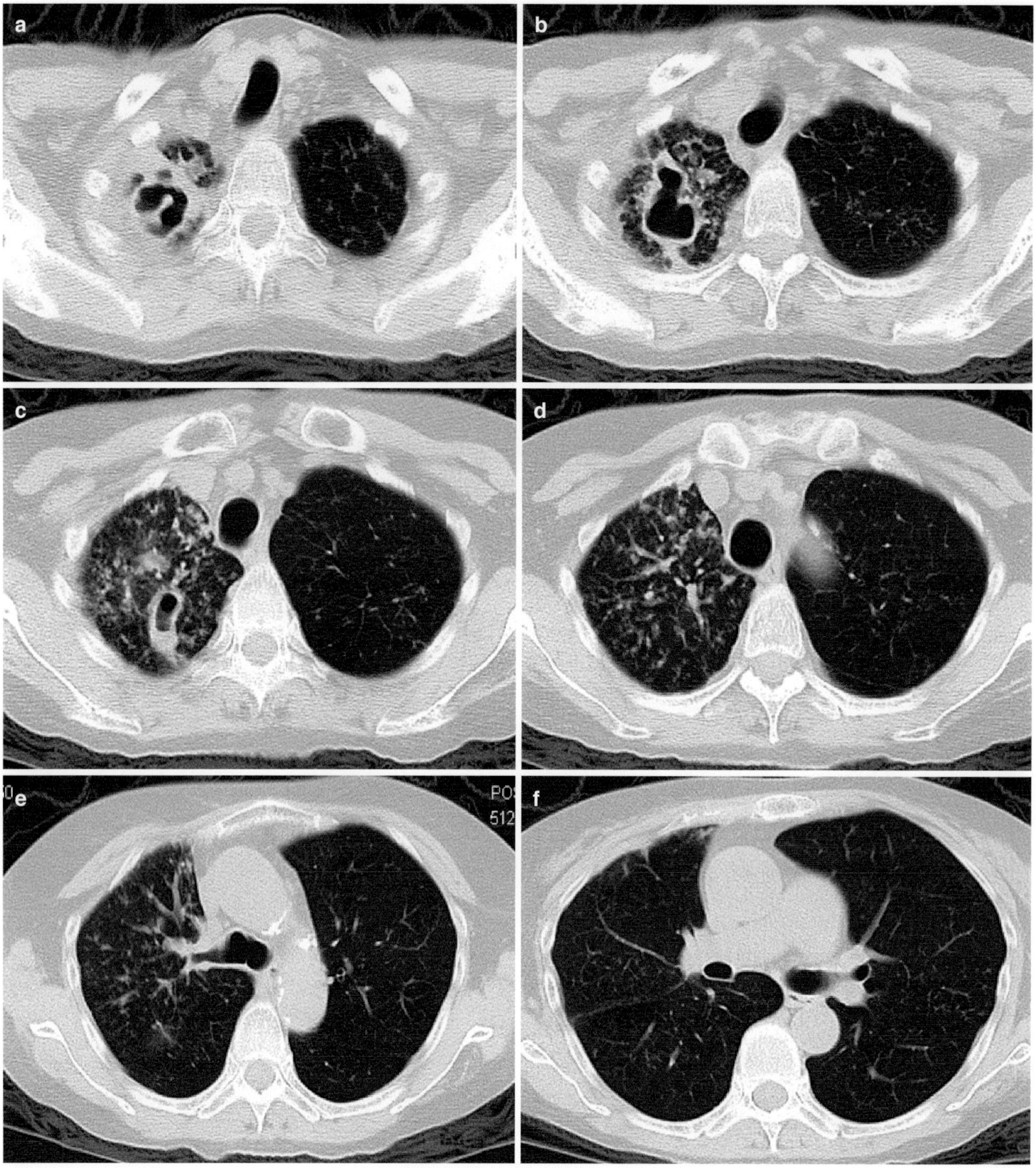

Fig. 7.10 (**a**–**r**) Primary poly-resistant TB in a 62-year-old woman, with resistance to isoniazid, levofloxacin, and moxifloxacin. Chief complaint of cough, expectoration, low fever, and hoarseness for more than 2 months. She had a history of diabetes for 5 years. (**a**–**h**) Chest CT scans on January 4, 2020, showed centrilobular nodules, tree-in-bud signs, and patchy opacities in both lungs, with thick-walled cavity in the right upper lobe; stenosis with thick wall was observed in the right upper bronchus, suggesting the presence of bronchial tuberculosis. (**i**–**p**) In comparison with CT scans on January 4, 2020, chest CT scans on March 24, 2020, showed the decreased number of lesions in both lungs, the decrease in the size of the cavity in the right upper lobe with the increased consolidation area around it, bronchial stenosis of the right upper bronchus with thicker wall was much more severe. (**q**, **r**) Fiberoptic bronchoscope showed bronchial tuberculosis in the right upper lobe (ulcerative necrotic type)

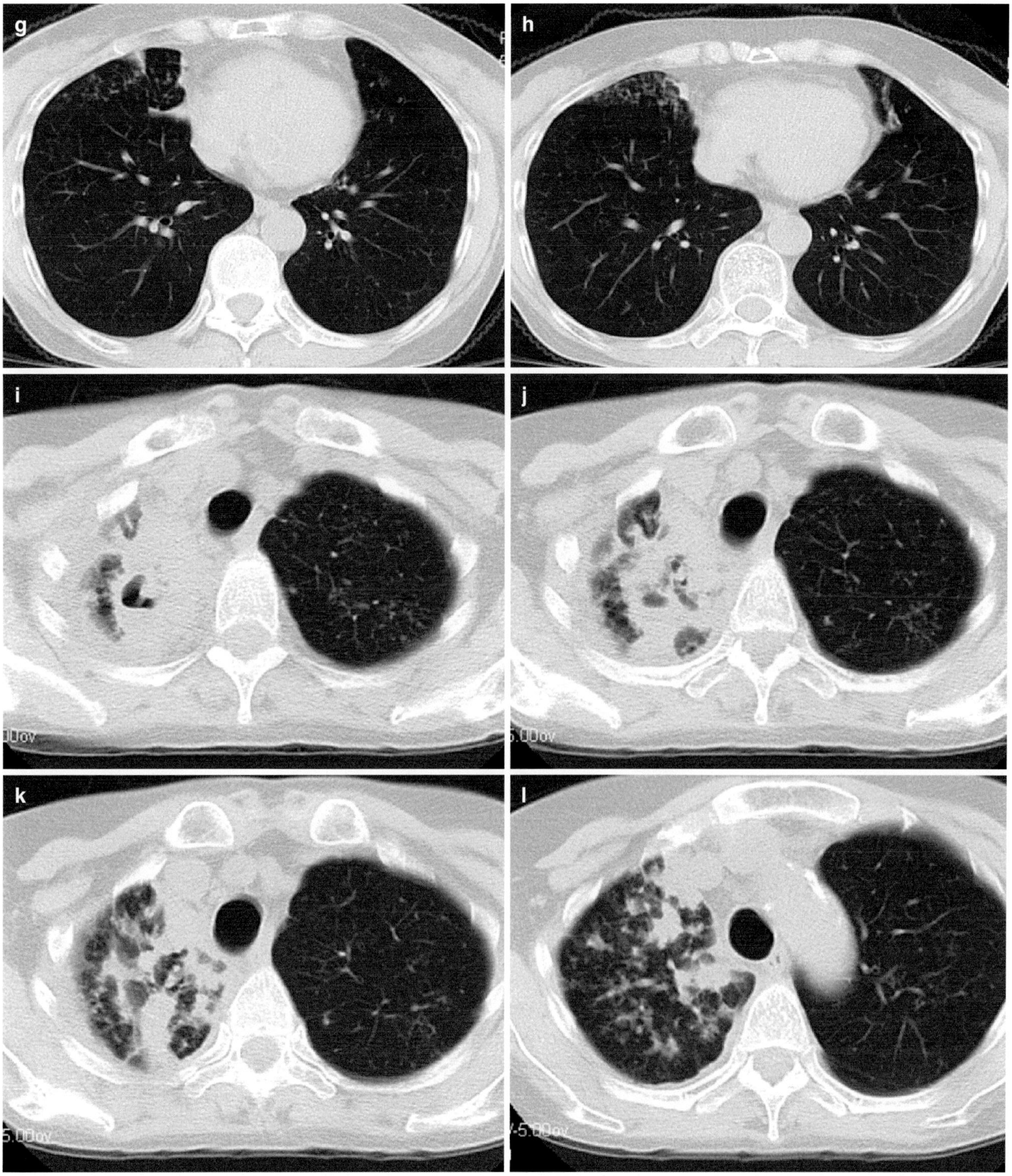

Fig. 7.10 (continued)

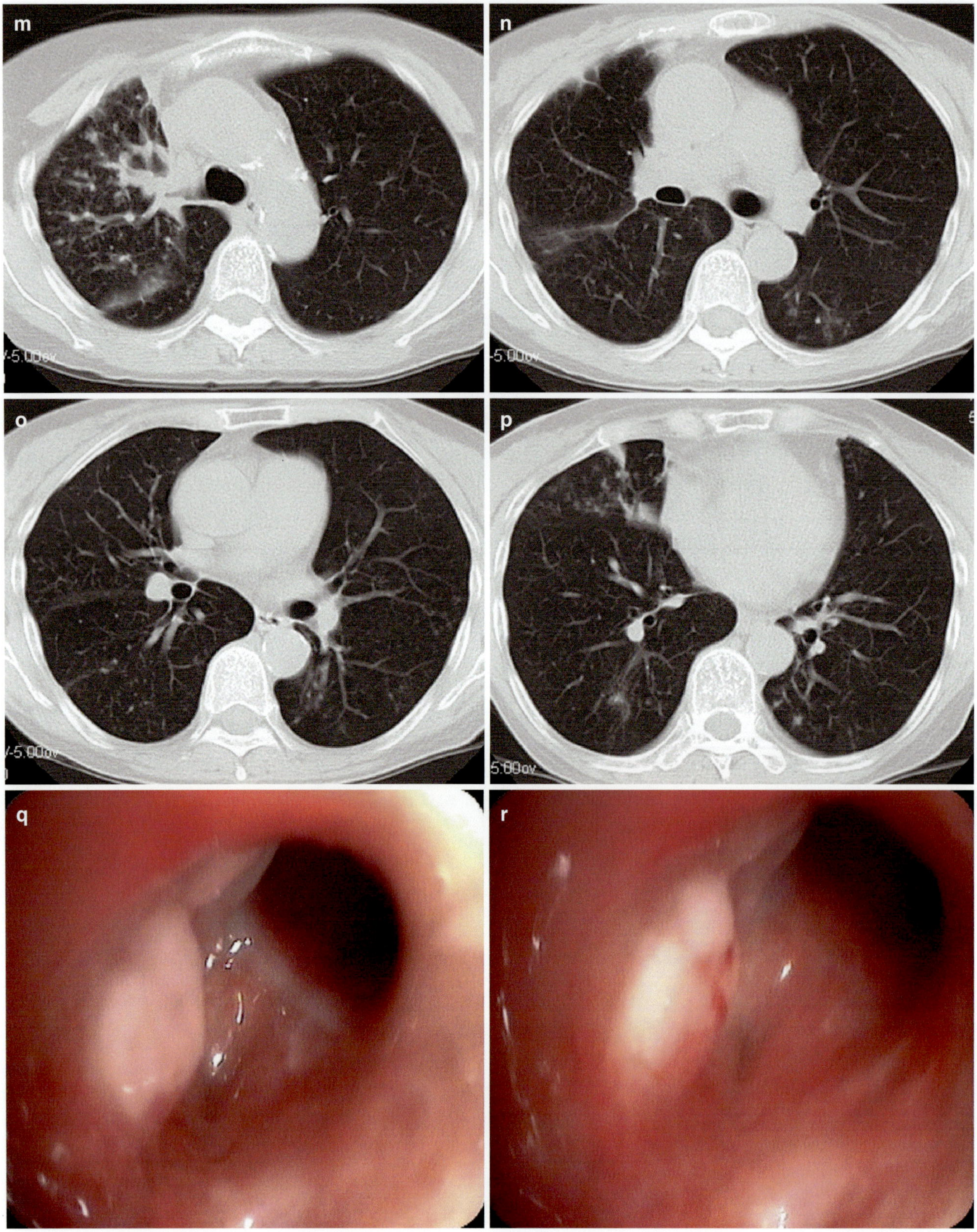

Fig. 7.10 (continued)

7.3 Introduction of Typical Cases of Poly-Resistant Pulmonary Tuberculosis

Case 1

Patient Guo XX, a 56-year-old-female, had paroxysmal cough without obvious inducement in April 2018, complicated with an expectoration of white sticky sputum. The patient did not seek systematic medical service. Since September, 2018, her cough had been aggravated significantly for 3 weeks in a row, complicated with shortness of breathe inducible even by slow walking, her amount of sputum had been increasing and the color of sputum had been turning yellow. Then she visited the local hospital for treatment and received Traditional Chinese Medicine treatment in the outpatient department, but there was no obvious amelioration of her symptoms, with exacerbation of her cough and short of breath. CT scans in the local hospital showed multiple lesions in both lungs with multiple cavities suspected to be pulmonary tuberculosis, and she was admitted into China Guangzhou Chest Hospital in October 2018. Since the onset of the disease, the patient has clear mind, good spirit, normal diet, good sleep, and normal urination and defecation. Her weight dropped by 4 kg during 6 months since April 2018. She had a history of diabetes for 12 years, without regular medication and blood glucose level controlled unsatisfactorily. She denied the history of cerebrovascular or mental diseases, and the history of blood transfusion. Her vaccination history was unknown, and she had no surgical trauma history or allergy history.

Physical examination at the admission in October 2018 showed the temperature of 36.5 °C, the pulse of 112 beats per minute, the respiratory rate of 22 per minute and the blood pressure of 127/90 mmHg. The chest seemed flat, with decreased respiratory sounds in both lungs and moist rales heard in both lower lungs. speech transmission was normal, without pleural friction sound in both lungs.

Blood-gas analysis at admission in October 2018 showed that partial pressure of oxygen was 7.81 kpa ↓, partial pressure of carbon dioxide was 5.18 kpa with pH value of 7.452 ↑, actual bicarbonate was 26.6 mmol/L, and blood residual alkali was 2.5 mmol/L. Blood routine: leukocyte 15.96×10^9/L ↑, neutrophil percentage 85.80% ↑, neutrophil count 13.69×10^9/L ↑, hemoglobin 110.0 g/L ↓. Procalcitonin <0.16 ng/mL; high sensitivity C-reactive protein <1.28 mg/L. CD4/CD8/CD3 cytology examination: normal.

Chest CT scans on October 9, 2018, suggested secondary pulmonary tuberculosis in both lungs with cavities in the right upper and lower lobes, and right pleurisy (right interlobular fissure effusion). Sputum smear: 3+ in Mycobacterium tuberculosis. Drug susceptibility test suggested the resistance to rifampicin, rifabutin, levofloxacin, and moxifloxacin. A regimen containing INH, EMB, PZA, and Pto was given.

However, the patient withdrew her medication by herself from her discharge to her admission for the second time in November 2020, during which she had recurrent symptoms including cough, expectoration, and short of breath.

Chest CT scans on April 11, 2019, showed the increase in lesions in the right middle lobe and anterior segment of the left upper lobe, the absorption of lesions in the right lower lobe, the apical posterior segment and lingual segment of the left upper lobe, the decreased size of the cavity in the right lung with thinner wall and the absorption of the right pleural effusion, in comparison with CT scans on April 11, 2019.

On October 20, 2020, she had cough and more expectoration than before without obvious inducement, the sputum was yellowish white without any odor. The patient felt shortness of breath after mild activity, but no chest pain, hemoptysis, or fever. The patient did not pay attention to it. Later, she felt severer shortness of breath than before for 4 days since November 7, 2020, with shortness of breath at rest, though she could lie down in supine position, with no nocturnal paroxysmal dyspnea, edema, palpitation, dizziness, headache, nausea, or vomiting. On November 11, 2020, she visited our hospital for emergent treatment and received treatment including anti-infection with "ceftriaxone tazobactam," diuresis, etc. However, her symptoms did not improve significantly and she was admitted to our hospital for further treatment. Examinations post to her admission included blood-gas analysis showing PO_2 9.96 KPa, PCO_2 3.80 KPa, and pH 7.322, which suggested the presence of hypoxemia, so oxygen inhalation was given. Blood routine showed WBC 23.43×10^9/L, NE% 89.10%, NE# 20.88×10^9/L, HGB 90.0 g/L, PLT 765.0×10^9/L, hs-CRP 116.69 mg/L, and PCT 8.21 ng/mL. No obvious abnormality was observed for CEA, AFP or coagulation routine. BUN: 20.29 mmol/L, CREA: 232.00 μmol/L, MYO μg/L, TNIU: 0.22 μg/L, PRO-BNP: 7617.00 pg/mL, GLU: 10.50 mmol/L, and BQDS: 0.40 mmol/L. Sputum smear showed 4+ for acid fast bacilli. Genetic detection for resistance in Mycobacterium tuberculosis showed the resistance to isoniazid, rifampicin, rifabutin, levofloxacin and moxifloxacin. So this case was a MDR-TB transformed from PDR-TB.

Chest CT scans on November 14, 2020, showed the significant increase in lesions in both lungs, enlargement of the cavity in the right lower lobe with liquid level inside, as compared with CT scans on April 11, 2019. After admission, the patient received anti-infection treatment with meropenem, together with expectorant, kidney protection, hypoglycemics, reduction of blood pressure, amelioration of circulation, and anti-heart failure therapy, plus an anti-tuberculosis treatment containing "H, Z, E, Pto, and Cfz", and her symptoms were ameliorated.

The patient insisted on regular treatment after this discharge, and chest CT scans on her return visit on October 22, 2021, showed (in comparison with scans on November 14,

2020): obvious absorption of pulmonary lesions and the general absorption of the right pleural effusion.

Discussion about Case 1

Brief history: the patient was an old female with a history of diabetes for 15 years, with glucose level control unsatisfactorily. Her history at the first admission into our hospital was episodic cough without obvious inducement half a year before, showing exacerbation for last three weeks complicated with progressive short of breath, with a proposed diagnosis of "pulmonary tuberculosis" by another hospital based on chest CT scans. The examination at admission included blood-gas analysis showing type I respiratory failure, and blood routine showing the increase in leukocyte, neutrophil percentage and neutrophil count, indicating the complication with bacterial infection, and the slight decrease in hemoglobin, suggesting the presence of anemia. Chest plain CT scans on October 9, 2018, showed multiple nodules, tree-in-bud signs, consolidation and ground glass exudation in both lungs, with one large thick-walled cavities, respectively, in the right upper and lower lobes. The lobar and segmental bronchi of the right upper lobe became narrow, and multiple mild mediastinal lymphadenectasis were found. There was effusion in the right pleural cavity. Susceptibility test result suggested resistance to rifampicin, rifabutin, levofloxacin and moxifloxacin, based on which a regimen was formulated by the attending physician, containing INH, EMB, PZA and Pto. Her disease was ameliorated post to treatment, and she was discharged. After discharge, however, the patient discontinued voluntarily his medication, resulting in recurrent cough, expectoration and shortness of breath. Chest CT scans on April 11, 2019, showed the increased number of lesions in the right middle lobe and the anterior segment of the left upper lobe, the decreased number of the rest of lesions, the shrinkage of cavities in the right lung, and the decreased effusion in the right pleural cavity, in comparison with CT scans on October 9, 2018.The patient was admitted again into our hospital by emergency department in November 2020, with a chief complaint of cough, increased expectoration and exacerbation of shortness of breath. Examination at admission: blood-gas analysis indicated hypoxemia, and blood routine examination indicated the presence of bacterial infection and moderate anemia. In addition, the results of laboratory examination indicated also that the patient had elevated blood glucose and cardiac and renal dysfunction. Compared with her previous results, Mycobacterium tuberculosis increased in the sputum (4+), and the results of drug resistance gene detection of Mycobacterium tuberculosis showed that there emerged isoniazid-resistant gene on the basis of the original drug resistance. Results of chest CT scans on November 14, 2020, in comparison with the scans on April 11, 2019 showed the number of lesions in both lungs increased significantly, cavitation newly occurred in the right middle lobe and the left upper lobe, the cavity in the right lower lung was enlarged with the emergence of liquid level inside, the cavity in the right upper lobe decreased in size and the bronchial lumen of the right upper lung was narrower than before. The patient post to admission received treatment including resisting infection, reducing phlegm, protecting the kidney, lowering blood sugar, lowering blood pressure, improving circulation, and resisting heart failure, plus the anti-tuberculosis treatment containing "H, Z, E, Pto, and Cfz", and she was discharged after her symptoms were relieved. The patient insisted on regular treatment after discharge. On October 22, 2021, she returned to the hospital for chest CT scanning with the results showing that (compared with the CT scans on November 14, 2020): the lesions in the lung were absorbed obviously, there was the collapse of distal pulmonary tissue of the right upper lung, the right pleura became thinner than before, and the right pleural effusion was absorbed basically.

Poly-resistant tuberculosis (PDR-TB) is defined as the mycobacterium tuberculosis infecting a pulmonary tuberculosis patient and confirmed by drug susceptibility testing (DST) in vitro to be resistant simultaneously to more than 1 anti-tuberculosis drugs not including simultaneously isoniazid (INH) and rifampicin (RFP). The result of drug susceptibility test at her first admission in this case showed resistance to rifampicin, rifabutin, levofloxacin and moxifloxacin, which was consistent with the diagnosis of PDR-TB. According to the medical history of the patient, the course of disease was long with extensive pulmonary lesions, which caused severe chronic invasion and damage to the bronchus. The clinical symptoms of the patient, therefore, are mainly symptoms of irritation of respiratory tract, i.e., cough and expectoration [25], complicated with symptoms such as obvious shortness of breath. Because the patient had a prolonged history of diabetes with her blood glucose controlled poorly and she did not adhere to the regular treatment of PDR-TB after discharge, the clinical symptoms were recurrent and she was admitted into our hospital for several times due to cough and expectoration with aggravation of shortness of breath. As reported in literature, diabetes not only increases the risks of active tuberculosis, but also correlates to drug-resistant tuberculosis, which is probably related to metabolism, molecular immunity and gene polymorphism [26]. Moreover, because of the poorly controlled diabetes, obvious bacterial infection was complicated in this patient as confirmed by laboratory test at her every admission into the hospital. Multiple pulmonary infections complicated with anemia resulted in obvious shortness of breath and type I respiratory failure as confirmed by blood-gas analysis. The patients did not adhere to the regular treatment of PDR-TB in the early stage, which also led to the continued mutation of drug resistance genes, with the newly added target genes for resistance to isoniazid and the transformation from the former PDR-TB into multidrug-resistant tuberculosis (abbreviated as MDR-TB as follows), suggesting further that insufficient treatment is an important pathogenic factor of drug-resistant tuberculosis [27].

The chest CT findings of the patient were characteristic PDR-TB.

1. It had the common characteristic of all smear-positive pulmonary tuberculosis: results of multiple CT re-examinations before the end of the treatment showed dominantly the typical manifestations of active pulmonary tuberculosis including centrilobular nodules, tree-in-bud signs, consolidations, multiple cavities, bronchial wall thickening with lumen stenosis and dilatation (Figs. 7.11a–h, 7.12a–h and 7.13a–h). There were fewer calcified foci. In CT scans of 2018, 2019, and 2020, the mediastinal window showed no definite calcified foci in the pulmonary lesions. The last CT scans showed that under the condition of significant amelioration of pulmonary lesions, a few calcified foci appeared within the pulmonary lesions (Fig. 7.14g, h).
2. Lesions in pulmonary tuberculosis was extensive and involved all lung lobes, including sites not commonly involved by tuberculosis, such as the anterior segment of the right upper lobe, the right middle lobe, the basal segments of both lower lungs, the lingual segment and anterior segment of left upper lung, which was considered to be caused by extensive intra-pulmonary dissemination due to the high load of Mycobacterium tuberculosis in the sputum (3+ ~ 4+), the prolonged course of disease, and the recurrent disease. According to literatures [28, 29], pulmonary tuberculosis patients complicated with diabetes in comparison with those without this complication have a higher risk of emergence of lesions in lower pulmonary lobes, especially in patients with their blood glucose controlled poorly. Pulmonary dissemination in this patient not only occurred in the common sites for pulmonary tuberculosis such as both upper lobes and the dorsal segments in the lower lobes, but also involved extensively the right middle lobe, the lingual segment in the left upper lobe, and basal segments of both lower lobes in the inferior lung field, which was consistent with literatures.
3. There are many cavities (>3), and all of them are thick wall cavities, consistent with literatures reported [17–22]. The risk of drug resistance in pulmonary tuberculosis is related closely to the bacterial load, and high concentration of bacterial load increases the possibility of the establishment of drug-resistant bacterial population, thereby promoting spontaneous gene mutation to produce drug resistance. The high load of Mycobacterium tuberculosis in the tuberculous cavity is an important way for the dissemination of Mycobacterium tuberculosis and is also considered to be the biological basis to generate drug resistance in pulmonary tuberculosis [30]. It has been pointed out [28, 29] that the risk of cavitation increases in diabetes patients with their glucose level controlled poorly. Our case was also a patient with her blood glucose controlled poorly, so multiple thick-walled cavities appeared in both lungs, which was consistent with the literatures. Multiple cavities in the lung led to not only the continuous bacterial excretion and wide dissemination in the lung but also the high Mycobacterium tuberculosis load (3+ ~ 4+) in the sputum of the patient. As a result of the continuous high bacterial load in the patient, a new target gene for isoniazid resistance emerged in the late stage of disease development, with a transformation from PDR-TB to MDR-TB. It can be inferred that tuberculosis cavitation is one of the important factors resulting in drug resistance, and diabetes is one of the vital conditions promoting the genesis and development of this factor.
4. Bronchial stenosis with bronchiectasis. The patient did not undergo bronchoscopy during the treatment, but her CT scan findings showed thickening of the wall in each lobar and segmental bronchus in both lungs, with bronchial stenosis, pulmonary consolidation and reduction of volume in the right upper lobe, basal segments in the right lower lobe (Fig. 7.11b, j, 7.12a, b, 7.13c, f, g), considering probably the complication of bronchial tuberculosis based on image findings. Multiple scattered bronchiectases were seen in both lung lesions, which was considered to be the reason for the prolonged course of disease, delayed healing, presence of multiple pulmonary lesions and persistent high excretion of bacteria, resulting in chronic invasion and severe damage to the bronchus. Airway injury is an important risk factor, as shown by study [31], for drug-resistant pulmonary tuberculosis to happen in patients. At the same time, it is considered that drug resistance is related to thickening and stenosis of trachea and bronchus. Thickening and stenosis of bronchial wall may cause poor sputum excretion, and Mycobacterium tuberculosis multiplying continuously will increase the quantity of bacteria and raise the probability of drug resistance. The emergence of drug-resistant bacteria which cannot be eradicated will aggravate further airway injury. So these two factors may be reciprocal causation.
5. Waxing and waning of pulmonary lesions. Due to the failure to receive treat as required, the chest CT scans of this PDR-TB patient with diabetes in April 2019 in comparison with the CT scans in October 2018 showed that the number of some lesions in lung tissues increased, some pulmonary lesions were absorbed, and pleural effusion decreased; CT scans in November, 2020 showed an obvious increase in the number of pulmonary lesions, the raised number of cavities and the stenosis of bronchial

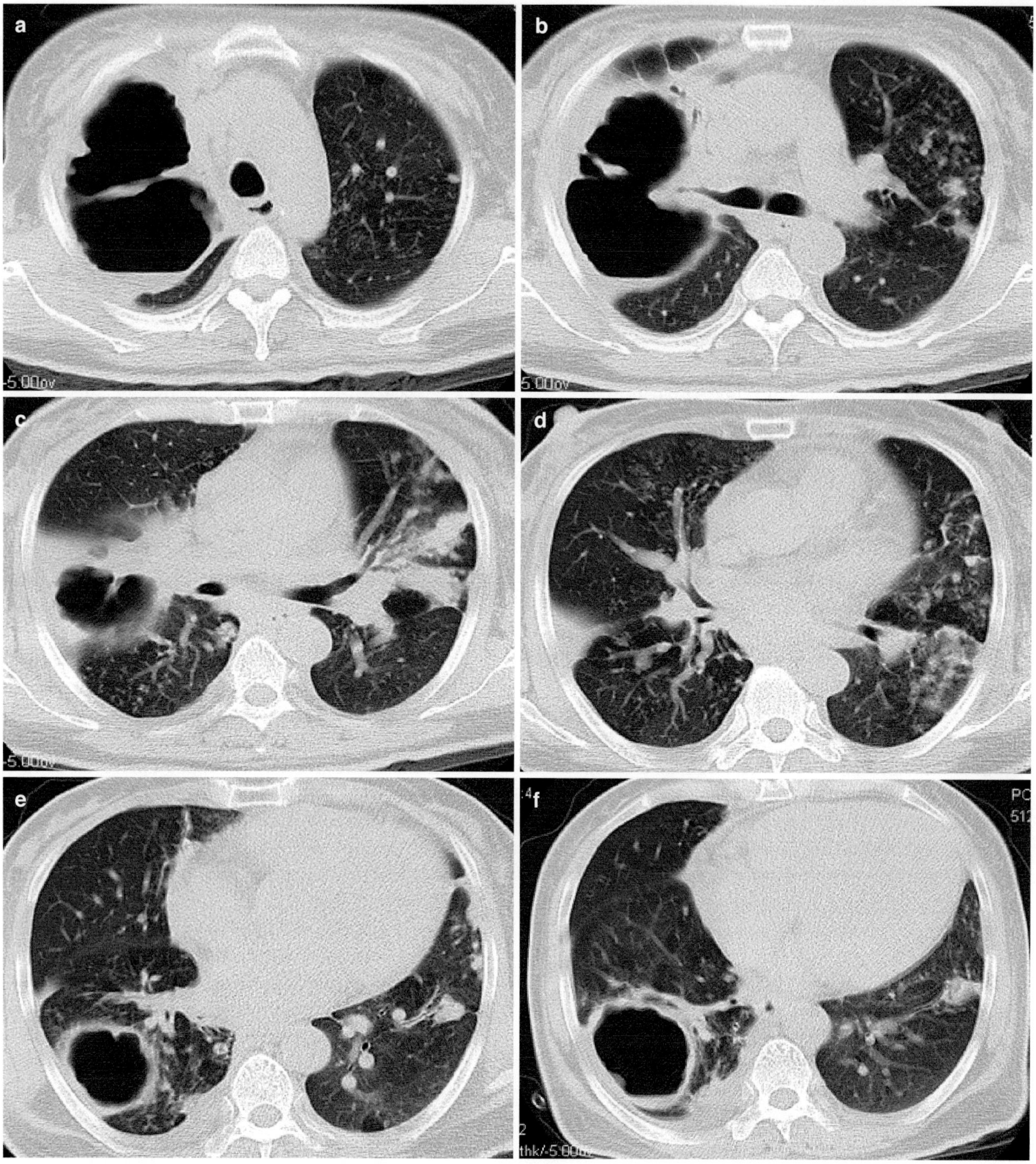

Fig. 7.11 (**a**–**j**) Chest CT scans on October 9, 2018, showed multiple nodules, tree-in-bud signs, consolidations, and ground glass opacities in both lungs, with one large cavity, respectively, in the right upper and lower lobes. The stenosis was observed for lobar and segmental bronchi in the right upper lobe. Multiple mild lymphadenectasis within mediastinum, with their shorter diameter <1.3 cm. Effusion was observed for the right pleural cavity, with the slightly widened right interlobar fissure

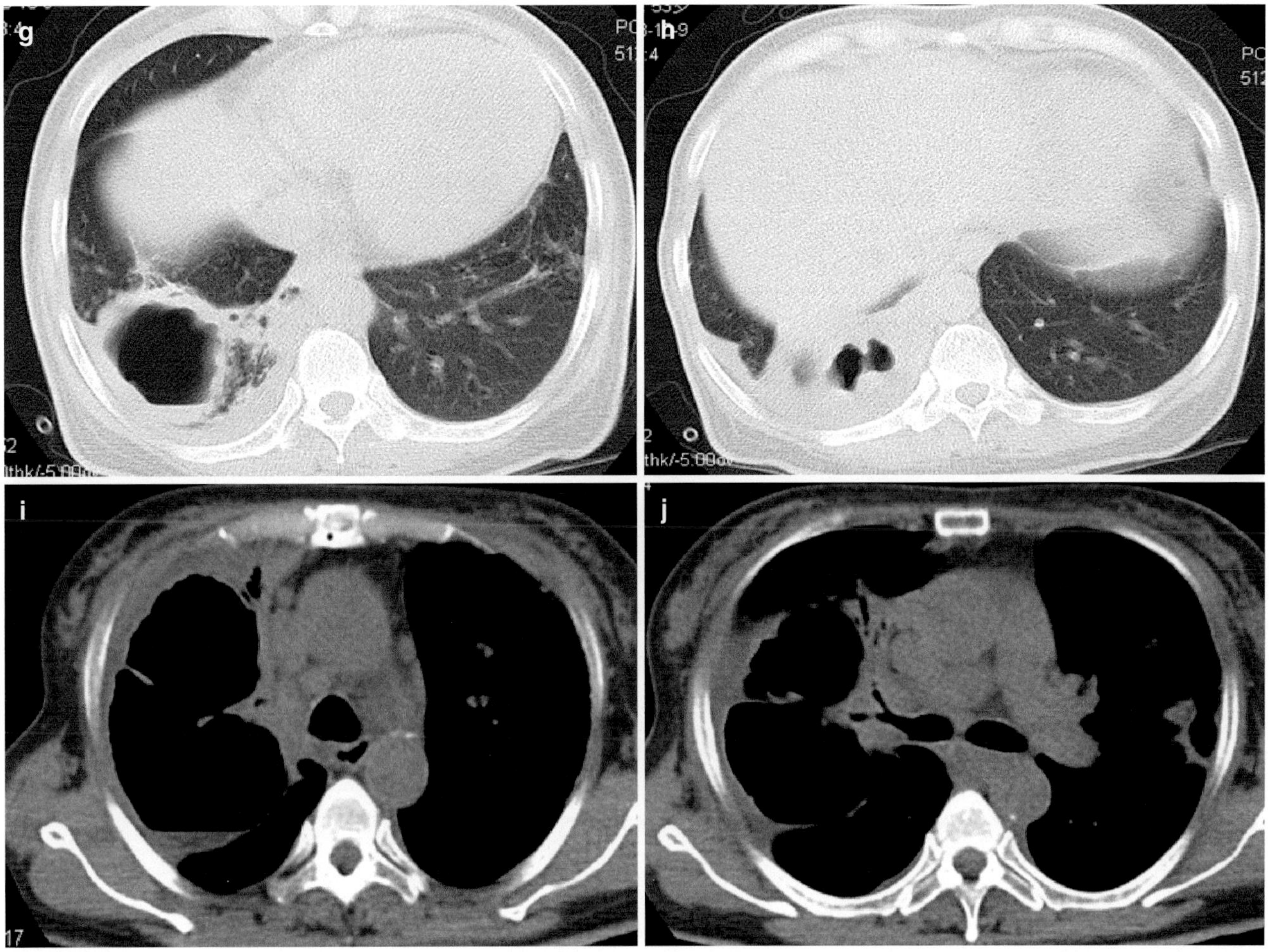

Fig. 7.11 (continued)

lumen than before. After receiving her regular treatment in 2021 as required by the regimen confirmed by susceptibility test with blood glucose level controlled, on the contrary, the lesions in the lung were obviously absorbed, most of the cavities disappeared, and the wall of the diseased bronchial tube became thinner and smoother than before. Therefore, PDR-TB has the possibility of being cured through regular treatment using regimen based susceptibility test and active control of blood glucose.

6. Among several CT scans for this patient, the scans in 2018 showed multiple lymphadenectasis with the shorter diameter <1.3 cm without calcification in mediastinum and at both hila, while CT scans from 2019 to 2021 showed only small lymph nodes with the shorter diameter <1 cm without calcification in mediastinum and both hila, which was consistent with characteristics of image findings of PDR-TB that we summarized before.

Experience in diagnosis based on clinical, laboratory and imaging features: PDR-TB patients are characterized in prolonged disease course, easily recurrence, vulnerability to multiple infections if complicated with diabetes, severe clinical symptoms, and high load of Mycobacterium tuberculosis in sputum. Image findings of PDR-TB patients complicated with diabetes are characterized in: (1) manifestations of active tuberculosis such as centrilobular nodules, tree-in-bud signs, consolidations, multiple cavities, and thickening of bronchial wall with stenosis and expansion of the lumen, (2) extensive tuberculosis lesions, involving easily the lower lung fields; (3) multiple cavitations with thick-walled cavities, and consolidations with cavities; (4) airway involvement easily observed, and vulnerability to bronchial stenosis and bronchiectasis; (5) tendentiousness of waxing and waning or progressive increase in number of pulmonary lesions if the regimen is not based on susceptibility test results. Golden standard of diagnosis for PDR-TB, however, is to be established upon result of susceptibility test for sputum tubercle bacillus.

Case 2

Chen xx, a 34-year-old male, was diagnosed as bronchial tuberculosis with (+) in sputum smear with a chief complaint

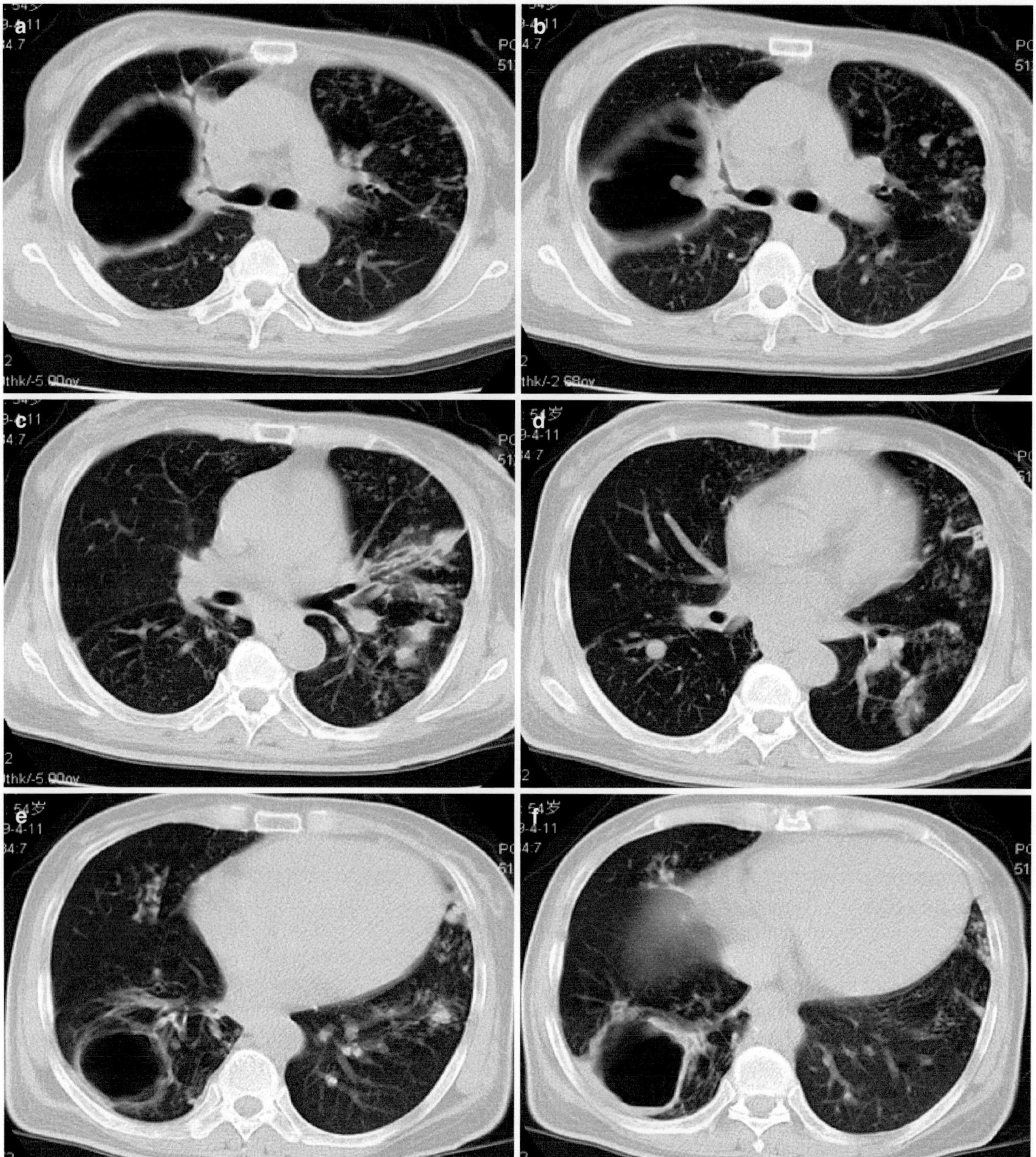

Fig. 7.12 (**a**–**h**) Chest CT scans on April 11, 2019, showed tuberculosis in both lungs, with cavities in the right upper and lower lobes and the right pleurisy, complicated with infection in the right lower lobe. Chest CT scans on April 11, 2019, showed the increase in lesions in the right middle lobe and anterior segment of the left upper lobe, the decrease of number of nodules, tree-bud-signs and consolidation in the right lower lobe, the apical posterior segment and lingual segment of the left upper lobe, the decreased size of the cavity in the right lung with thinner wall and the absorption of the right pleural effusion, in comparison with CT scans on April 11, 2019

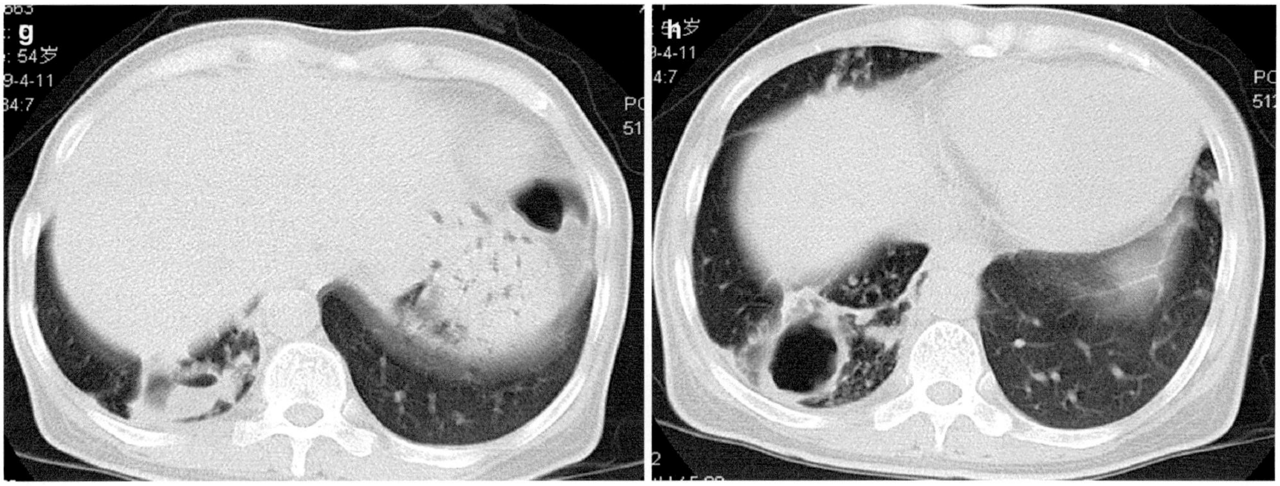

Fig. 7.12 (continued)

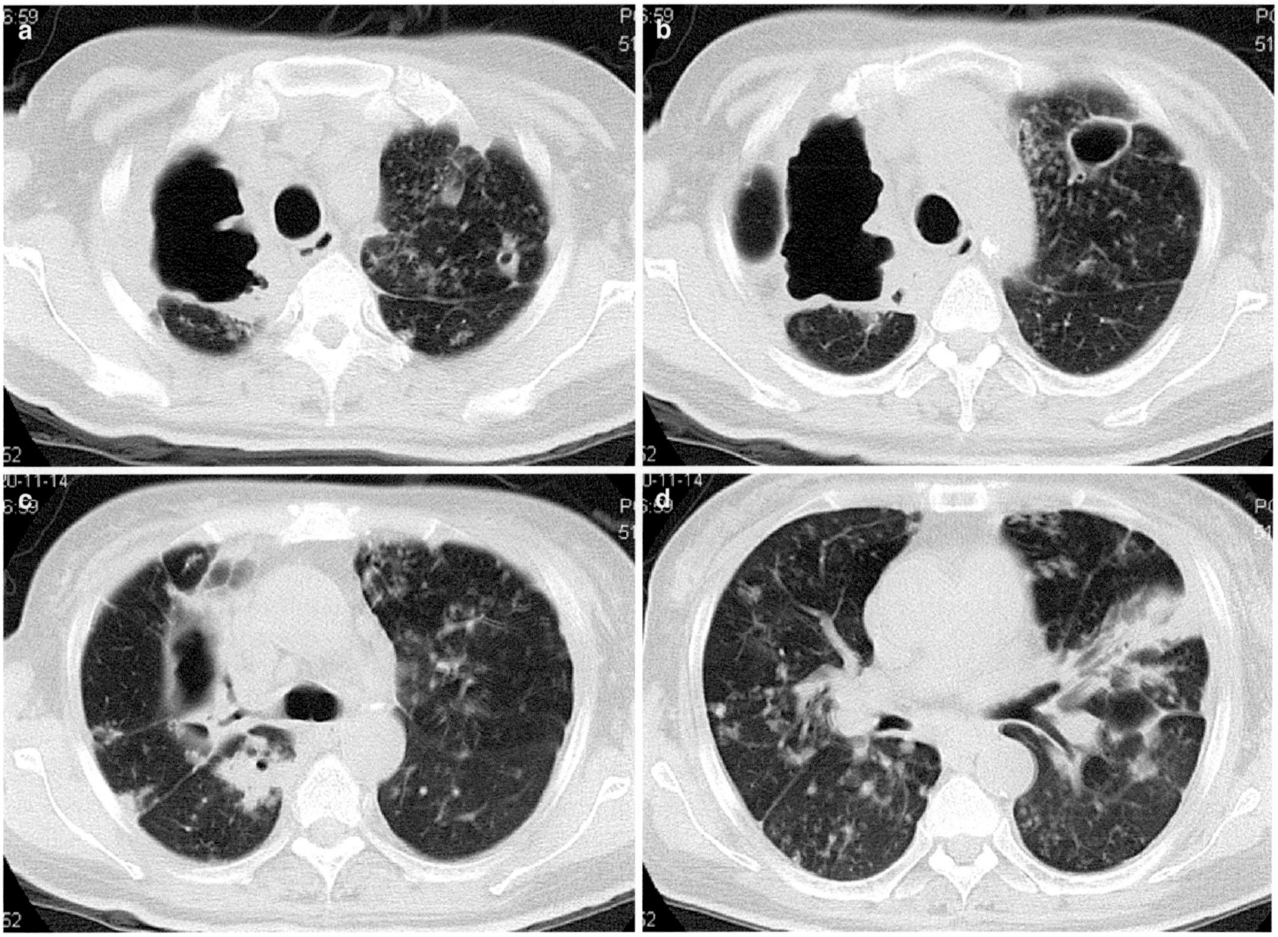

Fig. 7.13 (**a**–**h**) Compared with CT scans on April 11, 2019, chest CT scans on November 14, 2020, showed the significant increase in lesions in both lungs including nodules, tree-in-bud signs and consolidations, new emergence of cavities in the right middle lobe and the left upper lobe, enlargement of the cavity in the right lower lobe with liquid level inside, the shrinkage of the cavity in the right upper lobe, and narrowing of the bronchial lumen with thinner wall in the right upper lobe

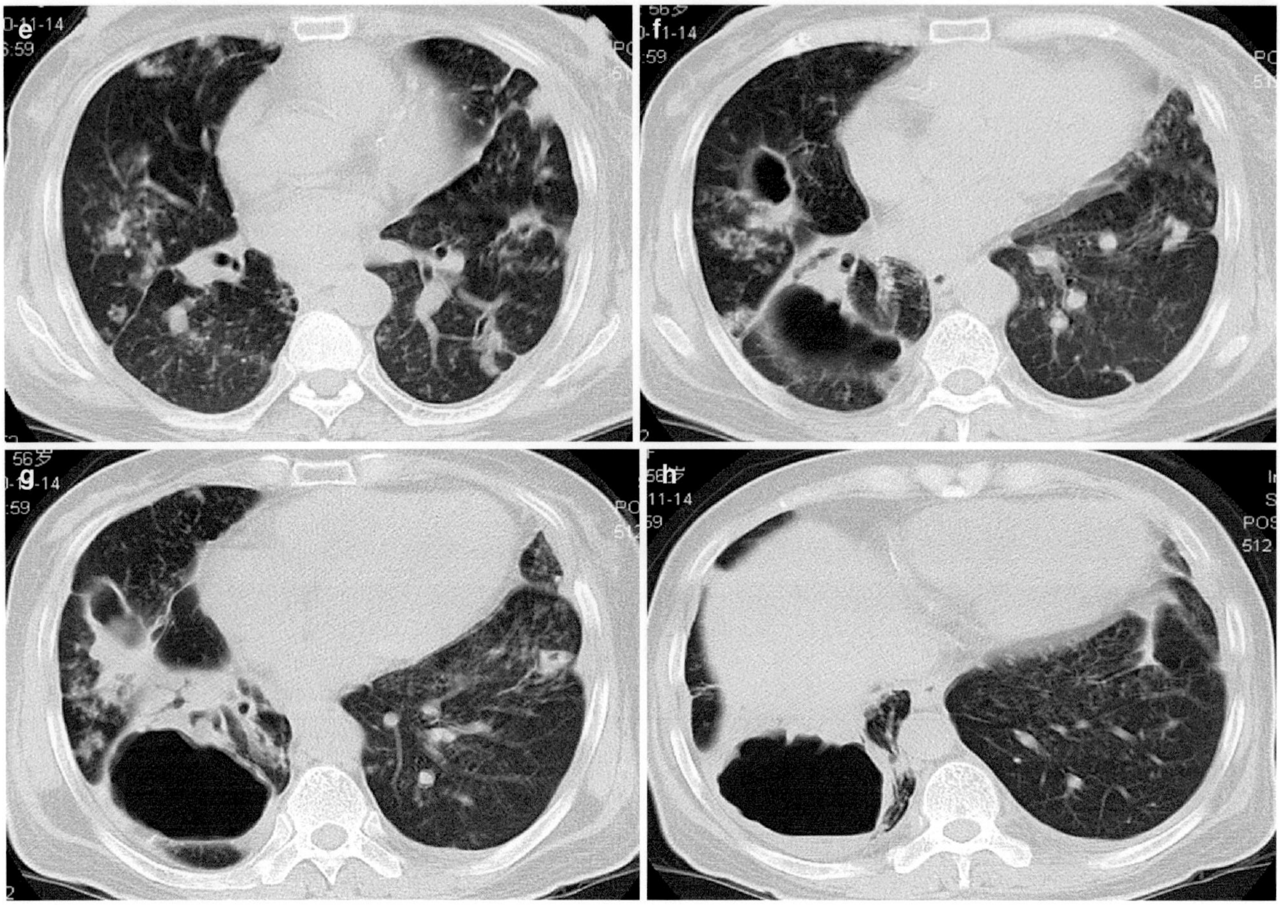

Fig. 7.13 (continued)

of cough with shortness of breath in March 2013, and an anti-tuberculosis treatment of HRZE plus levofloxacin was launched on March 5, 2013.

Since the onset of the disease, the patient had clear mind, good spirit, normal diet, good sleep, normal urination and stool, without significant change in body weight. The patient was a carrier of hepatitis B virus with a history of diabetes for 2 years. At present, he received the treatment using "Yilikang" that he purchased by himself, and the glucose level was not controlled well. Unknown vaccination history; he denied the history of hypertension or coronary heart disease. He denied the history of "hepatitis or tuberculosis" and any other infectious diseases, the history of trauma or operation, the history of blood transfusion, the history of food and drug allergy. Born and living in the country of origin, he had no history of exposure to epidemic water or radioactive substances, and no history of long-term exposure to dust. He had been addicted to smoking for 18 years consuming about 2 packs/day and addicted to beer for 2 years consuming about 4–5 bottles/day, and had given up more than 1 year before. He denied the history of venereal diseases.

Physical examination at admission in March 2013 showed normal thorax and costal space, with bilateral symmetrical breasts, without obvious abnormality; normal respiratory movement with normal rhythm. Normal speech tremor, no pleural friction or subcutaneous twisting sensation. There was no sternal percussion pain, with clear percussion of both lungs. The lower boundary of the left lung was located in the 6th intercostal space along the middle clavicular line, the 8th intercostal along of the middle axillary line, and the 10th intercostal space of the scapular line. The percussion of the lower boundary of the right lung was unclear, with the movement of the lower boundary of the lung between 6 and 8 cm. The breath sounds of both lungs were slightly harsh, and wet rales were heard in the upper and lower lobes of the right lung, without dry rales. The speech conduction was normal, and pleural friction sound was heard in the right lower lung. Body temperature was 36.5 °C, pulse 85 beats/min, respiration 19/min, and blood pressure 120/80 mmHg. Normal development, moderate nutrition, appearance of chronic disease, active posture, consciousness, normal expression, and cooperative in physical examination.

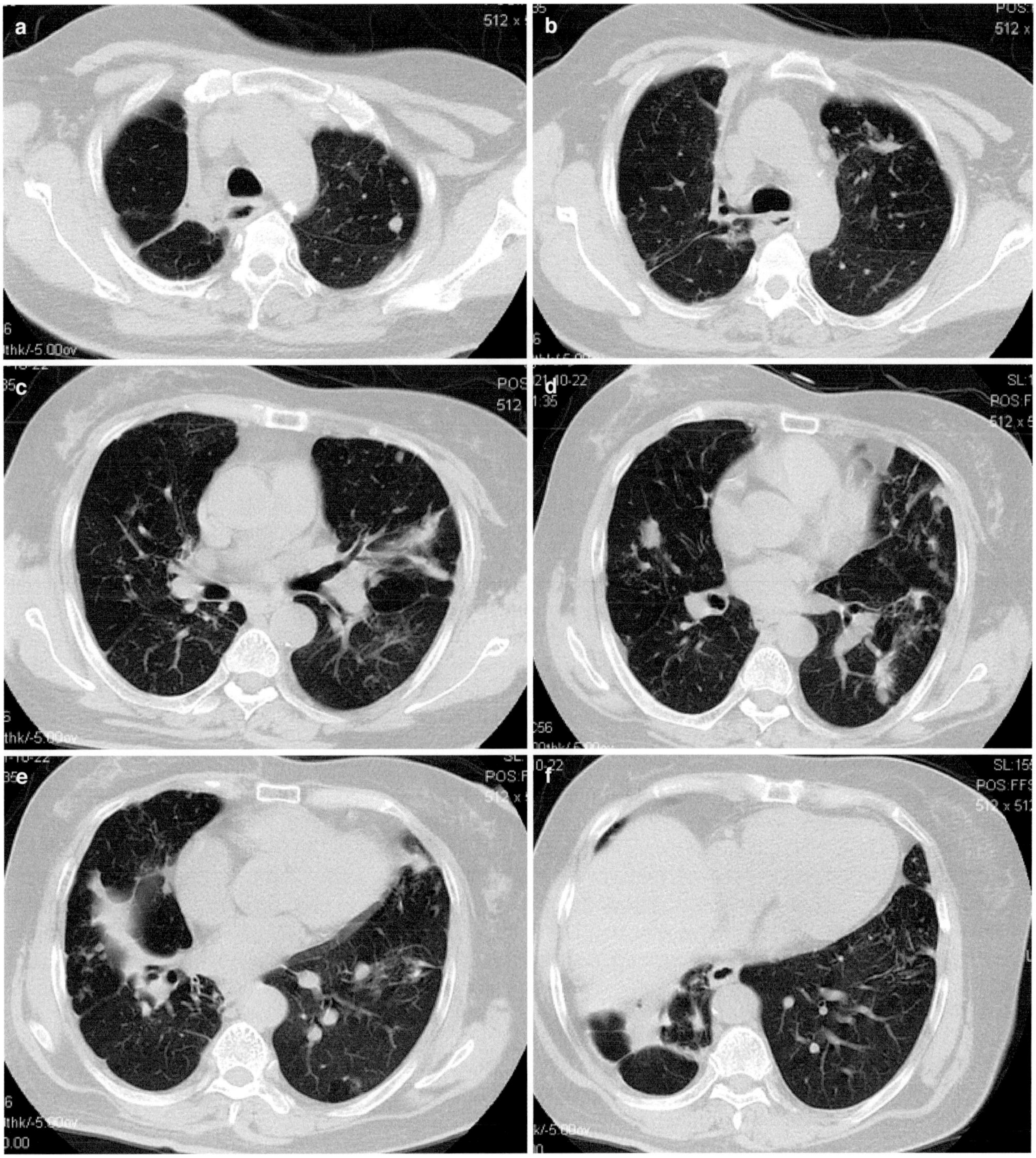

Fig. 7.14 (**a**–**h**) Chest CT scans on October 22, 2021, showed (in comparison to scans on November 14, 2020): obvious absorption of lesions in both lungs, including the narrowing of the right upper bronchus with collapse of distal pulmonary tissue in the right upper lobe, disappearance of intra-pulmonary cavities, the emergence of calcification within some of lesions in the left lung, and general absorption of the right pleural effusion was observed

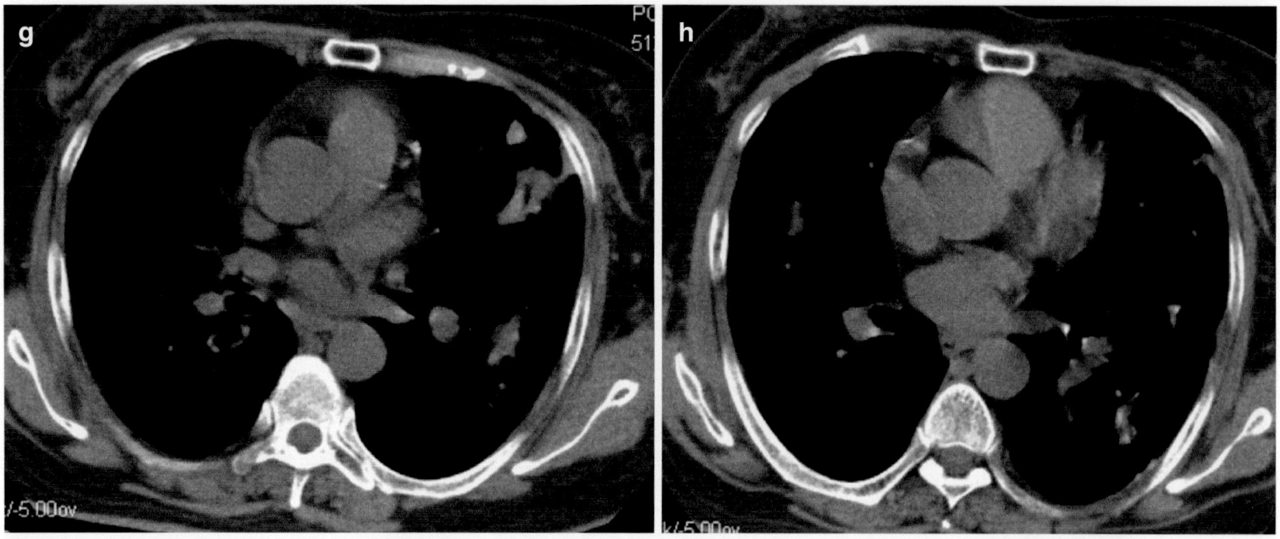

Fig. 7.14 (continued)

Examinations were completed in March 2013, including blood routine: white blood cells [WBC] 10.00 × 10^9/L ↑, Lymphocyte count [LY#] 0.79 × 10^9/L ↓, monocyte ratio [MO%] 10.30% ↑, neutrophil ratio [NE%] 80.50%↑, neutrophil count [NE#] 8.05 × 10^9/L ↑, hemoglobin [HGB] 120.0 g/L ↓, hematocrit [HCT] 0.354 ↓, mean corpuscular volume [MCV] 79.2fl ↓, immature granulocyte count 0.030 × 10^9/L ↑, and blood sedimentation [ESR] 62 mm/h ↑. Biochemistry: C-reactive protein [CRP] 86.00 mg/L ↑, uric acid [UA] 199 μmol/L ↓, total protein [TP] 62.3 g/L ↓, albumin [ALB] 33.0 g/L ↓, prealbumin [PA] 100.0 mg/L ↓, transferrin [TRF] 128.1 mg/dL ↓, sodium [NA] 130.5 mmol/L ↓, chlorine [CL] 95.0 mmol/L ↓, glucose (random) [GLU] 23.70 mmol/L ↑. Determination of glucose (fasting) + serum β- Hydroxybutyric acid determination: glucose [GLU] 14.30 mmol/L ↑, glycosylated hemoglobin [HbA1c] 12.65% ↑; blood gas and coagulation were generally normal. Antigen/antibody examination of hepatitis B showed positiveness in HBsAg, HbeAb and HbcAb. Positiveness (4+) was confirmed for acid fast bacteria in sputum smear, with positiveness in sputum TB-RNA, but negativeness in sputum TB-DNA.

Chest CT scans on March 8, 2013, showed bilateral pulmonary tuberculosis with multiple cavities, infections, mild mediastinal lymphadenectasis, and bilateral pleuritis.

Fiberoptic bronchoscopy on April 15, 2013, showed right upper bronchial tuberculosis, with cicatricial stenosis in the apical and frontal segmental subbronchi of the right upper lobe.

The drug susceptibility result on March 16, 2013, showed resistance to isoniazid, pyrazinamide and streptomycin, and susceptibility to rifampicin, ethambutol, rifabutin, amikacin, levofloxacin, moxifloxacin, pasiniazide, and isonicotinamide propionate, and the patient was diagnosed as pulmonary tuberculosis (poly-resistant), bronchial tuberculosis, and carriers of hepatitis B virus. He received an anti-tuberculosis regimen containing pasiniazide + amikacin + levofloxacin + ethambutol + rifabutin, and the concomitant hypoglycemic therapy with insulin and Acarbose Tablets and was discharged after his symptoms were relieved.

The patient did not adhere to regular anti-tuberculosis treatment, however, as prescribed by the physician, and he had recurrent cough and shortness of breath. He re-visited our outpatient department when his symptoms became severe, and sputum bacteria showed persistent positiveness. He received anti-tuberculosis, anti-inflammation and symptomatic treatment. In September 2014 the patient had recurrent shortness of breath again, which aggravated especially after the exertion, with intermittent cough and less sputum, but without chest tightness, chest pain, palpitation, fever or night sweats, but the patient did not paid attention to and did not receive any treatment. On December 20, 2014, the patient had obvious shortness of breath when he climbed the stairs to the second floor, then he visited our outpatient department and was admitted for further treatment. Since the onset of the disease, the patient had clear mind, good spirit, normal diet, good sleep, normal urination and stool, without significant change in body weight. Body temperature was 36.5 °C, pulse 85 beats/min, respiration 19/min, and blood pressure 120/80 mmHg. Normal development, moderate nutrition, appearance of chronic disease, active posture, consciousness, normal expression, and cooperative in physical examination. The breath sounds of both lungs were slightly harsh, and wet rales were heard in the upper and lower lobes of the right lung , without dry rales. The speech conduction was normal, and pleural friction sound was heard in the right lower lung.

Re-examination of chest CT scans on February 3, 2015, showed bilateral pulmonary tuberculosis with multiple cavities and infections in both lungs, mediastinal lymphadenectasis and bilateral pleurisy. In comparison with CT scans on December 30, 2014, lesions in both lungs were absorbed, the size of the cavities shrank, and lumen of each segmental bronchus in the right upper lobe became slightly narrower.

Fiberoptic bronchoscopy on January 4, 2015, showed that the mucosa of each segmental bronchus in the right upper lobe was congested and swollen, with the cicatricial stenosis at the opening of the apical segment and the opening of the anterior subbranch branch, and the stenosis aggravated than before.

After discharge, the patient still did not receive regular anti-tuberculosis treatment as prescribed by the physician. In April 2017, he was admitted again. After discharge, the patient withdrew the medicine on his own, and his cough and expectoration were still obvious.

In March 2020, the shortness of breath of the patients aggravated again and kept becoming worse, which might occur when going upstairs or taking bath and might be relieved after rest in supine position. He could lie flat without night paroxysmal dyspnea. With intermittent cough, he had expectoration with more yellow sticky sputum, which was not easy to expectorate. He had no chills, fever, chest pain, or hemoptysis, and then he was admitted for further treatment. In comparison with images on January 5, 2017, re-examination of chest CT scans on July 8, 2020, showed the obvious absorption of lesions in both lungs, and a residue cavity was observed in the right upper lobe with an aspergilloma formed inside. The rest of the pulmonary cavities disappeared.

As of press time, he is still under regular treatment, but the effect was unsatisfactory.

Discussion

The patient, a middle-aged male, had a history of diabetes for 2 years with his blood glucose controlled unsatisfactorily. The results of drug susceptibility of sputum Mycobacterium tuberculosis in the first admission showed the resistance to isoniazid, pyrazinamide, and streptomycin, so this case was consistent with the diagnosis of PDR-TB. With a prolonged course of the disease, the patient had the dominant clinical symptoms including cough and short of breath, considered to be related to extensive distribution of pulmonary lesions, high load of tubercle bacillus in sputum, which predisposed bronchi and pulmonary tissues to prolonged invasion. The patient was often complicated with bacterial infection due to poorly controlled blood glucose and lowered value of CD4/CD8/CD3 lymphocytes.

Evolution of chest CT scans for the drug-resistant pulmonary tuberculosis of this patient had the characteristics as follows:

1. CT scans prior to treatment (March 8, 2013) showed active pulmonary tuberculosis in both lungs including multiple consolidations/exudation, centrilobular nodules, tree-in-bud signs, cavities and consolidations with cavities (Fig. 7.15a–j), with mild enhancement of pulmonary lesions (Fig. 7.15k, l). The lumen of the anterior and apical bronchi in the right upper lung was slightly narrowed, with their inner wall not so smooth, without bronchiectasis sign in both lungs. The right pleura was slightly thickened, with effusion in the right pleural cavity. These findings indicated that the patient's pulmonary foci at this stage were in an acute exudative phase. Through observation, we found that the consolidation/exudation and consolidation with cavities in lungs of the patient accounted for a high percentage during this period and were scattered in lobes of both lungs. A study [24] explained that the reasons for the above manifestations may be the number of CD4 + CD25 + Foxp3 + T lymphocytes and levels detected for transforming growth factor β1 (TGF-β1) and interleukin-10 (IL-10), which were much higher in drug-resistant pulmonary tuberculosis patients than in those with nondrug-resistant disease. As a result, the cellular immunity of the body was weakened, and the invasiveness of DR-TB patients against drug-resistant tuberculosis bacteria was suppressed. It caused the invasion of drug-resistant TB bacteria to the lung tissue and then caused bronchial tuberculosis. Bronchial tuberculosis leads to airway obstruction and then caused fatty and caseous necrotizing pneumonia at different stages, which predisposed the lesions to the formation of lobar or segmental consolidation, liquefaction necrosis and mouth-eaten cavities [32]. The incidence of consolidation was even higher in researches on CT images in treatment-naive MDR-TB patients complicated with HIV positiveness or diabetes [30]. Therefore, incidence of pulmonary consolidation in drug-resistant pulmonary tuberculosis correlated to not only the mode to acquire the resistance, but also the presence of concomitant disease undermining immunity. Number of consolidations in lungs of this patient decreased obviously after the treatment with susceptible drugs in combination with hypoglycemic therapy.
2. The pulmonary tuberculosis lesions of PDR-TB patients were distributed widely, involving all lung lobes, including sites rarely invaded by pulmonary tuberculosis, such as the anterior segment of the right upper lobe, the right middle lobe, the basal segments of both lower lobes, and the lingual and anterior segments of the left upper lobe. Moreover, shadows of multiple cavities were observed in the lesions of each pulmonary lobe. Present studies [9, 20] have proved that tuberculosis cavity is an important factor resulting in drug resistance, while diabetes increases the risk of cavitation and the incidence of lesions in lower lung field, especially in young patients [28, 29]. After the regular treatment using the regime

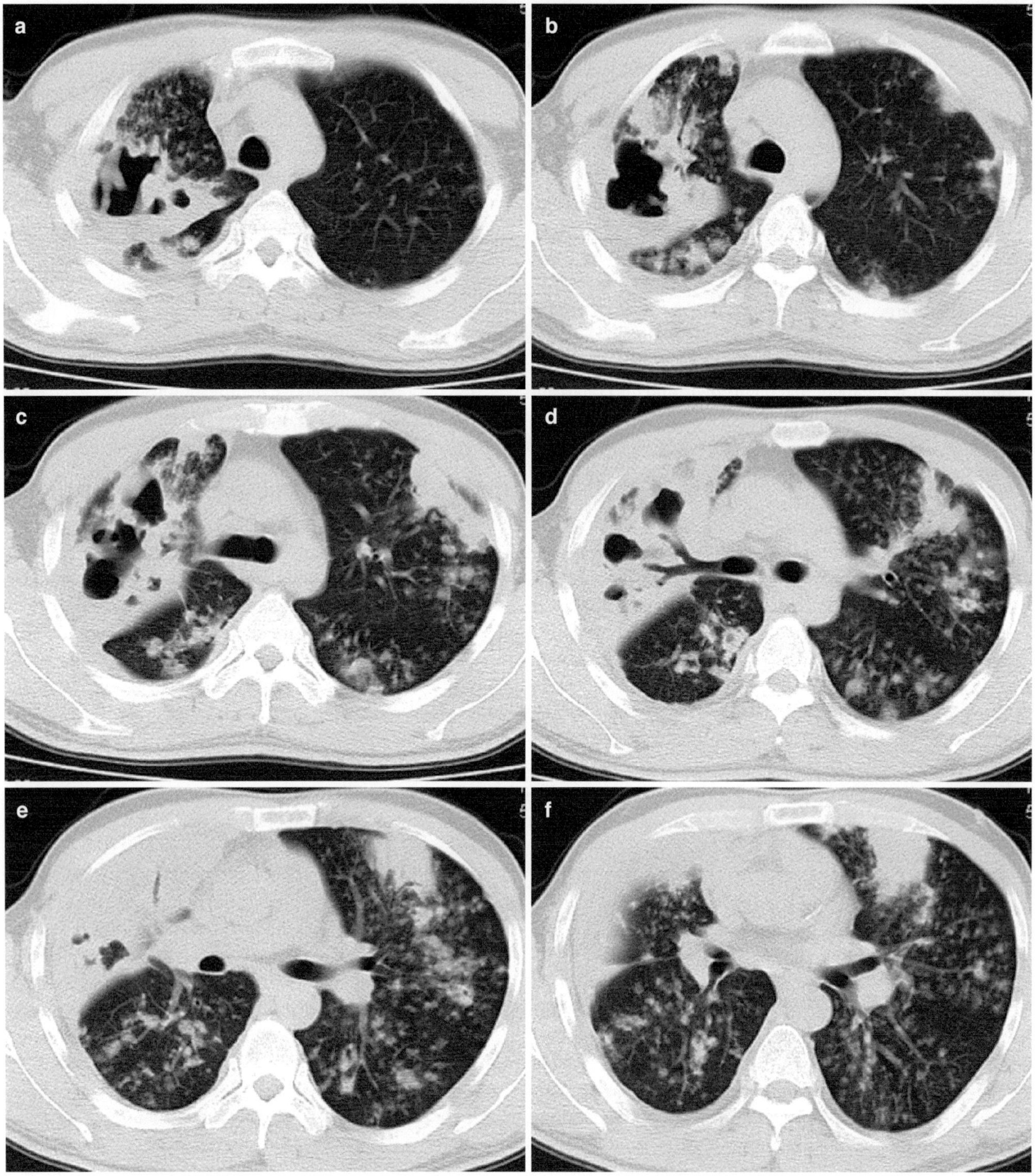

Fig. 7.15 (**a**–**n**) Chest CT scans on March 8, 2013, showed multiple consolidations/exudations, centrilobular nodules and tree-in-bud signs, multiple thick-walled cavities and consolidations with cavities. The big cavity in the right upper lobe had internal partitions inside. The decreased volume of the right upper lung was observed, with slight stenosis of lumen of the anterior and apical bronchi of the right upper lobe, with the interior wall not so smooth. Uneven enhancement was observed for pulmonary lesions, with patchy non-enhanced necrotic areas in lesions of both upper lobes. Slight enlargement was observed at posterior vena cava lymph nodes, with image of effusion in the right pleural cavity and slight thickening of the right pleura

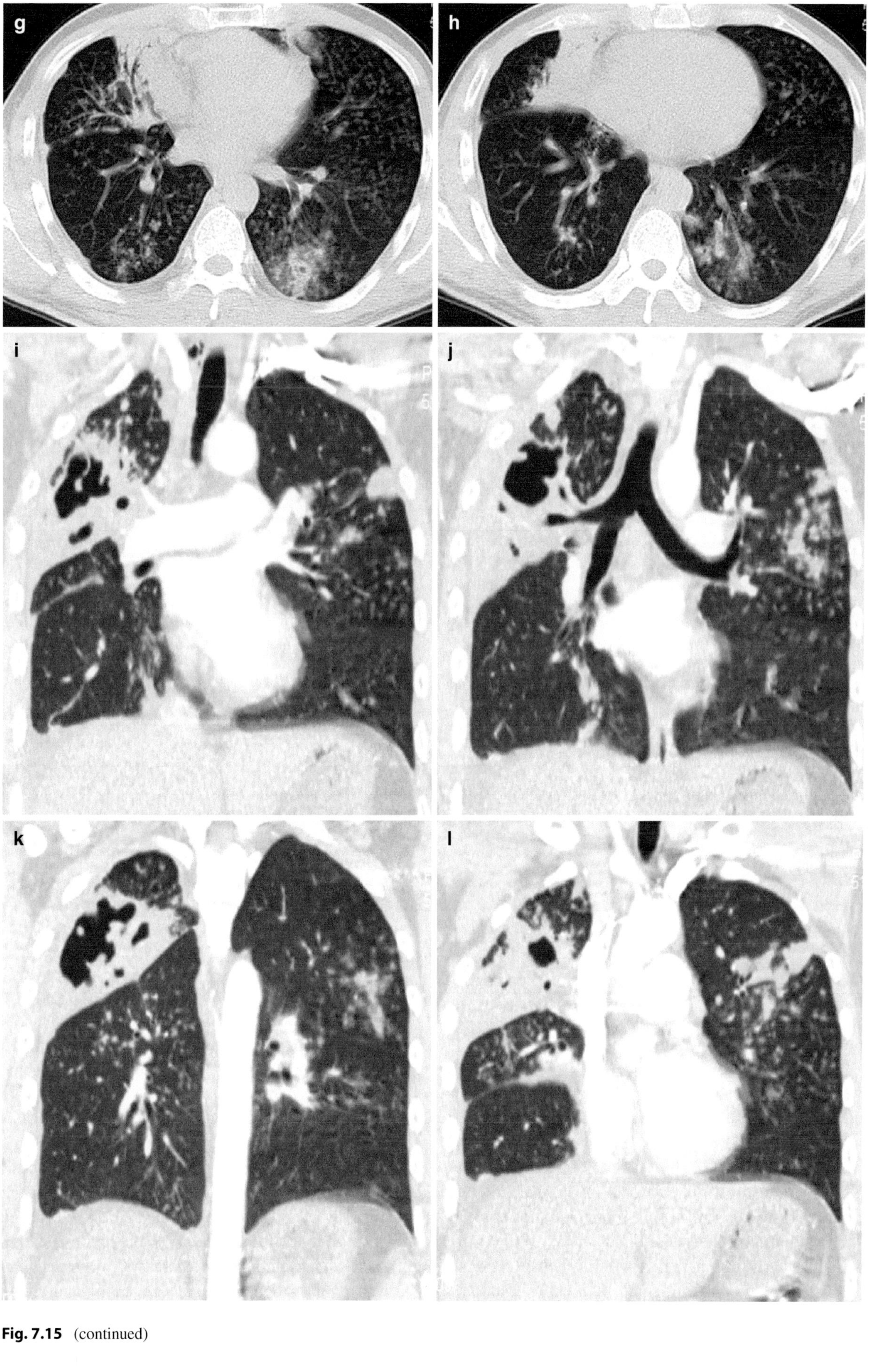

Fig. 7.15 (continued)

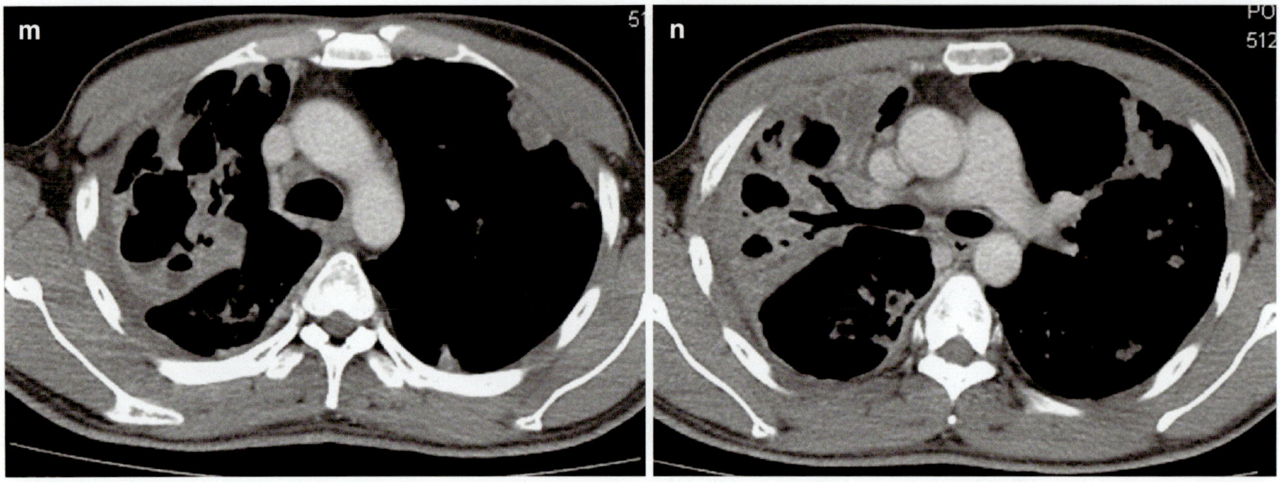

Fig. 7.15 (continued)

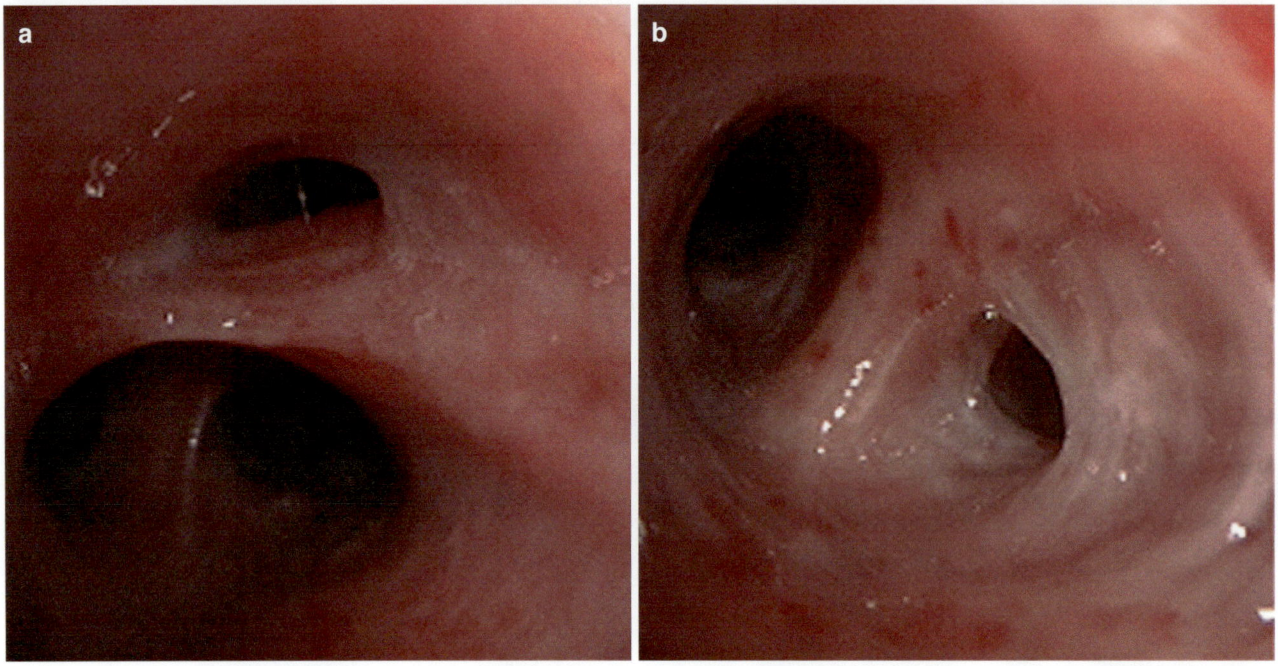

Fig. 7.16 (**a**, **b**) Cicatricial stenosis was observed for the apical and anterior segmental subbronchi under fiberoptic bronchoscope on April 15, 2013

based on drug sensitivity test in combination with hypoglycemic therapy, CT scans on July 8, 2020, showed that all lesions were absorbed with the cavities eradicated basically, except for the huge residual cavities with Aspergillus fungus balls inside, as observed in the upper and lower right lungs, which was consistent with the results in the literature [28]. This indicates that positive anti-tuberculosis treatment together with hypoglycemic therapy is an effective approach to cure pulmonary lesions in PDR-TB patients complicated with diabetes.

3. The CT findings of the patient at his first visit showed narrowing of the anterior and apical segmental bronchi of the right upper lung, which was confirmed to be bronchial tuberculosis based on bronchoscopy (Fig. 7.16a, b). In subsequent treatment, however, the change of the affected bronchi was not significant in the re-examination from 2014 to 2017, but images of multiple bronchiectasis appeared in lesions in both lungs, which was considered related to recurrent pulmonary lesions and persistent positiveness in sputum bacteria caused by absence of regular treatment in the early stage and repeated illness. Prolonged invasion into bronchi predisposed the bronchi to stenosis with obstructed excretion and increasing bacterial load [31], making the patient with diabetes as the underlying

disease vulnerable also to additional infections besides bronchiectasis, which was manifested in blood routine and image findings in his re-visits (Figs. 7.17, 7.18, 7.19, and 7.20). CT re-examination in 2020 showed the emergence of an Aspergillus ball that in the event of obvious absorption of the original pulmonary tuberculosis focus and disappearance of most of the pulmonary cavities, a large Aspergillus ball appeared in the cavity in right upper lobe and involved simultaneously the dorsal segment of the right lower lobe (Fig. 7.21). This situation was considered related to the significant drop of immunity post to chronic disease in the patient with impaired respiratory mucosal barrier, dramatic decrease in macrophages and neutrophils in airways, which resulted in infection by opportunistic pathogenic fungi such as aspergillus [33].

4. Intra-pulmonary lesions also showed waxing and waning before regular treatment against PDR-TB, as shown by re-examination in follow-up. Previous tuberculosis lesions in lungs were absorbed significantly. In addition, no definite calcified lesion was seen in intra-pulmonary lesions as shown by mediastinum window with mediastinal lymphadenectasis rarely observed from his first visit to his last re-visit, which seemed consistent with features in image findings in PDR-TB patients as we summarized above.

The similarities can be inferred between Case 2 and Case 1 as follows, based on their comparison: (1) both were PDR-TB patients with diabetes as the underlying disease and had severe clinical symptoms often complicated with bacterial infection; (2) CT at the first visit showed that there were extensive pulmonary lesions, consolidation/exudation, centrilobular nodules, tree-in-bud signs, multiple cavities and consolidations with cavities. After treatment, cavities increased in number or were absorbed slowly, while other pulmonary lesions could be absorbed; (3) There were signs of bronchial tuberculosis shown by the images, and signs of bronchiectasis appeared during the prolonged treatment; (4) There were few calcification in pulmonary lesions and mediastinal lymphadenectasis was rare; (5) With prolonged treatment, pulmonary lesions were prone to waxing and waning. Their differences included: (1) CD4/CD8/CD3 T lymphocytes count was lower in case 2, in comparison with the normal value in case 1 during the whole process of treatment; (2) both had a consolidation in the right upper lobe with a giant cavitation in their first visits. On the re-examination post to treatment against PDR-TB, however, an atelectasis of right upper lung appeared with the disappearance of cavity in case 1 in the event of the obvious absorption of the previous pulmonary tuberculosis lesion with clear boundary, while in case 2 an aspergillus ball appeared inside the giant cavity in the right upper lobe, which offered another proof that the old pulmonary tuberculosis with cavity is the risk factor of pulmonary aspergilloma [33].

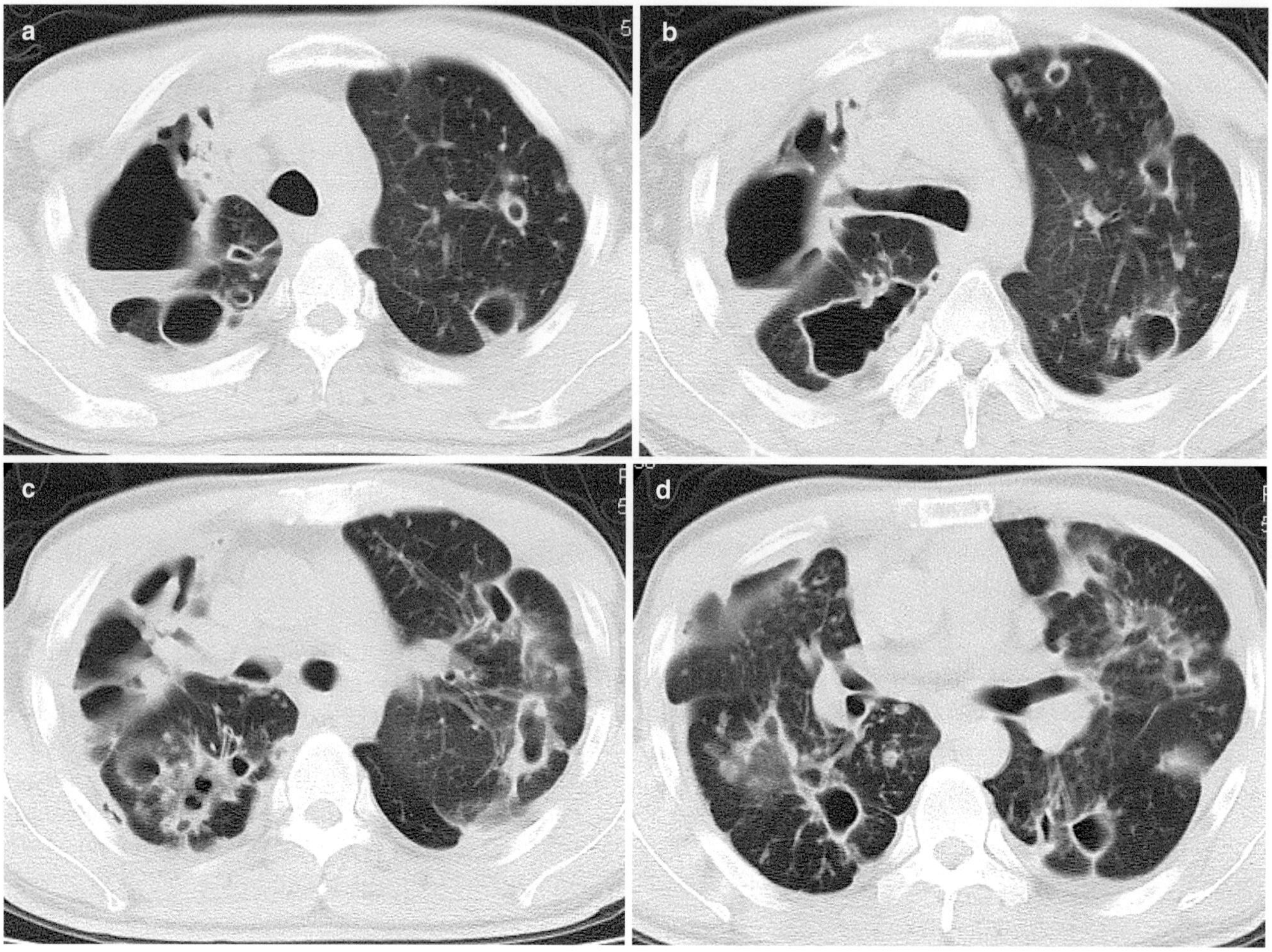

Fig. 7.17 (**a**–**h**) Chest CT scans on December 30, 2014, showed most of consolidations/exudation, centrilobular nodules, and tree-in-bud signs shown in the previous scans on March 8, 2013, were absorbed, but multiple irregular cavities, consolidation/exudative lesions and small nodules with unclear boundary emerged newly in lungs, with the appearance of a liquid level in the cavity in the right upper lobe. Multiple mild bronchiectases were observed in each lobe of both lungs. The right pleural effusion was basically absorbed, and each segmental bronchus in the right upper lung became less smooth than before

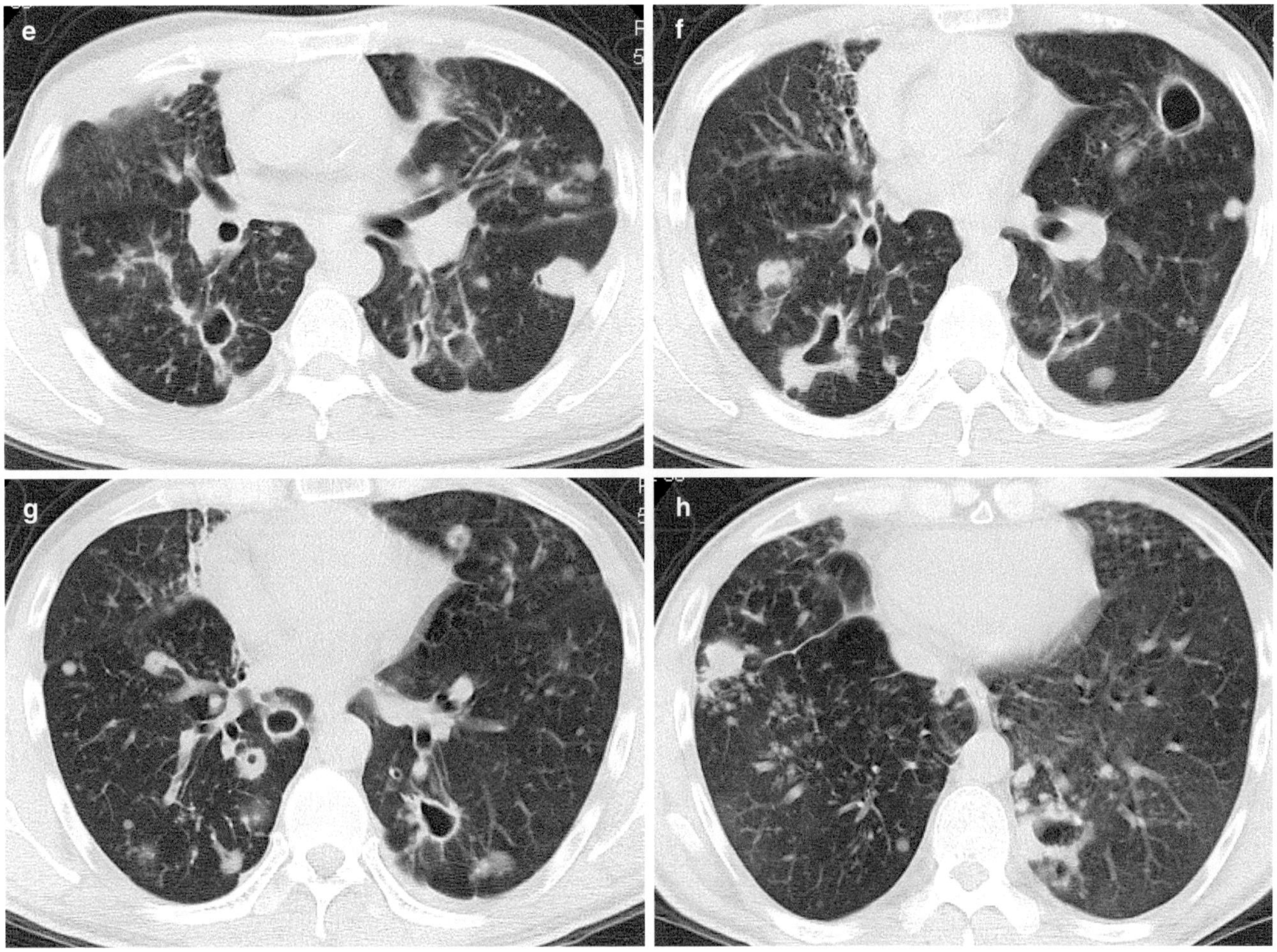

Fig. 7.17 (continued)

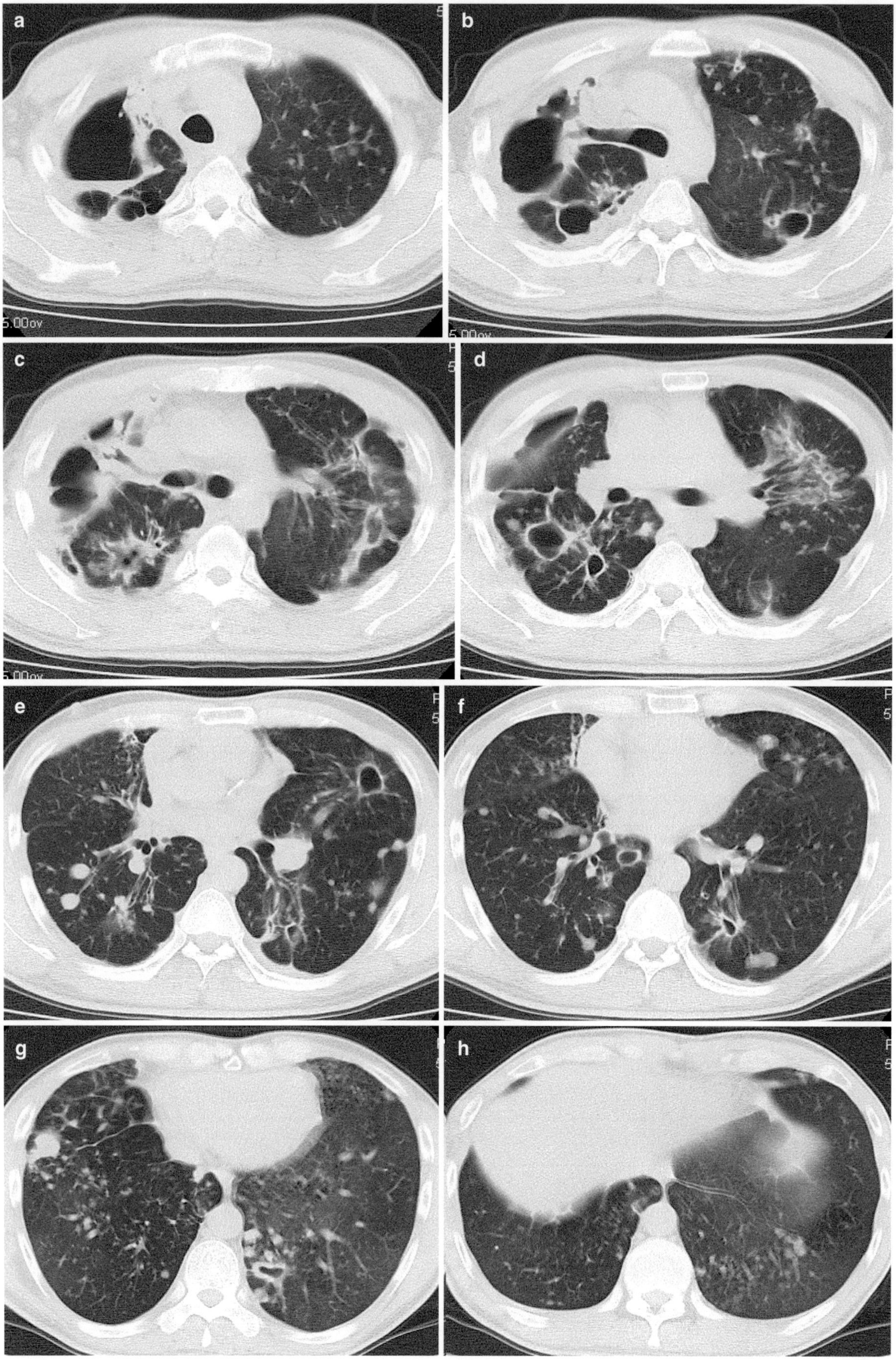

Fig. 7.18 (**a–l**) Chest CT scans on February 3, 2015, showed lesions in both lungs were absorbed, the cavities shrank, and lumen of each segmental bronchus in the right upper lobe became narrower than before, in comparison to CT scans on December 30, 2014

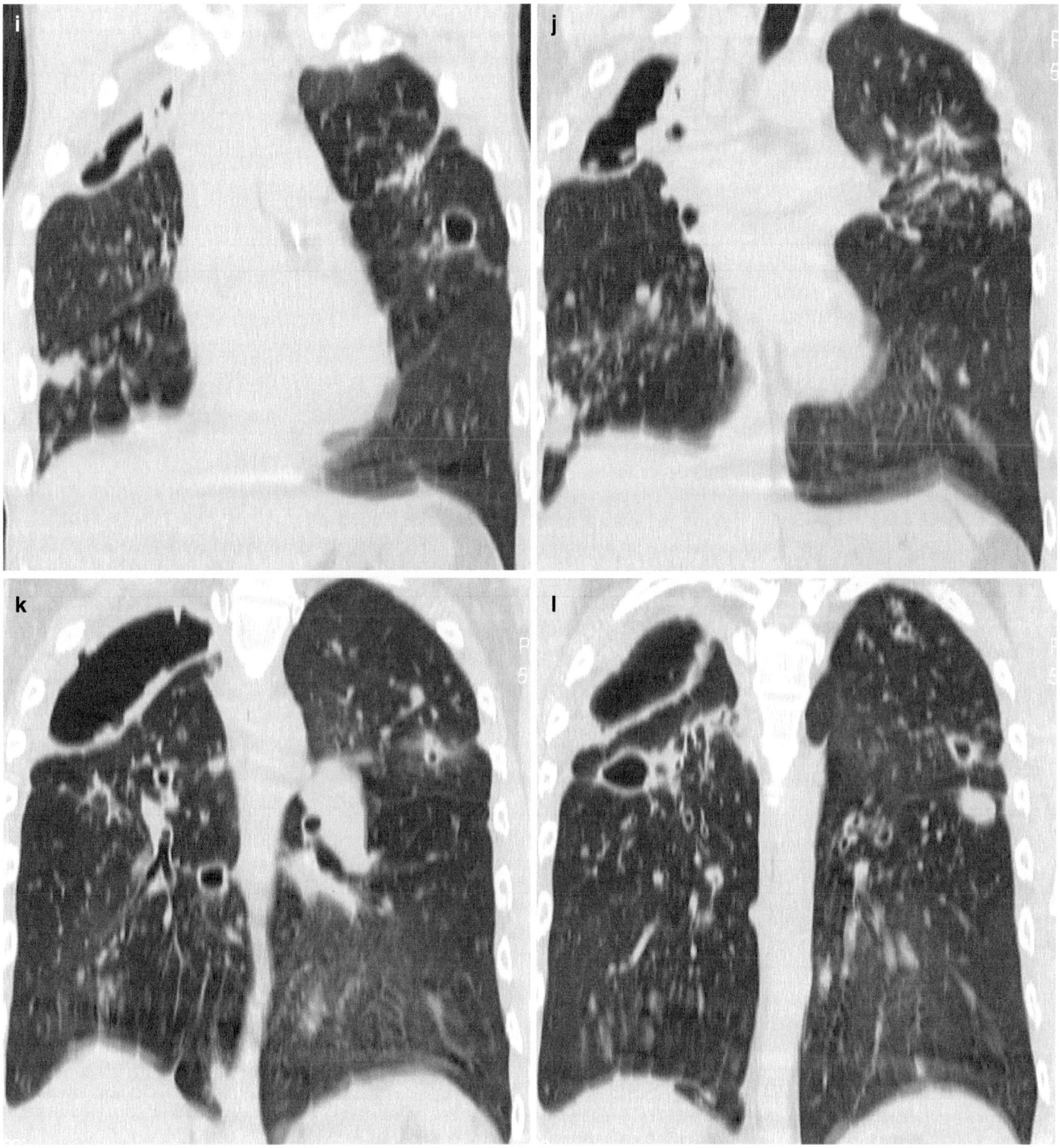

Fig. 7.18 (continued)

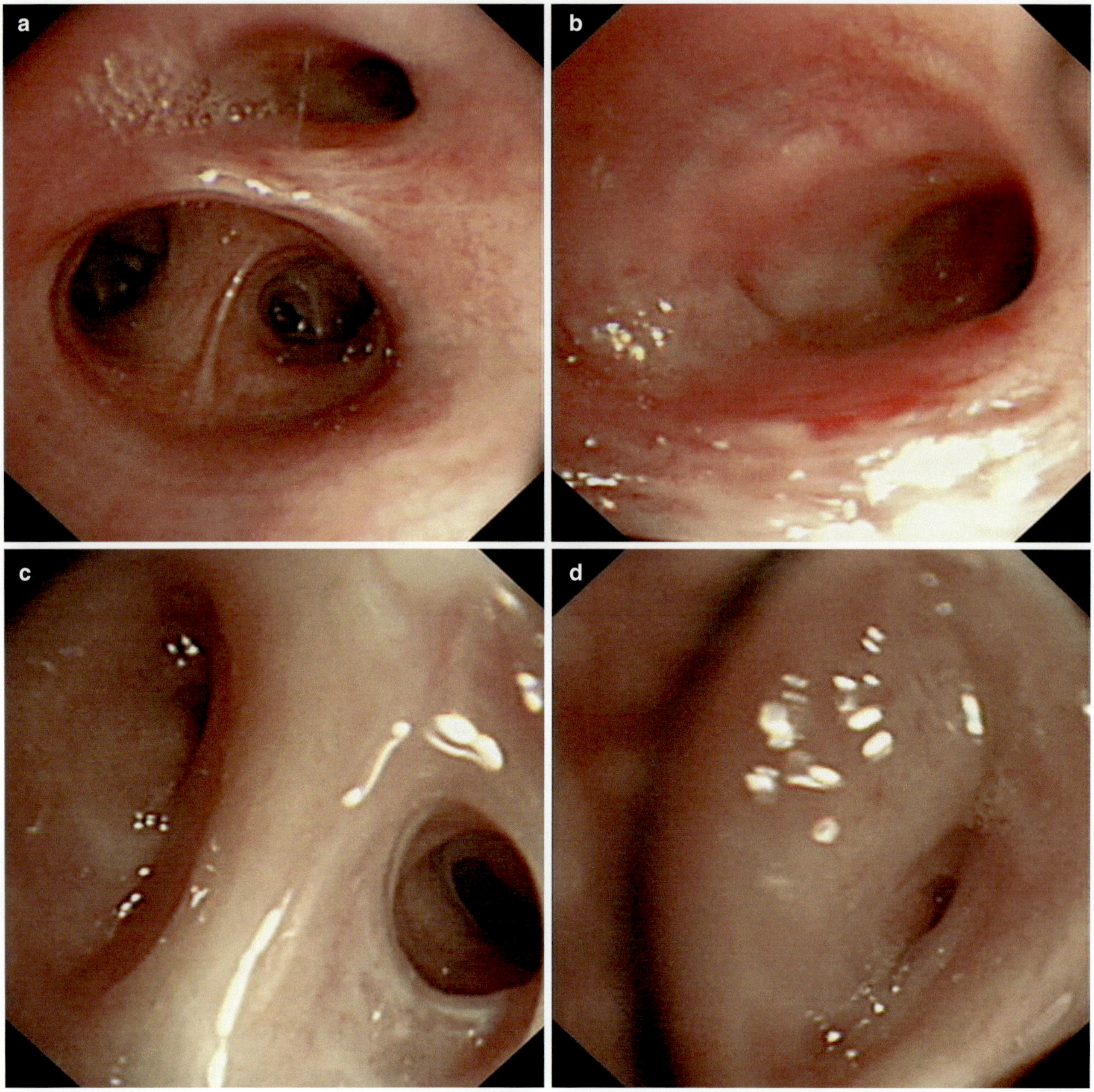

Fig. 7.19 (**a**–**d**) Fiberoptic bronchoscopy on January 4, 2015, showed mild hyperemia of the mucosa of the right bronchus with a little amount of white sticky secretions. Mild hyperemia with swelling was observed for mucosa in each segmental bronchus in the right upper lobe, with the cicatricial stenosis at the opening of the apical segment and the opening of the anterior subbranch branch, and the stenosis aggravated than before

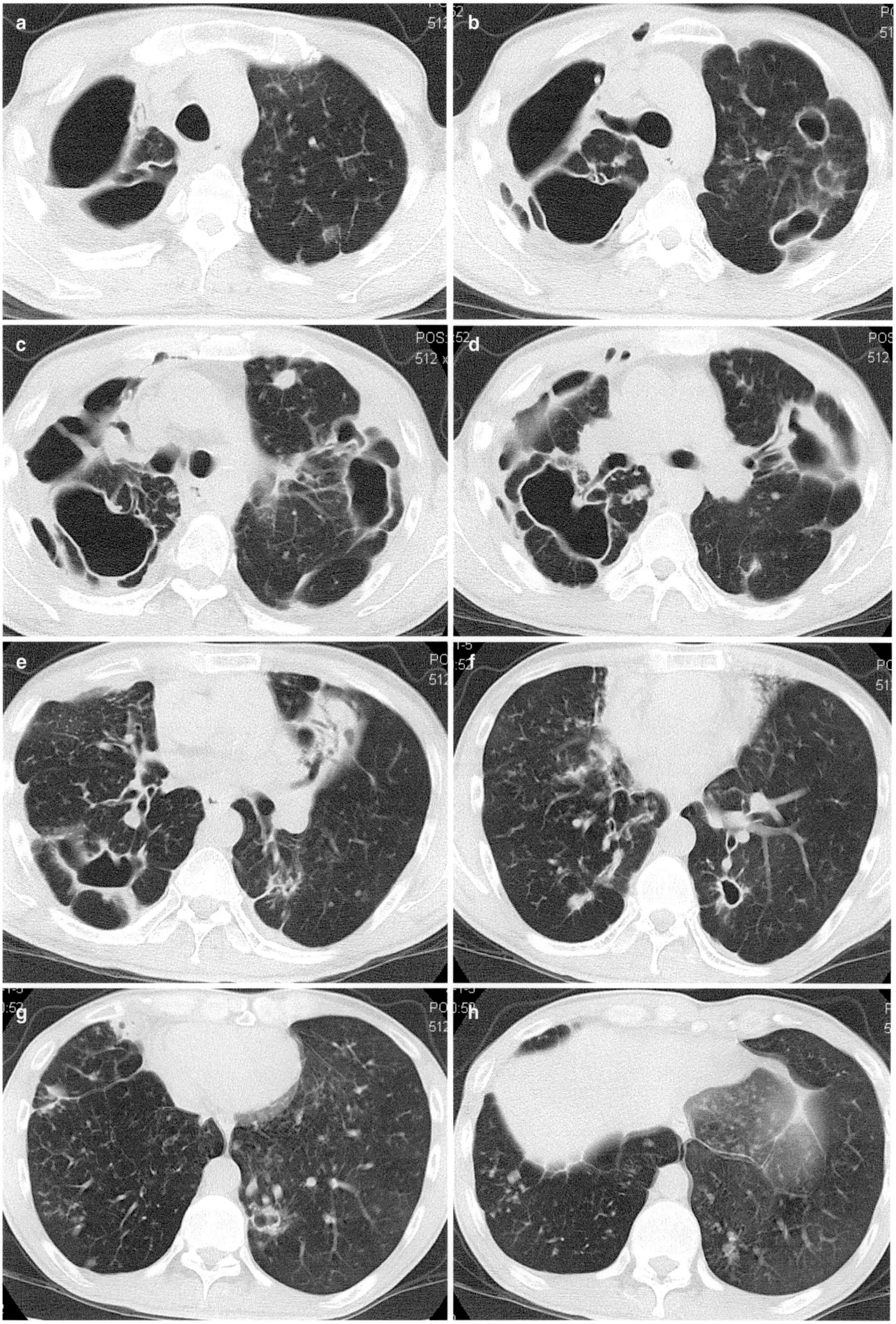

Fig. 7.20 (**a**–**h**) Re-examination of chest CT scans on January 5, 2017 showed emergence of multiple consolidation/exudation, centrilobular nodules and tree-in-bud signs, the cavities were enlarged in size with their wall thickened

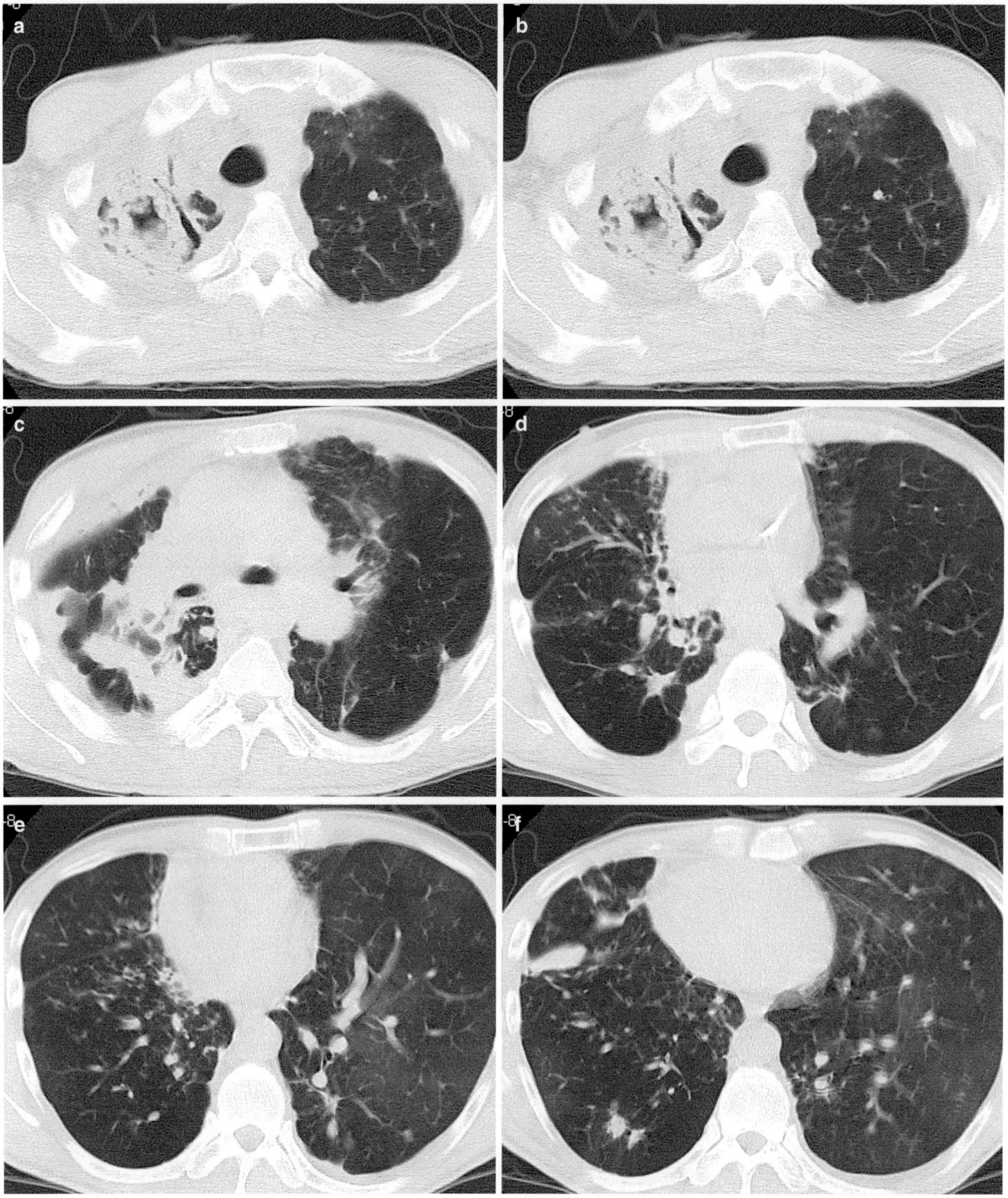

Fig. 7.21 (**a–j**) Chest CT scans on July 8, 2020, showed the obvious absorption of lesions in both lungs, and a residue cavity was observed in the right upper lobe with an aspergilloma formed inside. The rest of the pulmonary cavities disappeared, in comparison with images on January 5, 2017

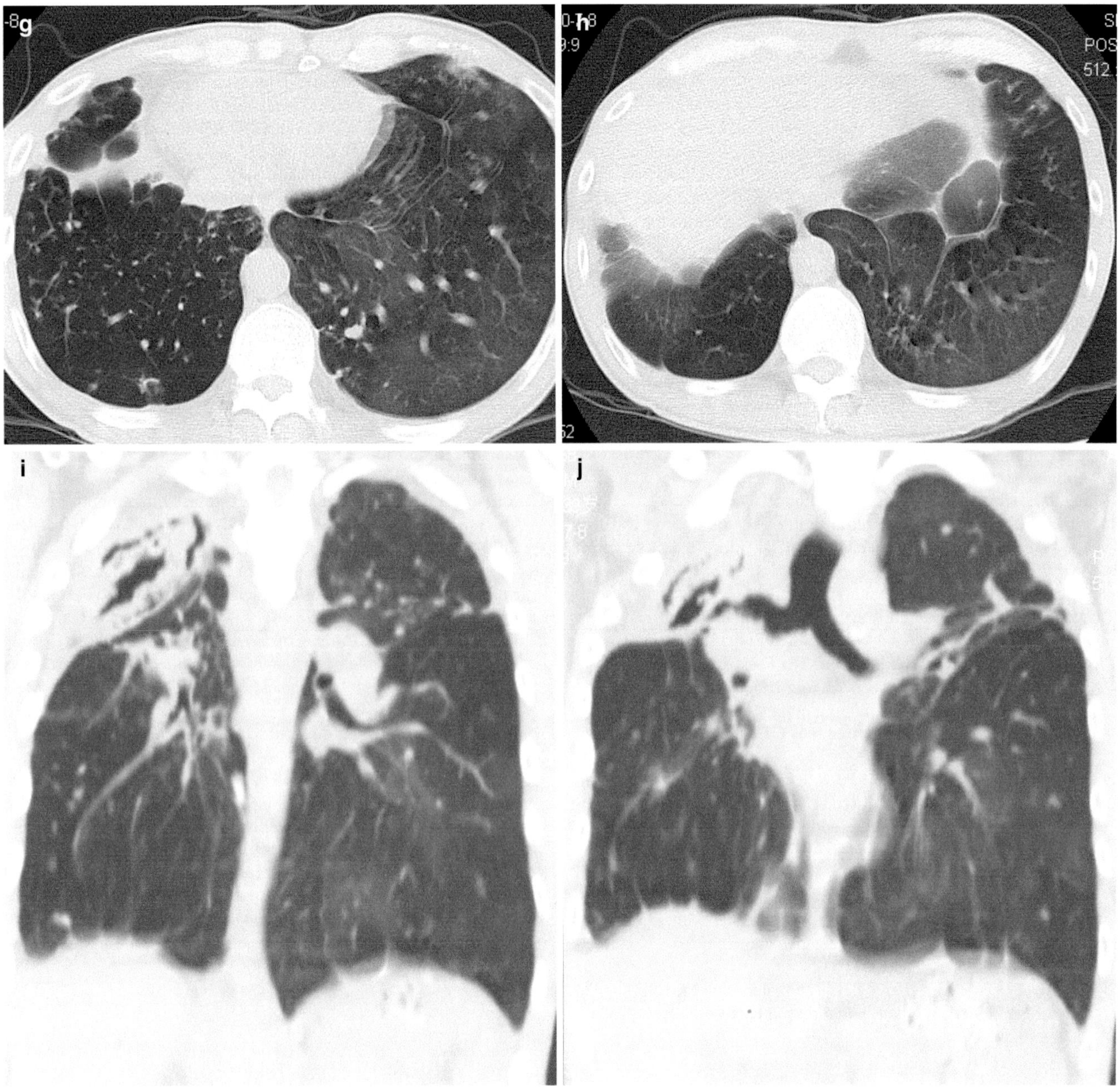

Fig. 7.21 (continued)

References

1. World Health Organization. Global tuberculosis report 2022 [EB/OL]. https://www.who.int/teams/global-tuberculosis-programme/tb-reports/global-tuberculosisreport-2022.
2. Qian H, Lin G, Lu L, et al. Monitoring and analysis of drug resistance in 244 patients in the high-risk population of drug-resistant pulmonary tuberculosis in Changshu from 2012 to 2016. Mod Prev Med. 2017;44(18):3334–6, 3345.
3. Han Z, Li J, Sun G, et al. A study on characteristics of drug resistance and transmission of mycobacterium tuberculosis in Jing'an district of Shanghai from 2010 to 2014 [J]. Chin Prev Med. 2017;18(9):680–4.
4. Yue H, Lu G, Gao X, et al. A monitoring study on drug resistance of mycobacterium tuberculosis in Handan City of Hebei Province [J]. J Med Pest Control. 2017;33(11):1150–15.
5. Li Y, Wang X, Chen M, et al. An analysis of drug resistance in mycobacterium tuberculosis during six years in Shan'xi region [J]. J Clin Pulm Med. 2017;22(8):1489–526.
6. Yang A, Zhou L, Xu Z, et al. A study on drug-resistance characteristics of four first-line anti-tuberculosis drugs for pulmonary tuberculosis and their influencing factors in Hunan Province [J]. Chin J Zoonoses. 2018;34(5):396–400.
7. World Health Organization. Global tuberculosis report 2021 [EB/OL]. https://www.who.int/publications/digital/global-tuberculosis-report-2021.

8. Ko JM, Park HJ, Kim CH, et al. The relation between CT findings and sputum microbiology studies in active pulmonary tuberculosis [J]. Eur J Radiol. 2015;84(11):2339–44.
9. Li Y, Wang B, Wen L, et al. Machine learning and radiomics for the prediction of multidrug resistance in cavitary pulmonary tuberculosis: a multicentre study [J]. Eur J Radiol. 2023;33(1):391–400.
10. Li D, He W, Chen B, et al. Primary multidrug-resistant tuberculosis versus drug-sensitive tuberculosis in non-HIV-infected patients: comparisons of CT findings [J]. PLoS One. 2017;12(6):e0176354.
11. Song Q, Guo X, Zhang L, et al. New approaches in the classification and prognosis of sign clusters on pulmonary CT images in patients with multidrug-resistant tuberculosis [J]. Front Microbiol. 2021;12:714617.
12. Song Q, Zhang G, Jiang H, et al. Imaging features of pulmonary CT in type 2 diabetic patients with multidrug-resistant tuberculosis [J]. PLoS One. 2016;11(3):e0152507.
13. Lv Y, Li C, Xie R, et al. A study on HRCT image findings in patients with treatment-naive secondary pulmonary tuberculosis [J/CD]. Chin J Exp Clin Infect Dis. 2015,9(5):643–8.
14. Li C, Shengxiu L, Wang H, et al. CT findings in multiple-resistance pulmonary tuberculosis patients and their relationship with CD4 cells [J]. Chin J Antituberc. 2017;39(6):597–603.
15. Luyao M, Qiuting Z, Lu P, et al. Pulmonary multi-drug resistant tuberculosis: a radiological review [J/CD]. Electr J Emerg Infect Dis. 2021;6(1):58–65.
16. Wang YXJ, Chung MJ, Skrahin A, et al. Radiological signs associated with pulmonary multi-drug resistant tuberculosis: an analysis of published evidences. Quant Imaging Med Surg. 2018;8(2):161–73.
17. Chung MJ, Lee KS, Koh WJ, Kim TS, Kang EY, Kim SM, et al. Drug-sensitive tuberculosis, multidrug-resistant tuberculosis, and nontuberculous mycobacterial pulmonary disease in non-AIDS adults: comparisons of thin-section CT findings. Eur Radiol. 2006;16(9):1934–41.
18. Kim HC, Goo JM, Lee HJ, Park SH, Park CM, Kim TJ, et al. Multidrug-resistant tuberculosis versus drug-sensitive tuberculosis in human immunodeficiency virus-negative patients: computed tomography features. J Comput Assist Tomogr. 2004;28(3):366–71.
19. Cha J, Lee HY, Lee KS, Koh WJ, Kwon OJ, Yi CA, et al. Radiological findings of extensively drug- resistant pulmonary tuberculosis in non-AIDS adults: comparisons with findings of multidrug-resistant and drug-sensitive tuberculosis. Korean J Radiol. 2009;10(3):207–16.
20. Kim W, Lee KS, Kim HS, et al. CT and microbiologic follow-up in primary multidrug-resistant pulmonary tuberculosis. Acta Radiol. 2016;57(2):197–204.
21. Rosenthal A, Gabrielian A, Engle E, et al. The TB portals: an open-access, web-based platform for global drug-resistant tuberculosis data sharing and analysis. J Clin Microbiol. 2017;5(11):3267–82.
22. Chung MJ, Lee KS, Koh WJ, et al. Drug-sensitive tuberculosis, multidrug-resistant tuberculosis, and nontuberculous mycobacterial pulmonary disease in non AIDS adults: comparisons of thin-section CT findings. Eur Radiol. 2006;16(9):1934–41.
23. Chuchottaworn C, Thanachartwet V, Sangsayunh P, et al. Risk factors for multidrug-resistant tuberculosis among patients with pulmonary tuberculosis at the Central Chest Institute of Thailand. PLoS One. 2015;10:e0139986.
24. Yi K, Yang L, Li Y, et al. A study on CD4+CD25+Foxp3+T lymphocytes inhibiting cellular immunity in patients with drug-resistant pulmonary tuberculosis [J]. Chin J Infect Control. 2012;11(5):328–31.
25. Drain PK, Bajema KL, Dowdy D, et al. Incipient and subclinical tuberculosis: a clinical review of early stages and progression of infection [J]. Clin Microbiol Rev. 2018;31(4):e00021–18.
26. Qu HQ, Rentfro AR, Lu Y, et al. Host susceptibility to tuberculosis: insights from a longitudinal study of gene expression in diabetes [J]. Int J Tuberc Lung Dis. 2012;16(3):370–2.
27. Yu W, Tan W, Luo Y, et al. 2018 WHO tuberculosis report: key data analysis for global and China [J/CD]. Electr J Emerg Infect Dis. 2018;3(4):229–34.
28. Chen-Yuan C, Jen-Jyh L, Shun-Tien C, et al. Glycemic control and radiographic manifestations of tuberculosis in diabetic patients [J]. PloS One. 2014;9(4):e93397.
29. Perez-Guzman C, Torres-Cruz A, Villarreal-Velarde H, et al. Progressive age-related changes in pulmonary tuberculosis images and the effect of diabetes [J]. Am J Respir Crit Care Med. 2000;162(5):1738–40.
30. Long R. Drug-resistant tuberculosis [J]. CMAJ. 2000;163(4):425–8. [32]
31. Kuang H, Tan S, Liang M, et al. A study concerning the concomitant tracheal and bronchial tuberculosis in patients with multiple-resistant pulmonary tuberculosis [J]. Chin J Antituberc. 2017;39(3):242–6.
32. Hunter RL. Pathology of post primary tuberculosis of the lung: an illustrated critical review. Tuberculosis. 2011;91(6):497–509.
33. Pan Y, Xiao H, Li Y, et al. An analysis on clinical features of 100 patients with pulmonary aspergilloma infection [J]. Int Med Health Guidance News. 2021;27(12):1750–3.

Extensively Drug-Resistant Tuberculosis

8

Sheng-xiu Lv, Chun-hua Li, Yu-feng Xu, Bu-dong Chen,
Ying-ying Deng, and Hong-zhou Lu

8.1 Summary of Extensively Drug-Resistant Tuberculosis

Extensively drug-resistant tuberculosis (XDR-TB) is defined as a tuberculosis of MDR/RR-TB plus resistant simultaneously to any one of fluoroquinolones and at least any one of bedaquiline and linezolid.

It was pointed out by Global Tuberculosis Report 2020 WHO that there were 889,000 TB cases in China based on statistics in 2019, with about 58,000 cases of MDR-TB and rifampicin resistant TB [1]. 4–20% of MDR-TB, however, are XDR-TB, having poorest responses to treatment among all tuberculosis, and both its unresponsiveness rate and mortality were higher than those of non-extensively drug-resistant MDR-TB [2, 3]. Despite the great effort in anti-tuberculosis treatment made by human being and the drop in certain degree of overall TB incidence, the evidences have not been discovered supporting the best treatment regimens for XDR-TB patients [4], and the treatment success rate of this disease is as low as 34% [5]. Diagnosis of XDR-TB is mainly based on sputum bacterial examination/identification and drug susceptibility test, but incubation lasts too long, usually several weeks. Image examinations, especially CT scans, are of great importance in diagnosis, treatment, and follow-up of tuberculosis.

S.-x. Lv (✉) · C.-h. Li
Department of Medical Imaging, Chongqing Public Health Medical Center, Chongqing, China

Y.-f. Xu
Department of Radiology, Peking University First Hospital, Beijing, China

B.-d. Chen
Department of Radiology, Beijing You'an Hospital, Capital Medical University, Beijing, China

Y.-y. Deng
Department of Radiology, Yantian District People's Hospital, Shenzhen, Guangdong, China

H.-z. Lu
Infectious Disease, The Third People's Hospital of Shenzhen, Shenzhen, China

However, XDR-TB patients have greater challenge in treatment, poorer responses, longer disease course, and severe injuries of pulmonary tissues and structures, in comparison with MDR-TB patients. Although both XDR-TB and MDR-TB are prone to lung consolidation, tree-in-bud sign, micro-nodule, lobular lung consolidation, cavitation, bronchiectasis, and emphysema, XDR-TB has lesions often involving more than three lung fields and is more prone to destroyed lungs, extensive airway spread, and lung consolidation. Compared with MDR-TB, XDR-TB has thicker wall, greater number, and larger size of cavities [6]. During anti-tuberculosis treatment, pulmonary disseminating lesions of XDR-TB keep increasing, with cavities increasing in number or in size or decreasing in size and lowered ratio of cavity closure, which reflects that XDR-TB responds poorly to treatment and is characterized in a continuous deterioration of pulmonary lesions. Having more types of drug resistance than MDR-TB does, XDR-TB shows severe non-susceptibility to anti-tuberculosis treatment, wider distribution of lesions in lungs, and greater vulnerability to multiple intra-pulmonary dissemination predisposing lesions to protracted course, progression, and evolution. XDR-TB does not differ significantly from MDR-TB in the way to illustrate findings in CT scans, and both may manifest intra-pulmonary infiltration, bronchial dissemination, multiple cavitations, destroyed lung, thickened pleura, bronchiectasis, etc. Severe damage with higher incidence, however, is observed for XDR-TB compared with MDR-TB, and number of involved pulmonary segments is greater than that of drug-susceptible tuberculosis [7].

8.2 Introduction of Typical Cases of XDR-TB

Case 1

The patient was a 48-year-old female with a chief complaint of cough and expectoration for 9 years, with exertional dyspnea for more than 2 years and a recurrence for 1 month.

P.-x. Lu et al. (eds.), *Diagnostic Imaging of Drug Resistant Pulmonary Tuberculosis*,
https://doi.org/10.1007/978-981-99-8339-1_8

Positiveness of Mycobacterium tuberculosis was observed in sputum smear and sputum culture on many occasions during 9 years, and a gradual progression from MDR-TB into XDR-TB was evidenced by multiple drug susceptibility tests. She had irregular medication with exposure to non-standardized anti-tuberculosis drugs and voluntary withdrawal of treatment, during this period she was hospitalized for many times due to repeated exaggeration of symptoms.

Having experienced a relief of her symptoms post to anti-tuberculosis treatment, she used voluntarily traditional Chinese medicine (TCM) herbs, and persistent positiveness was shown by sputum acid fast bacillus smear (Fig. 8.1).

Rapid drug susceptibility test on May 20, 2014, showed resistance to H, R, S, Pto, Pa, and Rfb, based on which an anti-tuberculosis treatment containing Pa, Z, E, Lfx, A, and Clr was given and continued until December 2014, and during this period results of multiple re-examinations of sputum bacteria were positive. Re-examination of chest CT scans on December 2, 2014, showed findings as follows (Fig. 8.2).

She received an anti-tuberculosis treatment consisting of "R-Z-E" at the local Tuberculosis Prevention and Control Institute in January 2015, and she had an onset of cough and expectoration complicated with hemoptysis and fever in May 2015. Sputum smear acid fast bacilli was positive on May 10, 2015, and rapid drug resistance test showed resistance to H, R,S, Ofx, Pa, Mfx, PAS, and RFB. An anti-tuberculosis regimen containing "Pa, Z, E, Lfx, A, and Clr" was given. Chest CT scans on June 5, 2015, showed findings as follows (Fig. 8.3).

The patient sticks to the anti-tuberculosis treatment using this regimen outside the hospital until March 2016, during which she took anti-tuberculosis drugs intermittently and adjuvant therapy with TCM herbs. Sputum culture for Mycobacterium tuberculosis remained positive at her intermittent follow-up visits at outpatient department. Chest CT examination was performed on March 28, 2016, with its findings as follows (Fig. 8.4).

The patient continued her intermittent anti-tuberculosis medication and TCM herbs, and there was no significant change in the patient's condition. Findings of re-examination of CT scans on June 3, 2016, are as follows (Fig. 8.5).

The patient experienced an aggravation of cough, with an expectoration of a large amount of yellow sticky phlegm and exertional dyspnea and shortness of breath, and there was no

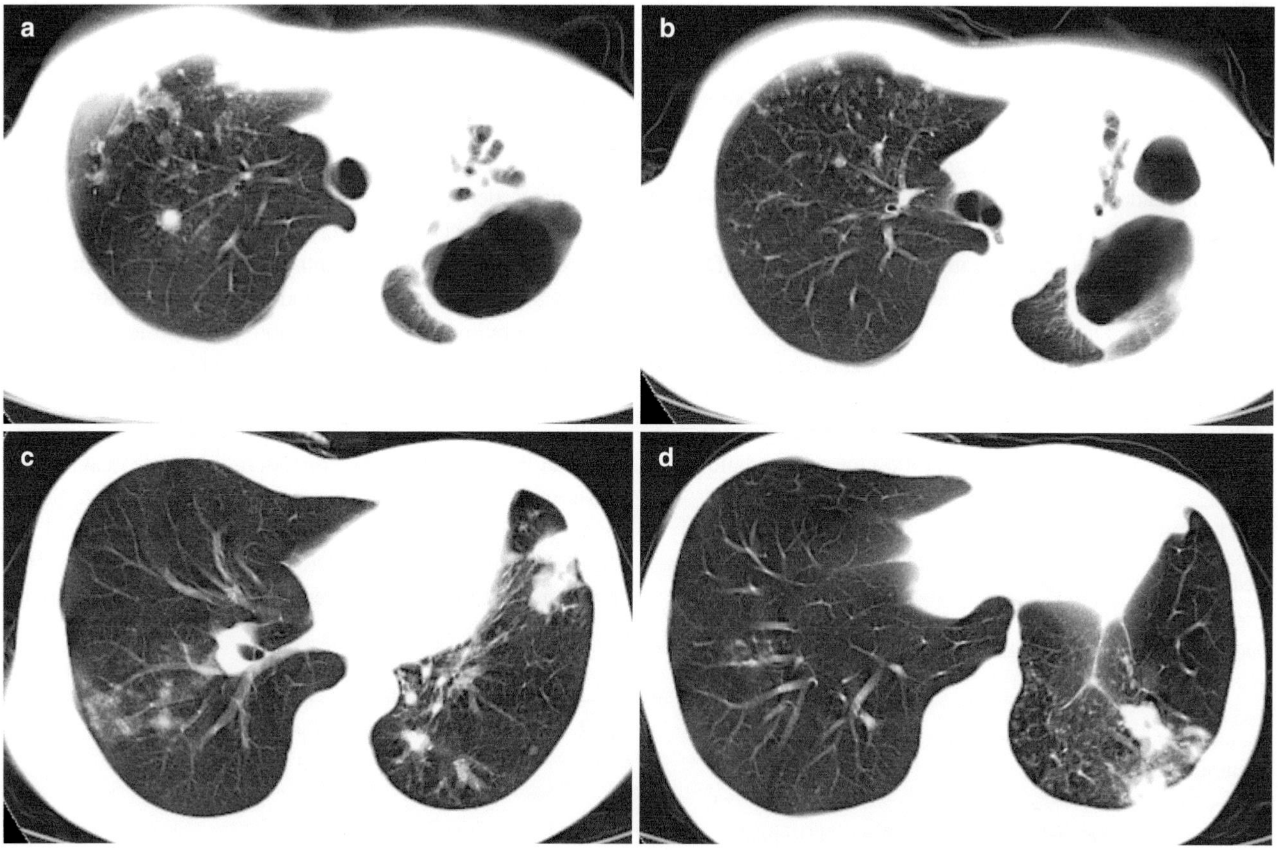

Fig. 8.1 (**a**–**d**) Chest CT scans on April 10, 2014, show the shrinkage of the left thorax with the left shift of the mediastinum. Both lungs are scattered with patchy, nodular, and centrilobular high-density opacities with uneven density, and some of them are in unclear border. Bronchiectasis exists in the left upper lobe, where thickened bronchial wall was observed, and the fusion of multiple cavities formed the destroyed chamber, with adhesion and thickening of adjacent pleura

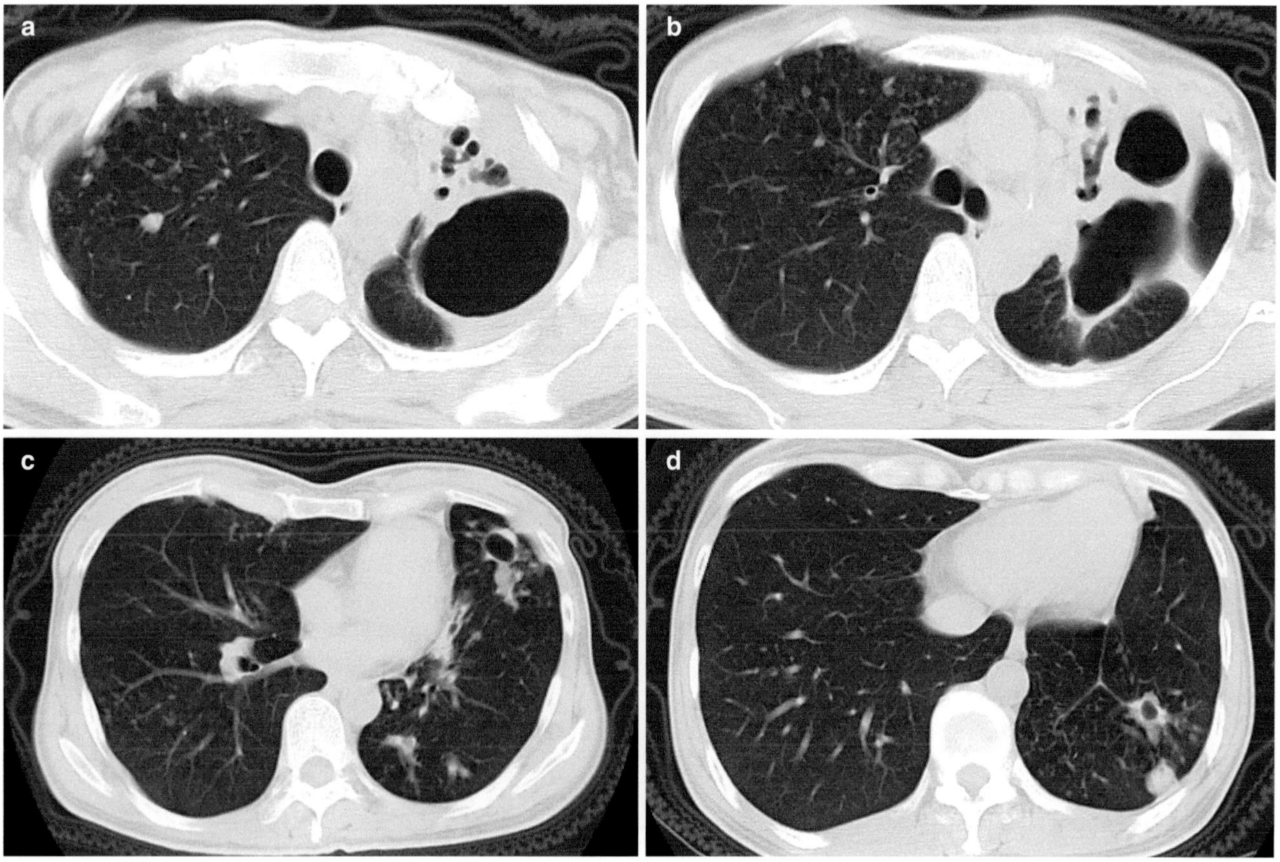

Fig. 8.2 (**a**–**d**) Chest CT scans on December 2, 2014, show the slightly enlargement for the cavity and for the destroyed chamber in the left upper lobe, absorption and amelioration of the rest of lesions scattering both lungs, absorption of lesions in the lingual segment of the left upper lobe and the basal segment of the left lower lobe, and the formation of a thin-walled cavity with dissolution and discharge of lesions

obvious amelioration after oral TCM herbs were given. Results of drug susceptibility test on November 7, 2016, showed the resistance to H, R, S, and Am. A treatment containing Cm, Lfx, and Z was launched only, because of her severe gastrointestinal reactions. She had performed chest CT examination on October 17, 2016 (Fig. 8.6).

In January 2017, the patient had diarrhea after taking self-purchased linezolid outside the hospital, without exposure to any other anti-tuberculosis drugs. She experienced repeated aggravation of her symptoms with dyspnea for 10 days, and then she was admitted into our hospital for the fourth time to undergo an anti-tuberculosis treatment containing Pa-Pto-C-Lfx-Z-PAS-E. Sputum culture in April 2017 showed positiveness in Mycobacterium tuberculosis, and Lowenstein–Jensen drug susceptibility test showed the resistance to H, R, Pto, Pa, E, L, Lfx, and Sm. Findings of CT re-examination on June 13, 2017 are as follows (Fig. 8.7).

During the treatment, she has exacerbation of cough and expectoration complicated with dyspnea and fever for 1 month. Sputum culture and Lowenstein–Jensen drug susceptibility test on March 31, 2018, showed the resistance to H, R, E, L, Am, Lfx, Cm, Pto, and Pa, and the susceptibility only to PAS. She underwent an anti-tuberculosis treatment with a regimen of "Pa-Pto-Cm-Lfx-Z-E," and her disease ameliorated (Fig. 8.8).

During the treatment, the patient experienced nausea, vomiting, and upper abdominal discomfort and withdrew voluntarily her anti-tuberculosis medication. Again, she had the onset of cough, expectoration, asthma, and expectoration of yellow purulent sputum in February 2019. She was admitted again on March 12, 2019, when blood routine showed white blood cell count of 7.71×10^9/L, hemoglobin 107.00 g/L ↓, platelet 375×10^9/L; ESR 27 mm/h ↑; c-reactive protein 33.80 mg/L; fungal D-glucan quantification (74.7 pg/m); TB golden label and protein chip showed positiveness in TB antibody IgG (golden label), TB gene LAM (antibody), and TB gene 38 KDa (antibody); acid fast bacilli smear microscopy was positive (direct smear; 4+), and Mycobacterium fluorescent staining was also positive (4+). Findings of CT re-examination are as follows (Fig. 8.9).

The final diagnosis and outcome: The secondary pulmonary tuberculosis positive in smear and culture, with extensive drug resistance to H, R, Am, and Lfx with a protracted course.

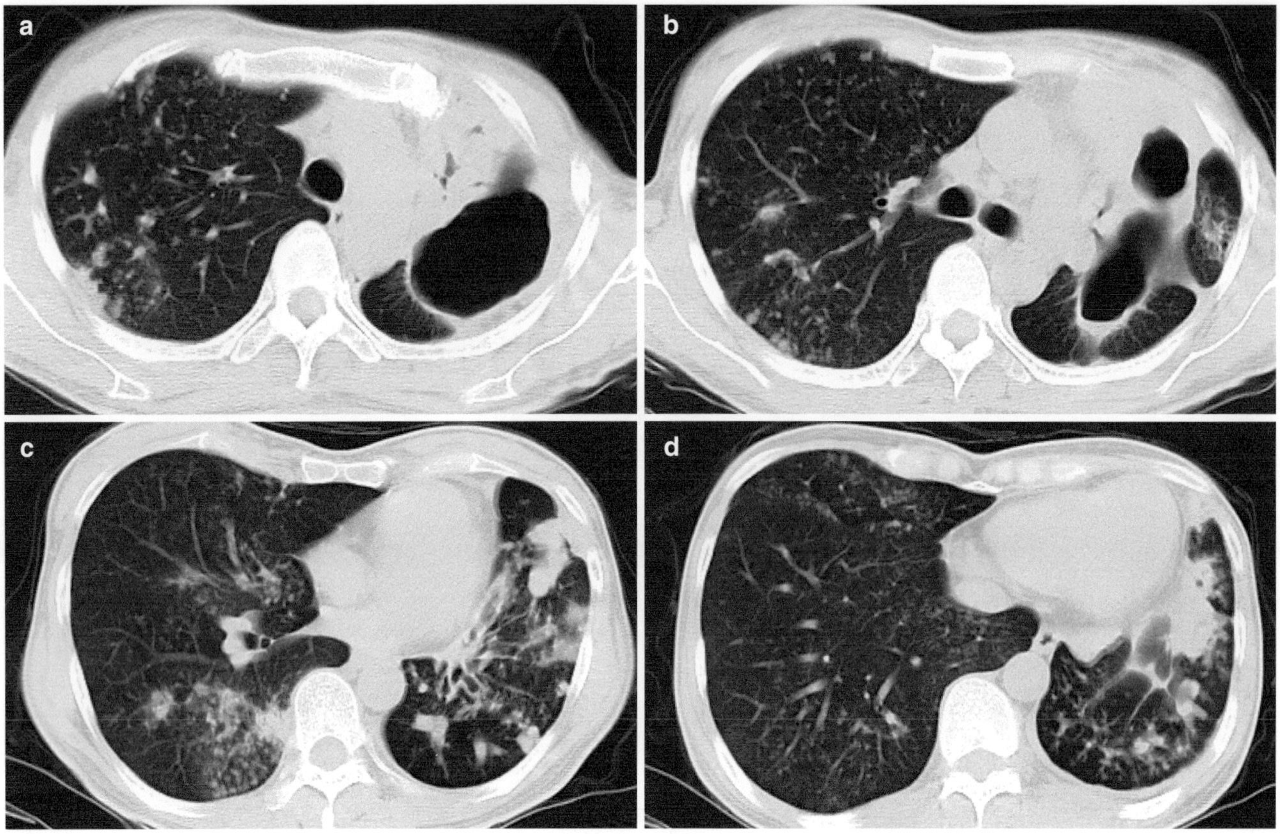

Fig. 8.3 (**a**–**d**) Chest CT scans on June 5, 2015: the cavity in the left upper lobe shrinks slightly and the rest lesions in both lungs increase, with newly emergence of patchy and centrilobular nodules as well as tree-in-bud signs compared with CT scan findings on December 2, 2014. The lesions have blurred boundaries and the consolidation in the apical posterior segment in the left upper lobe seems more obvious than before. The cavity in the lingual segment of the left upper lobe shows a filling with increased contents

Discussion

The patient had been receiving intermittent anti-tuberculosis treatment out of the hospital for 4 years before visiting out hospital, but the disease responded poorly to the treatment. Drug susceptibility test was not done during her treatment out of hospital, and her compliance was not good, which made her tuberculosis prone to drug resistance. At the beginning of her diagnosis and treatment in our hospital, MDR-TB was confirmed by sputum culture. During subsequent treatment, however, the patient withdrew arbitrarily her medication on many occasions or received TCM herbs in other hospitals voluntarily due to severe gastrointestinal reactions caused by medication and poor economic affordability and repeatedly returned to our hospital for treatment after her condition worsened. The irregular medication stimulated and aggravated the further development of drug resistance of tubercle bacillus, thereby leading to the final development of XDR-TB. Pulmonary CT findings in this patient correlated to her irregular medication to a certain extent during her treatment in our hospital, manifesting a slowed progression of lesions and even absorption with amelioration of some of them in case of her good compliance, in contrast to the progression with further exacerbation in case of her irregular medication or after her discontinuation of treatment. Moreover, no effective anti-tuberculosis drugs were available due to the inherent attribute of XDR-TB that she suffered from, so it was hard to inhibit the progression of tubercle bacillus in vivo, and the destruction caused by proliferation of tubercle bacillus in lungs would be enhanced to result in further aggravation of her disease. Positiveness was shown, therefore, in results of multiple sputum smears and sputum cultures, and pulmonary CT findings showed progressive disease with an increase in disseminated lesions, the fusion of cavities, and aggravation of lung destruction.

Despite the vital role that sputum culture and drug susceptibility test play in the diagnosis of patients, imaging examination has an important value for both the diagnosis and evaluation of responsiveness to treatment before the results of laboratory tests become available, especially CT scans having an irreplaceable effect for diagnosis and response evaluation during treatment and follow-up for bacterial negative pulmonary tuberculosis. MDR-TB manifests often centrilobular nodules, tree-in-bud sign, lobular consolidation, consolidation, cavitation and bronchiectasis

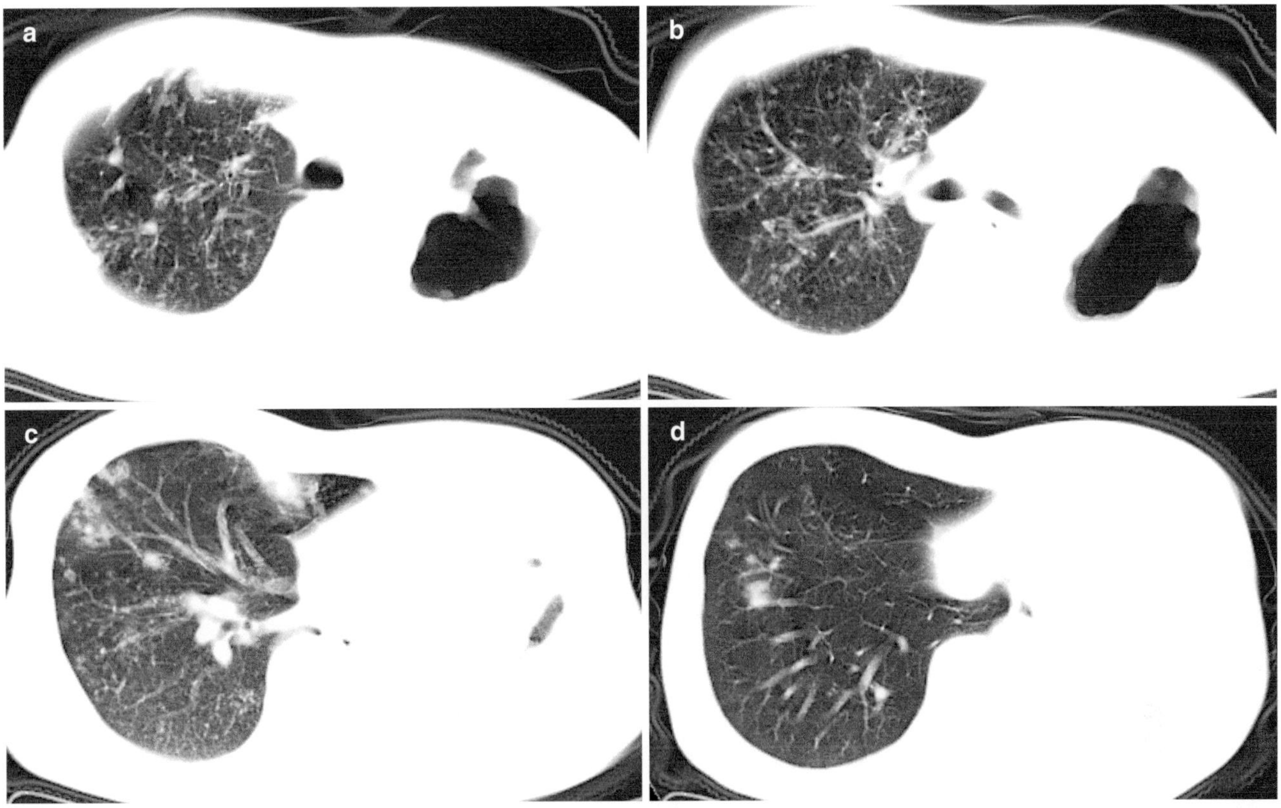

Fig. 8.4 (**a**–**d**) Chest CT scans on March 28, 2016: the collapse of the left thorax seems more obvious than the findings of the previous CT scans on June 5, 2015. Lesions in the right lower lobe showed absorption and amelioration, but an increased number of lesions were observed in the right upper and middle lobes, with an enlargement of the destroyed chamber in the left lung. A large consolidation appeared in the lower lobe of the left lung, and no normal lung tissue was found

in pulmonary CT findings. It has been reported by literature that centrilobular nodules and tree-in-bud sign are the most common image findings in XDR-TB and MDR-TB patients, with an incidence up to 100% [2]. The centrilobular nodules and tree-in-bud sign appearing in all CT examinations of this patient are the most common CT manifestations reflecting the evolution of the disease. Despite their high incidence in patients with XDR-TB or MDR-TB, these manifestations are not typical ones for either of them, nor the signs unique to XDR-TB to distinguish from MDR-TB. XDR-TB patients have severer clinical manifestation, more extensive lesions, and broader parenchyma damages shown by CT scans in comparison with MDR-TB patients, due to stronger invasiveness in XDR-TB than in non-extensive drug-resistant tuberculosis or a weaker eradication achieved by anti-tuberculosis drug against drug-resistant tuberculosis. Centrilobular nodules and tree-in-bud sign are related to bronchial dissemination of caseous necrotic substances, which implies most XDR-TB patients are sufferers of an active pulmonary TB and may explain the repeated occurrence of positiveness in sputum bacteria in this patient during her 9-year anti-tuberculosis treatment.

Moreover, high incidence of cavitation and emergence of multiple cavities are also important features of XDR-TB [2], which has an incidence of cavitation up to 85%, higher than that in MDR-TB patients. Studies [8–10] have shown that presence of multiple cavities is another major feature of XDR-TB patients and even the only specific manifestation. In case of the number of pulmonary tuberculosis cavities is more than three, the diameter of the cavity is larger than 30 mm, and the area where the cavity exists is more than two lung fields, it is related to pulmonary MDR -TB [9], nevertheless, the incidence of cavitation is higher in XDR-TB patients than in those with MDR-TB. The more cavities there are, the more foci spread to the lungs through the bronchi and aggravate further the extent of pulmonary lesions. Thickness of cavities and their average diameter are larger in XDR-TB patients than in MDR-TB patients [11], and their thickened wall acts as a barrier against the entry of anti-tuberculosis drugs into the cavity. In addition, the increased concentration of Mycobacterium tuberculosis inside the cavity with an insufficient plasma concentration raises the risk for the bacteria to progress into a drug-resistant colony [11, 12]. Cavitation is the biological basis of MDR and XDR-TB, and what's more, the thickness of its wall is related to drug resistance [11]. Caseous sub-

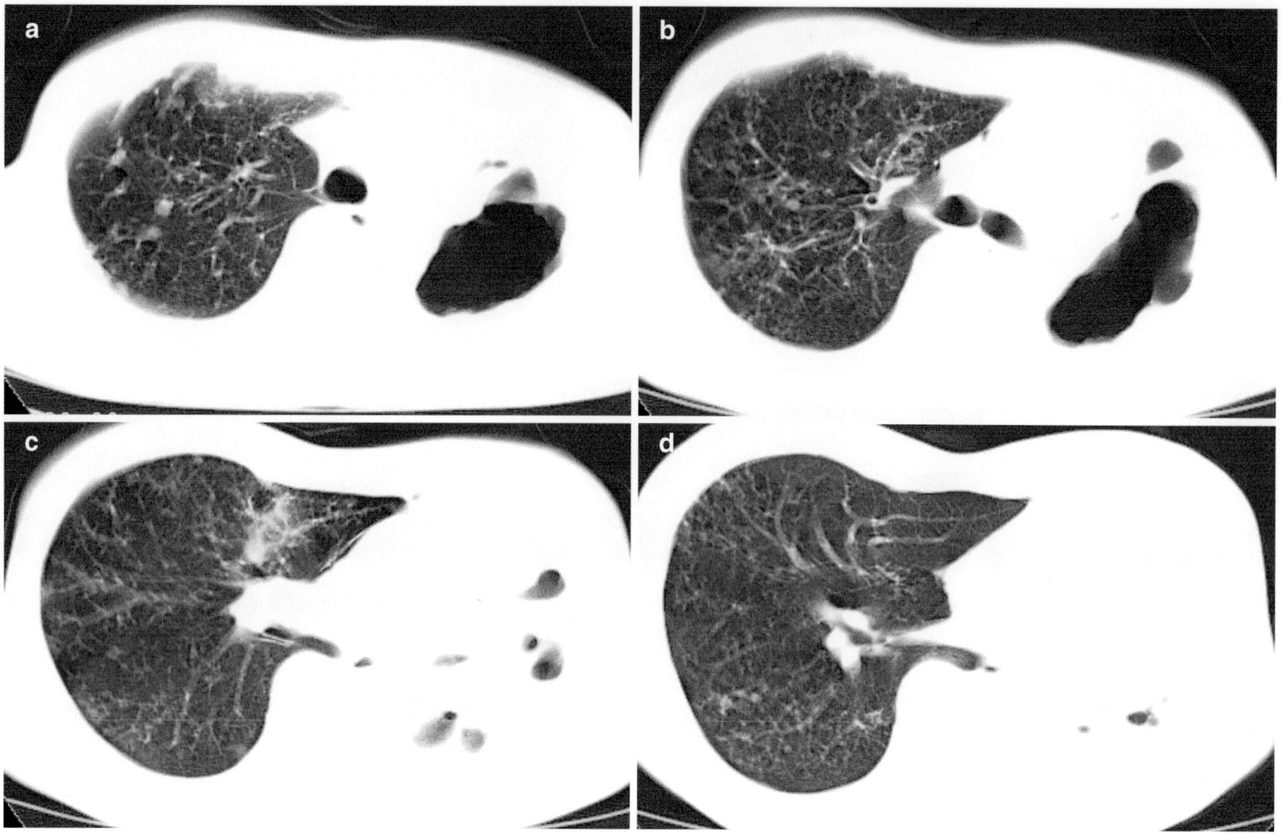

Fig. 8.5 (**a**–**d**) Chest CT scans on June 3, 2016, show an amelioration of the patchy, nodular, and strip opacity compared with CT findings on March 28, 2016, with a further deterioration of the destroyed left lung. The number of mouth-eaten cavities inside the consolidation in the left lower lobe increases compared with previous image findings

stances in lesions in the lingual segment of the left upper lobe and the basal segment in the left lower lobe were dissolved and discharged, followed by new cavitation in this patient, under a circumstance that the concurrent lesions had been absorbed during the treatment. The pre-existing cavity in the left lung, however, kept increasing in size with fusion, and the lung destruction aggravated further. Meanwhile, the consolidation in the left lower lobe became increasingly obvious, with persistent increase in caseous necrosis and liquidation inside the consolidation in later phase, leading finally to complete destruction of the left lung. The increased number of cavities, in addition, resulted in bronchial dissemination more easily, and therefore a vicious cycle was started. That was also one of the reasons predisposing this patient to the increasing number of disseminated lesions in the right lower lobe during the treatment. Among patients with cavitation, XDR-TB manifested more pulmonary lobes containing cavities compared with MDR-TB, resulting in broader extent and greater severity of intra-pulmonary disseminating lesions in XDR-TB than in MDR-TB [2].

A possibility of XDR-TB should be considered, in case of multiple cavitations, broad tree-in-bud signs and centrilobular nodules as shown by findings of CT scans. It is worth noting, however, that there is considerable overlap of CT findings between XDR-TB and MDR-TB, and a differentiation between MDR-TB and XDR-TB can be hardly based on CT findings alone, thereby necessitating laboratory tests including sputum culture and drug susceptibility tests.

Case 2

The patient was a 29-year-old female complaining recurrent cough with fever and night sweat for 1 and half year, and anorexia for 10 days. One and a half years before (January 2017), the patient had cough and expectorated a small amount of white sticky sputum which was hard to discharge without obvious inducement, complicated with night sweat and fever (mainly on the afternoon and during the night) with the highest temperature about 38.5 °C. No significant amelioration of symptoms was observed post to self-administered treatment against "cold." She sought medical service in People's Hospital at the local county in April 2017, and chest CT scans showed "the secondary pulmonary tuberculosis in both lungs, with cavitation in the right upper lobe," suggesting a diagnosis of pulmonary tuberculosis. An anti-tuberculosis treatment of combined drugs in blister pack was launched on April 16, 2017, but after that she still had cough

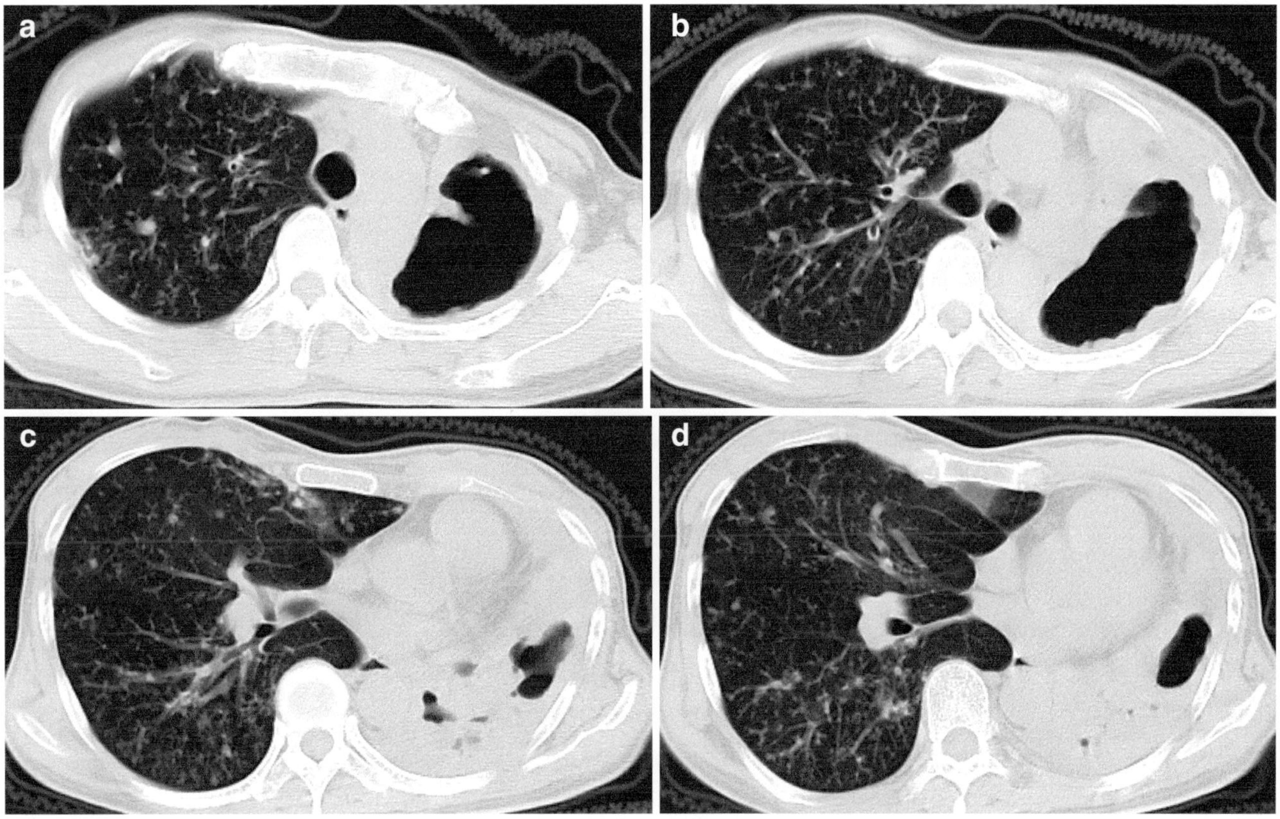

Fig. 8.6 (**a**–**d**) Chest CT scans on October 17, 2016: The number of subpleural lesions in the right upper lobe and the lesions in the right lower lobe increase than before, and there is emergence of patchy opacities and bronchial disseminating lesions, while an absorption and amelioration are observed for lesions in the right middle lobe, in comparison with findings of CT scans on June 3, 2016. Mouth-eaten cavities in the left lower lobe were enlarged gradually and fused, aggravating further the destruction of the left lung

with fever. On June 15, 2017, she was transferred to the Hospital of Infectious Diseases for hospitalization.

Physical examination: Emaciation, a facial feature of chronic disease, coarse breath sound in both lungs, no obvious wheezes or moist crackles were heard. Blood routine: hemoglobin 72 g/L. Renal function: uric acid 610 μmol/L. No abnormality was observed for flow cytometry or hepatic function. Positiveness (4+) was shown in sandwich cup acid fast bacillus smear on June 15, 2017. Mycobacterium tuberculosis culture with modified Lowenstein–Jensen test: positive (3+). Identification of Mycobacterium species (MPB64): positive. Fluorescent PCR and GeneXpert MTB/RIF test: positive (a great quantity). Test of tuberculosis drug resistance genes (INH + RFP): resistance to INH and RFP (Fig. 8.10).

Acid fast bacillus smear on July 21, 2017, showed positiveness (4+). Drug susceptibility test on July 23, 2017, showed resistance to S, H, R, E, Lfx, Am, Cm, Pto, Mfx, Clr, and Rfb.

Negativeness was shown for smear and sandwich cup. Mycobacterium culture (modified Lowenstein–Jensen test): positive (1+). Identification of Mycobacterium species (MPB64): positive. Fast Mycobacterium BD960 culture: positive. Identification of Mycobacterium species (PCR) on September 21, 2017: complex of mycobacterium tuberculosis. Lowenstein–Jensen susceptibility test plus fast drug susceptibility test on October 9, 2017: resistance to S, H, R, RFT, Pto, E, PAS-Na, Lfx, and Cm. Results of re-examination of CT scans on October 9, 2017, are as follows (Fig. 8.11).

The original regimen was continued until December 14, 2017, and the patient had no obvious discomforts. Re-examined hepatic and renal functions revealed no obvious abnormality. Results of re-examination of CT scans on December 18, 2017, are shown below (Fig. 8.12).

Sandwich cup acid fast bacillus smear was negative (−) on January 22, 2018. Mycobacterium BD960 rapid culture: positive. Identification of Mycobacterium species (MPB64): positive. Lowenstein–Jensen susceptibility plus fast susceptibility on March 5, 2018, showed resistance to S, H, R, Pto, Rfb, E, PAS-Na, and Lfx, and a treatment containing Am-Cs-Lzd-Cfz-Mfx-Z-Pa was given.

Sandwich cup acid fast bacillus smear was negative (−) on April 24, 2018. Mycobacterium culture (modified Lowenstein–Jensen method): negative. Identification of Mycobacterium species (MPB64): no mycobacterium was found. Mycobacterium BD960 rapid culture: negative. A treatment

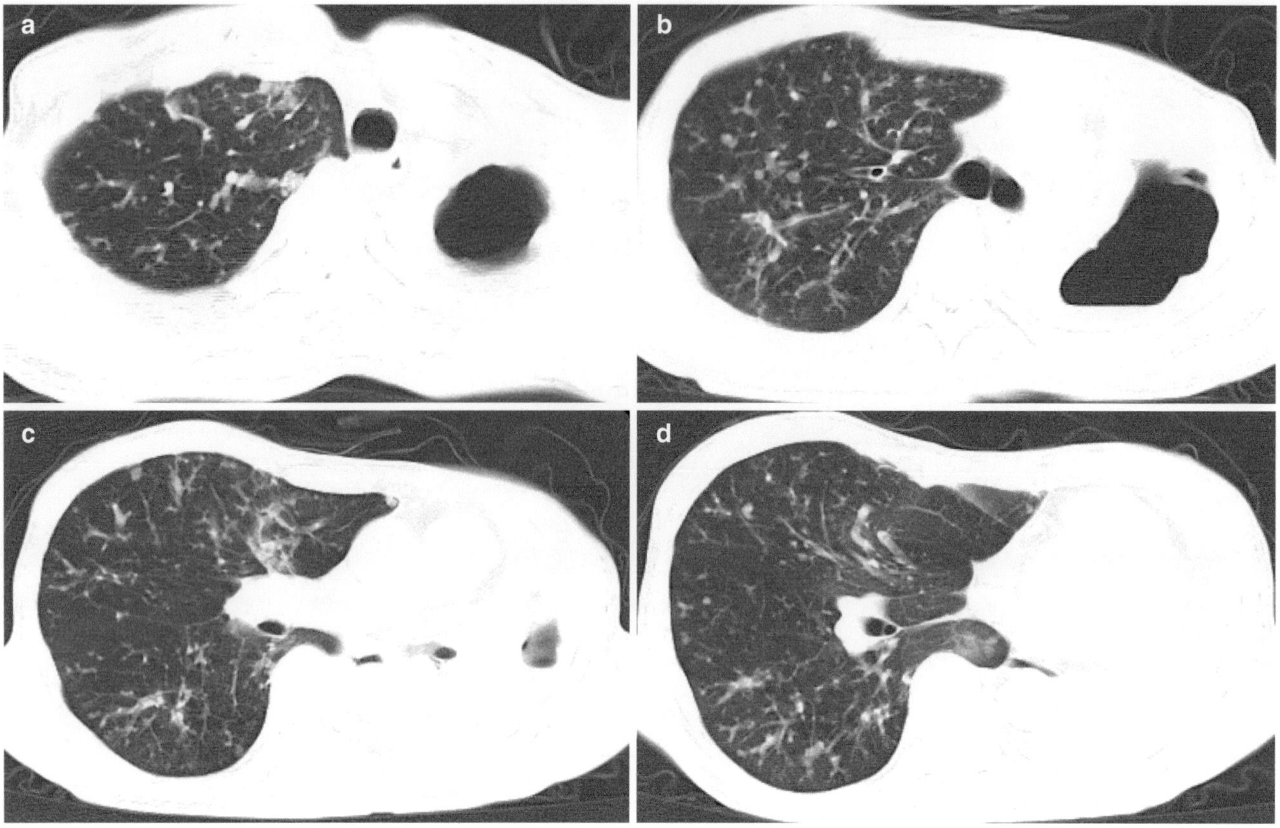

Fig. 8.7 (**a**–**d**) Chest CT scans on June 13, 2017, show an absorption and amelioration of lesions in the right lower lobe in comparison with findings of CT scans on October 17, 2016. A gas/liquid interface is formed in destruction chamber in the left upper lobe, the cavity in the left lower lobe shows a filling with the increased contents, and the bronchial stenosis in the left lower lobe becomes more obvious than before

containing Cs-Lzd-Cfz-Mfx-Z-Pa was given on April 15, 2018. Re-examination of chest CT scans was performed on May 9, 2018, with findings shown below (Fig. 8.13).

Mycobacterium tuberculosis culture (modified Lowenstein–Jensen method) on July 11, 2018, and in August: negative. Identification of Mycobacterium species (MPB64): no mycobacterium was found. Mycobacterium BD960 rapid culture: negative. Re-examination of chest CT scans on May 9, 2018, showed findings as follows (Fig. 8.14).

The anti-tuberculosis treatment was continued, and the patient had no obvious discomfort. Results of chest CT scans on December 11, 2018, are as follows (Fig. 8.15).

The patient had no obvious discomfort. Sandwich cup acid fast bacillus smear shows negativeness on March 13, 2019. Mycobacterium culture (modified Lowenstein–Jensen method): negative. Identification of Mycobacterium species (MPB64): no Mycobacterium was found. Mycobacterium BD960 rapid culture: negative. Rifampicin incubation (100ug/ml): negative. Re-examination of chest CT scans manifested findings as below (Fig. 8.16).

Discussion

It took only 3 months for the disease in these patients evolving from the onset of symptoms to the diagnosis of pulmonary tuberculosis. Moreover, the presence of cavities was found in her first consultancy with positiveness in sputum bacterium. After a diagnosis of cavitary tuberculosis was established, an anti-tuberculosis treatment of combined drugs in blister pack was continued for 2 months, but symptoms of the patient showed no relief. After hospitalization on June 15, 2017, sputum smear and sputum culture showed the presence of Mycobacterium tuberculosis, and the bacterial content was great (sputum smear acid fast bacilli 4+). Rapid gene detection showed resistance to both rifampicin and isoniazid, while the exposure to anti-tuberculosis drugs had lasted only 2 months, exceeding the time range of 1 month as defined for the primary drug resistance. According to the results of drug susceptibility test after admission, the range of the drug susceptibility test in the patient was wide, with a resistant almost to most of the drugs, exceeding further the definition of XDR-TB. According to the severity of drug resistance and the duration of anti-tuberculosis treatment, it was extremely unbelievable that such a widespread drug resistance occurred due to gene mutation of Mycobacterium tuberculosis caused by the use of ant-tuberculosis drugs lasting such a short period of only 2 months. It was reasonable to believe, therefore, that the extensive drug resistance in this

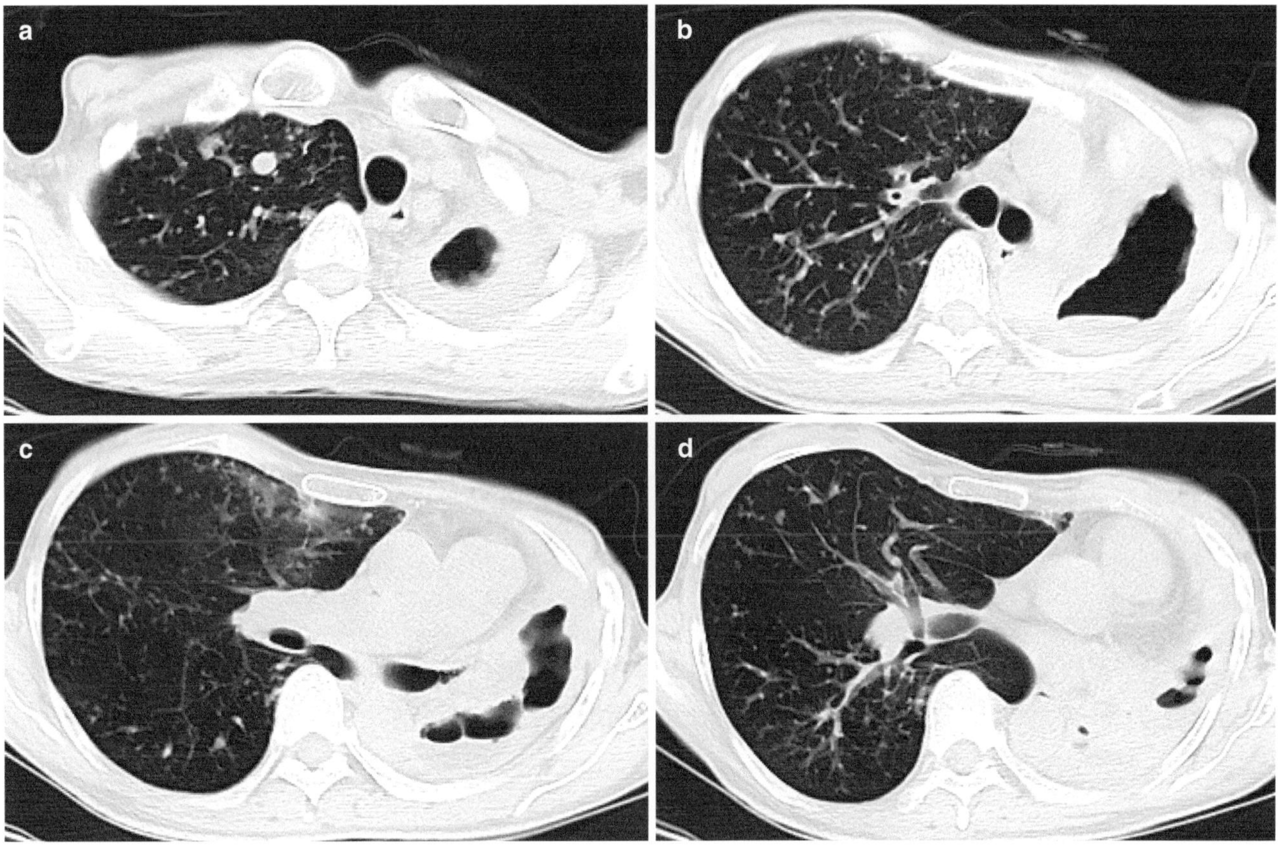

Fig. 8.8 (**a–d**) Chest CT scans on August 28, 2018, show an increased number of lesions in the apical segment of the right upper lobe and in the lateral segment of the right middle lobe, with a discharge of contents from the destruction chamber in the left lung and the shrinkage of the destruction chamber in the left upper lobe than before, as compared with CT scans on June 13, 2017

patient is the primary rather than the acquired. Meanwhile, the disease of this patient ameliorated gradually post to an anti-tuberculosis treatment based on her actual susceptibility, and sputum culture decreased gradually from bacteria positiveness (4+) to negativeness, which persisted up to the last sputum culture. Gradual absorption of intra-pulmonary lesions was also shown by multiple CT scans, together with shrinkage and closure of the cavities. Despite non-complete absorption of lesion as shown by the final CT scans, there was no enlargement of lesions or an emergence of new disseminated lesions. No matter from the clinical, laboratory, or CT examination results, the patient was in an evolving process of continuous improvement. This also showed that the treatment of this patient was very effective.

The chest CT findings of this patient, characterized in consolidations in both lungs, lobular consolidations, centrilobular nodules and tree-in-bud signs, as well as multiple cavities in both lungs, seem consistent with the CT findings of multi-resistant pulmonary tuberculosis or extensively drug-resistant tuberculosis [5, 13]. Despite the persistent absorption and amelioration of pulmonary lesions post to active treatment based on multiple drug susceptibility tests, the post-treatment absorption in this patient was still distinguishable from that in drug-susceptible pulmonary tuberculosis characterized in obvious absorption as early as month 3 post to the start of anti-tuberculosis treatment, an absorption of most of or all lesions in most patients within half a year, and smaller extent of residual proliferative fibrotic lesions with minor influence on patients. XDR-TB patients, however, have prolonged treatment cycle, high expenditure, and side reactions of the drug, making the ratio lower than 26% for patients completing successfully the whole treatment [14]. This also resulted in lower rate and lower speed in negative conversion of sputum bacteria in XDR-TB patients with slow absorption of lesions. In the course of treatment, there are often new disseminated lesions or the expansion of the original ones, and repeated destruction of pulmonary tissue causes easily the prolonged non-closure of the cavities or the increase and the fusion of enlarged cavities to form a destruction chamber. Despite the persistent amelioration achieved for this patient, a hidden risk of recurrence still remained because of prolonged duration of treatment with still presence of many lesions post to the absorption of cavities. Although the stable lesions were shown by the last a few CT scans, regular X-ray examination and follow-up should be continued and the vigilance should never languish because

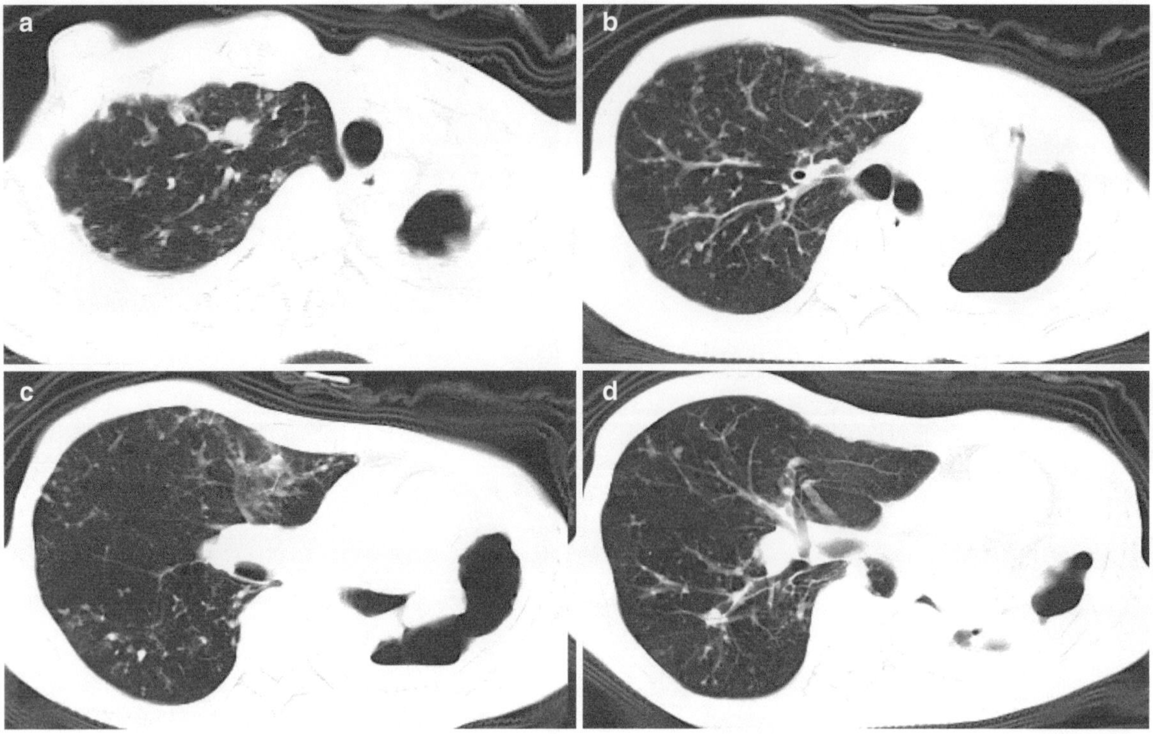

Fig. 8.9 (**a**–**d**) Chest CT scans on March 13, 2019, show a shrunk size of the nodular opacity in the right middle lobe, an increase in number of lesions with enlarged area in the right upper and lower lobes, a more obvious bronchial stenosis in the left lower lobe, and a further enlargement of the destruction chamber in the left lung, as compared with CT scans on August 28, 2018

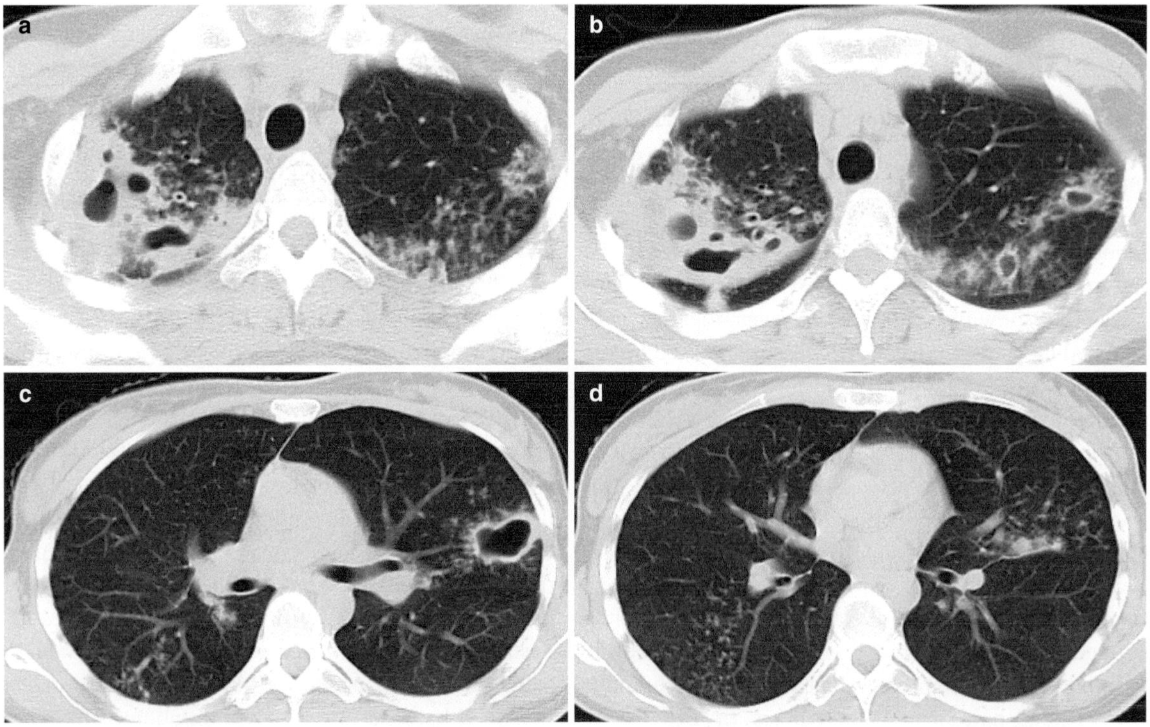

Fig. 8.10 (**a**–**d**) Chest plain CT scans on June 15, 2017, show both lungs are scattered with patchy consolidations, small dotty opacities, centrilobular nodules, and tree-in-bud signs, which seem obvious in both upper lungs. Multiple mouth-eaten cavities are shown inside the consolidation in the right upper lobe. Bronchiectasis is observed for the apical segment in the right upper lobe with thickening of the wall. Multiple thin-walled cavities are seen in the right upper lobe with smoother interior wall, and satellite lesions are noticed around the cavities

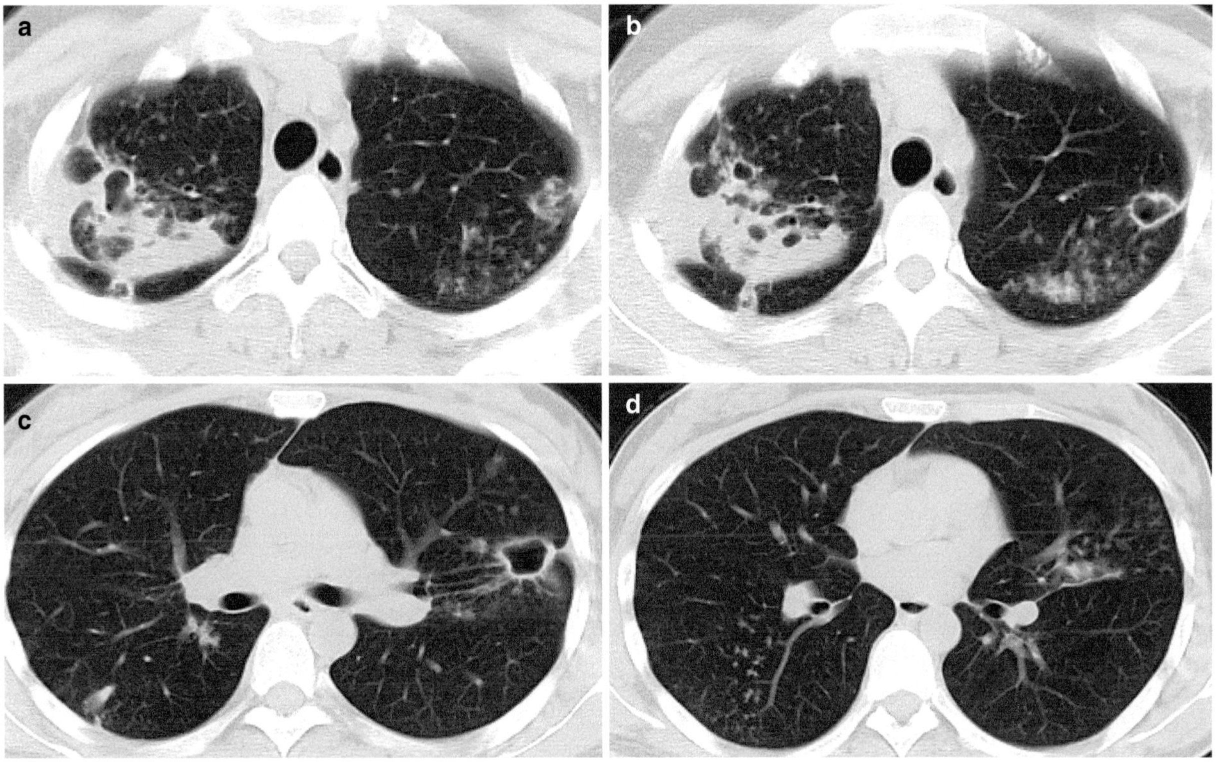

Fig. 8.11 (**a**–**d**) Chest CT scans on October 9, 2017: multiple cavities in both upper lobes shrink after anti-tuberculosis treatment, with absorption and amelioration of centrilobular nodules in the dorsal segment of the right lower lobe

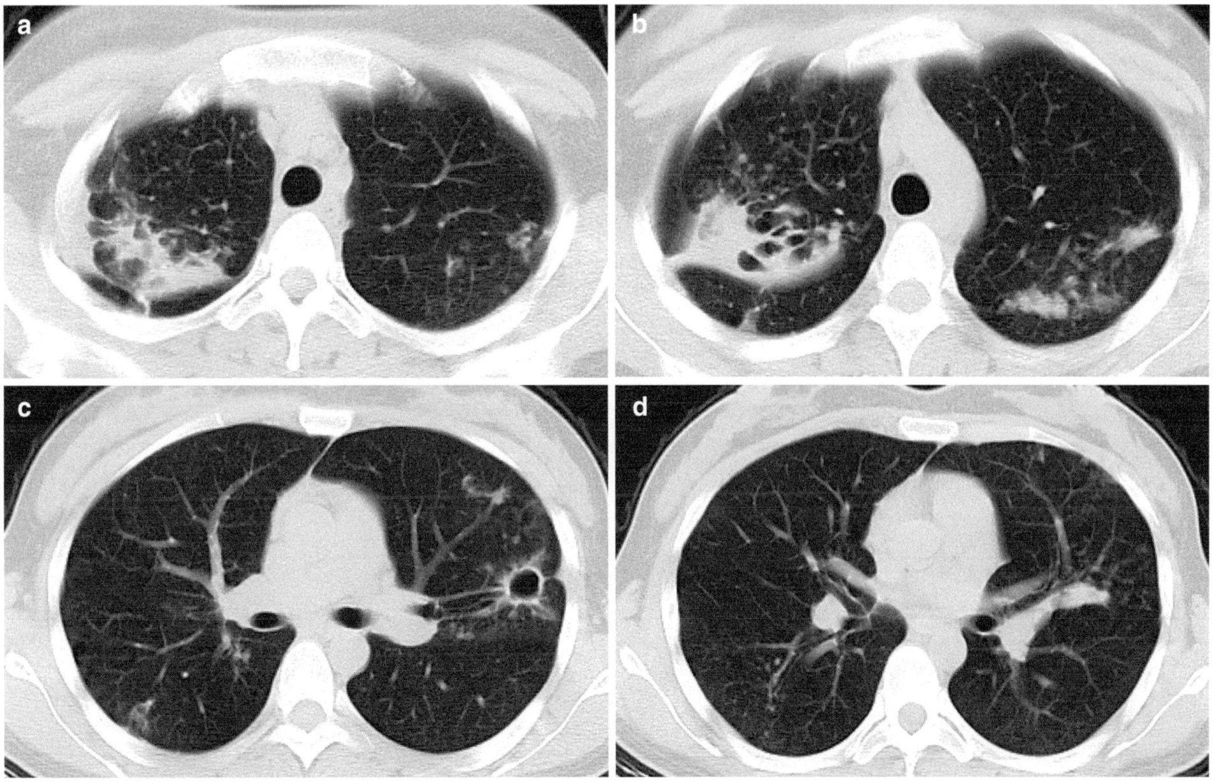

Fig. 8.12 (**a**–**d**) Chest plain CT scans on December 18, 2017: absorption and amelioration are observed for lesions in both lungs, with decreased extent of the consolidation, shrinkage, and closure of cavities in both upper lobes, and significantly decreased number of centrilobular nodules and tree-in-bud signs in both lungs, in comparison with findings of CT scans on June 15, 2017

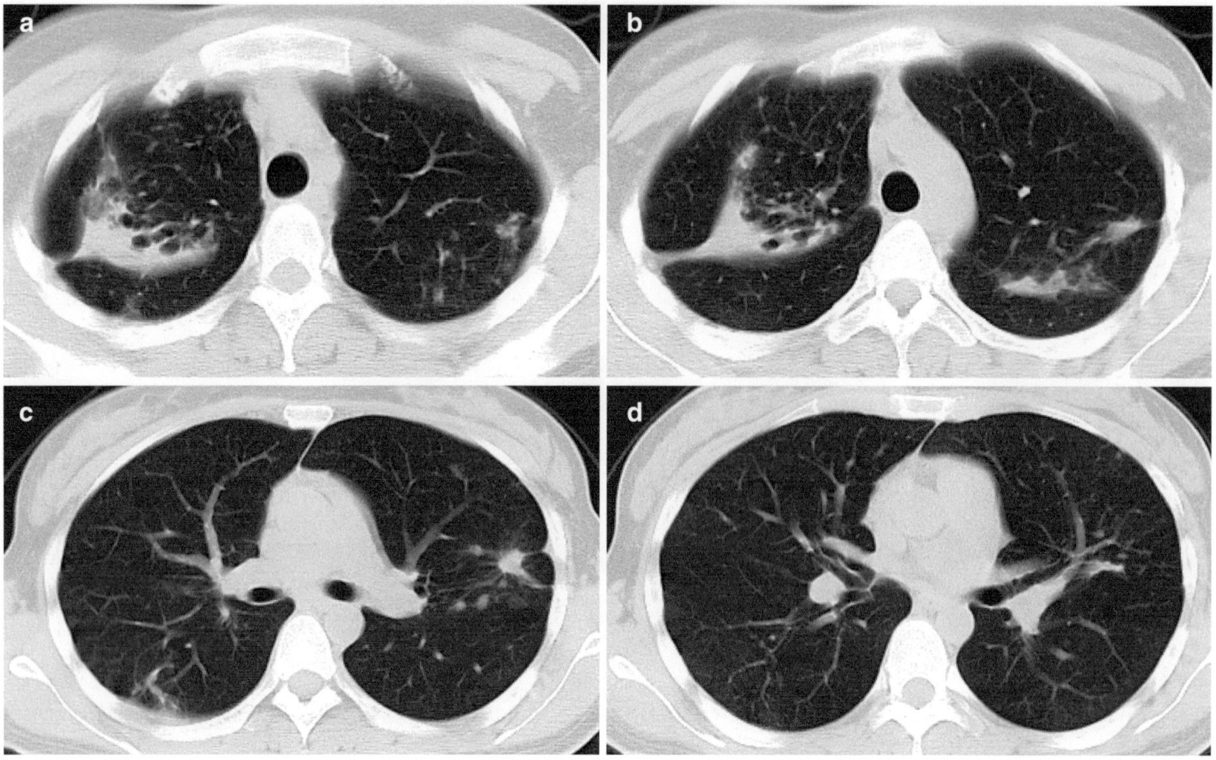

Fig. 8.13 (**a–d**) Chest plain CT scans on May 9, 2018: further absorption and amelioration are observed for lesions in both lungs, with decreased extent of consolidation, thinning of the previously thickened bronchial wall in the right upper lobe, a gradual decrease in the extent of lesions in the left upper lobe, and the closure of the cavity in the left upper lobe

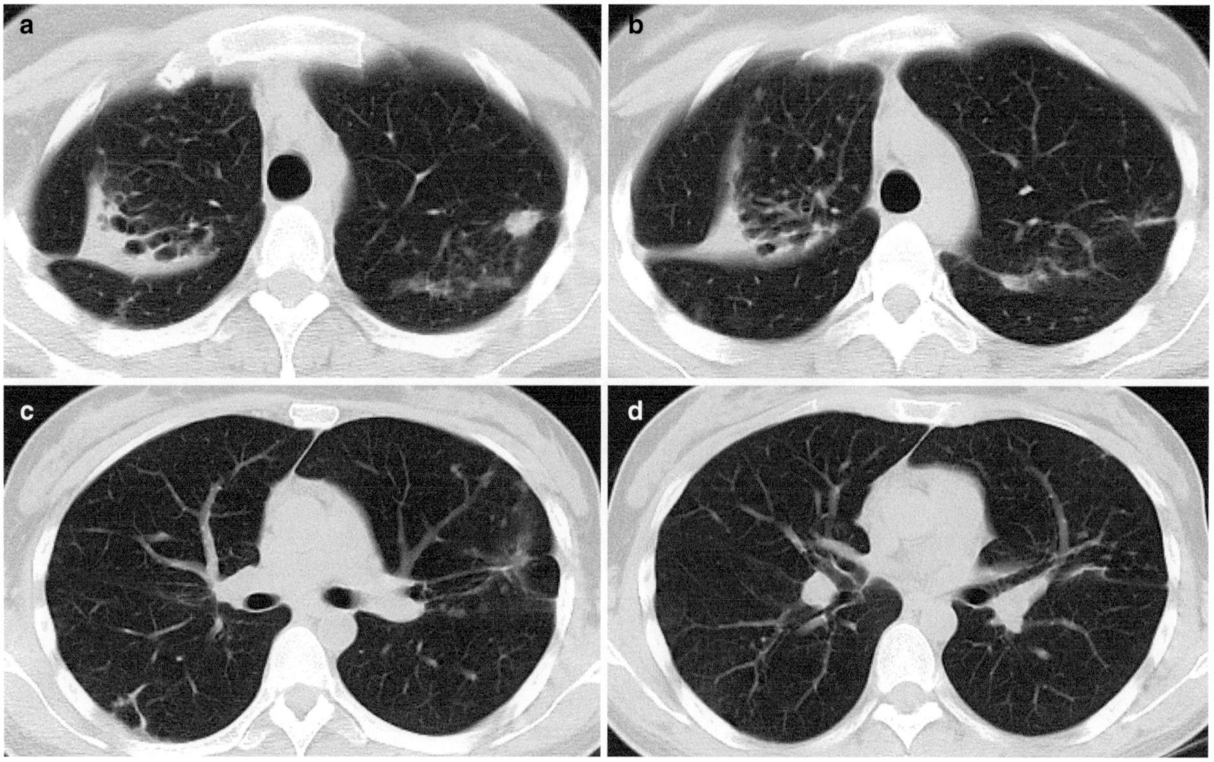

Fig. 8.14 (**a–d**) Chest CT scans on September 25, 2018: lesions in the apical segment in the left upper lobe are further absorbed, while the nodules shrink with clearer border and some of them form fibrous cord opacities

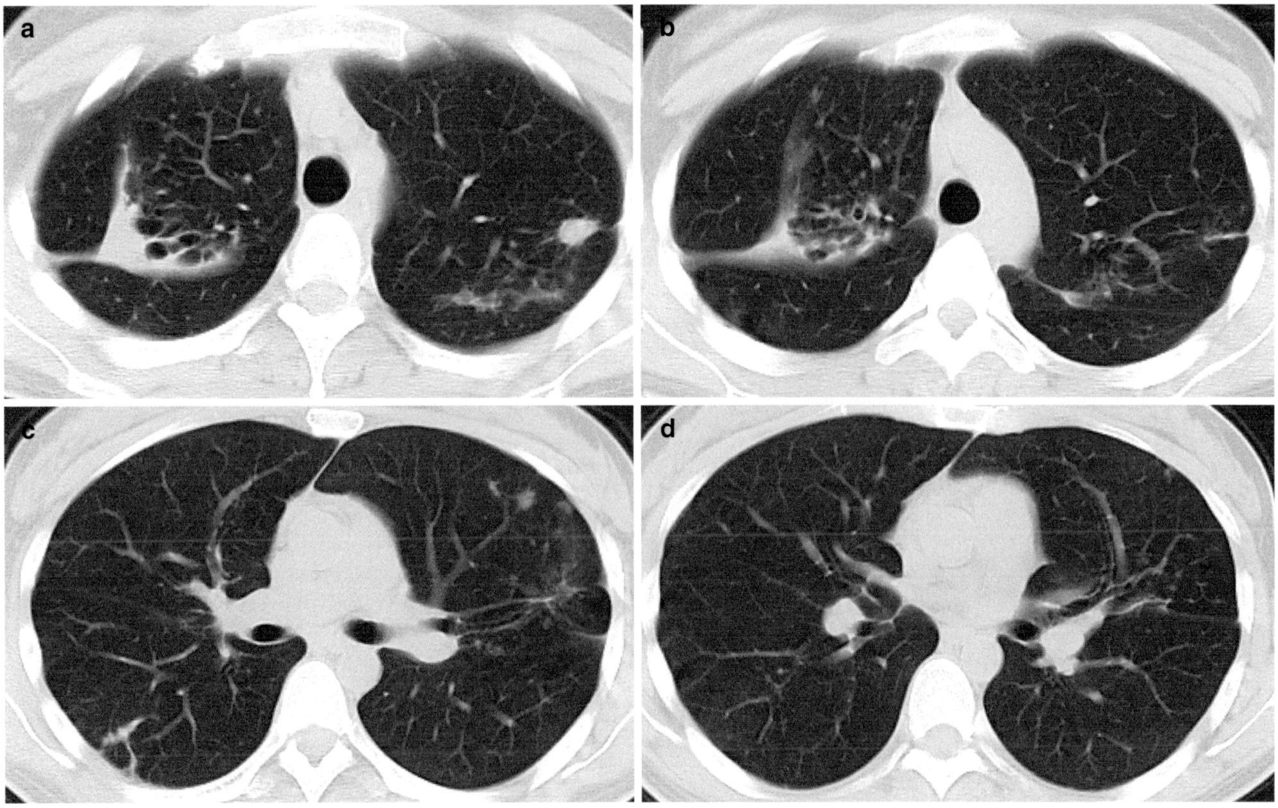

Fig. 8.15 (**a**–**d**) 2018.12.11 Chest CT plain scan: Compared with 2018.9.25CT, both lung lesions were stable. Still proliferation fibrotic changes

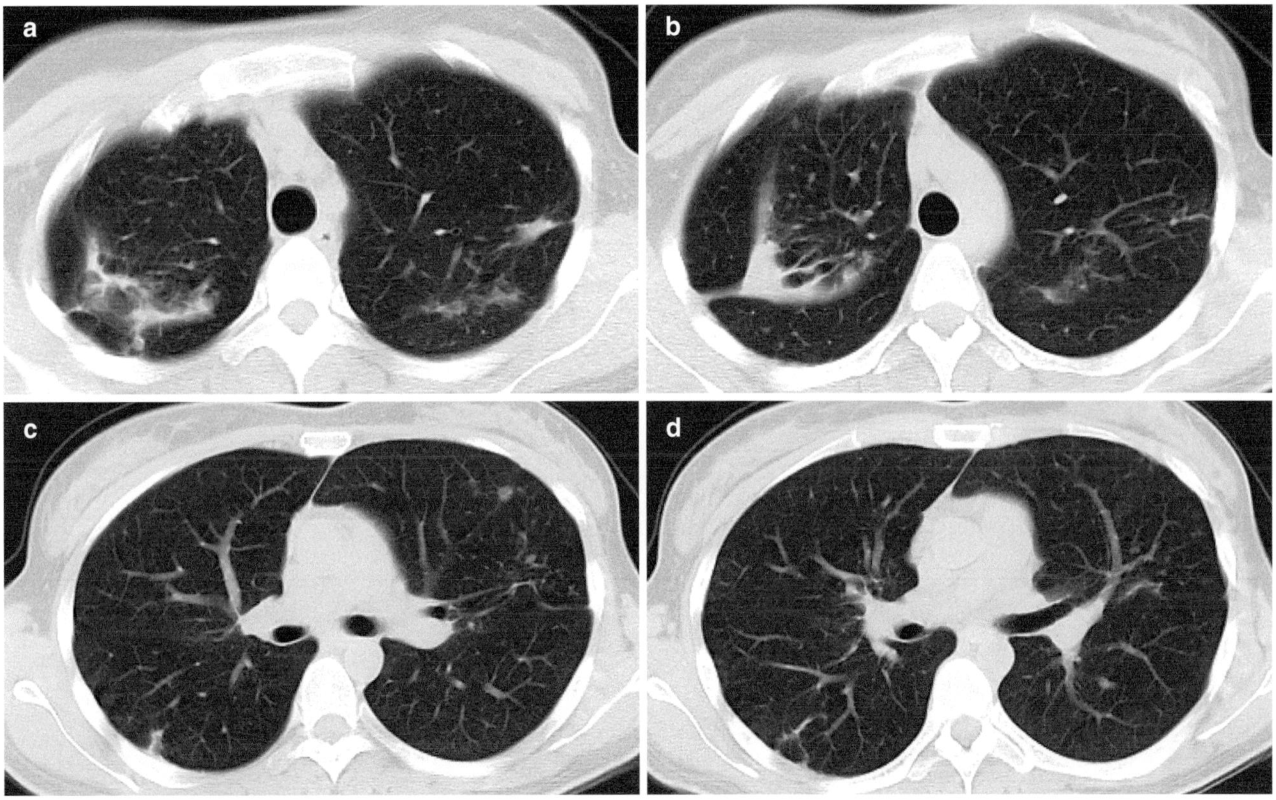

Fig. 8.16 (**a**–**d**) Chest CT scans on March 13, 2019: further absorption of lesions in both lungs is observed, while the lesions have clear borders and are dominated by mainly proliferation and fibrotic changes

the recurrence rate was significantly higher in XDR-TB patients than in drug-susceptible TB patients.

References

1. Tantan R, Lu P, Guofang D. 2020 WHO tuberculosis report: key data for China and the whole world [J/CD]. Electr J Emerg Infect Dis. 2020;5(4):280–4.
2. Lee ES, Park CM, Goo JM, et al. Computed tomography features of extensively drug-resistant pulmonary tuberculosis in non-HIV-infected patients [J]. J Comput Assist Tomogr. 2010;34(4):559–63.
3. Migliori GB, Besozzi G, Girardi E, et al. Clinical and operational value of the extensively drug-resistant tuberculosis definition [J]. Eur Respir J. 2007;30(4):623–6.
4. Nie L, Chu N. Interpretation of guidelines for planning and management of drug resistant tuberculosis 2011 update [J]. Chin J Clinicians. 2013;41(3):6–8.
5. Yu W, Tan W-g, Lu P-x. Classification and imaging manifestations of drug-resistant pulmonary tuberculosis [J/CD]. Electr J Emerg Infect Dis. 2019;4(1):42–7.
6. Wang Y-x, Chung MJ, Skrahin A, et al. Literature analysis of radiological signs related to multidrug-resistant tuberculosis [J/CD]. Electr J Emerg Infect Dis. 2018;3(2):244–53.
7. Cha J, Lee HY, Lee KS, et al. Radiological findings of extensively drug-resistant pulmonary tuberculosis in non-AIDS adults: comparisons with findings of multidrug-resistant and drug-sensitive tuberculosis [J]. Korean J Radiol. 2009;10(3):207–16.
8. Chuchottaworn C, Thanachartwet V, Sangsayunh P, et al. Risk factors for multidrug-resistant tuberculosis among patients with pulmonary tuberculosis at the central chest institute of Thailand [J]. PLoS One. 2015;10(10):e0139986.
9. Joshi AR, Mishra S, Sankhe AP, et al. HRCT spectrum of pulmonary multidrug-resistant tuberculosis in HIV negative patients: a study in Indian population [J]. Int J Sci Res. 2017;6(4):596–600.
10. Kim HC, Goo JM, Lee HJ, et al. Multidrug-resistant tuberculosis versus drug-sensitive tuberculosis in human immunodeficiency virus negative patients: computed tomography features [J]. J Comput Assist Tomogr. 2004;28(6):366–71.
11. Cheon H. Comparison of CT findings of between MDR-TB and XDR-TB: a propensity score matching study [J]. Imaging Med. 2017;9(5):125–9.
12. David HL. Probability distribution of drug resistant mutants in unselected populations of mycobacterium tuberculosis [J]. Appl Microbiol. 1970;20(5):810–4.
13. Li D, He W, Chen B, et al. Primary multidrug-resistant tuberculosis versus drug-sensitive tuberculosis in non-HIV-infected patients: comparisons of CT findings [J]. PLoS One. 2017;12(6):e0176354.
14. Wilson JW, Tsukayama DT. Extensively drug-resistant tuberculosis: principles of resistance, diagnosis, and management [J]. Mayo Clin Proc. 2016;91(4):482–9.

Drug-Resistant Bronchial Tuberculosis

9

Guan-qiao Jin, Fang-jun Wei, Jie-qi Luo, Pu-Xuan Lu, Hong-zhou Lu, and Yi Xiang J. Wang

9.1 Summary of Drug-Resistant Bronchial Tuberculosis

Tracheobronchial tuberculosis (TBTB), defined as a tuberculosis occurring at mucosa, submucosa, smooth muscle, cartilage, and/or adventitia of trachea or bronchi [1], is one type of pulmonary tuberculosis. About 10–40% of pulmonary tuberculosis patients are complicated with tracheobronchial tuberculosis, and its prevalence keeps rising little by little with the gradual application of bronchoscopy during recent years [2]. The absence of specific early clinical manifestations in tracheobronchial tuberculosis results in misdiagnosis and missed diagnosis in many patients. The diagnosis of TBTB relies on bronchoscopy, which is capable of detecting promptly lesions in tracheobronchial lumen, such as intimal congestion, purulent secretion, swelling, membranous matter and granuloma, and the most characteristic microscopic finding is white or milky caseous substances covering diffusely bronchial mucosa [3]. TBTB can be categorized into six types based on findings under tracheoscopy: inflammatory infiltration (type I), ulcerative necrosis (type II), granulation proliferation (type III), cicatricial stenosis (type IV), softening of tracheobronchial wall (type V), and lymph node fistula (type VI) [1]. Bronchoscopic brush biopsy, having increased significantly the positiveness rate of acid fast bacilli in bronchial tuberculosis patients, provides a basis for pathogenic diagnosis. In addition, imaging examination is the first option for examining bronchial tuberculosis, and CT scans when used to examine bronchial tuberculosis may define not only the location of bronchial lesions, but also the situation of bronchial lumen, such as obstruction or stenosis and atelectasis. Bronchial stenosis, interruption, and deformation shown by chest CT scans are evidences supporting the diagnosis of bronchial tuberculosis. Main modalities for treating tracheobronchial tuberculosis are anti-tuberculosis medications, and the cure rate in treated patients is about 75% with an amelioration rate of about 24% [4].

As reported by WHO, there was estimated to be about 0.558 million cases of newly diagnosed multidrug-resistant tuberculosis (MDR-TB) worldwide in 2017. There were 58,000 MDR/rifampicin-resistant patients with 12% of new rifampicin-resistant cases and 108,000 relapse rifampicin-resistant cases (69%) among all pulmonary TB cases in bulletin China in this year. In addition, there were also 13,000 laboratory confirmed cases of MDR/rifampicin resistance. Patients starting to receive the second-line treatment against MDR/rifampicin-resistant tuberculosis in 2015 in China witnessed a treatment success rate of about 41% [5]. It was found by researchers based on a set of data in China that the incidence of DMR/TB complicated with TBTB was as high as 70.56% among all ordinary pulmonary TB with concurrent TBTB, higher than the 53.28% reported by our research for drug-susceptible bacterial-positive TB patients complicated with TBTB, and even much higher than the 14.30% reported by previous investigation for all TB patients with concurrent TBTB [5]. Cases of MDR complicated with TBTB were dominated by the types of inflammatory infiltration and cicatricial stenosis, accounting for 43.43% and 41.14%, respectively [6]. MDR-TB complicated with the

G.-q. Jin (✉)
The Affiliated Cancer Hospital of Guangxi Medical University, Guangxi, China
e-mail: jinguanqiao77@gxmu.edu.cn

F.-j. Wei · J.-q. Luo
Department of Radiology, The Third People's Hospital of Shenzhen, Shenzhen, Guangdong, China

P.-X. Lu
Diagnostic Imaging, Shenzhen Center for Chronic Disease Control, Shenzhen, China

H.-z. Lu
Infectious Disease, The Third People's Hospital of Shenzhen, Shenzhen, China
e-mail: luhongzhou@shphc.org.cn

Y. X. J. Wang
Department of Imaging and Interventional Radiology, Faculty of Medicine, The Chinese University of Hong Kong, New Territories, Hong Kong SAR

P.-x. Lu et al. (eds.), *Diagnostic Imaging of Drug Resistant Pulmonary Tuberculosis*,
https://doi.org/10.1007/978-981-99-8339-1_9

infiltration and cicatricial stenosis, i.e., the two types of TBTB, will affect airway discharge and ventilation to various extent and will cause obstructive pneumonia and atelectasis in severe cases due to failure in timely treatment and even endanger lives of patients [7]. Early local intrabronchial drug injection through electronic bronchoscope for MDR-TB patients on the basis of core chemotherapeutic regimens may increase the early sputum negative conversion rate and promote the absorption of lesions [8]. There is no authoritative data report, however, concerning incidence and cure rate of bronchial drug-resistant tuberculosis either domestic or abroad, because the realization of precise diagnosis and local intervention requires vital procedures including bronchofibroscopy to determine the sites of lesions, categorization based on bronchofibroscopic findings, etiological examination of bronchofibroscope lavage fluid and local interventional therapy under bronchofibroscope, in addition to examinations required by the diagnosis of drug-resistant tuberculosis, such as the etiological laboratory examination, drug sensitivity test related to Mycobacterium tuberculosis, and imaging examination [9]. High-resolution CT scans and three-dimensional reconstruction are of great importance for evaluating comprehensively tracheobronchial lesions and observing their responses [10–12].

9.2 Image Findings of Drug-Resistant Bronchial Tuberculosis

With the continuous development of equipment and technology needed by CT scans and wide application of CT diagnosis, HRCT plays an increasingly important role in the clinical diagnosis, differential diagnosis, and response evaluation of tracheobronchial tuberculosis and/or drug-resistant tuberculosis. (1) Tracheobronchial wall, stenosis or expansion of lumen, stump occlusion, and presence/absence of calcification can be displayed fully through three-dimensional reconstruction technology, using, respectively, CT virtual bronchoscopy (CTVB), surface shaded display (SSD), maximum intensity projection (MIP), minimum intensity projection (min IP), and multi-planar reconstruction (MPR) [13]. (2) Transverse, sagittal, and coronal images of HRCT may show the morphology of trachea and bronchi, their stenosis degree, the extent of involvement along the long axis of the wall, the invasion outside the wall, and the location of the lesions, based on which a comparison can be made between CT findings and branchofiberoscope findings/pathology to establish a precise diagnosis. (3) By means of axial images of CT scans, lesions in the lungs are observed, including their location, shape, size, distribution, and density, as well as presence/absence of invasion of pleura, pericardium, and mediastinum. (4) Re-examination of CT is performed in follow-up, in order to evaluate responses and guide the treatment.

There is a certain difficulty in using chest X-ray to evaluate tracheobronchial lesions in patients with tracheobronchial tuberculosis and/or drug-resistant tuberculosis. HRCT can show mucosal edema, lumen stenosis, and roughness/thickening of tracheal and bronchial wall [14], while CT examination can understand accurately tracheal/bronchial pathogenetic location, as well as the number of affected bronchi and their severity. Bronchofibroscope can be used to observe directly the situation in the tracheobronchial lumen, including the presence of congestion, edema, erosion, ulcer, tumor-like protrusion, granuloma formation, and necrotic caseous matter and whether tubercles are under the bronchial mucosa. Some limitations exist, however, in bronchofibroscope if used to evaluate extra-bronchial and intra-pulmonary lesions. Using CT scans, we not only understand the basic lesions in the bronchial lumen based on a three-dimensional reconstruction of images but also realize a limited evaluation of the lesions in bronchial wall and in lungs. Therefore, the systematic combination of these two approaches is of great significance for establishing accurate diagnosis.

Most patients with tracheobronchial tuberculosis are complicated with pulmonary tuberculosis, and cases of pure tracheobronchial tuberculosis occupy about 5–10%. It is vital, therefore, to understand intra-pulmonary lesions through CT scans for patients with tracheobronchial tuberculosis and/or drug-resistant tuberculosis [15]. Mycobacterium tuberculosis having involved with the trachea and bronchi may spread to pulmonary bronchioles and alveolar tissue, thereby inducing corresponding pulmonary manifestations. Meanwhile, mucosal congestion, edema, erosion, ulcer, or granuloma formation caused by bronchial tuberculosis may result in lumen stenosis, thereby inducing obstructive pneumonia, emphysema, or lobar/segmental atelectasis. The above pathological process leads to chest CT findings manifesting either patches, strips, nodules, and tree-in-bud signs distributed in both lungs, or obstructive inflammatory changes or consolidations in various degrees in lobes or segments of both lungs.

Anti-tuberculosis responses can be evaluated accurately using follow-up with CT scans for patients during their treatment, based on which a clinical guidance is performed to modify timely therapeutic regimen. Therefore, the improvement of cure rate and reduction of complications necessitate the dynamic observation of images. The principle of standard imaging follow-up for drug-resistant tracheobronchial tuberculosis is an evaluation based on a low-dose CT examination post to one-month anti-tuberculosis treatment. The absorption of the lesions as anticipated indicates a satisfactory response. Subsequently, chest CT scans should be performed, respectively, at month 3 and 9 after anti-tuberculosis treatment is launched, and their results will be evaluated to decide whether to end the anti-tuberculosis treatment [15, 16].

9.3 Introduction of Typical Cases of Drug-Resistant Bronchial Tuberculosis

Poly-Resistant Bronchial Tuberculosis (Treatment-Naive)

Patient XX Yin, a 14-year-old female, visited a primary hospital with a chief complaint of cough with expectoration for 1 month, where chest CT scans showed patchy shadows in both upper pulmonary lobes (Fig. 9.1). On February 8, 2018, she was referred to and inhospitalized in a specialized hospital with a clinical diagnosis of infiltrative pulmonary tuberculosis with bronchial tuberculosis without bacteriological or histological tests.

Physical examinations at admission: no sternum tenderness; symmetrical respiratory movement; no significant increase or decrease in tactile fremitus in both lungs. Resonance in percussion in percussion and coarse respiratory sound heard for both lungs, without wheezes or moist crackles; no pleural friction rub.

Blood routine: White blood cell count 9.52×10^9/L, monocyte percentage 10.4%, erythrocyte count 5.52×10^{12}/L, hemoglobin concentration 149 g/L, platelet count 423×10^9/L, cytokeratin normal. Results were normal for liver and kidney functions, electrolytes, blood lipids, blood glucose, PCT, coagulation function, ESR, T-lymphocyte subsets, and glycosylated hemoglobin. Negativeness in syphilis, hepatitis B, hepatitis C and HIV. AFB (+) in alveolar lavage fluid.

The patient underwent bronchoscopy on February 12, 2018, under local anesthesia, with the findings revealing a patchy ulcerative necrosis in the parietal mucosa on the left of a sharp tracheal carina, without obvious abnormality in epiglottis, glottis, or trachea. The mild stenosis was observed in the lumen of the left main bronchus, the segmental

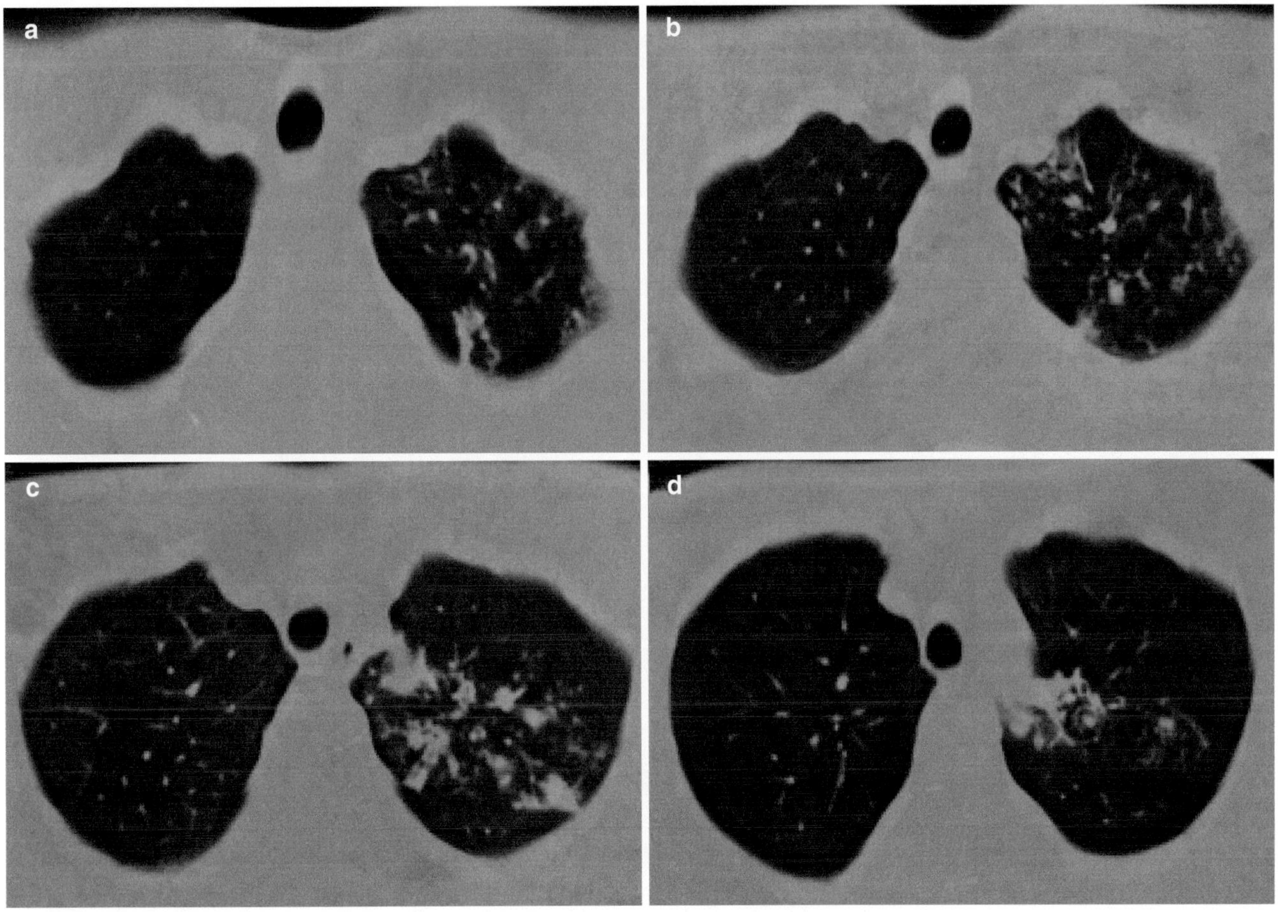

Fig. 9.1 (**a**–**k**) The first chest CT scans on February 8, 2018. (**a**–**d**) The lung window shows patchy and punctiform opacities with increased density and unclear boundaries in the left upper lung. (**e**–**h**) The lung window shows strip-like, nodular, and patchy opacities with various sizes, irregular shapes, and increased density in the right lower lobe, wherein Fig. **f** shows the mild stenosis in the left main bronchus and in the left superior bronchus. (**i**–**k**) Coronal view of the three-dimensional reconstruction shows patchy, punctiform, nodular, and strip-like opacities with increased density in the left upper lobe and the right lower lobe

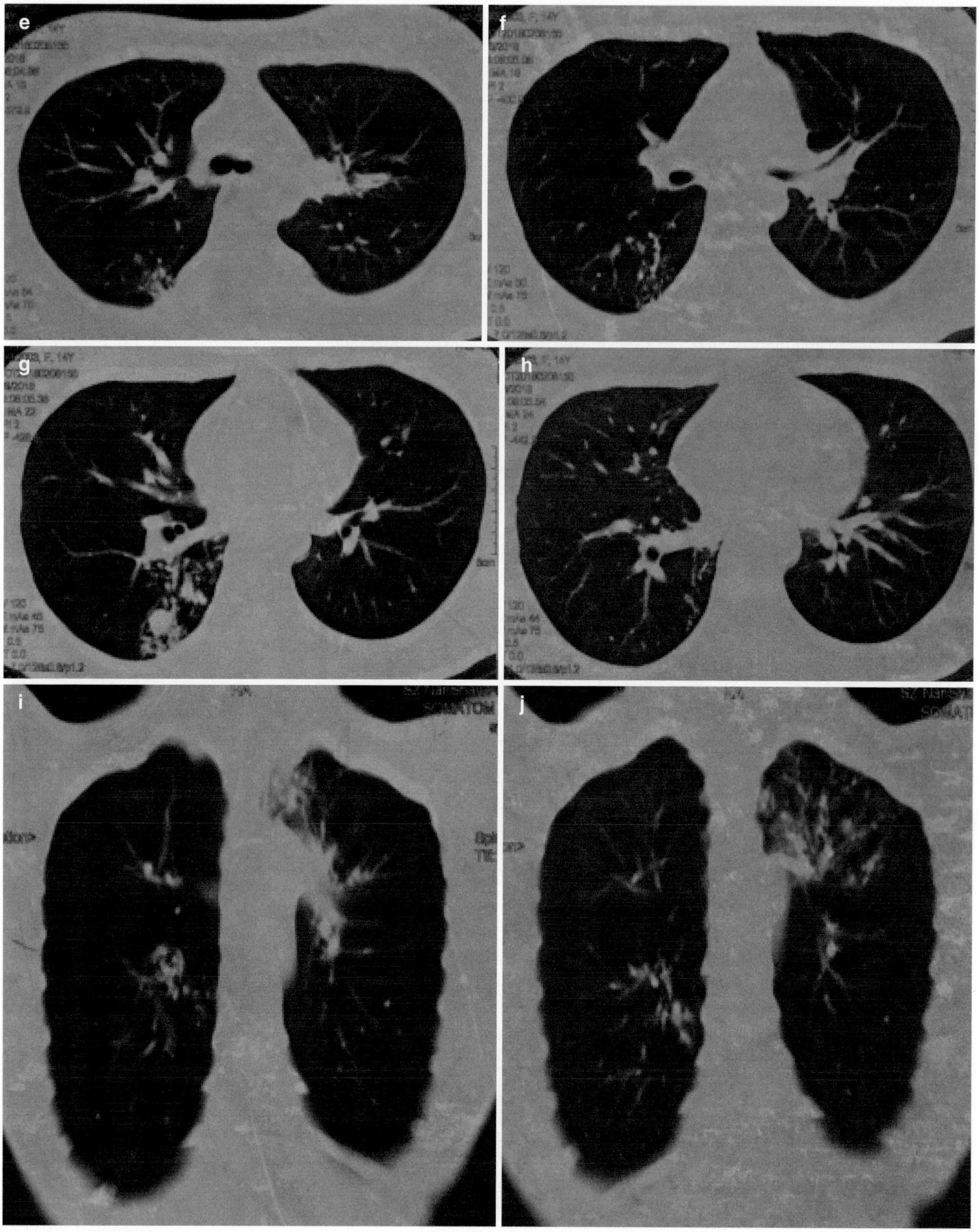

Fig. 9.1 (continued)

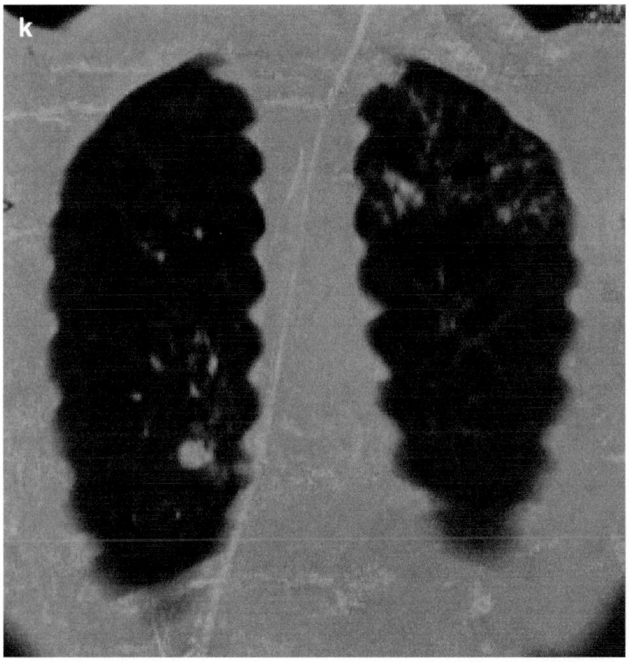

Fig. 9.1 (continued)

bronchus propria in the left upper lobe, the left lingual bronchus, and the left lower lobar bronchus, with an outer diameter of 4.9 mm, and the bronchoscope could pass through. The mucosa was swollen and thickened, with a large amount of white phlegm in the lumen of the bronchus propria in left upper lobe. The right main bronchus and each lobar/segmental bronchus seemed unobstructed, without any congestion of the mucosa. The anterior segment of the bronchoscope was inserted into the segmental bronchus propria of the left upper lobe, and a lavage was performed using 15 mL of normal saline with fractionated injection, followed by an etiological examination on about 15 mL of lavage fluid recovered. Bronchoscopy diagnosis: tracheal tuberculosis, and the left main bronchial and the left upper lobar bronchial tuberculosis; the ulcerative necrosis type (Fig. 9.2).

Results of human Mycobacterium tuberculosis showed resistance to amikacin (AK), capreomycin (CAP), and isoniazid (INH). An anti-tuberculosis treatment was launched immediately, consisting of isoniazid, rifampicin, ethambutol, and pyrazinamide, with concurrent liver protection and pulverization inhalation. On March 30, 2018, i.e., at month 1.5 of the anti-tuberculosis treatment, the pediatric patient was in a good condition and experienced an amelioration of symptoms such as cough. Re-examination of chest CT scans showed an obvious absorption of lesions in the left upper lobe and the right lower lobe (Fig. 9.3).

The general condition of the pediatric patient was generally good on June 1, 2018, post to 3.5-month anti-tuberculosis treatment, without obvious symptoms such as cough. Re-examination of chest CT scans showed a significant absorption of lesions in the left upper lobe and the right lower lobe (Fig. 9.4).

The patient underwent re-examination of bronchoscopy on June 4, 2018, revealing that the tracheal carina, the right main bronchus, and each lobar and segmental bronchus were unobstructed, without mucosal hyperemia. A mild cicatricial stenosis was observed at the left main bronchus with an exterior diameter of 4.9 mm, and the bronchoscopy could pass through. The mucosa seemed smooth without abnormal excretions, and a mild scarring was observed in the lumen of posterior segmental bronchus propria in the left upper lobe, without obvious abnormality in the rest of bronchi. The anterior segment of the bronchoscope was inserted into the segmental bronchus propria of the left upper lobe, and a lavage was performed using 30 ml of normal saline with fractionated injection, followed by an etiology examination on about 15 mL of lavage fluid recovered. Bronchoscopy diagnosis: scarring at the left main bronchus and at bronchus propria of the left lobe (Fig. 9.5).

The general condition of the pediatric patient was generally good on September 7, 2018, post to 7-month anti-tuberculosis treatment, without obvious symptoms such as cough. Re-examination of chest CT scans showed a somehow absorption of lesions in the left upper lobe and the right lower lobe (Fig. 9.6).

The general condition of the pediatric patient was generally good on December 9, 2018, post to 10-month anti-tuberculosis treatment, without obvious symptoms such as cough. Re-examination of chest CT scans showed a significant absorption of lesions in the left upper lobe and the right lower lobe (Fig. 9.7).

Bronchial lavage was performed for segmental bronchus propria in the left upper lobe on June 4, 2018, revealing the negativeness in acid fast bacillus smear. Result of RNA of acid fast bacillus was negative on June 6, 2018. Negativeness was shown for culture of Mycobacterium tuberculosis on October 12, 2018, and on December 9, 2018. Image findings on December 9, 2018, seemed consistent with changes of secondary tuberculosis in both lungs, with scarring in the left main bronchus and the bronchus propria of the left upper lobe. The patients reported no discomfort on February 3, 2019, post to 12-month anti-tuberculosis treatment.

Final diagnosis and outcome: (1) Initial drug-resistant tuberculosis; (2) Multi-resistant bronchial tuberculosis, the ulcerative necrosis type; (3) Cured.

Discussion

No case has been reported so far for treatment-naïve polyresistant bronchial tuberculosis. The pediatric patient was 14 years old, and there was evidence that the source of infection was her father. After her consultancy, she underwent chest CT scans confirming strip-like and patchy opacities in

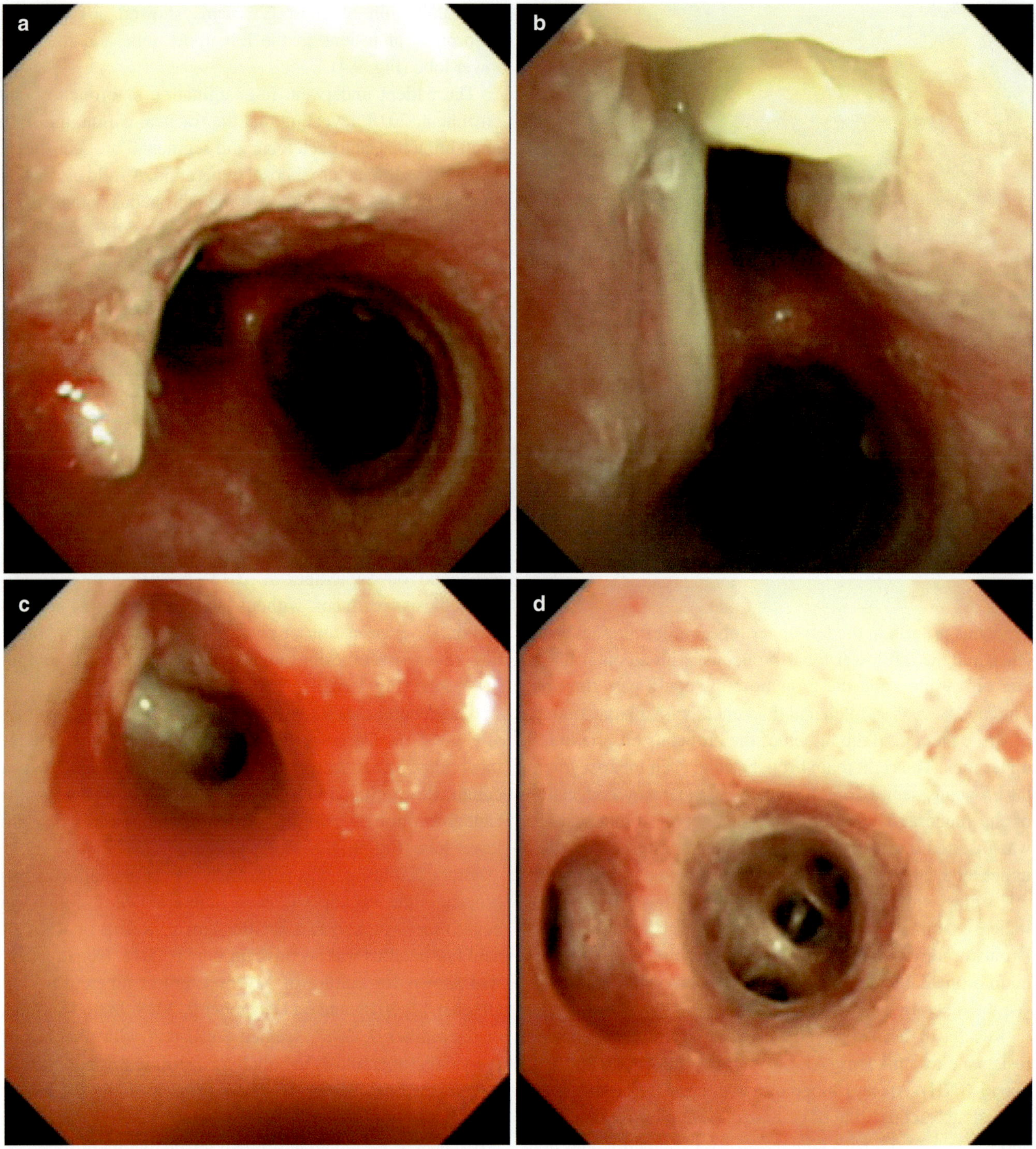

Fig. 9.2 (**a–d**) The bronchoscopy was performed on February 12, 2018, under local anesthesia, showing tracheal tuberculosis, and the left main bronchial and the left upper lobar bronchial tuberculosis; the ulcerative necrosis type. (**a**) The patchy ulcerative necrosis in the parietal mucosa on the left of the tracheal carina. (**b**) A mild stenosis in the lumen of the left main bronchus, with swollen and thickened mucosa. (**c**) A mild stenosis in the lumen with swollen and thickened mucosa in the left upper lobar bronchus, with a great amount of white phlegm in the lumen of the bronchus propria in left upper lobe. (**d**) A mild stenosis in the lumen of the left lower bronchus, with swollen and thickened mucosa, and a great amount of white phlegm in a lumen

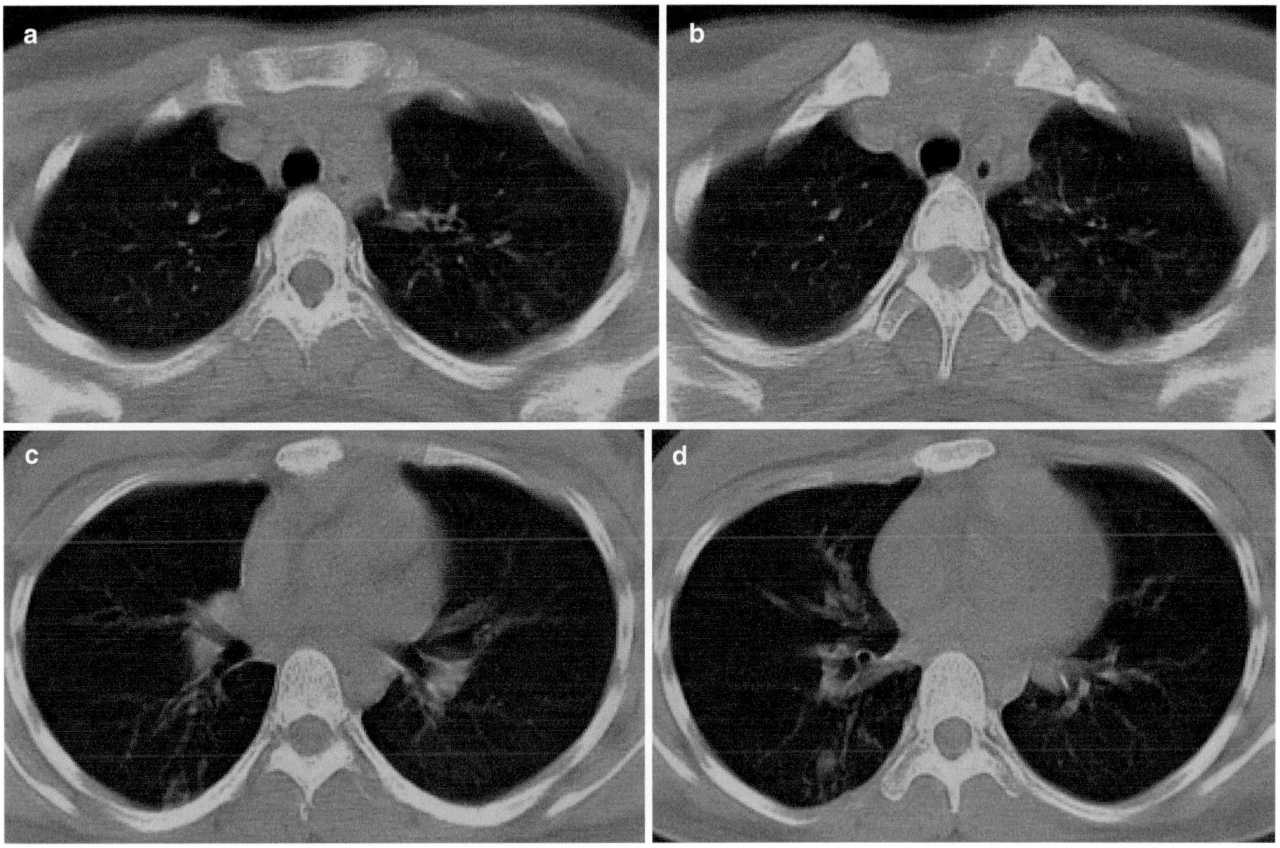

Fig. 9.3 (**a**–**d**). Re-examination of chest CT on March 30, 2018. (**a**, **b**) Lung window of CT scans shows small punctiform opacities with increased intensity in the left upper lobe. (**c**, **d**) Small punctiform and patchy opacities are observed in the right lower lobe. The comparison with the first chest CT scans on February 8, 2018, shows obvious absorption and amelioration of lesions in both lungs

both lungs, bronchofibroscope and laboratory etiological detection with drug susceptibility test. Bronchoscopy showed a patchy ulcerative necrosis in the parietal mucosa on the left of the tracheal carina, a mild stenosis of lumen with swollen and thickened mucosa in the left main bronchus and in the bronchus of the left upper lobe, a great amount of white sticky sputum in the lumen of bronchus propria in the left upper lobe, and a mild stenosis of lumen with swollen and thickened mucosa in the left lower lobar bronchus containing a great amount of white sticky sputum. The diagnosis was tracheal tuberculosis, the left main bronchial and the left upper lobar bronchial tuberculosis; the ulcerative necrosis type. Mycobacterium tuberculosis was identified in the laboratory etiological culture, which showed resistance to three anti-tuberculosis drugs including amikacin (AK), capreomycin (CAP), and isoniazid (INH). This pediatric patient belonged to the ulcerative necrosis type of initial polyresistant bronchial tuberculosis, based on the Guideline of Diagnosis and Treatment of Tracheobronchial Tuberculosis and the latest grouping criteria for drug-resistant pulmonary tuberculosis [1, 10].

In addition, the patient manifested also clinical symptoms and signs dominated by cough and expectoration, the typical manifestations commonly observed in patients with ordinary pulmonary tuberculosis. The prolonged cough with expectoration in this patient, however, might correlate to the long duration needed for tissue repair in the specifically vulnerable sites, such as trachea and bronchi infected by tubercle bacillus. These may also be one of the clinical features of bronchial tuberculosis, based on which this disease is made distinguishable from pulmonary tuberculosis. The dominant lesions were in the left upper and the right lower lobes, as revealed by her first CT scans, were related to the involvement of the tracheal carina and the left main bronchus. The manifestations were dominantly strip-like, patchy, and nodular opacities, which were consistent with image findings of tracheobronchial tuberculosis or drug-resistant pulmonary tuberculosis [11, 12]. A gradual absorption of lesions was shown in the image findings post to effective anti-tuberculosis treatment, though this absorption was prolonged up to 10 months before the general disappearance of lesions in both lungs.

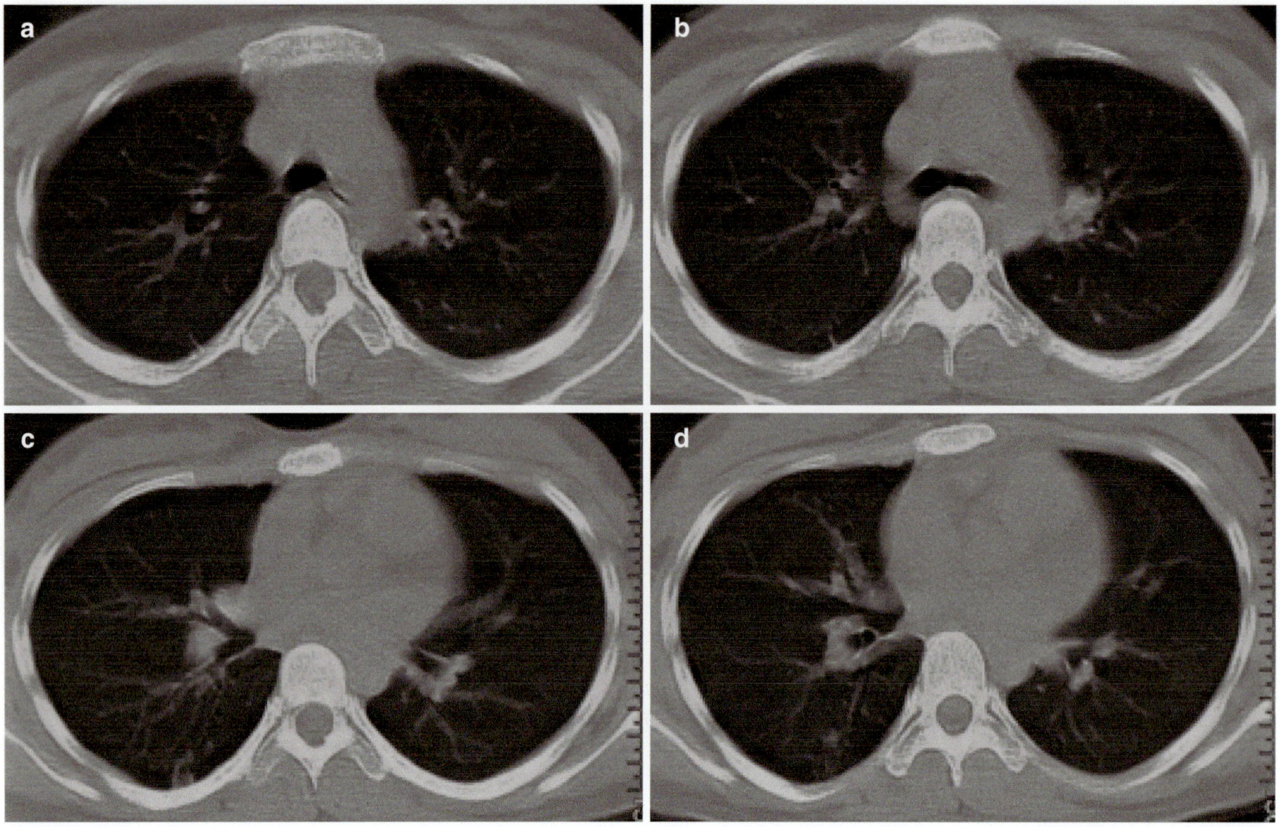

Fig. 9.4 (**a**–**d**) Re-examination of chest CT scans on June 1, 2018. (**a**, **b**) Patchy high-density opacities are observed in para-aortic region in the left upper lobe and in the left hilar region in the lung window. (**c**, **d**) Continuation of absorption is observed for the tubercles in the right lower lobe

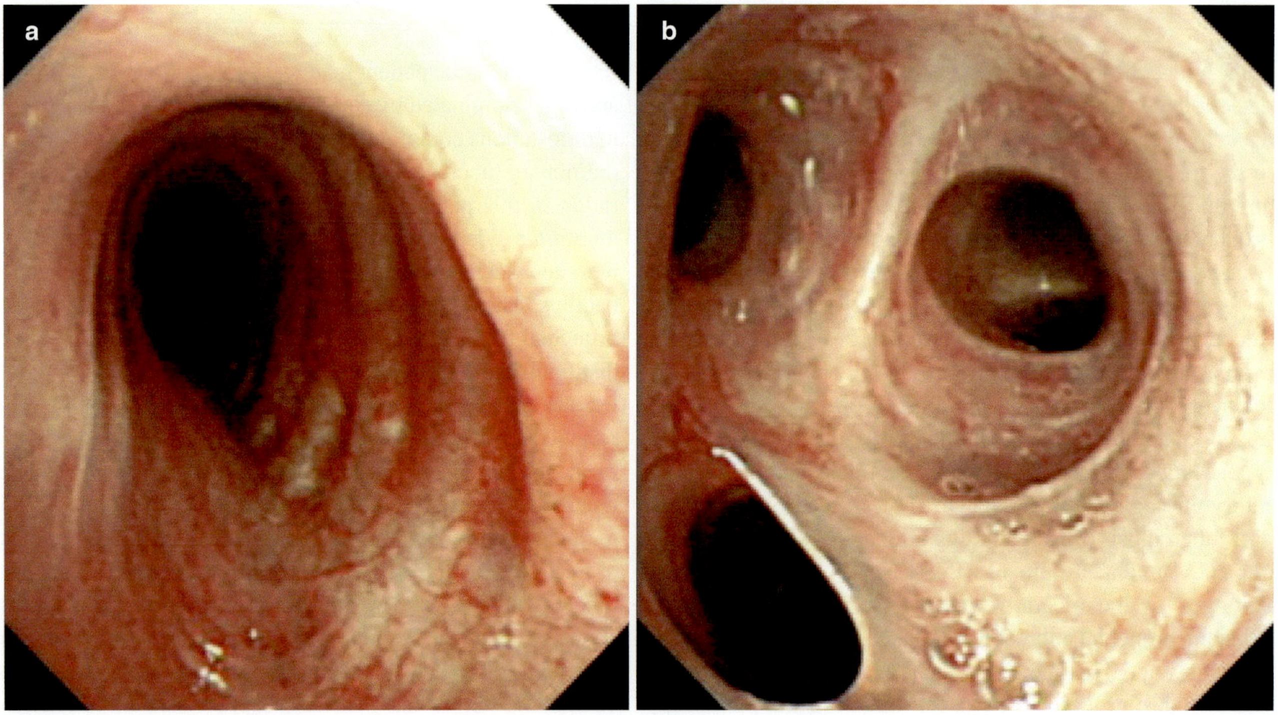

Fig. 9.5 (**a**, **b**) Re-examination of bronchoscopy on June 4, 2018, revealing the left bronchial tuberculosis. (**a**) A mild cicatricial stenosis at the left main bronchus. (**b**) A mild scarring at bronchus propria of the left upper lobe

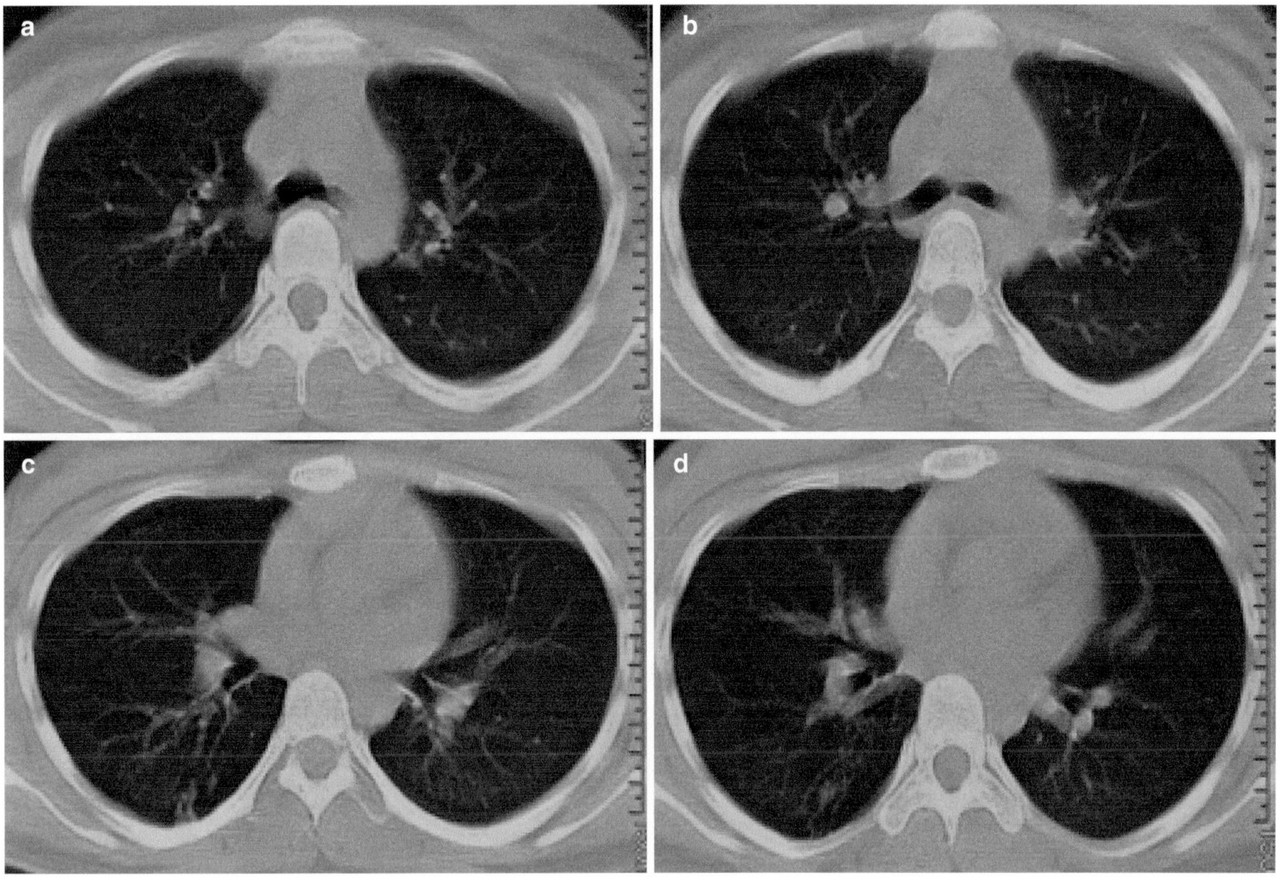

Fig. 9.6 (**a**–**d**) Re-examination of chest CT scans on September 7, 2018. (**a**, **b**) High-density strip-like opacities are observed in para-aortic region in the left upper lobe and in the left hilar region. (**c**, **d**) Small nodular opacities are shown in the right lower lobe, with some strip-like opacities adhered to the right inferior posterior pleura. The absorption is noticed for lesions in both lungs in comparison to images of CT scans on June 1, 2018

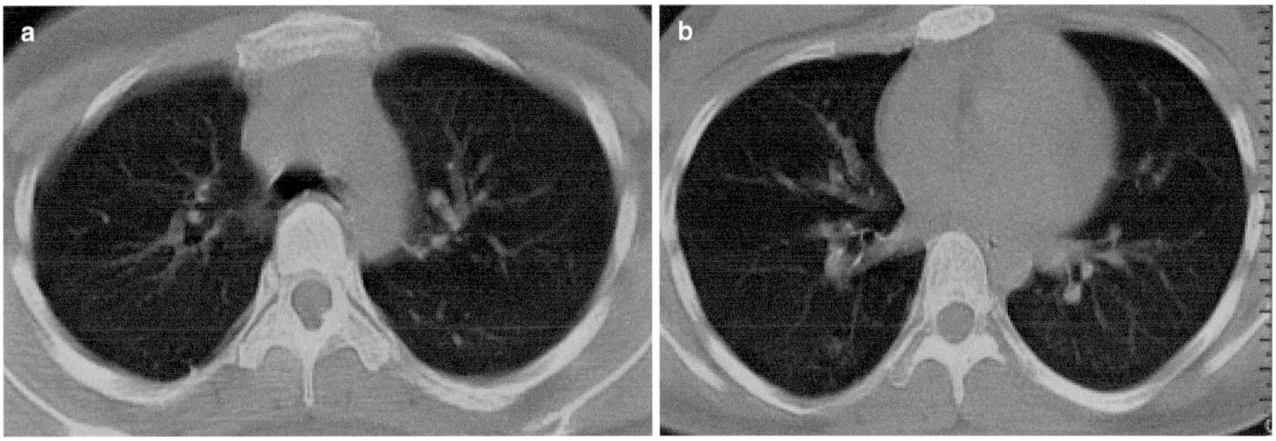

Fig. 9.7 Re-examination of CT scans on December 9, 2018. (**a**, **b**) Strip-like high-density opacities are shown in the left upper lobe by the lung window, with small nodular opacities in the right lower lobe. A significant absorption is observed in comparison with CT scans on September 7, 2018

The tuberculosis lesions were located in this case through bronchofibroscope. Based on pathological morphology of lesions and their variation, a discussion has been made by authors concerning bronchoscopic types of bronchial tuberculosis including inflammatory infiltration, ulcerative necrosis, granulation proliferation, cicatricial stenosis, softening of tracheobronchial wall and lymph node fistula [1, 6]. The accurate typing achieves the goal of precise diagnosis, with a certain importance and value in guiding clinical treatment. This case belonging to the type of ulcerative necrosis showed a significant absorption and amelioration and became the type of cicatricial stenosis, as suggested by the second bronchofibroscopy post to the treatment. This suggests that this typing criteria is not a fast rule, and the responses decide the outcome of the disease. During the treatment of this patient, standardized dynamic imaging and bronchofibroscope were performed, which was of great importance for evaluating the disease and monitoring responses.

References

1. Editorial board of Chinese journal of tuberculosis and respiratory diseases, tuberculosis branch of Chinese Medical Association. Guideline of diagnosis and treatment of tracheobronchial tuberculosis (trial draft) [J]. Chin J Tuberc Resp Dis. 2012;35(8): 581–7.
2. Wei M, Liu L, Wei H, et al. An analysis on clinical manifestations and diagnosis/treatment of patients with tracheobronchial tuberculosis [J]. Med J Western China. 2017;29(8):1122–4, 1128.
3. Tang S, Xue Q. An research on the value of CT and pathology/histopathology of bronchoscopic biopsy applied to the diagnosis of bronchial tuberculosis [J]. Chin J CT MRI. 2017;15(9):70–3.
4. Chen L. An analysis on clinical features of 520 patients with tracheobronchial tuberculosis [J]. J Aerospace Med. 2018;29(4):413–4.
5. Global tuberculosis report 2018 [EB/OL]. Geneva: World Health Organization; 2018. http://www.who.int/tb/publications/global_report/en/.
6. Kuang H, Liang M, Yuan Y, et al. An analysis on endoscopic features of multi-resistant pulmonary tuberculosis complicated with tracheobronchial tuberculosis [J]. China J Endoscopy. 2017;23(12):32–5.
7. Kuang HB, Tan SY, Liang MQ, et al. Study of tracheobronchial tuberculosis complicated with multidrug-resistant pulmonary tuberculosis [J]. Chin J Antituberc. 2017;39(3):242–6.
8. Liu H, Zhang XG, An HJ, et al. Analysis of multidrug resistant pulmonary tuberculosis treated by electronic bronchoscope drug-injection combined with chemotherapy [J]. Int J Resp. 2015;35(4):261–4.
9. Ye T-s, Zhang P-z, Zeng X, et al. Analysis of the effect of the treatment of lymph node fistula bronchial tuberculosis by bronchoscope [J/CD]. Electr J Emerg Infect Dis. 2018;3(4):202–5.
10. Yu W, Tan W-g, Lu P-x. Classification and imaging manifestations of drug-resistant pulmonary tuberculosis [J/CD]. Electr J Emerg Infect Dis. 2019;4(1):42–7.
11. Wang Y-x, Chung MJ, Skrahin A, et al. Literature analysis of radiological signs related to multidrug-resistant tuberculosis [J/CD]. Electr J Emerg Infect Dis. 2018;3(2):244–53.
12. Fishman JE, Sais GJ, Schwartz DS, et al. Radiographic findings and patterns in multidrug-resistant tuberculosis [J]. J Thorac Imaging. 1998;13:65–71.
13. Xiong M, Zhang W, Wang D, et al. An appraisal of effects of spiral CT three-dimensional imaging in diagnosing tracheobronchial diseases [J]. J Clin Radiol. 2000;19(12):766–869.
14. Guo X. The value of 64-row spiral CT in diagnosing endobronchial tuberculosis [J]. Chin Commun Doctors. 2017;33(8):97–8.
15. China National Association for Prevention of Tuberculosis. Guideline of chemotherapy against drug-resistant tuberculosis [S]. Chin J Antituberc. 2015;37(5):421–69.
16. Cen W, Chen P, Liao C, et al. An analysis on clinical features and treatment in 320 patients with tracheobronchial tuberculosis [J]. Guangdong Med J. 2013;34(16):2508–10.

10 Pediatric Drug-Resistant Pulmonary Tuberculosis

Wei-jun Fang, Min Song, Yuan-yuan Han, Chuan-jun Xu, Yong-xiang Yi, and Shui-hua Lu

10.1 Summary of Pediatric Drug-Resistant Pulmonary Tuberculosis

It was pointed out by WHO global tuberculosis report 2022 [1] that there were about 10.6 million newly diagnosed cases of tuberculosis worldwide in 2021, 1.2 million of which were children, accounting for 11%. 217,000 children died of tuberculosis in the same year, accounting for about 14% of the world's deaths due to tuberculosis. The greater proportion of pediatric deaths than the estimated proportion suggests that children with tuberculosis have a lower chance to establish the diagnosis and acquire treatment. The report also pointed out that, the cumulative number of pediatric MDR/RR-TB patients registered for treatment between 2018 and 2021 was 17,700, only 15% of the global 5-year target of 115,000 from 2018 to 2022, which was set by the United Nations High level Conference. Some studies [2] have pointed out that there have been about 25,000–32,000 newly increased pediatric MDR-TB cases worldwide per year and the actual prevalence may be 12 times of the existing patients with confirmed diagnosis, through evaluating the incidence of pediatric MDR-TB by using MDR-TB risk model based on the integration of various global data. Pediatric drug-resistant tuberculosis tends to raise the rate of severe cases and mortality, especially in infants and young children (below 3 years old) prone to miliary tuberculosis and/or tuberculosis meningitis, and it would progress very easily from infection with tubercle bacillus because of their immaturely developed immune organs [3]. Characterized by high expenditure and multiple drugs required by the prolonged medication with adverse reaction commonly observed [4–6], pediatric drug-resistant tuberculosis can also become an important infectious source of drug-resistant tuberculosis [7]. Fortunately, the treatment success rate can reach to 78–90% [4, 8, 9], if the drug-resistant tuberculosis can be diagnosed in the early stage with treatment provided timely, owing to the low TB load in children. Diagnosis in early stage, therefore, seems to be the key link to cure pediatric drug-resistant tuberculosis. However, difficulties in acquiring etiological evidences for this disease predispose its diagnosis to a great challenge, making image examination become extremely important and likely the unique method, especially CT scans endowed with an overwhelming significance in clinical imaging diagnosis, differential diagnosis, and evaluation of responses and prognosis in pediatric population with this disease [10].

10.1.1 Epidemiology of Pediatric Drug-Resistant Tuberculosis Worldwide

A great limitation exists in the data of research and surveillance on pediatric tuberculosis around the world due to difficulties in diagnosing this disease. Adong Shen et al. [11] analyzed the data of researches on pediatric tuberculosis both domestic and abroad and found that in 2014 the multi-resistance rate was 3.3% in globally newly diagnosed cases and 20% in relapse cases, and 9.7% of multi-resistant patients were those with extensively drug resistance. Nations with extremely serious MDR-TB situation include India, China and Russia, embracing their MDR-TB cases accumulated together accounting 54% of the total MDR-TB cases in the world [12]. The lack of monitoring data relevant to pediatric

W.-j. Fang (✉) · M. Song · Y.-y. Han
Department of Radiology, Guangzhou Chest Hospital, Guangzhou, Guangdong, China

C.-j. Xu
Department of Radiology, The Second Hospital of Nanjing, Nanjing University of Chinese Medicine, Nanjing, China

Y.-x. Yi
Hepatobiliary Surgery, Nanjing Drum Tower Hospital, Nanjing, China

S.-h. Lu
Department of Tuberculosis, The Third People's Hospital of Shenzhen, Shenzhen, Guangdong, China

P.-x. Lu et al. (eds.), *Diagnostic Imaging of Drug Resistant Pulmonary Tuberculosis*, https://doi.org/10.1007/978-981-99-8339-1_10

tuberculosis has led to the uncertainty of drug-resistant tuberculosis in children around the world. As pointed out by the Global Tuberculosis Report 2012, pediatric MDR rate was 1–13% [13] among 37 countries that provided the prevalence of MDR-TB stratified by age. Some researchers made statistics on the surveillance data of tuberculosis in 85 countries reported to WHO from 1994 to 2011 [14], revealing that 35 countries among them reported cases of pediatric MDR-TB. An analysis on drug resistance in correlation to age in TB cases from these countries revealed a similar multi-resistance rate in pediatric population and in the adults in most of these countries, in contrast to countries with high prevalence of HIV such as Namibia and South Africa, where pediatric tuberculosis was observed in a close correlation to MDR, illustrating likely the overwhelming challenge imposed by tuberculosis transmission onto these countries. Moreover, the incidence of multi-resistant tuberculosis has also been reported to be higher in pediatric populations than in adults in developed countries such as Germany, UK, and USA, which may be explained by their mature system capable of identifying earlier the pediatric tuberculosis sufferers with a history of the exposure to MDR-TB patients when the system is used to follow up populations exposed to tuberculosis patients.

10.1.2 Epidemiology of Pediatric Drug-Resistant Tuberculosis in China

The baseline survey report on drug resistance in tuberculosis in China from 2007 to 2008 showed that among the total smear-positive pulmonary tuberculosis patients in China, the rate of overall resistance, multi-resistance, and extensive resistance were 37.8%, 8.3%, and 0.7%, respectively, based on which the number of newly diagnosed MDR-TB patients per year is estimated to be about 120,000, with about nearly 10,000 cases of extensively resistant pulmonary TB patients. Pediatric patients younger than 15 years, however, were not covered by this investigation, resulting in an uncertainty concerning present condition of drug resistance in pediatric tuberculosis in China [15].

Based on an analysis on drug resistance in Mycobacterium tuberculosis originating from China (including 100 strains in the pediatric cohort and 191 strains in adult cohort), Jiao et al. [16] found an overall drug resistance rate of 55% and a multi-resistance rate of 22% in pediatric population with tuberculosis, which seemed similar to their counterparts of 60.2% and 30.9%, respectively, in adult tuberculosis patients, suggesting the severe present status of drug resistance in Chinese pediatric tuberculosis necessitating the high attention. Zhe Peng et al. [17] found the overall- and multi-resistance rate were 20.9% and 6.5%, respectively, based on an analysis on drug resistance in 139 strains of Mycobacterium tuberculosis in Children's Hospital Affiliated to Chongqing Medical University, while Tao Li and Shuihua Lu [18] analyzed clinical isolates from 61 pediatric tuberculosis patients under the age of 15 in Shanghai from 2010 to 2011, revealing 32.8% and 4.9%, respectively, for these two rates. In addition, an investigation by Qing Huang et al. [19] on 458 pediatric patients with sputum smear-positive in acid fast bacillus in Wuhan China showed the overall resistance rate of 28.4%, wherein the multi-resistance rate and extensive resistance rate were 7.4% and 3.9%, respectively.

The discrepancies in the rates of pediatric drug-resistant tuberculosis suggested by above studies might be caused mainly by the different regions where strains originated from and by difference among hospitals. Although these hospital-based epidemiological investigations cannot represent drug-resistant level in Chinese pediatric tuberculosis, they reflect from one respect the serious situation in pediatric drug-resistant tuberculosis in China, thereby suggesting that the surveillance on epidemiology and drug resistance of pediatric tuberculosis should be strengthened in controlling tuberculosis in China.

10.1.3 Developing Trend of Drug Resistance Rate in Pediatric Drug-Resistant Tuberculosis

The fluctuation of drug resistance level in pediatric tuberculosis during nearly recent 10 years was analyzed by Tao et al. [20] through collecting Mtb clinical isolates from 784 cases of newly diagnosed pediatric tuberculosis from 2006 to 2015, revealing the overall drug resistance rate rising from 14.7% to 27.5% and the multi-resistance rate rising from 1.3% to 15.4%.

29 cases of pediatric drug-resistant pulmonary tuberculosis diagnosed from January 2015 to December 2019 by China Guangzhou Chest Hospital were collected retrospectively. These patients included 14 boys and 15 girls and were aged between 0.25 and 14 years, comprising 14 patients with the history of exposure to active tuberculosis, 11 with tuberculosis resistant to multiple tuberculosis drugs (2 poly-resistances, 8 multi-resistances, and 1 extensive resistance), 18 with single-resistant pulmonary tuberculosis, 21 with rifampicin-resistant tuberculosis (these 21 patients consisted of 12 with single rifampicin-resistant tuberculosis and the other 9 complicated with resistance to other drugs (such as isoniazid)), 23 with newly diagnosed drug-resistant tuberculosis, and 6 with relapse drug-resistant tuberculosis. All pediatric patients in this research were negative in HIV, without any other underlying diseases undermining immunity.

Data provided by the group in China Guangzhou Chest Hospital showed that the pediatric tuberculosis patients with poly-resistance, multi-resistance, and extensive resistance occupied 37.93% among all drug-resistant patients, suggesting that refractory drug-resistant tuberculosis occupied a very high percentage in all pediatric drug-resistant patients. Among pediatric drug-resistant patients, however, the ratio of those complicated with a severe extra-pulmonary tuberculosis, such as intracranial, intestinal, or spinal tuberculosis, was up to 51.72%. The reduction of the severe case rate and mortality of pediatric drug-resistant children, therefore, necessitate continuous improvement of examination technology and diagnostic level for clinical practitioners, so as to achieve the purpose of early diagnosis and early treatment.

10.1.4 Summary of Resistance Rate to the First-Line Anti-Tuberculosis Drugs

Attaching increasing importance to pediatric tuberculosis, scholars from various countries have carried out a series of researches and surveillance on drug resistance in pediatric tuberculosis. A Mexican investigation on 90 strains collected from 2002 to 2003 from pediatric tuberculosis patients below 18 years old from 19 states showed an overall rate of 26.7% for the resistance to the first-line anti-tuberculosis drugs, and the mean rate of 23.3% and 11.1%, respectively, for the resistance to isoniazid and rifampicin in pediatric patients [21]. An analysis by Nelson et al. [22] on 11,480 pediatric tuberculosis patients registered in National Tuberculosis Surveillance System USA from 1993 to 2001 showed the rate of 15.2% for the resistance to the first-line anti-tuberculosis drugs, 1.6% for the multi-resistance rate, and 7.3% for the isoniazid resistance, and the drug resistance rate in pediatric tuberculosis higher in patients born abroad than in those born in USA. A research in South Africa on 1317 pediatric tuberculosis patients under 14 years old revealed the rate of 14.2% for isoniazid resistance, of 8.8% for multi-drug resistance, and of 53.9% and 52.1% for co-infection with HIV, respectively, in children infected with the multi-resistant strain and those infected with susceptible one [23].

10.1.5 Diagnosis of Pediatric Drug-Resistant Tuberculosis

Based on diagnosis criteria of pediatric drug-resistant tuberculosis [24], the criteria for diagnosing suspected pediatric drug-resistant tuberculosis includes: (1) the history of close contact with any patient with confirmed diagnosis of drug-resistant tuberculosis; (2)the history of close contact with any patient with suspected drug-resistant tuberculosis (e.g., the source of infection is any patient unresponsive to treatment, any relapse patient or any patient having recently died from tuberculosis); (3) unresponsiveness to the first-line anti-tuberculosis treatment (excluding irrational medication); (4) any recurrent case. The suspected cases require susceptibility test or gene test on drug resistance, and those showing positiveness are diagnosed as confirmed drug-resistant tuberculosis.

The lower smear rate and positiveness rate in pediatric tuberculosis patients make it harder to diagnose drug-resistant tuberculosis. Therefore, the isolation of drug-resistant strain with its resistance confirmed by susceptibility test is the unique approach to diagnose the drug-resistant tuberculosis. However, we should be vigilant of drug-resistant tuberculosis in case of [24]: (1) a definite history of exposure to any drug-resistant tuberculosis patient; (2) a history of exposure to any suspected drug-resistant tuberculosis patient (e.g., any patient with treatment failure or undergoing re-treatment, or with a history of exposure to any patient having recently died from tuberculosis); (3) any child persisting in the first-line anti-tuberculosis treatment but showing unresponsiveness to treatment; (4) any child with recurrence post to anti-tuberculosis treatment. Susceptibility test should be carried out as soon as possible, once drug-resistant tuberculosis is suspected. The specificity of lower bacterial load in children predisposes them to greater challenge in drug resistance test than adults.

10.1.6 Treatment of Pediatric Drug-Resistant Tuberculosis

A regimen against pediatric drug-resistant tuberculosis should be formulated according to the results of drug susceptibility testing (DST) in children or DST results in an adult contact with drug-resistant tuberculosis and the history of anti-tuberculosis treatment and contain at least five effective anti-tuberculosis drugs. In 2016 WHO updated the regimens suitable for treating drug-resistant tuberculosis in adults and children, including the regimen of RR-TB. As for RR-TB, MDR-TB regimen is recommended no matter whether there is resistance to isoniazid or any other anti-tuberculosis drugs. The updating of the composition of the second-line anti-tuberculosis drugs based on the latest research data proposes that the second-line treatment should be centered at linezolid, which shows good therapeutic effect in both adults and children, and is especially suitable for MDR-TB, XDR-TB and patients not tolerating other drugs. The adverse reactions, however, must be monitored closely when linezolid is chosen, including lactic acidosis, optic neuropathy, thrombocytopenia, and anemia, of which the parents of children should be informed through a full communication before the treatment is launched. Zhen Guo et al. [25] discussed the short-term efficacy of cycloserine in treating pediatric drug-resistant tuberculosis. 48 children with drug-resistant tuberculosis treated in Tuberculosis Prevention and Treatment Hospital of Shanxi Province from February 2015 to February 2017 were selected as subjects and divided into a control and an observation group with 24 for each based on their different treatment regimens. Negative conversion at month 3, 6, 9, and 12 as well as response and adverse reactions at month 12 post to treatment were evaluated for the observational group treated with pyrazinamide, levofloxacin, amikacin sulfate, isonicotinamide, propionate, and cycloserine in comparison with the control treated with pyrazinamide, levofloxacin, amikacin sulfate, isonicotinamide propionate, and para-aminosalicylic acid. The negative conversion rate at these timepoints was marginally higher in the observational group than in the control, though this difference showed no statistical significance. The observational group had an overall response rate of 87.50%, significantly higher than the data in the control (62.50%; $P < 0.05$). The incidence of liver dysfunction was significantly lower in observational group than in the control ($P < 0.05$), while no statistical significance was revealed for adverse events including gastrointestinal discomfort, leucopenia, and renal dysfunction between the two groups. Cycloserine was shown by these results to be capable of improving effectively the negative conversion rate of Mycobacterium tuberculosis in pediatric drug-resistant tuberculosis patients with significant clinical efficacy and minor harm to liver function, and worthy of generalization and application.

10.1.7 Prevention from Pediatric Drug-Resistant Tuberculosis

The prevention is the focus in controlling pediatric drug-resistant tuberculosis, with the measures including: (1) the pediatric patients once confirmed should be isolated from patients with drug-susceptible patients to receive treatment until negative conversion is achieved; (2) DST test should be performed as early as possible to understand the drug resistance in local tuberculosis patients and avoid prolonged exposure to improper empirical therapeutic regimens, thereby preventing from further aggravation of drug resistance; (3) the compliance of children should be improved by regular medication and avoiding the newly induced drug resistance.

Despite the lowered incidence of tuberculosis to some extent during recent years, medical burden imposed by this disease worldwide keeps increasing. The challenge caused by pediatric drug-resistant tuberculosis that becomes increasingly prominent all over the world, and it predisposes the control of pulmonary tuberculosis to difficulties increasing gradually in contrast to continuously elevated requirement [26]. The popularity and detection efficiency of DST technology, therefore, should be improved to achieve the early diagnosis, aiming to formulate a personalized treatment regimen suitable for children with shorter course and less toxicity, and guarantee the complete control of pediatric drug-resistant tuberculosis.

10.2 Image Findings in Newly Diagnosed and Relapsing Pediatric Drug-Resistant Tuberculosis

A description will be provided for pediatric patients divided into two different age groups (<5 years and 5–14 years), based on the difference on susceptibility to tuberculosis and disease progression in children aged below 5 years (including infants younger than 1 year) compared with older children [26], and diverse features observed in pulmonary tuberculosis children in different age groups concerning clinical symptoms, anatomy, and image manifestations including morphology and distribution of lesions [10].

10.2.1 Image Findings of Drug-Resistant Tuberculosis in Young Children Aged Below 5 Years

The most common morphological manifestations in CT scans for intra-pulmonary lesions in pediatric drug-resistant patients aged below 5 years are multiple tubercles (including miliary ones; Fig. 10.1), followed by hilar and mediastinal lymphadenectasis and pulmonary consolidation (Fig. 10.2). That is because, as implied by researches available at present [27], pediatric pulmonary tuberculosis is often complicated with hilar and mediastinal lymphadenectasis (Fig. 10.3). Pediatric patients younger than 5 years old complicated with bronchial tuberculosis are seldom observed, possible due to the low bacterial load in children where drug-resistant bacteria cannot be induced spontaneously, and therefore pediatric drug-resistant tuberculosis strain derives mainly from infectious spread from adult tuberculosis patients [28]. The mechanism for drug resistance emerging in adult tuberculosis patients lies in the mutation of chromosomal genes encoding drug targets and relevant metabolic enzyme [6], which makes drug-resistant Mycobacterium tuberculosis with strong adaptability become the dominant flora replacing the highly destructive and toxic susceptible stains eradicated by improper treatment, while bronchial tuberculosis cannot emerge due to the inability of lesions in lymph nodes to invade through bronchial wall, possibly because of the genetic mutation undermining toxicity and destructive force of the drug-resistant bacteria in the background of low immunity in children showing insufficient systemic response to tuberculosis. In addition, the low incidence of pleural effusion and of pleural thickening also confirms the point of view of the undermined toxicity and destructive force in these drug-resistant bacteria [29].

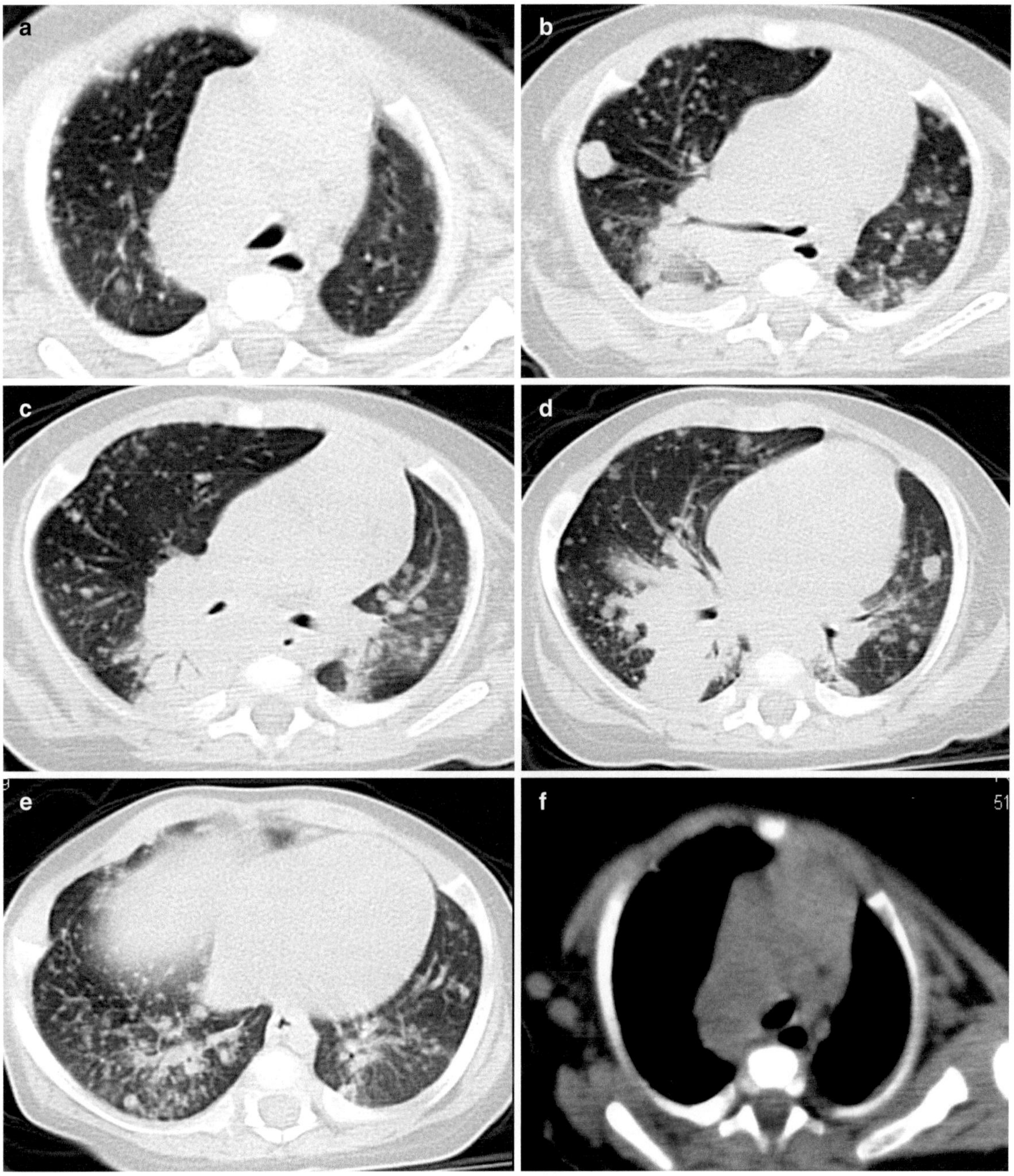

Fig. 10.1 (**a**–**g**) Primary multidrug-resistant TB in a 5-month-old baby, with resistance to isoniazid, rifampicin, and streptomycin. Chief compliant of fever for more than 2 months with crying and left strabismus of both eyes for 2 days. The baby's mother had pelvic tuberculosis for more than 2 years (**a**–**e**). Lung window of a transverse CT scan shows multiple nodules, consolidations, which are distributed extensively in both lungs. (**f**, **g**) Mediastinal window shows mediastinal and hilar lymphadenectasis with the compression of the right main bronchus and bilateral axillary lymphadenectasis

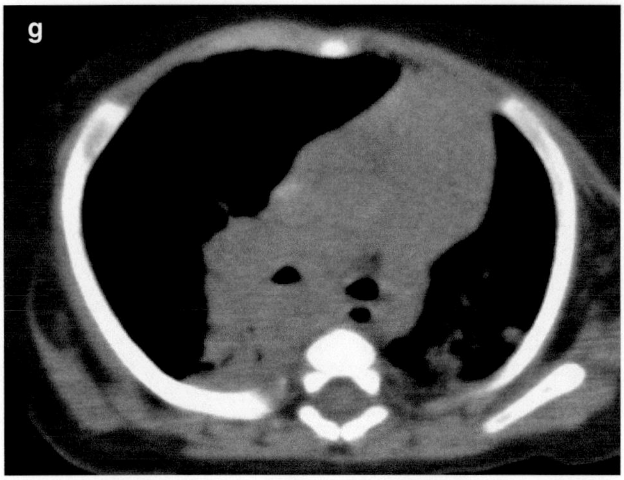

Fig. 10.1 (continued)

10.2.2 Image Findings in the Group of Drug-Resistant Tuberculosis Patients Aged 5–14 Years

Lesions involving all lobes in both lungs show a high incidence, as far as the distribution of pulmonary tuberculosis is concerned, though areas with concentrated distribution of pulmonary lesions are relatively limited and the most common areas include mainly the posterior segment of the right upper lobe, the dorsal segment of the right lower lobe, and the posterior apical segment and the lingual segment of left upper lobe, followed by the apical segment of the right upper lobe, and the dorsal segment of the left lower lobe. The most common morphological CT findings of pulmonary lesions include multiple tubercles, patches, consolidations, hilar and mediastinal lymphadenectasis (Fig. 10.4) and bronchial tuberculosis (see introduction of classical cases), followed by tree-in-bud opacities, cord-like opacities, masses, cavities, and local pleural thickening. Increased incidence of morphological manifestations including tree-in-bud opacities, cord-like opacities, mass and cavities predisposes CT findings for drug-resistant tuberculosis in older children to multiform changes in higher ratio compared with this disease in younger children (Fig. 10.4). Manikkam et al. [29] investigated X-ray findings in 45 pediatric multi-resistant pulmonary tuberculosis, revealing consolidation to be the most common manifestation (Fig. 10.5), followed by lymphadenectasis, tree-in-bud sign, and cavities.

The incidence of intra-pulmonary cavities, including mouth-eaten cavities, thick-walled cavities and multiple cavities, was higher obviously in the group of elder pediatric drug-resistant pulmonary tuberculosis than that of pediatric non-resistant pulmonary tuberculosis [30] (Fig. 10.6). Despite the elevated incidence of cavitation facilitates the discharge of a great amount of tuberculosis bacteria through bronchi, the cavity wall consists of collagen outside the cavity, caseous substances inside the cavity and granulation tissue in the middle, which are the hypovascular tissues not easily penetrated by anti-tuberculosis drugs and make blood drug concentration at a low level in the cavity wall where a great amount of hidden Mycobacterium tuberculosis is kept alive [10], thereby resulting in persistent presence of drug-resistant bacteria in pediatric patients or the secondary mutation inducing the emergence of new drug-resistant bacterial colony. Therefore, the ratio of cavities seems high for poly-, multi- and extensively resistant pediatric patients in elder children, while the incidence of pleural infusion is lower in this group than in non-resistant pulmonary tuberculosis patients.

In summary, the common CT features in pediatric drug-resistant pulmonary tuberculosis include multiple tubercles, consolidations, hilar and mediastinal lymphadenectasis. The difference of CT manifestations between the elder and younger groups of drug-resistant tuberculosis: (1) drug-resistant tuberculosis in children younger than 5 years shows a wide distribution of intra-pulmonary lesions, and most of them have no bronchial tuberculosis, cavities, or pleural effusion; (2) children aged from 5 to 14 years have lesions distributed mainly in the apical posterior segments of the both upper lobes, the dorsal segments of both lower lobes and the lingual segment of the left upper lobe, with a high incidence of bronchial tuberculosis and cavitation, in contrast to the lower incidence of pleural effusion; (3) pediatric RR-TB cases cause easily intra-pulmonary and systemic dissemination, and lesions in RR-TB pediatric patients without nonhematogenous dissemination are distributed mainly in the apical posterior segments of both upper lobes, the dorsal segments of both lower lobes, the right middle lobe and the lingual segment of the left upper lobe, with a high incidence of cavitation but a lower incidence of pleural effusion.

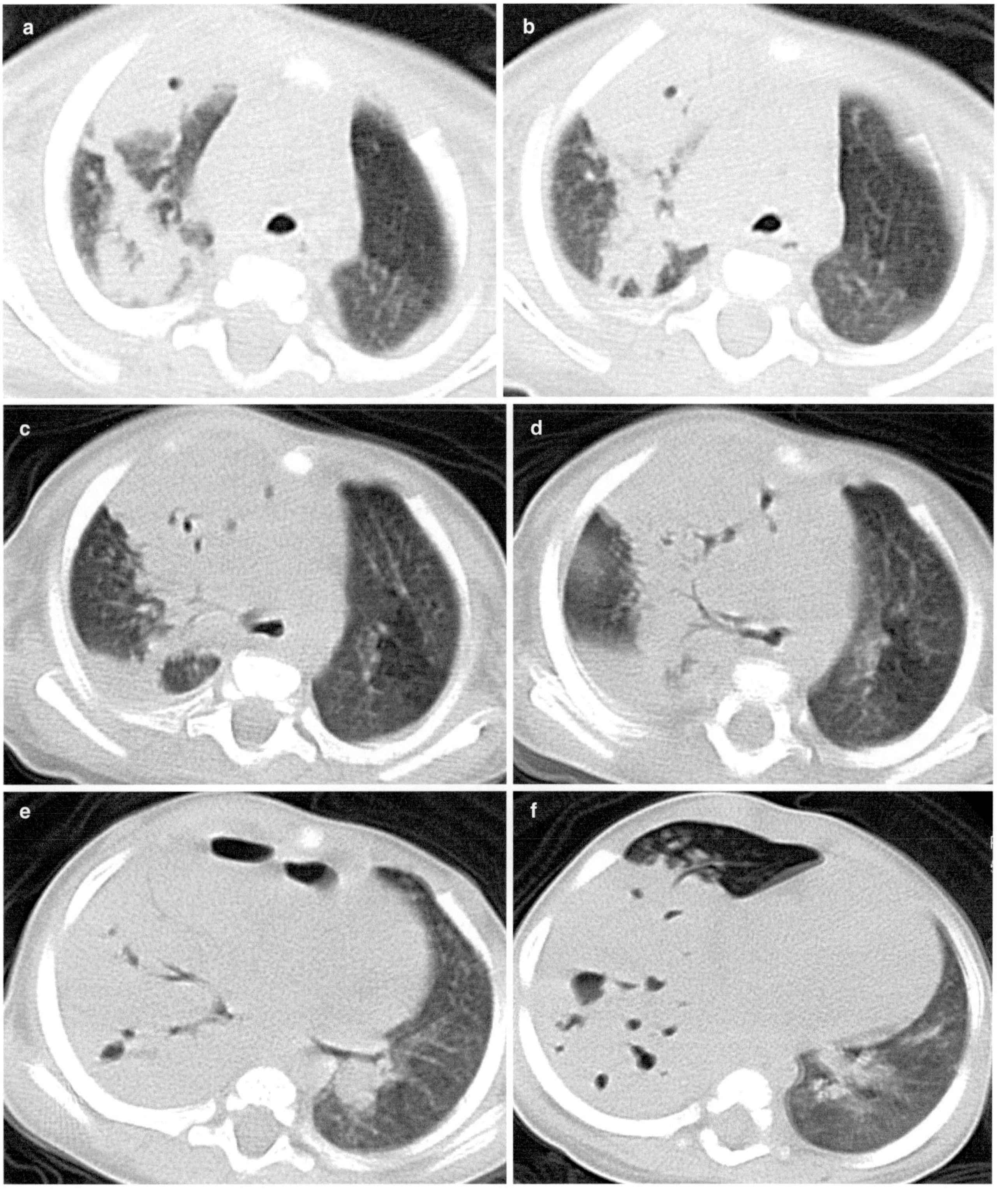

Fig. 10.2 (**a**–**j**) Primary multidrug-resistant TB in a seven-month-old baby with resistance to rifampicin and isoniazid. Chief complaint of episodic monophonic cough for 4 months with phlegm sound heard at the throat. She was complicated with shortness of breath, cyanosis and fever showing the highest temperature of 39.3 °C. Her father had smear-positive pulmonary tuberculosis. (**a**–**g**) Chest CT scans show large consolidations with cavities in the right lung complicated with multiple nodules in two lungs, thickening wall and stenosis can be seen in the right main bronchus, lobar and segmental bronchi in the right lung, which considered to be bronchial tuberculosis. The left axillary lymphadenectasis is observed. (**h**–**j**) Head MRI shows multiple intracranial tubercles, and post-contrast images show circular enhancement in multiple tubercles

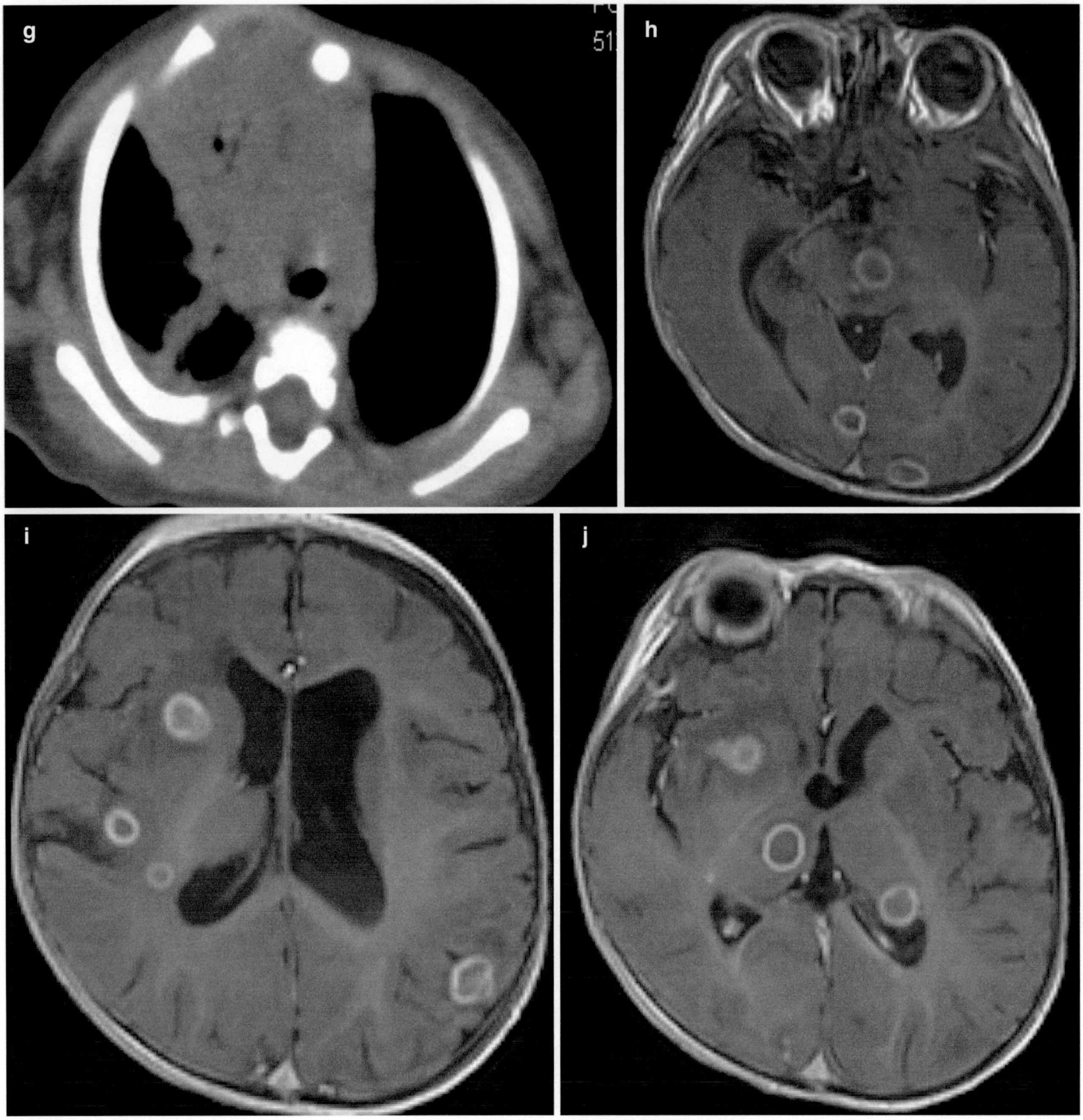

Fig. 10.2 (continued)

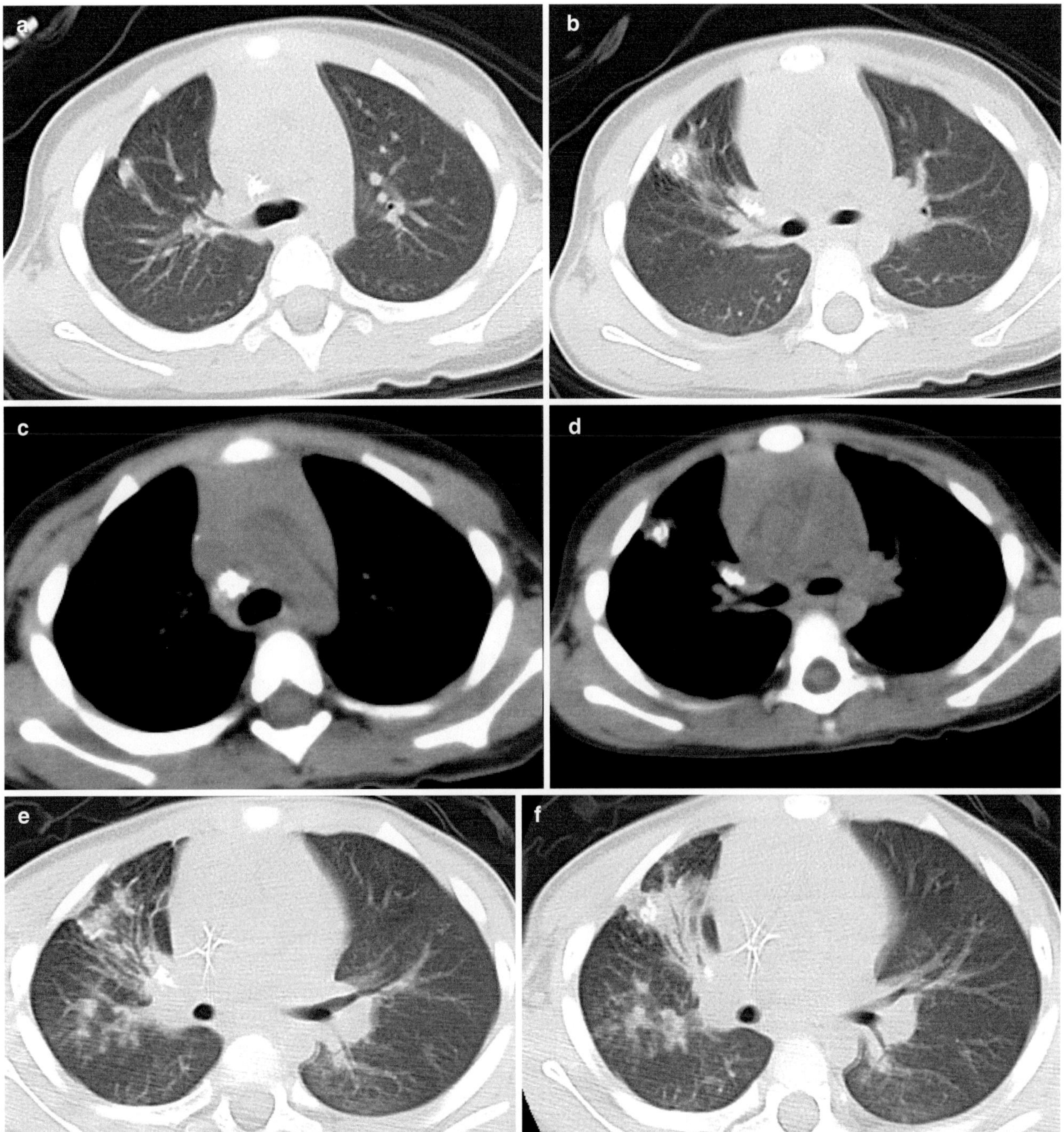

Fig. 10.3 (**a**–**f**) Primary multidrug-resistant TB in a 2-year-old baby, with resistance to isoniazid and rifampicin. Chief compliant of the swelling of the right thigh for more than 1 month. (**a**–**d**) Chest CT scans on March 1, 2019, show a high-density nodular opacity in the right upper lobe with mediastinal and the right hilar lymphadenectasis, and calcification can be observed in all lesions above. (**e**, **f**) Re-examination of chest CT scans on June 4, 2019, shows an increased number of lesions in the right lung and the left lower lobe in comparison with chest CT scans on March 1, 2019, suggesting that drug-resistant tuberculosis of the patient had not been effectively controlled

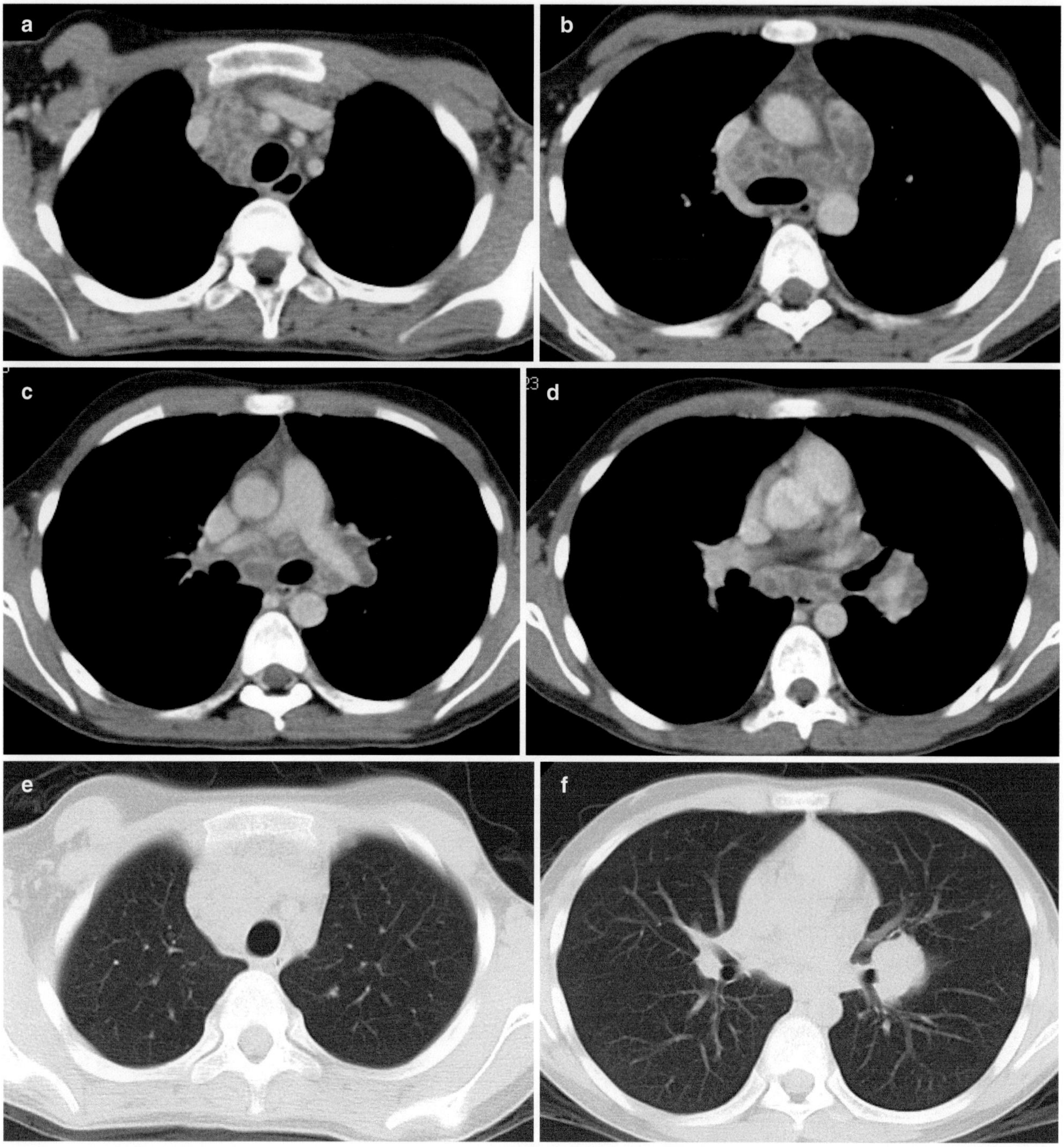

Fig. 10.4 (**a**–**r**) Primary rifampicin-resistant TB in a 12-year-old boy, with single resistance to rifampicin. Chief complaint of recurrent fever for 1 month and a half. (**a**–**f**) Chest CT scans on May 1, 2018, show multiple lymphadenectasis in mediastinum and the left hilum with circular or compartmentalized enhancement. Some nodules are seen in the left upper lobe, with heterogeneous density and clear margin. (**g**–**l**) Chest CT scans on August 20, 2018, show fused lymphadenectasis with increased size at the mediastinum and the left hilum, with the increased number of lesions in the apical posterior segment of the left upper lobe and the emergence of new lesion in the dorsal segment of the left lower lobe. (**k**–**r**) Chest CT scans on March 20, 2019, show the absorption of the lesion in the left lung and the shrinkage of the left hilar and mediastinal lymphadenectasis

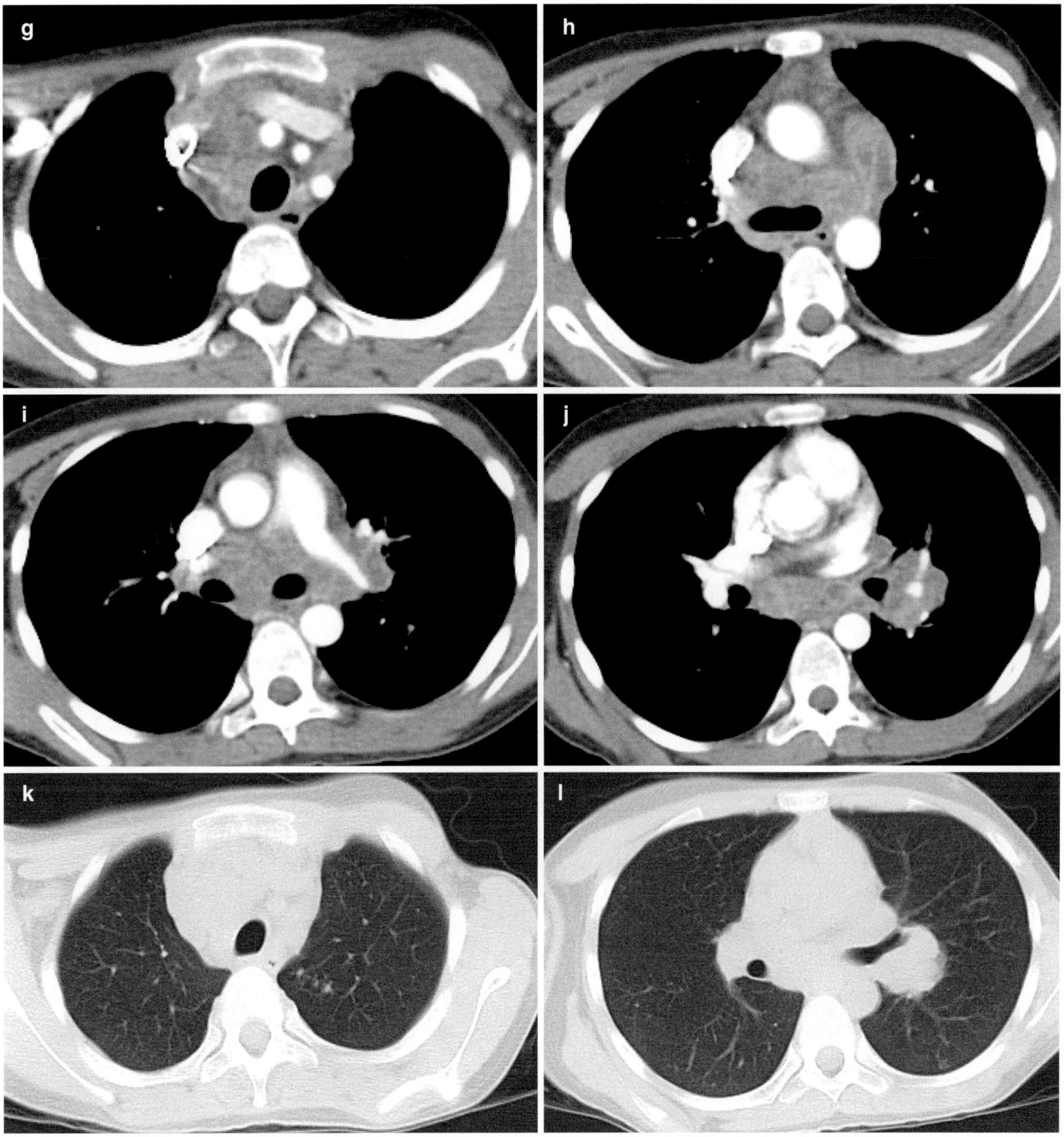

Fig. 10.4 (continued)

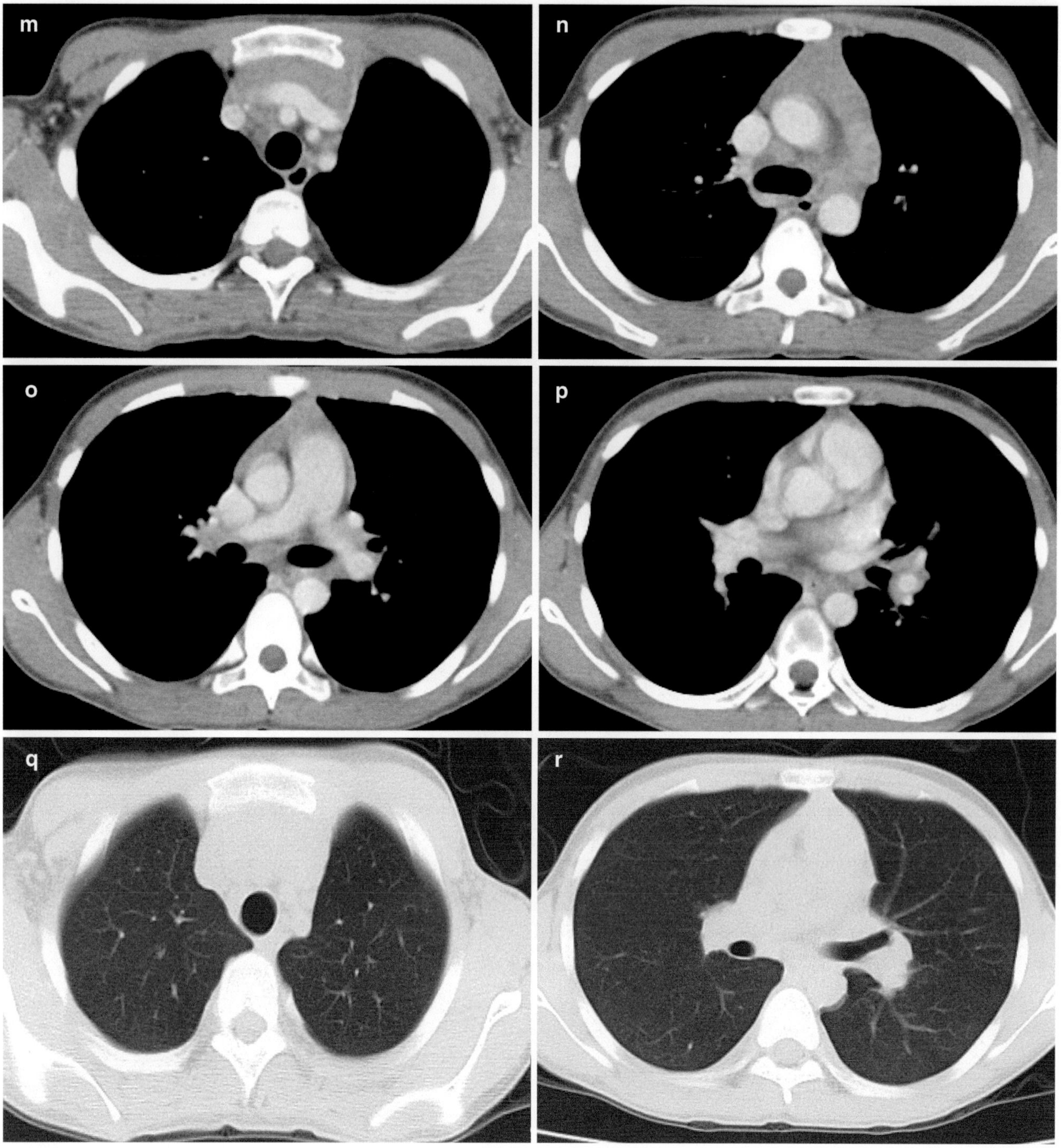

Fig. 10.4 (continued)

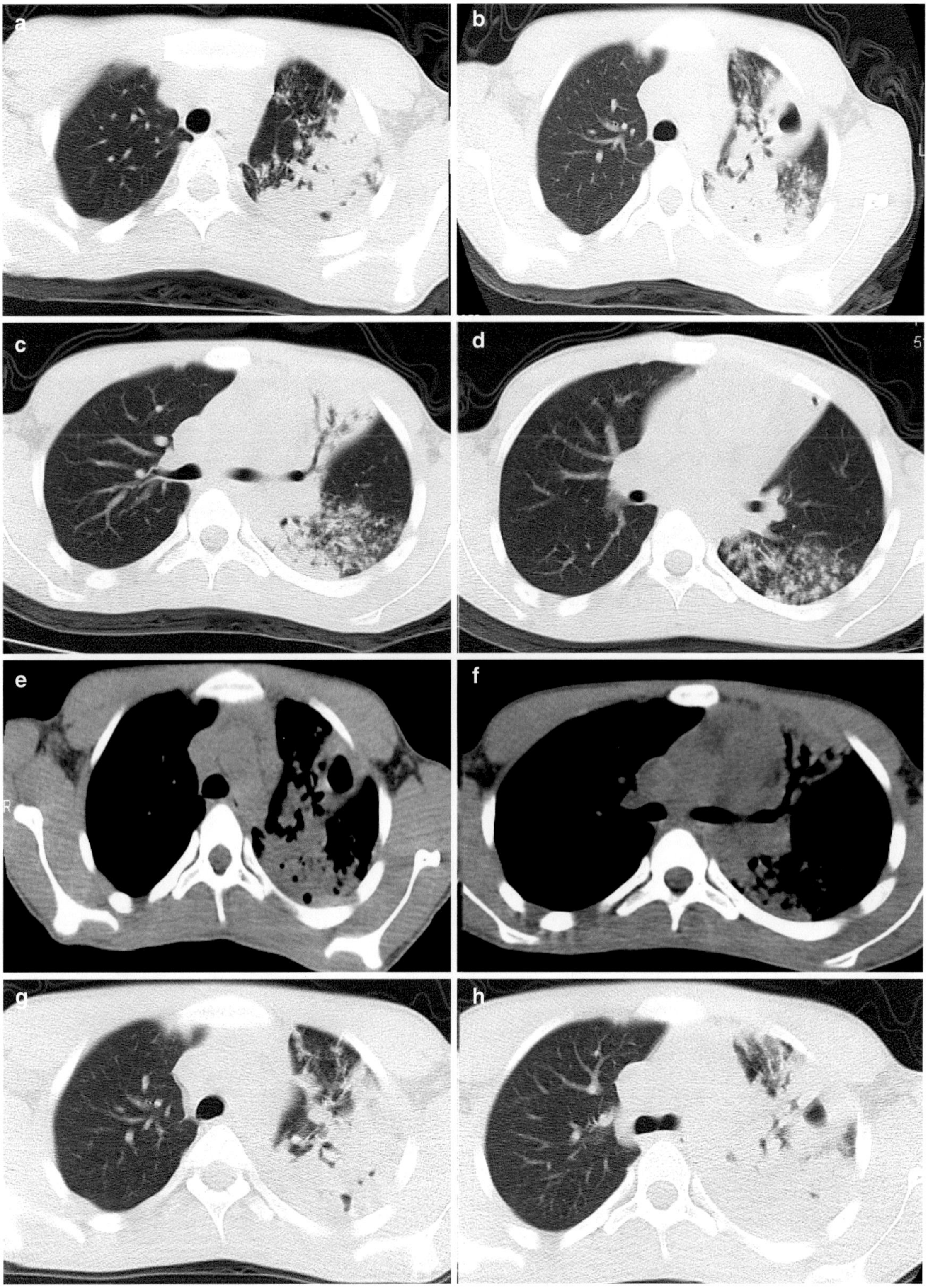

Fig. 10.5 (**a–q**) Primary poly-resistant TB in a 13-year-old boy, with resistance to isoniazid and moxifloxacin. Chief complaint of cough, expectoration, and fever for more than 1 month. (**a–f**) Chest CT scans on March 10, 2018, show multiple nodules, consolidations, tree-in-bud opacities, patchy opacities in lobes of left lung. A thick-walled cavity and consolidation with cavities were shown in the left upper lobe, and the interior wall of the left upper bronchus seems not so smooth with atelectasis of lingual segment. (**g–l**) In comparison with chest CT scans on March 10, 2018, chest CT scans on March 22, 2018, show the wider area of consolidations in lobes of the left lung and the emergence of patchy opacities in the dorsal segment of the right lower lobe. (**m–q**) Chest CT scans on May 24, 2018, show an absorption of the lesions in the left upper lobe, in contrast to the bigger area of consolidations in both lower lobes, in comparison with chest CT scans on March 22, 2018 (**q**)

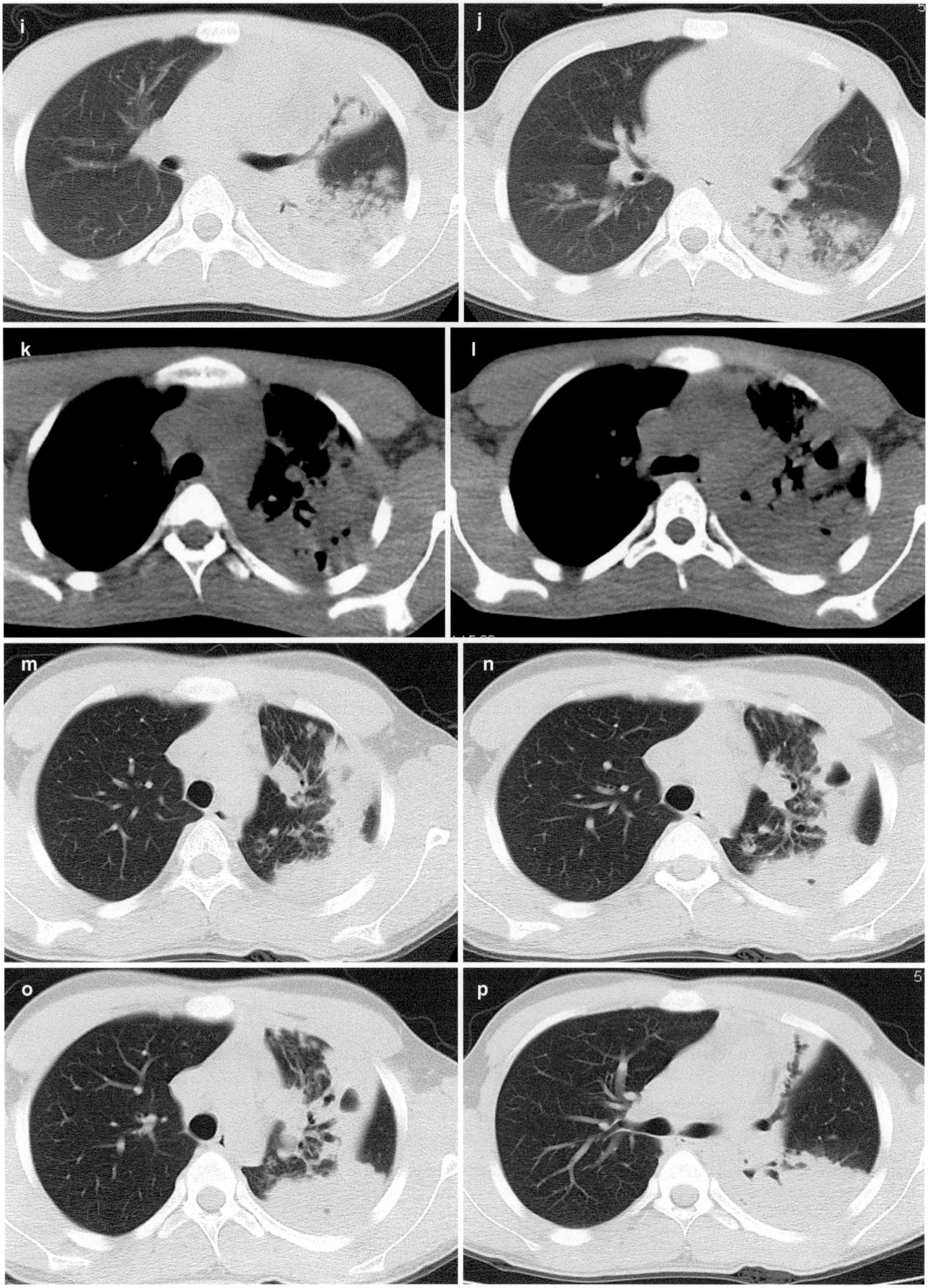

Fig. 10.5 (continued)

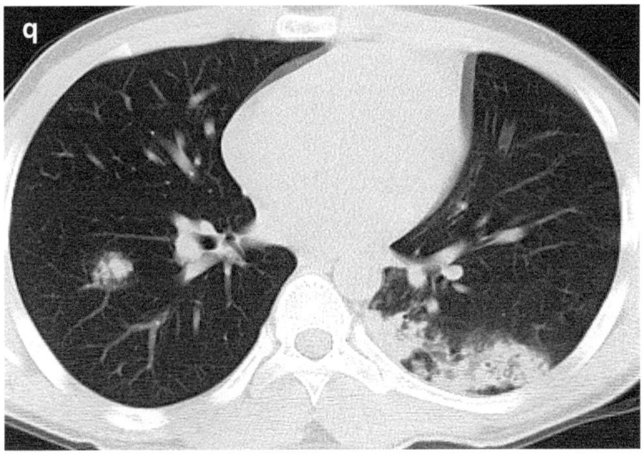

Fig. 10.5 (continued)

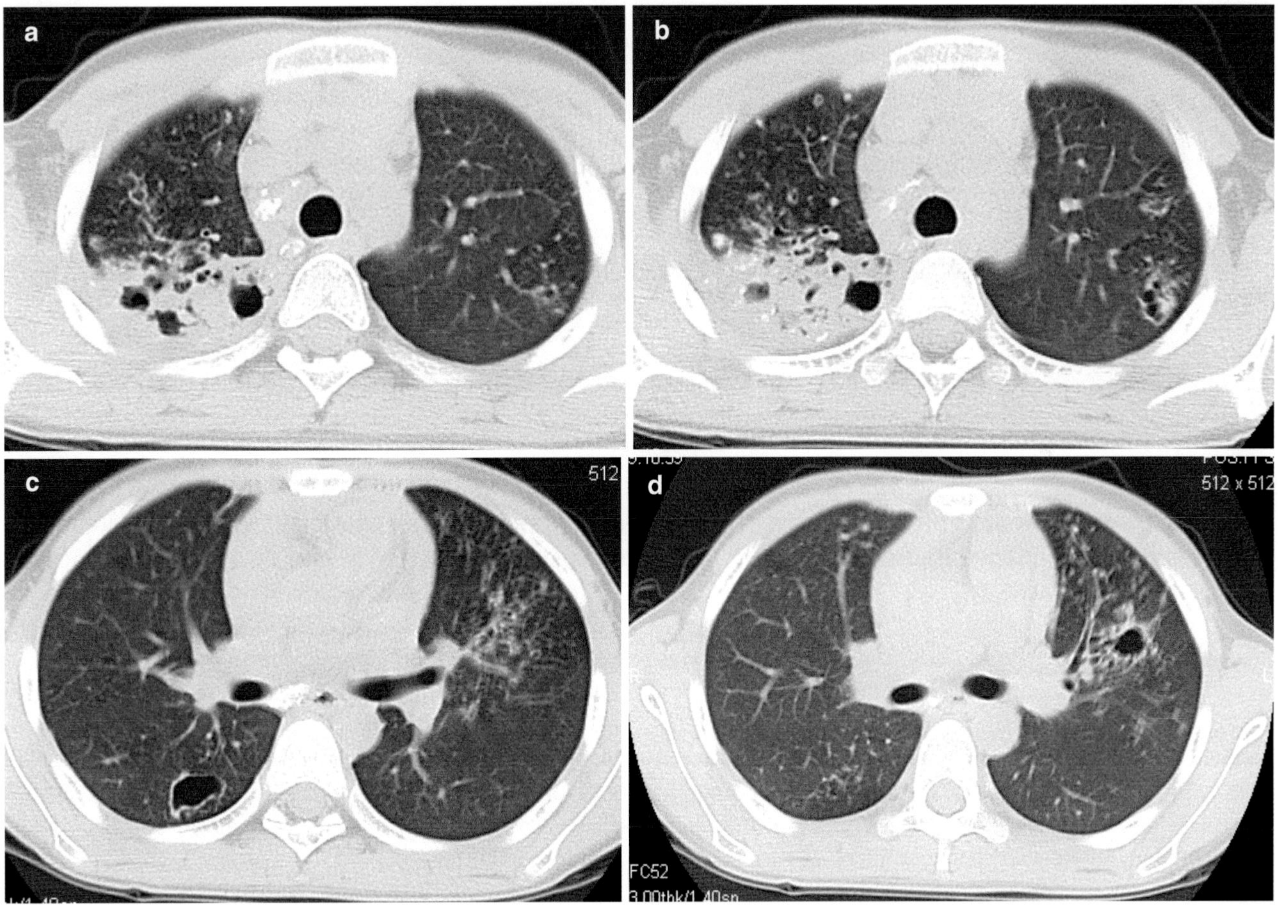

Fig. 10.6 (**a**–**h**) Relapsing rifampicin-resistant TB in a 9-year-old girl, with resistance to rifampicin. Chief complaint of cough and expectoration more than 1 month. (**a**–**f**) Lung window of chest CT scans show multiple nodules, consolidations, cavities, and consolidation with cavities in both lungs, with multiple calcifications in the lesions above and bronchiectasis in the right upper lobe and the lingual segment of the left upper lobe. (**g**, **h**) Mediastinal window shows consolidation with cavities as well as punctiform and patchy calcifications in the right lung, with calcified lymphadenectasis in the mediastinum

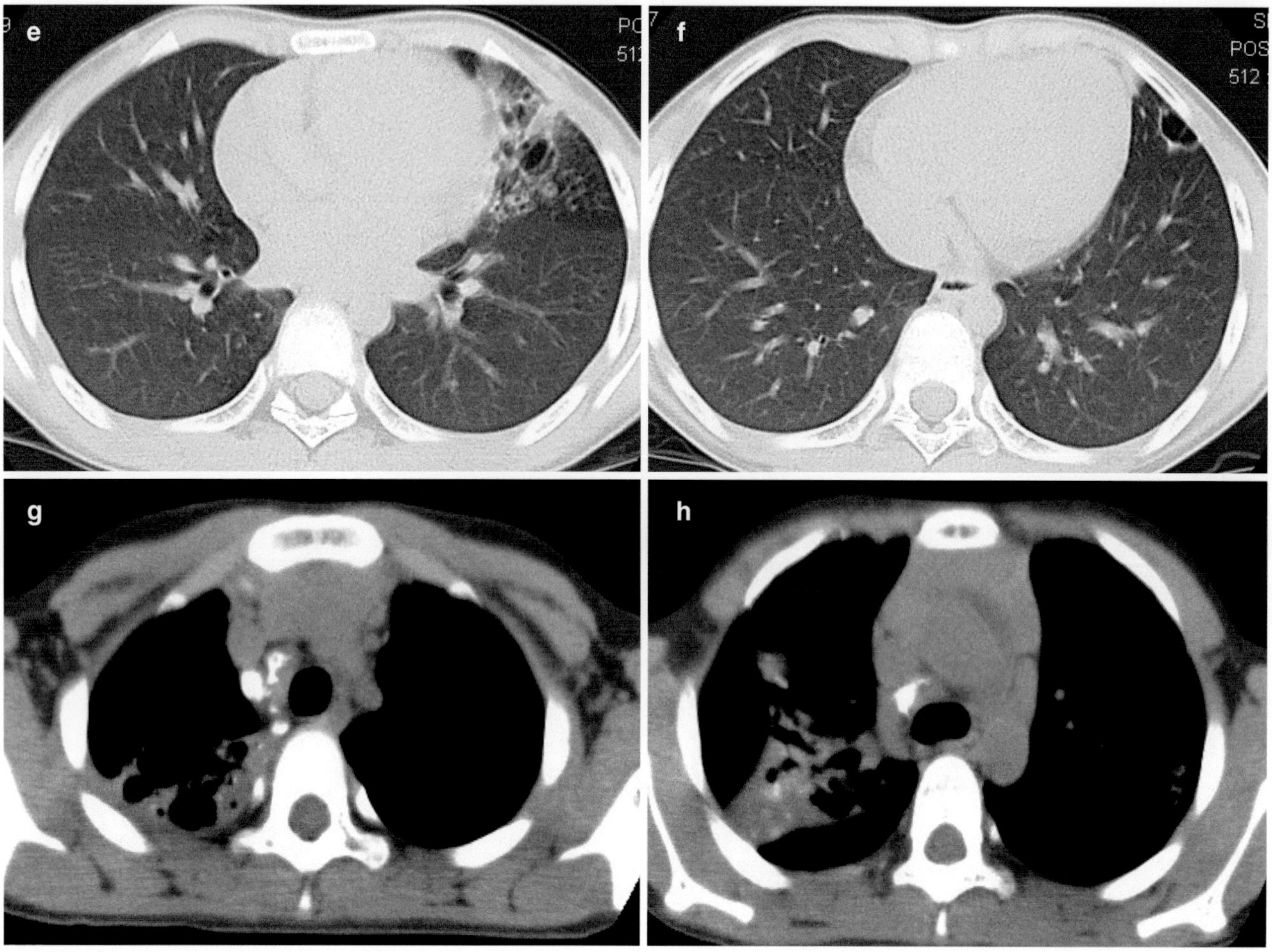

Fig. 10.6 (continued)

10.3 Introduction of Typical Cases of Pediatric Drug-Resistant Tuberculosis

Patient XX Qiu, a 13-year-old boy, had an onset of cough since January 2018, complicated with the expectoration of a small amount of white sticky sputum. He was admitted for several times in a local hospital and had recurrent fever and cough during his in hospitalization. Chest CT scans showed multiple lumpy foci with abnormal density in the mediastinum and at the right hilum, with obvious compression and narrowing of adjacent trachea and esophagus. Multiple tubercles were also observed in both lungs, with the right middle lobar atelectasis (the middle lobar bronchial occlusion) and local thickening of the right posterior inferior pleura. Tracheoscopy showed that the right main bronchus and intermediate bronchus were compressed and narrowed, and a great deal of caseous obstructions could be seen at the opening of the middle lobar bronchus, with bloody secretions observable in the lavage, suggesting the suspected endobronchial tuberculosis. IGRAs in peripheral blood and TB-DNA in bronchial lavage fluid were negative. Biopsy pathology at the right middle lobar bronchial mucosa showed caseous necrosis, which was considered to be tuberculosis. He received anti-tuberculosis treatment using HRZE regimen together with an anti-infection therapy and was discharged after his symptoms ameliorated. Thereafter the patient had recurrent cough and fever, so he was referred to Guangzhou Chest Hospital in July 2018, where he was inhospitalized for further treatment.

Physical examination after admission: no tenderness in the sternum, symmetrical bilateral respiratory movements, no significant increase or decrease in the tactile fremitus of both lungs, clear percussion sound in both lungs, weakened bilateral respiratory sound, no dry rale or moist crackle in both lungs, and no pleural friction sound.

Blood routine: WBC 7.63 × 10^9/L, NE% 87.50%, RBC 4.70 × 10^{12}/L, HGB 85.0 g/L, and PLT 437.0 × 10^9/L; Blood biochemistry: ALT 155.50 U/L, AST 279.20 U/L, TP 49.00 g/L, RBP 8.0 mg/L, K 3.30 mmol/L, CA 2.04 mmol/L, P 0.86 mmol/L, HDL 0.20 mmol/L, and LDL 2.17 mmol/L. Coagulation function: D2 2.88 mg/L, Hs-CRP 46.42 mg/L and PCT 0.63 ng/mL; ESR: abnormal; Syphilis, hepatitis B, hepatitis C, HIV: negative.

Chest X-ray after admission showed multiple nodular and patchy opacities in middle and lower fields of both lungs with a cavity in the right middle lobe and right pleural effusion, considered to be pulmonary tuberculosis with right pleurisy. Chest CT scans (Fig. 10.7) show: (1) pulmonary

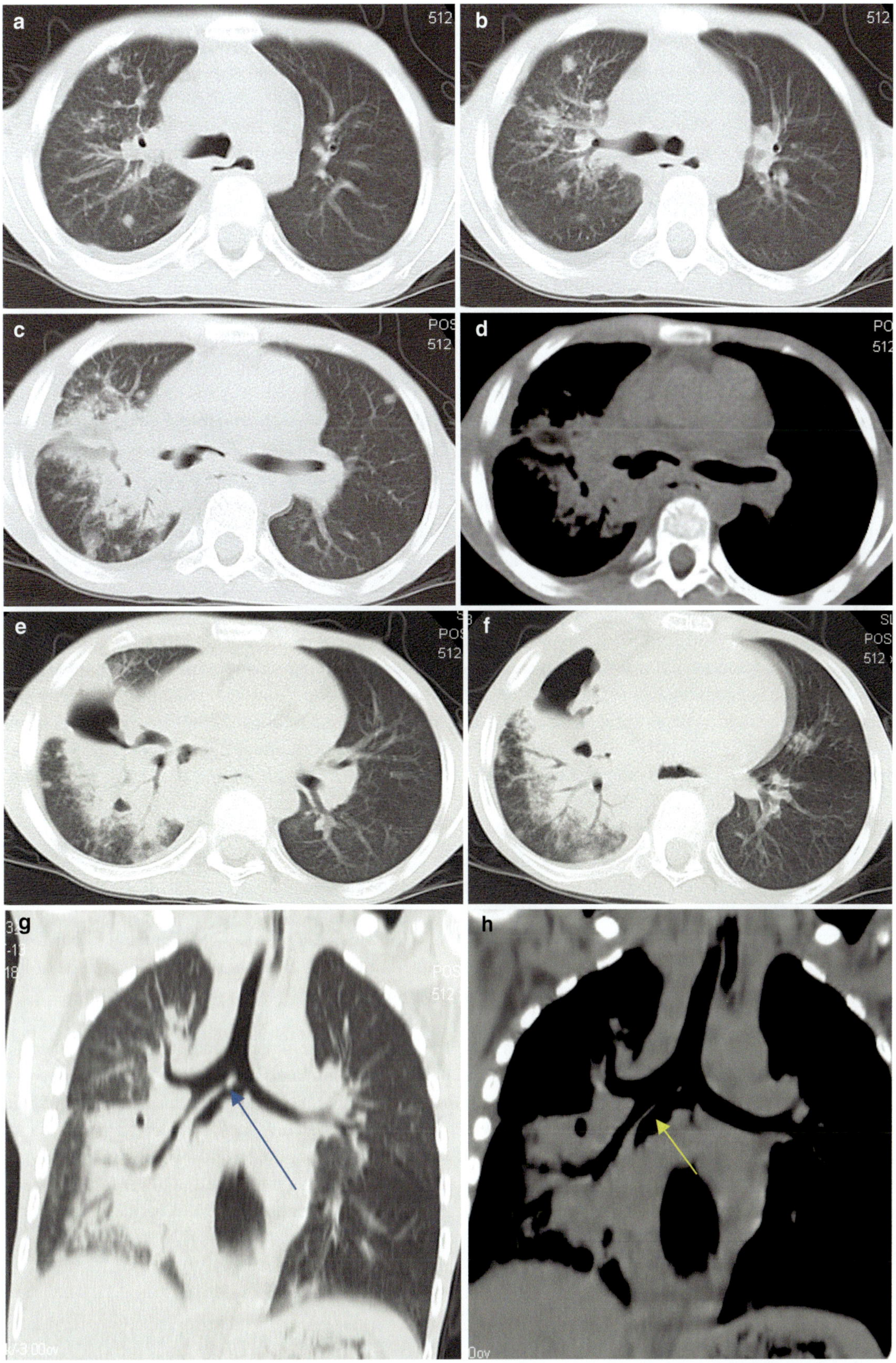

Fig. 10.7 (**a**–**h**) The first chest CT scans on July 13, 2018, after admission. Lung window shows multiple nodules, consolidations, consolidation with cavities, patchy opacities in both lungs, a fistula is observed inferior the carina and linked to bilateral main bronchi; with narrowing of the right main bronchus, the right intermediate bronchus, and the right middle and lower lobar bronchi (**c**–**h**)

tuberculosis in both lungs with cavities in the right middle and lower lobes; (2) bronchial tuberculosis including the right main bronchus, the right intermediate bronchus, and the right middle and lower lobar bronchi; (3) the right pleural effusion; (4) multiple lymphadenectasis in the right supraclavicular fossa, bilateral hila, and mediastinum.

Bronchoscopy performed under local anesthesia on July 13, 2018, revealed that the carina mucosa was congested and swollen, and the carina angle became blunt. The tracheal lumen was unobstructed and the cartilage ring seemed clear. The mucosa of the left main bronchus was found congested and swollen with a fistula observed to the carina communicating with the main bronchus, and a mild congestion was seen for bronchial mucosa of each segment of the left upper and lower lobes, with a small amount of white viscous secretions noticeable, but without any stenosis, neoplasia, or bleeding in the left bronchi. The mucosa of the right main bronchus was congested and swollen, and on its left wall there was a great deal of granulomatous hyperplasia and necrosis, with a fistula observed communicating with the left main bronchus. The opening of each segmental bronchi of the right upper lobe was unobstructed, with a small amount of white viscous secretions observed. The bronchi of the right middle and lower lobes were deformed, and the mucosa was obviously congested and swollen. White necrotic substances were seen in the lateral branch of the middle lobe, the dorsal segment and the anterior basal segment in the lower lobe (Fig. 10.8).

Bronchial lavage on July 14, 2018, showed positiveness in Gene Xper, in extremely low concentration, with resistance to rifampicin.

The sputum culture for the patient in another hospital showed methicillin-resistant Staphylococcus aureus, so a strengthened anti-infection therapy was given with the supplement of vancomycin and azithromycin after the admission. Both blood IGRAs and sputum smears in our hospital were negative, but tracheoscopy and chest CT showed the presence of pulmonary lesions with positive Gene Xper in bronchial lavage fluid. hs-CRP and PCT then seemed elevated than before.

The proposed diagnosis: pulmonary tuberculosis (bronchial tuberculosis). An anti-tuberculosis medication was launched on July 16, 2018, consisting of levofloxacin, cycloserine, linezolid, amikacin and propionate isonicotinic acid, with concurrent liver protection and pulverization therapy.

The pediatric patient was in good condition on November 1, 2018, post to 3.5-month treatment, without any symptom such as fever and cough. Re-examination of chest CT scans showed an obvious absorption of pulmonary lesion, the shrinkage of hilar and mediastinal lymph nodes, and smoother interior wall of the right main bronchus and lobar and segmental bronchi in the right lung than before (Fig. 10.9).

Bronchoscopy was done under local anesthesia on May 24, 2019. Findings under bronchoscope showed that the glottis was normal, active, and well aligned, and the carina was smooth, sharp and located at the middle. Tracheal lumen seemed unobstructed with clear image of cartilage rings. A mild congestion was noticed at the left bronchial mucosa, with a small amount of foam-like secretions, and the healed fistula was observed, which was situated on the medial wall of the left main bronchus adjacent to the carina, without any necrotic substance or granulation. Lumen of each lobar, segmental and sub-segmental bronchus seemed unobstructed, without stenosis, neoplasm or bleeding. Mild congestion and swelling were observed at the right bronchial mucosa, with medium amount of white foam-like and purulent secretions. The healed fistula was observed, which was situated on the medial wall of the right main bronchus adjacent to the carina and once communicating with the left main bronchus, and a slight narrowing due to twisting and deformation was observed at each bronchial opening of the right middle and lower lobes, without any neoplasm or hemorrhage (Fig. 10.10). Bronchoscopic diagnosis: (1) Tuberculosis of the right middle and lower lobar bronchus. (2) Occluded fistulae of the right and the left main bronchi.

The anti-tuberculosis treatment had been continued so far for this patient, who was then in good condition without cough or expectoration.

The final diagnosis: (1) Treatment-naive drug-resistant tuberculosis. (2) Bronchial tuberculosis (type of lymph node fistula).

Discussion

The pediatric patients manifested the clinical symptoms and signs dominated by cough, expectoration, and fever, and the recurrent cough and fever during the early stage of treatment might be correlated to infected trachea and bronchi. Based on the congestion and swelling in the right main bronchus and in the right middle and lower lobar bronchi revealed by the first bronchoscopic examination for this patient with a

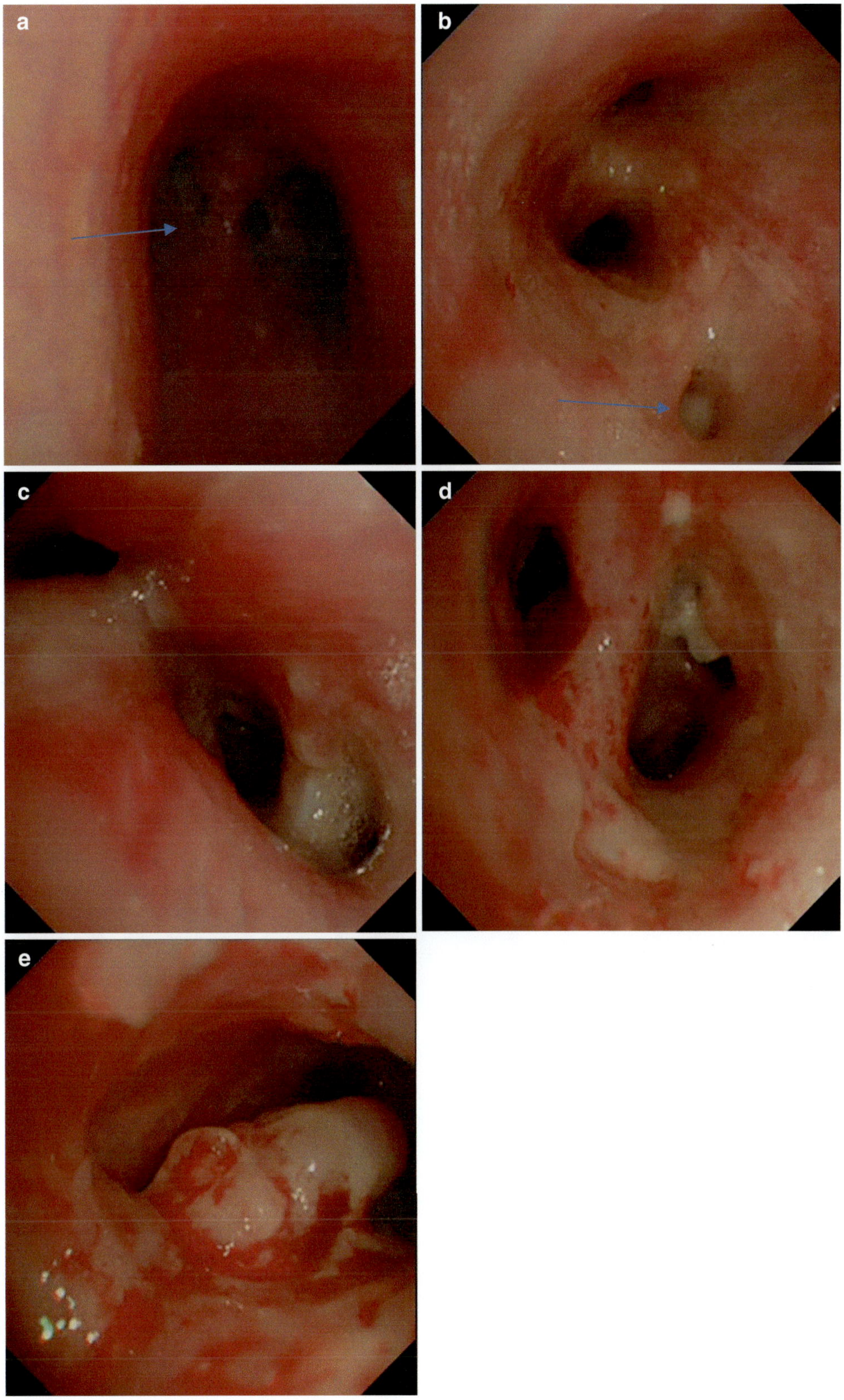

Fig. 10.8 (**a**–**e**) Bronchoscopy performed under local anesthesia on July 13, 2018: Figure **a** shows a fistula located at the right wall inferior to the carina communicating with the right main bronchus, with the formation of the right and the left main bronchial fistula (indicated by the arrow in Figure **a**). Figure **b** shows an obvious congestion and swelling at the mucosa of the right main bronchus under the bronchoscopy, and a fistula can be seen inferior to the carina (as indicated by the arrow in Figure **b**). Figure **c** shows obvious congestion and swelling in mucosa of bronchi of the right middle lobe and dorsal segment in the right lower lobe, with white necrotic substances observable. Figures **d**, **e** show bronchial mucosa illustrated by the image of the bronchial lumen of the anterior segment in the right lower lobe was congested and swollen, with a great deal of granulomatous hyperplasia and white necrotic substances

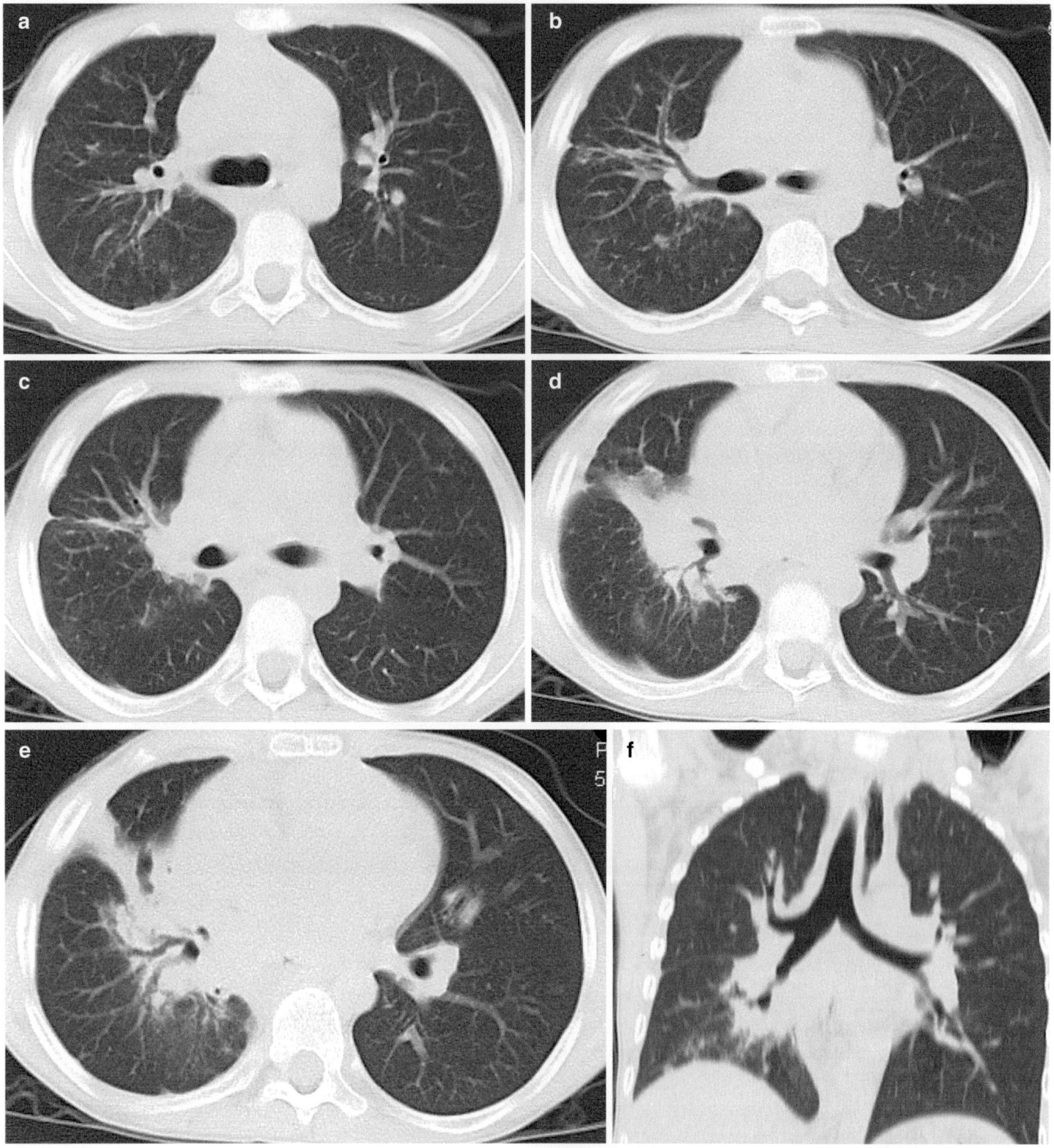

Fig. 10.9 (**a**–**f**) Re-examination of chest CT scans on November 1, 2018, compared with CT scans on July 13, 2018, lung window shows the obvious absorption of lesion in both lungs, smoother interior wall of the right main bronchus and lobar and segmental bronchi in the right lung than before, and the occlusion of the fistula inferior to the carina

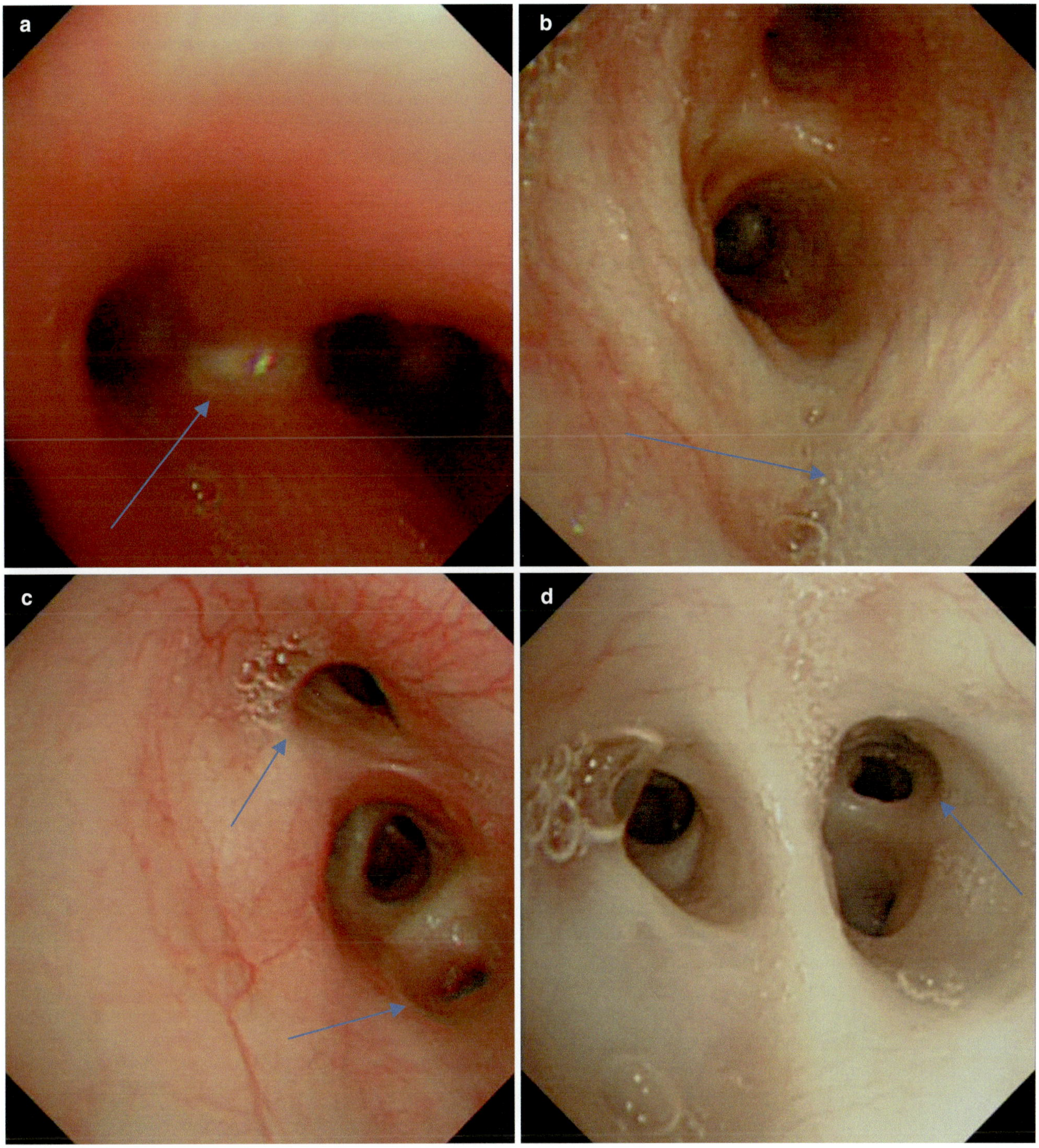

Fig. 10.10 (**a**–**d**) Bronchoscopy on May 24, 2019, under local anesthesia. Figure **a** shows the occluded fistulae at the right and the left main bronchi, inferior to the carina. Figure **b** shows a cicatricial stenosis of the right intermediate bronchus in the image of the opening of the right main bronchus. Figure **c** shows constricted bronchial opening of the right middle lobe and the dorsal segment in the right lower lobe, with cicatricial stenosis. Figure **d** shows that the great amount of granulation hyperplasia and white necrotic substances existing previously in the anterior segmental bronchial lumen in the right lower lobe has been absorbed

great deal of granulation hyperplasia, white necrotic substances and the fistulae in the right and the left main bronchi, and considering also multiple mediastinal lymphadenectasis shown by chest CT scans, the pediatric patient was diagnosed as bronchial tuberculosis in the type of lymph node fistula. Re-examination post to effective anti-tuberculosis treatment for 3 months and a half showed the obvious absorption of lesions in both lungs, shrinkage of hilar and mediastinal lymph nodes, and smoother interior wall of the right main bronchus and the lobar and segmental bronchi in the right lung than before. The occlusion was observed for the previous fistulae at the right and the left main bronchi in re-examination of bronchoscopy post to 10-month treatment, showing also a repair for the previous tuberculosis at the right main bronchus and the right middle and lower lobar bronchi compared with the previous images.

Tracheobronchial tuberculosis is caused by Mycobacterium tuberculosis invading tracheobronchial mucosa and sub-mucosa or destroying further the elastic fiber network and muscular layer, and scar that heals finally results in tracheobronchial stenosis. The pathology of bronchial tuberculosis is based on a series of pathological evolution during which tubercle bacillus invades the surface of bronchial mucosa, causing its congestion, edema, rupture, granulation tissue hyperplasia and fibrous cicatrization. Clinically, a small number of mediastinal lymph node tuberculosis located adjacent to the carina may compress the bronchial wall to induce ulceration, thereby penetrating their wall and causing fistula of bronchial lymph nodes. A discussion has been made by some scholars on grouping of bronchial tuberculosis based on bronchofibroscope findings to divide this disease into six types, including inflammatory infiltration, ulcer necrosis, granulation hyperplasia, cicatricial stenosis, wall softening type and lymph node fistula [31]. Precise diagnosis can be achieved by accurate grouping, with a certain significance and value in guiding clinical treatment. This case belonged to the type of lymph node fistula of bronchial tuberculosis, with the second bronchofibroscope post to the treatment showing the occluded fistulae at the right and the left main bronchi, the repair of the tuberculosis of the right main bronchus and the right middle and lower lobar bronchial tuberculosis in comparison with previous images, and a twisted deformation with a slight narrowing at the opening of middle and lower lobar bronchi of the right lung. CT re-examination and bronchofibroscope were performed during the treatment for this pediatric patient, which was of great importance in evaluating the disease and monitoring responses.

Bronchoscopy plays an important role in diagnosing and treating pediatric pulmonary tuberculosis complicated with bronchial tuberculosis. If allowed by the general condition, pediatric children with primary pulmonary tuberculosis should receive routinely bronchoscopy, through which the removal of caseous substances and granulation tissue in the trachea can improve significantly their clinical symptoms, and this cannot be replaced by medication. Therefore, it is suggested to strengthen intervention under bronchoscope for pediatric patients with drug-resistant pulmonary tuberculosis, so as to shorten the therapeutic cycle of anti-tuberculosis treatment and improve the cure rate.

Positiveness in smear and culture of Mycobacterium tuberculosis is the golden standard for diagnosing pulmonary tuberculosis. Positiveness rate of sputum smear and culture, as revealed by researches, seems low in pediatric tuberculosis patients. Both blood IGRAS and sputum smear were negative in these patients, suggesting the diagnosis of pediatric drug-resistant tuberculosis early detected should also be confirmed through XperMTB/RIF and detection of phenotypic drug resistance in Mycobacterium tuberculosis culture. XperMTB/RIF, one of the genotypic DST methods recommended by WHO, is capable of identifying simultaneously Mycobacterium tuberculosis DNA and detecting genetic mutation related to rifampicin resistance. Gene Xper in this case showed positiveness in bronchial lavage in an extremely low concentration with rifampicin resistance confirmed, which provided the basis for effective treatment launched as early as possible.

References

1. World Health Organization. Global tuberculosis report 2022 [EB/OL]. http://www.who.int/teams/global-tuberculosis-programme/tb-reports/global-tuberculosisreport-2022.
2. Jenkins HE, Yuen CM. The burden of multi-drug resistant tuberculosis in children [J]. Int J Tuberc Lung Dis. 2018;22(5):3–6.
3. Donald PR, Marais BJ, Barry CE. Age and the epidemiology and pathogenesis of tuberculosis [J]. Lancet 2010;375(9729):1852–1854.
4. Harausz EP, Garcia-Prats AJ, Law S, et al. Treatment and outcomes in children with multidrug-resistant tuberculosis: a systematic review and individual patient data meta-analysis [J]. PLoS Med. 2018;15(7):e1002591.
5. Li J, Shen A. The burden and harm of pediatric drug-resistant tuberculosis [J]. Chin J Antituberc. 2018;40(9):989–92.
6. Marquez L, Starke JR. Diagnosis and management of TB in children: an update [J]. Expert Rev Anti Infect Ther. 2011;9(12):1157–68.
7. Yang C, Luo T, Shen X, et al. Transmission of multidrug-resistant mycobacterium tuberculosis in Shanghai, China: a retrospective observational study using whole-genome sequencing and epidemiological investigation [J]. Lancet Infect Dis. 2017;17(3):275–84.
8. Dheda K, Gumbo T, Maartens G, et al. The epidemiology, pathogenesis, transmission, diagnosis, and management of multi-drug resistant, extensively drug-resistant, and incurable tuberculosis [J]. Lancet Respir Med. 2017;5(4):291–360.
9. Liao Q, Tan S, Zhu Y, et al. Clinical characteristics of pediatric drug-resistant tuberculosis and analysis of the effect of the second-line anti-tuberculosis treatment [J]. Chin J Pediatrics. 2017;55(2):100–3.

10. Yu W, Tan W-g, Lu P-x. Classification and imaging manifestations of drug-resistant pulmonary tuberculosis [J/CD]. Electr J Emerg Infect Dis. 2019;4(1):42–7.
11. Shen A, Jiao W. Status of epidemics and drug resistance in pediatric tuberculosis [J]. Chin J Appl Clin Pediatrics. 2016;31(4):269–71.
12. World Health Organization. Global tuberculosis report 2012 [M]. Who/HTM/TB/2012.6. Geneva: WHO Press; 2012. p. 49.
13. World Health Organization. Global Tuberculosis Report 2015 [M]. Who/HTM/TB/2015.22. Geneva: WHO Press; 2015. p. 32.
14. Zignol M, Sismanidis C, Falzon D, et al. Multidrug-resistant tuberculosis in children: evidence from global surveillance [J]. Eur Respir J. 2013;42(3):701–7.
15. Zhao Y, Xu S, Wang L, et al. National survey of drug resistant tuberculosis in China [J]. N Engl J Med. 2012;366(23):2161–70.
16. Jiao WW, Liu ZG, Han R, et al. Prevalence of drug resistant mycobacterium tuberculosis among children in China [J]. Tuberculosis (Edinb). 2015;95(3):315–20.
17. Peng Z, Liu R, Li Q, et al. An analysis of drug resistance status and risk factors of pediatric tuberculosis [J]. Chin J Microecol. 2011;23(7):644–6.
18. Li T, Lu S. Analysis of pediatric drug-resistant tuberculosis [C]. Chongqing: Tuberculosis Branch of Chinese Medical Association; 2013.
19. Huang Q, Li K, Yu Z, et al. An analysis on epidemiological and drug-resistance characteristics in 458 cases of pediatric tuberculosis in Wuhan from 2013 to 2015 [J]. Pract Prev Med. 2017;24:1511–3.
20. Ning-Ning T, Xiao-Chun H, Xian-Xin Z, et al. Drug-resistant tuberculosis among children, China, 2006–2015 [J]. Emerg Infect Dis. 2017;23(11):1800–5.
21. Macias Parra M, Kumate Rodriguez J, Arredondo Garcia JL, et al. Mycobacterium tuberculosis complex genotype diversity and drug resistance profiles in a pediatric population in Mexico [J]. Tuberc Restreat. 2011;2011(2011):7–15.
22. Nelson LJ, Schneider E, Wells CD, et al. Epidemiology of childhood tuberculosis in the United States, 1993-2001: the need for continued vigilance [J]. Pediatrics. 2004;114(2):333–41.
23. Fairlie L, Beykis NC, Reubenson G, et al. High prevalence of childhood multi-drug resistant tuberculosis in Johannesburg, South Africa: a cross sectional study [J]. BMC Infect Dis. 2011;11:28.
24. World Health Organization. Guidance for national tuberculosis programmes on the management of tuberculosis in children [M]. 2nd ed. Geneva: World Health Organization; 2014. p. 65–74.
25. Guo Z. Observation on the recent efficacy of cycloserine in pediatric drug-resistant tuberculosis [J]. Contemp Med. 2019;24(19):102–4.
26. Marais BJ, Gie RP, Schaaf HS, et al. The natural history of childhood intra-thoracic tuberculosis: a critical review of literature from the pre-chemotherapy era [J]. Int J Tuberc Lung Dis. 2004;8(4):392–402.
27. Wang Y, Zhao S, Yu T, et al. An analysis on clinical features of pediatric tuberculosis based on CT typing method [J]. Chin J Antituberc. 2018;9:940–3.
28. Wan C. Diagnosis and treatment of drug-resistant mycobacterium tuberculosis infection in children [J]. J Appl Clin Pediatrics. 2010;25(10):703–6.
29. Manikkam S, Archary N, Bobat R. Chest X-ray patterns of pulmonary multidrug-resistant tuberculosis in children in a high HIV-prevalence setting [J]. SA J Radiol. 2016;20(1):1–6.
30. Xin D, Xin J. An analysis of CT manifestations of pediatric secondary pulmonary tuberculosis [J]. Chin J Antituberc. 2018;40(9):1003–6.
31. Cen W, Chen P, Liao C, et al. An analysis on clinical features and treatment in 320 cases of tracheobronchial tuberculosis [J]. Guangdong Med. 2013;34(16):2508–10.

11 AIDS Complicated with Drug-Resistant Pulmonary Tuberculosis

Yi-bo Lu, Kui Huang, Xin-nian Wen, Hong-zhou Lu, Yong-xiang Yi, and Pu-Xuan Lu

11.1 Summary of AIDS Complicated with Drug-Resistant Pulmonary Tuberculosis

Pulmonary tuberculosis (PTB), defined as a tuberculosis occurring in pulmonary tissue, trachea, bronchi, and pleura [1], is an infectious disease induced by Mycobacterium tuberculosis (MTB, abbreviated as tubercle bacillus) transmitted through respiratory tract. Tuberculosis is one of the major infectious diseases endangering human health in the world today. Due to the impact of COVID-19, as shown by Global Tuberculosis Report 2021 [2] released by WHO, WHO modified the method for estimating tuberculosis epidemics in 2020, based on which 9.9 million newly added cases (95% CI: 8.9–11 million) of tuberculosis patients were estimated in 2020, equivalent to 127 cases per 100,000 people (range: 114–140 cases). In 2020, patients co-infected with tuberculosis and HIV accounted for 8% of all tuberculosis cases. This co-infection had its highest proportion in African countries and exceeded 50% in some regions of southern Africa. It was estimated that the global death caused by tuberculosis in 2020 was about 1.5 million, including 1.3 million (range: 1.2–1.4 million) deaths negative in HIV and 214,000 (range: 187,000–242,000) newly added deaths positive in HIV, higher, respectively, than 1.2 million (range: 1.1–1.3 million) and 209,000 (range: 178,000–243,000) in 2019 [2, 3].

Drug-resistant tuberculosis (DR-TB) is defined as the tuberculosis induced by drug-resistant Mycobacterium tuberculosis [4]. There are various taxonomies for drug-resistant tuberculosis. Based on the Report of Global Project of Monitoring the Resistance to Anti-Tuberculosis Drugs (the 3rd Edition) implemented by the World Health Organization/International Union Against Tuberculosis and Lung Disease (WHO/IUATLD) [5], this disease can be categorized into the new drug-resistant tuberculosis (NDR-TB) and relapsing drug-resistant tuberculosis (RDR-TB), respectively, for patients without and with previous exposure to anti-tuberculosis medication. In China, however, it is categorized into 5 types, including mono-resistant tuberculosis (MR-TB), multidrug-resistant tuberculosis (MDR-TB), poly-resistant tuberculosis (PR-TB), extensively drug-resistant tuberculosis (XDR-TB), and rifampicin-resistant tuberculosis (RR-TB). In data report on drug-resistant pulmonary tuberculosis in its Global Tuberculosis Report 2018, WHO emphasized three types including PR-TB, XDR-TB, and RR-TB. A description based on these three types of drug-resistant tuberculosis emphasized by WHO may have a greater clinical significance. Recent years have been witnessing a trend of the slow rising of newly diagnosed cases of AIDS complicated with tuberculosis, along with the increasing infection rate of human acquired immunodeficiency virus and the ascending population mobility, and tuberculosis has become one of the most common opportunistic infectious pathogens and causes of death in the population infected with HIV, with mutual influence and mutual promotion between these two infections [6, 7]. HIV/PTB co-infection predisposes tuberculosis to untypical manifestations

Y.-b. Lu (✉)
Department of Radiology, The Fourth People's Hospital of Nanning, Nanning, Guangxi, China

K. Huang
Infectious Diseases Department, Chest Hospital of Guangxi Zhuang Autonomous Region, Liuzhou, Guangxi, China

X.-n. Wen
Department of Medical Imaging, Chest Hospital of Guangxi Zhuang Autonomous Region, Liuzhou, Guangxi, China

H.-z. Lu
Infectious Disease, The Third People's Hospital of Shenzhen, Shenzhen, China
e-mail: luhongzhou@shphc.org.cn

Y.-x. Yi
Hepatobiliary Surgery, Nanjing Drum Tower Hospital, Nanjing, China

P.-X. Lu
Diagnostic Imaging, Shenzhen Center for Chronic Disease Control, Shenzhen, China

P.-x. Lu et al. (eds.), *Diagnostic Imaging of Drug Resistant Pulmonary Tuberculosis*,
https://doi.org/10.1007/978-981-99-8339-1_11

[8], challenge in early diagnosis [9], and insufficiency and delay in treatment, thereby causing emergence and epidemics of MDR/XDR-TB. The emergence of AIDS complicated with drug-resistant tuberculosis will bring new challenges to the world, threatening the achievements in controlling HIV/TB during past decades.

11.2 Image Findings for AIDS Complicated with Drug-Resistant Pulmonary Tuberculosis

AIDS, i.e. acquired immunodeficiency syndrome (AIDS), manifests impaired or defective immune function often complicated with various opportunistic infections (OIS), with the lung as the most common target organ. PTB is a common opportunistic infection in AIDS patients, and the incidence of PTB patients with concurrent AIDS is 34.73%, as shown by the epidemiological survey in Guangxi, China [10]. CD4+ T lymphocyte count during the early stage of AIDS is normal or slightly decreased. After the patient is infected with Mycobacterium tuberculosis, image findings of the chest X-ray and CT scans show no significant difference in comparison with ordinary pulmonary tuberculosis. In AIDS patients in the middle and late stage, however, Mycobacterium tuberculosis multiplies in human body with circulatory dissemination along with the continuous reduction of CD4+ T lymphocyte count, and its imaging findings are characterized in atypicality and diversity. Image findings show diversified morphology in lesions involving multiple pulmonary lobes and segments and manifesting usually atypical infiltrative lesions and miliary lesions in lungs with mediastinal lymphadenectasis and pleural effusion, in comparison to those findings rarely observed, such as pulmonary cavitation, pulmonary nodules, obsolete fibrotic pulmonary lesions, and calcified lymph nodes [11, 12].

Image findings of AIDS complicated with DR-TB correlates to drug-resistant strains to some extent. MDR-TB is an acquired resistance to drugs, characterized in prolonged course, recurrent disease, intra-pulmonary dissemination, complicated and diverse CT findings, and in most cases, the involvement of no less than 3 lobes [13, 14]. The most distinct feature of MDR-TB is the emergence of multiple cavities in image findings [9] and has a ratio of about 70%, as shown by researches, with the average number no less than 3 for cavities in MDR-TB patients with cavitation [15]. A large number of Mycobacterium tuberculosis hidden in the cavity may survive, leading eventually to drug resistance and making the patient prone to secondary tuberculosis [16]. Masses, consolidations, thick-walled and mouth-eaten cavities, mucus impaction, bilateral and multi-lobar involvement, large size of the cavities, and multiple cavitations are more common in MDR-TB, while consolidations, involvement of 6 lobes/segments and cavities with the number no less than 3 are independent predictors of MDR-TB [17].

XDR-TB is the most serious type among all pulmonary tuberculosis and involves in most cases no less than 3 pulmonary lobes, with its lesions manifesting mostly the nature of destroyed lungs, dissemination and complication of multiple cavities. Characterized in prolonged courses responding poorly to treatment with repeated damages of pulmonary tissues, XDR-TB patients are extremely prone to intra-pulmonary dissemination resulting in extensive pulmonary distribution of their lesions [18]. The unceasing increase in number of intra-pulmonary disseminated lesions in XDR PTB patients during their treatment, with increasing number and size of cavities in contrast to the low rate of their shrinkage or occlusion reflects fully the feature of this disease including its poor response to treatment and constant deterioration of pulmonary lesions.

11.3 An Introduction of a Typical Case of AIDS Complicated with Drug-Resistant Pulmonary Tuberculosis

Patient XX Wu, a 54-year-old male, complained recurrent fever, cough, and expectoration for 2 months. He had an onset of recurrent intermittent fever with the highest temperature up to 39 °C without obvious inducement 2 months before, with concurrent cough, expectoration of a small amount of white sticky sputum, poor appetite, and fatigue. He visited a local primary level hospital, with the diagnosis and treatment unknown, but no amelioration was achieved. Therefore, he visited a local People's Hospital on November 29, 2020, when chest CT scans showed an inflammation in the anterior segment of the right upper pulmonary lobe. XpertMTB/RIF test showed positiveness in MTB resistant to rifampicin, and he was referred to a Specialty Infectious Disease Hospital for further treatment on December 9, 2020. Past history: positiveness in HIV antibody was confirmed in August 2018, and he received HAART treatment in a district people's hospital, using a regimen consisting of zidovudine and lamivudine tablets plus efavirenz. HAART was discontinued voluntarily by the patient in May 2020.

Blood routine at admission: hemoglobin 114 g/L, red blood cell count 4.25 × 10^{12}/L, white blood cell count 2.52 × 10^9/L, platelet count 313 × 10^9/L, and neutrophil percentage 72.60%. Normal liver and kidney functions, electrolytes, blood lipids, blood glucose, PCT, and coagulation function. CD4+ T lymphocytes: 18 cells/μL. Sputum smear: positive in acid fast bacilli (2+), XpertMTB/RIF (December 11, 2020): positive in Mycobacterium tuberculosis complex, with resistance to rifampicin. Genetic detection for TB drug resistance (linear probe) on December 17, 2020: the flora was identified preliminarily as Mycobacterium tuberculosis complex, suggesting resistant to rifampicin and isoniazid. Based on consultation by the Ward of Drug-Resistant Tuberculosis, an anti-tuberculosis treatment was started on December 20, 2020, using a combined regimen consisting of 6Mfx, Lzd, Cs, Z, Am/12 Mfx, Lzd, Cs, and Z. Symptoms of cough and expectoration were relieved after treatment, and the body temperature was normalized. Sputum smear on January 5, 2021: positive in acid fast bacilli (1+) (Figs. 11.1 and 11.2).

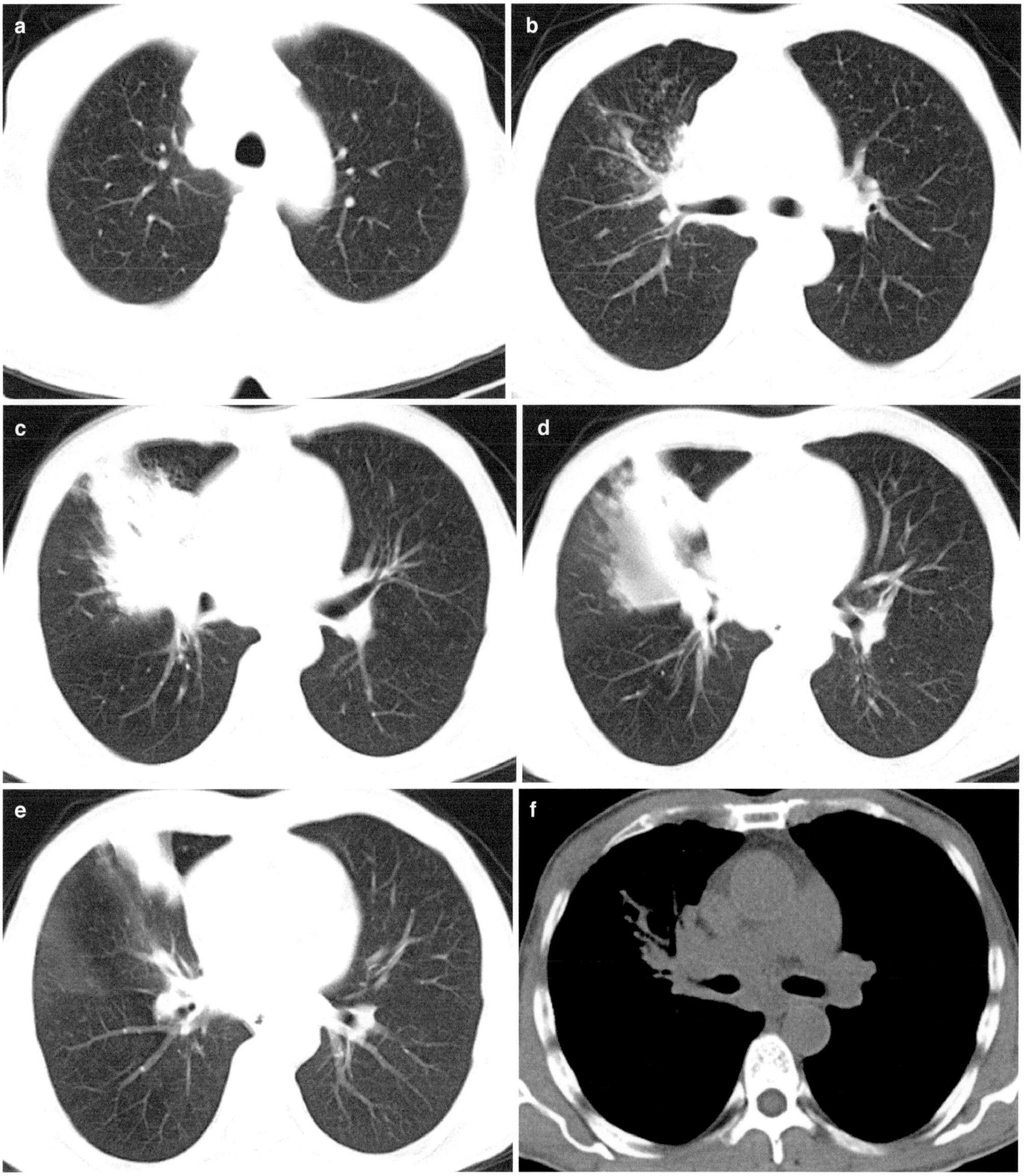

Fig. 11.1 (**a**–**h**) Chest CT scans in local People's Hospital were done on December 3, 2020. (**a**–**e**) Lung window shows mass, flaky, small nodular, and punctiform high-density opacities with blurred border in the right lung, and ground glass opacities in both lungs. (**f**–**h**) Mediastinal window shows multiple lymphadenectasis at the right hilum and in the mediastinum

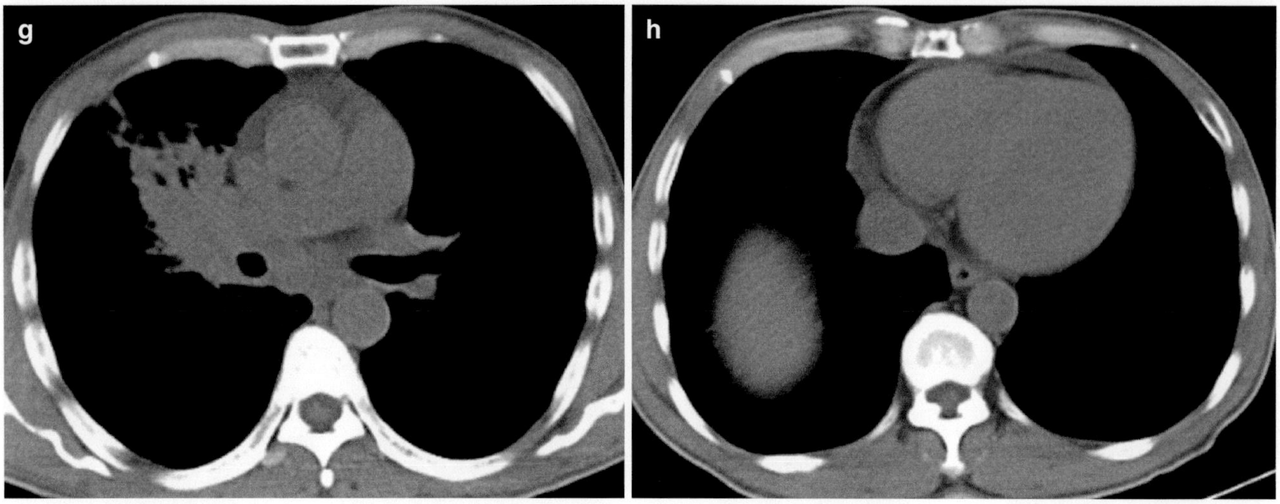

Fig. 11.1 (continued)

The former anti-tuberculosis regimen was continued and sputum smear showed negative in acid fast bacilli on January 12 and 19, 2021 (Fig. 11.3).

Mycobacterium tuberculosis in sputum culture was identified on February 3, 2021, and isolated on March 9, 2021, shown resistant to isoniazid, rifampicin, and ethambutol, and susceptible to ofloxacin, kanamycin, streptomycin, and capreomycin. The former regimen, therefore, was continued to treat tuberculosis. He was discharged on February 8, 2021, and came back to the local hospital to receive the former anti-virus treatment (Fig. 11.4).

The patient was followed up regularly every month with re-examinations. The patient had no obvious symptoms as of the press time, showing negativeness in sputum mycobacterium culture (−) on April 25, 2021, and in sputum smear of acid fast bacilli (−) in April, May, June, and July 2021, respectively. Then the patient continued his anti-tuberculosis treatment with follow-up.

His re-visit on August 31, 2021, showed no obvious symptoms, and re-examination of chest CT scans was performed (Fig. 11.5).

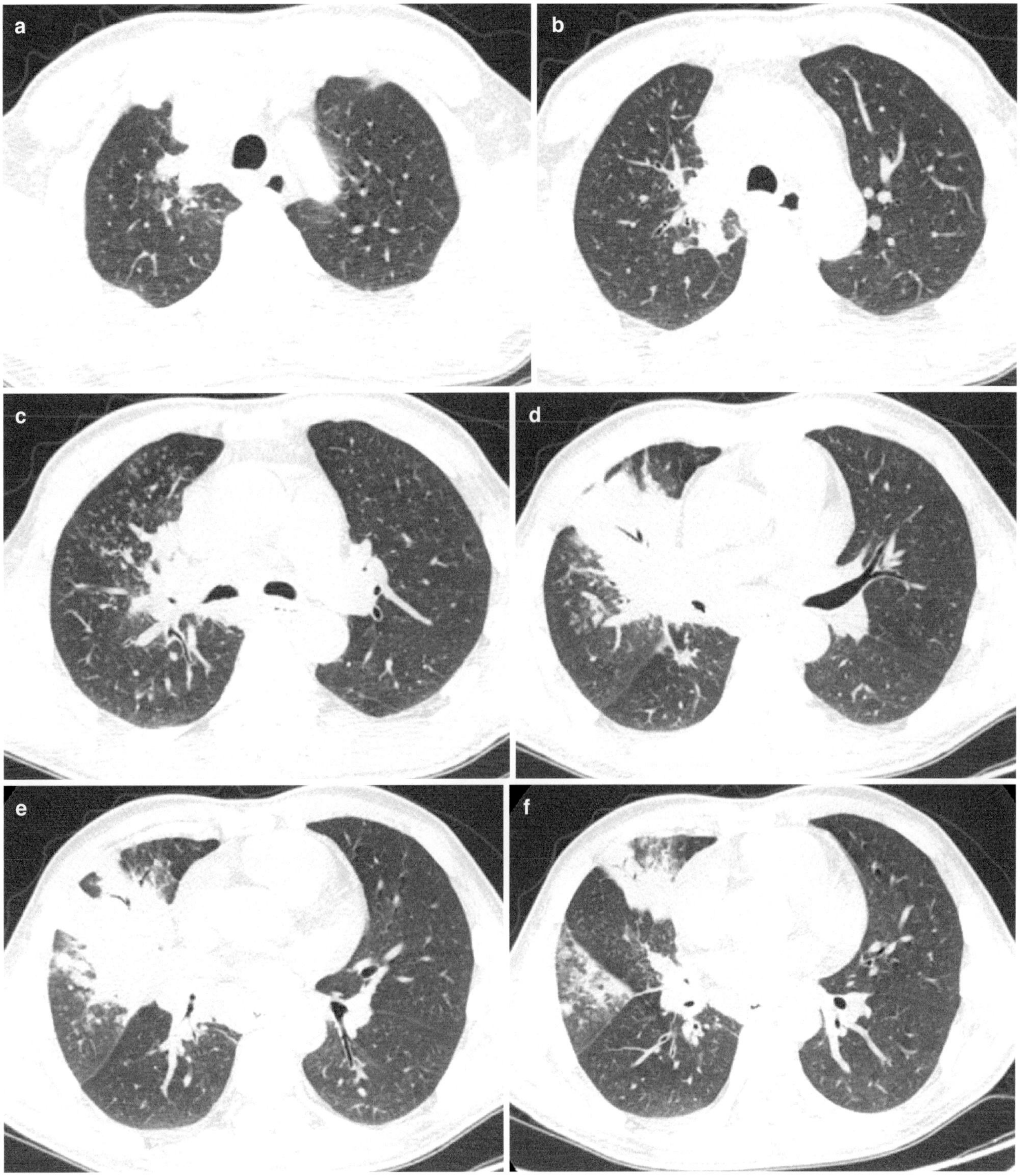

Fig. 11.2 (**a**–**i**) Re-examination of chest CT scans on January 6, 2021, shows the increased number of lesions in the right lung with a small amount of effusion in the right pleural cavity and in the pericardial cavity (I) in comparison with CT scans on December 3, 2020

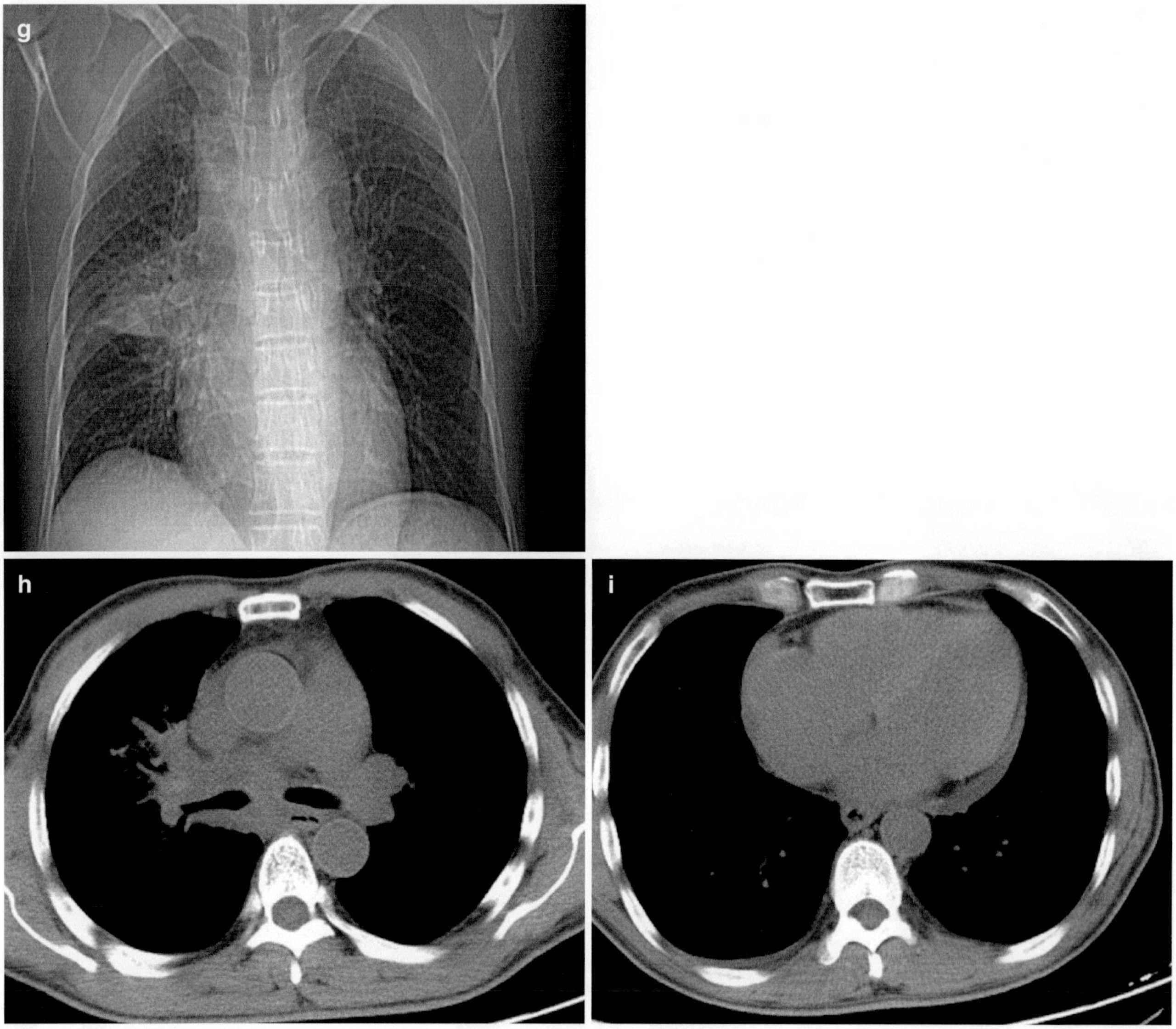

Fig. 11.2 (continued)

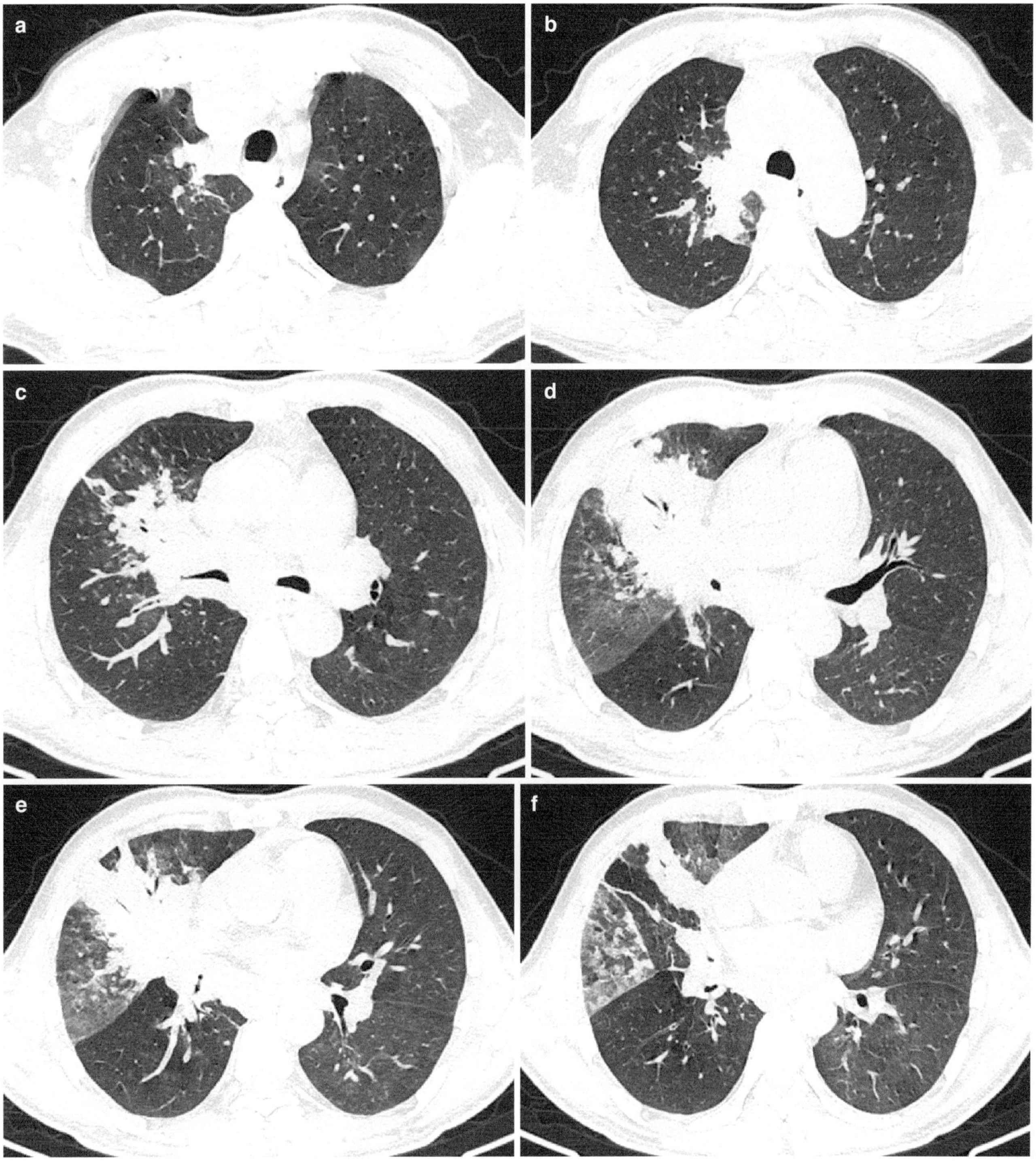

Fig. 11.3 (**a**–**i**) Re-examination of chest CT scans on January 18, 2021, shows the increased number of lesions in the right lung with decreased effusion in the right pleural cavity and in the pericardial cavity, in comparison with CT scans on January 6, 2021

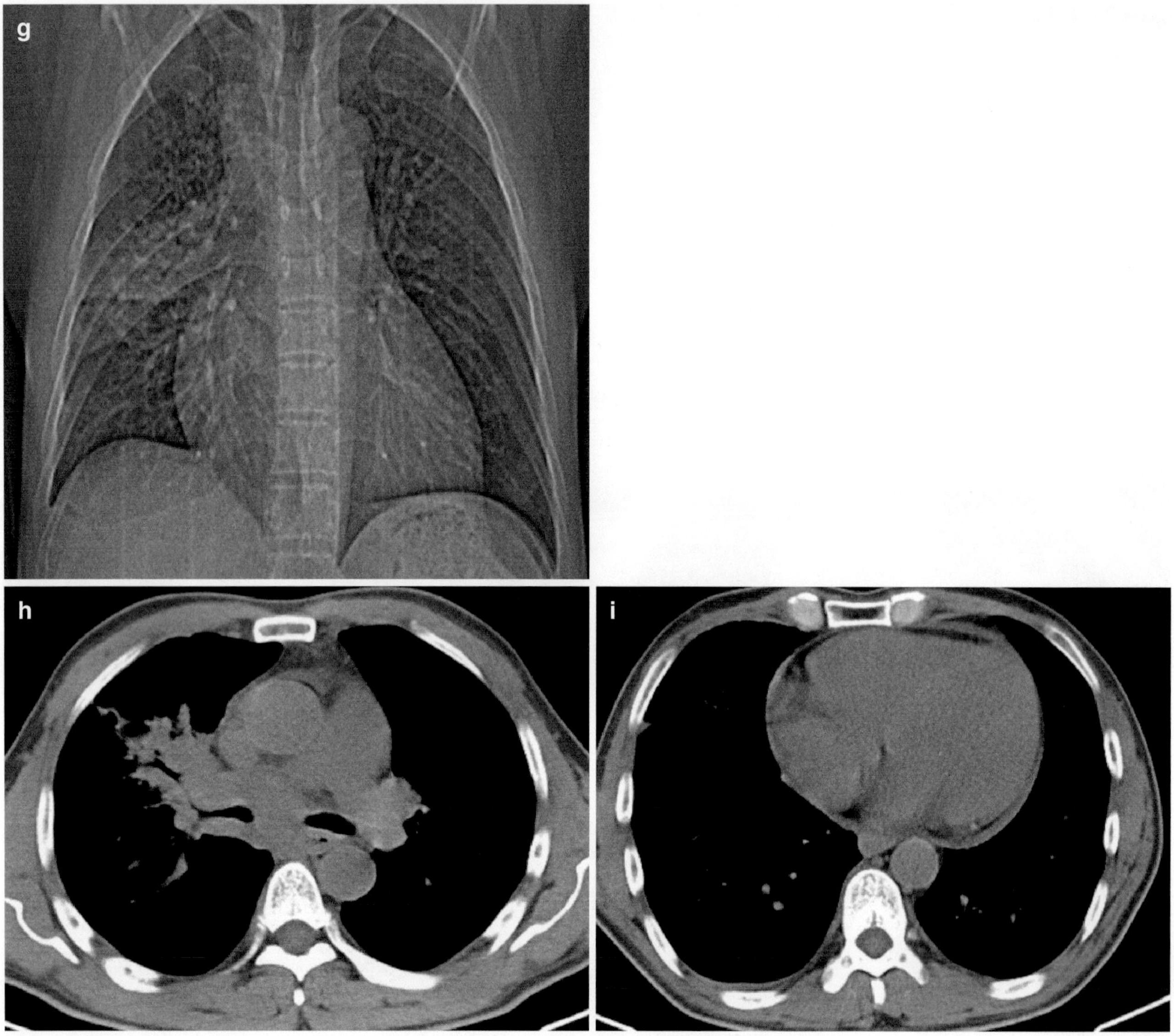

Fig. 11.3 (continued)

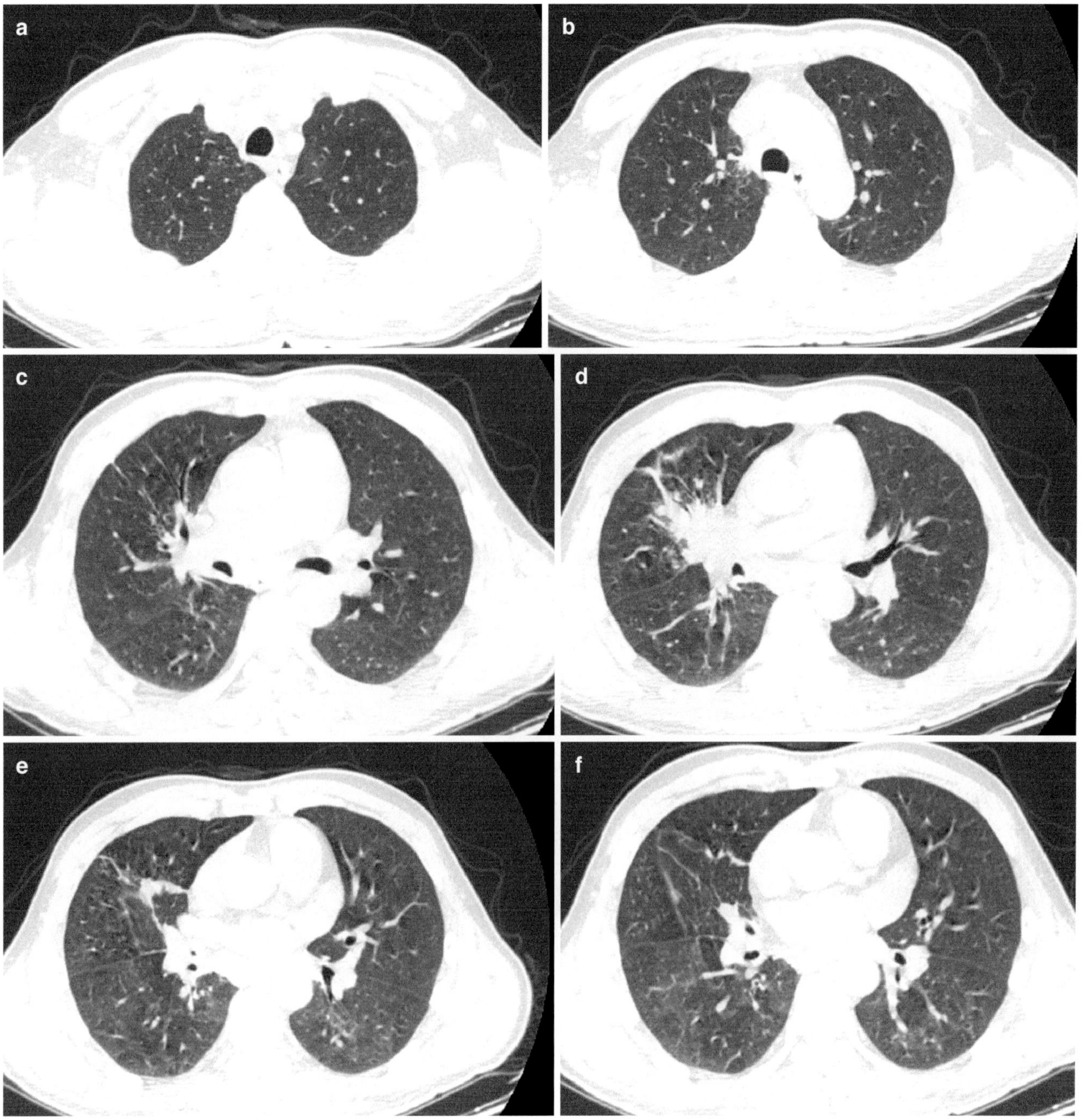

Fig. 11.4 (**a–i**) Re-examination of chest CT scans on April 8, 2021, shows the obvious absorption of lesions and the absorption of effusion in the right pleural cavity and in the pericardial cavity, as compared with CT scans on January 18, 2021

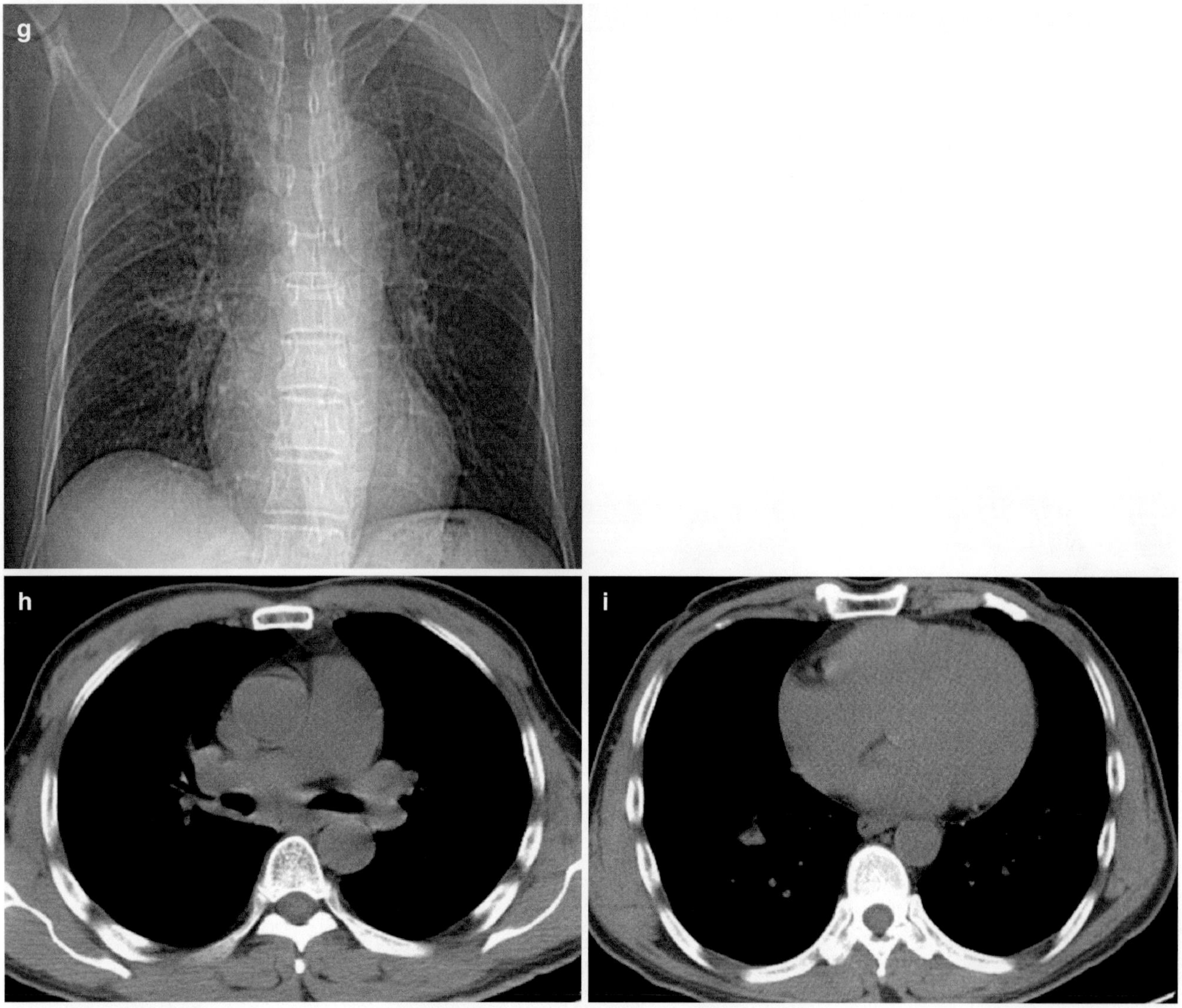

Fig. 11.4 (continued)

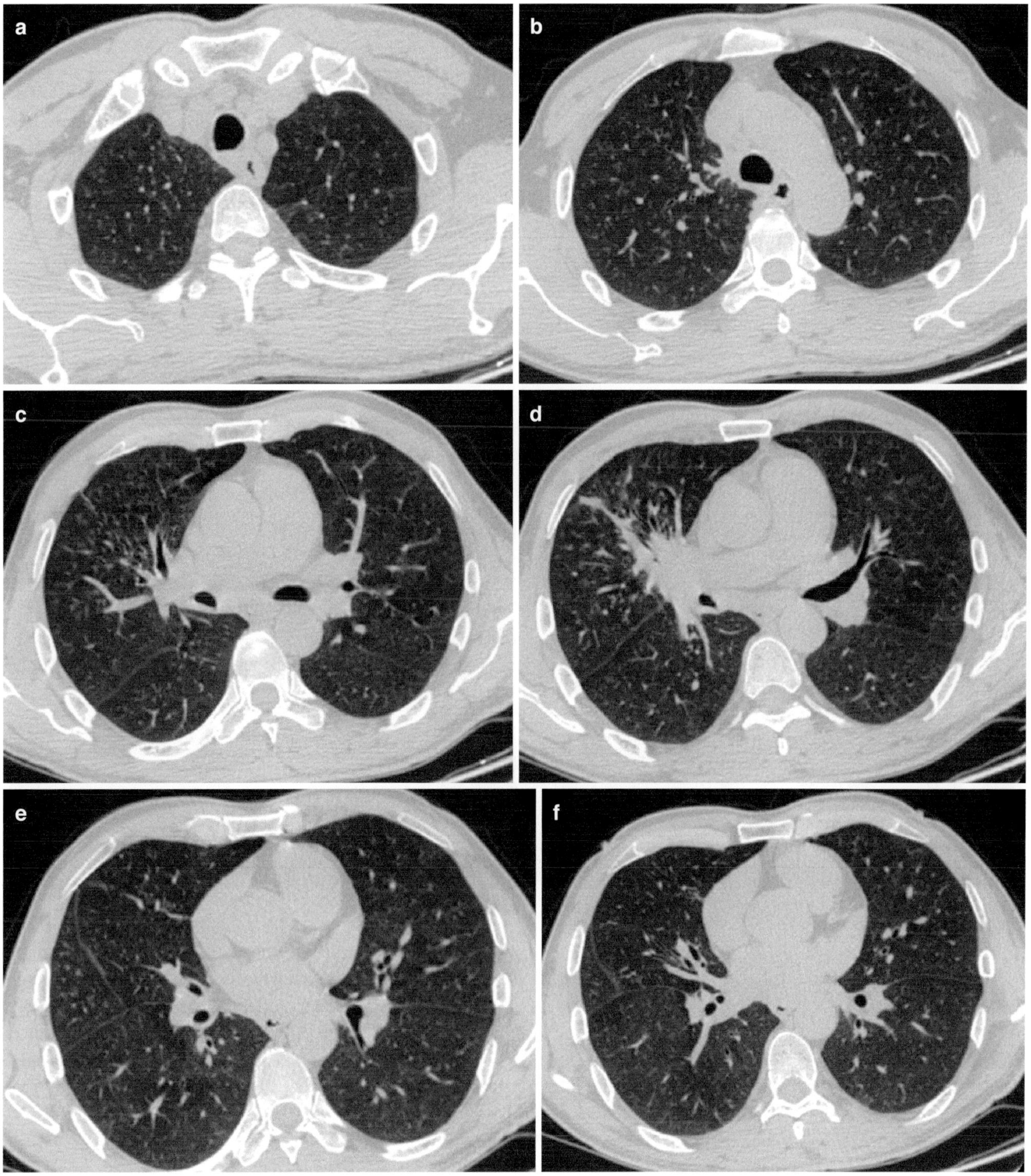

Fig. 11.5 (**a–i**) Re-examination of chest CT scans on August 31, 2021, shows an obvious absorption of lesions in comparison with CT scans on April 8, 2021

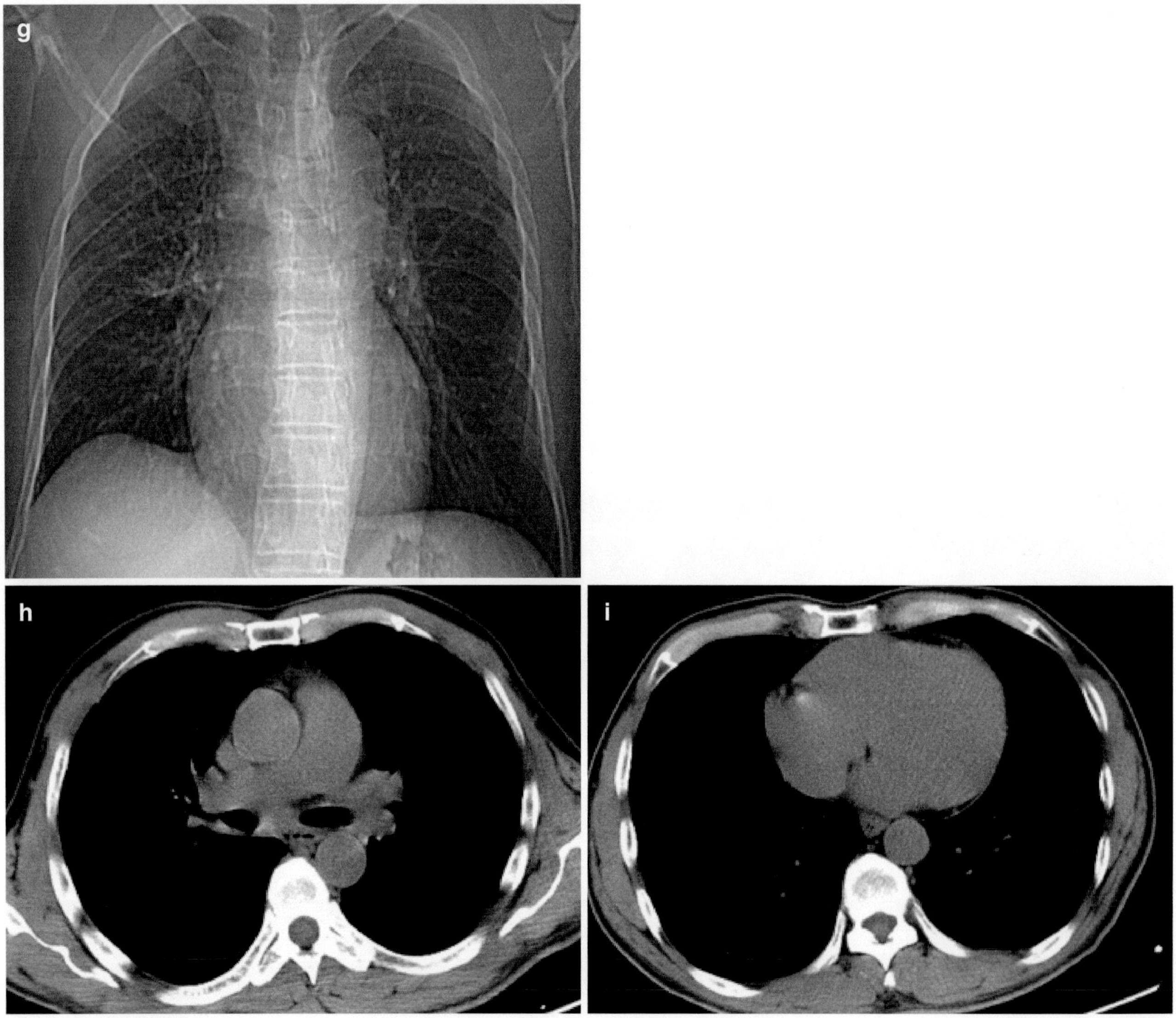

Fig. 11.5 (continued)

11.4 Discussion

Tuberculosis is one of the vital public health problems threatening human health. Among the estimated ten million cases of tuberculosis worldwide in 2017, there were 920,000 cases complicated with AIDS (accounting for 9%), and 558,000 cases of MDR-TB and rifampicin-resistant tuberculosis, wherein MDR-TB cases occupied 82%. In 2017, the estimated deaths were 300,000 caused by AIDS complicated with tuberculosis, and 230,000 caused by MDR and rifampicin-resistant tuberculosis [19]. China ranks the third around the world based on the severity in MDR-TB epidemiology and has its MDR-TB population accounting for 14% of global patients with this disease [20], while its primary multidrug-resistant rate is higher in tuberculosis patients co-infected with HIV than in those without HIV infection [21]. Therefore, the early detection of MDR tuberculosis co-infected with HIV and the effective treatment are the important measures to lower the incidence of MDR-TB complicated with HIV infection and decrease the mortality of AIDS patients.

The patient suffered from AIDS complicated with primary multidrug-resistant pulmonary tuberculosis, manifesting his CD4+ T lymphocyte count lower than 50/μL and lesions mainly located in the anterior segment of the right upper lobe, which was not the site vulnerable to tuberculosis. The lesions included mass, flaky, small nodular, and punctiform high-density opacities as well as ground glass opacities, with hilar and mediastinal lymphadenectasis, without cavitation. All these manifestations seemed consistent with image findings of AIDS complicated with drug-resistant pulmonary tuberculosis reported by Ying Zhu [9] and Peipei Liang et al. [22].

The diagnosis for drug-resistant tuberculosis, based on the definition of drug-resistant tuberculosis [1], necessitates culture of Mycobacterium tuberculosis and drug susceptibility test, while the former is time consuming and requires at least 2 months, predisposing the patient to delay in diagnosis and increased difficulties in treatment. A diagnosis of MDR-TB was established for this case by XpertMTB/RIF and genetic detection (linear probe) for drug-resistance TB within a few days after admission, which was consistent with that of drug susceptibility test 2 months later, and a treatment was carried out timely. Because of the limited financial affordability, the patient could not use bedaquiline (Bdq) and clofazimine (Cfz) but used alternative regimen consisting of 6mfx, LZD, Cs, Z, Am/12Mfx, Lzd, Cs, and Z instead, to which a good response was achieved less than 4 months. XpertMTB/RIF and genetic detection of drug-resistant tuberculosis are rapid methods for detecting multidrug-resistant tuberculosis with high accuracy [23], and the best approaches to establish the diagnosis in the early stage. The combination of Mfx, Lzd, Cs, Z, and Am is also a good alternative in treating drug-resistant tuberculosis to substitute for Bdq and Cfz if they are hardly affordable [24, 25].

References

1. National Health Commission of the People's Republic of China. Diagnostic criteria for tuberculosis (WS 288-2017) [J/CD]. Electr J Emerg Infect Dis. 2018;3(1):59–61.
2. World Health Organization. Global tuberculosis report 2021 [EB/OL]. https://www.who.int/publications/digital/global-tuberculosis-report-2021.
3. Chunrong L, Hongxia F, Lu P, et al. The global tuberculosis report 2021: key data analysis for China and the global world [J/CD]. Electr J Emerg Infect Dis. 2021;6(4):368–72.
4. Chinese Anti-Tuberculosis Association. Guidelines on chemotherapy against drug-resistant tuberculosis (simplified version 2019) [J]. Chin J Antituberc. 2019;41(10):1025–73.
5. World Health Organization. WHO consolidated guidelines on drug resistant tuberculosis treatment [M]. Geneva: World Health Organization; 2019.
6. WHO/IUATLD. Global project on anti-tuberculosis drug resistance surveillance. Anti-tuberculosis drug resistance in the world. Third report [R]. Geneva: WHO; 2004. p. 343.
7. Lian X. Progress in clinical research on HIV/AIDS complicated with tuberculosis [J]. Hainan Med J. 2013;24(15):2274–6.
8. Friedland G. Tuberculosis, drug resistance, and HIV/ AIDS: a triple threat [J]. Curr Infect Dis Rep. 2007;9(3):252–61.
9. Zhu Y, Zhang Z, Shi Y. Progress in imaging diagnosis of AIDS complicated with drug-susceptible multi-resistant and extensively drug-resistant tuberculosis [J]. Radiol Pract. 2011;26(9):941–3.
10. Wei L, Zhang T, Wu F, et al. Analysis of opportunistic infectious disease spectrum of HIV/AIDS inpatients in HAART era [J]. Chin J AIDS STD. 2018;24(5):454–7.
11. Lu P, Yu W, Zhu W, et al. Imaging characteristics of AIDS complicated with pulmonary tuberculosis and its correlation with CD4+T lymphocytes [J]. Chin J Tuberc Resp Dis. 2005;01:16–9.
12. Xiao G, Xiao Y, Chen H, et al. Clinicopathological features of opportunistic infectious diseases related to AIDS [J]. Acad J Guangzhou Med Univ. 2019;47(1):22–8.
13. Yu W-y, Tan W-g, Luo Y-t, et al. 2018 WHO tuberculosis report: key data analysis for global and China [J/CD]. Electr J Emerg Infect Dis. 2018;3(4):229–34.
14. Gao D, Wang S, Qiu L. An analysis on chest imaging in 86 patients with multi-resistant pulmonary tuberculosis [J]. J Clin Pulm Med. 2012;17(7):1265–6.
15. Li C, Lu S, Wang H, et al. CT findings in patients with multi-resistant pulmonary tuberculosis and its correlation to CD4 cells [J]. Chin J Antituberc. 2017;39(6):597–603.
16. Geng E, Kreiswirth B, Burzynski J, et al. Clinical and radiographic correlates of primary and deactivation tuberculosis: a molecular epidemiology study [J]. JAMA. 2005;293(22):2740–5.
17. Dong X, Chen H, Hong J, et al. Features of high resolution CT findings in multi-resistant secondary pulmonary tuberculosis [J]. Chin J Clin (Electr Ed). 2013;7(21):9494–7.
18. Sun H, Tang S, Gu J, et al. Chest CT features of extensively drug-resistant pulmonary tuberculosis [J]. Chin J Antituberc. 2011;33(2):123–5.
19. World Health Organization. Global tuberculosis report 2018 [EB/OL]. [2018-09-18]. http://www.who.int/tb/publications/global_report/en/.
20. World Health Organization. Global tuberculosis report 2019 [R/OL]. (2019-10-17). [2020-03-18]. https://www.who.int/tb/publications/global_report/en/.
21. Chen Y, Liu X, Wang Y, et al. An analysis on initial drug resistance in mycobacterium tuberculosis in patients with HIV/TB complicated with infection in Henan Province [J]. Chin J AIDS STD. 2021;27(1):14–6.
22. Liang P, Shen Y, Liu L, et al. A clinical epidemiological study on 359 cases of acquired immunodeficiency syndrome complicated with pulmonary tuberculosis [J]. Chin J Infect Chemother. 2017;17(3):233–7.
23. Tao C, Wang Y, Junfeng Z, et al. Diagnostic reliability of Xpert MTB/RIF with rifampicin resistance detected at very low bacterial level: a retrospective analysis [J/CD]. Electr J Emerg Infect Dis. 2021;6(4):319–22.
24. Liangzi Y, Tantan R, Xiangdong F, et al. Bedaquiline in the treatment of pulmonary drug-resistant tuberculosis: safety and efficacy [J/CD]. Electronic Journal of Emerging Infectious Diseases. 2021;6(4):302–5.
25. Le-Cai JI, Yu W-y, Tan W-g, et al. Clinical observation and adverse reactions analysis of linezolid in the treatment of severe multi-drug resistant pulmonary tuberculosis [J/CD]. Electr J Emerg Infect Dis. 2019;4(4):217–9, 234.

12 Diagnosis and Treatment of Drug-Resistant Cervical Tuberculous Lymphadenitis

Hai-jiang Wang, Hong-zhou Lu, Yong-xiang Yi, Zhe-huang Luo, and Yu-lin He

12.1 Clinical Classification and Image Findings of Drug-Resistant Cervical Tuberculous Lymphadenitis

Tuberculosis, a chronic disease induced by infection of mycobacterium tuberculosis (MTB), is one of main diseases endangering human health. Tuberculosis may affect almost all organs and tissues in the body. Clinically, it can be divided into pulmonary tuberculosis and extra-pulmonary tuberculosis according to the different sites infected in patients. Among all extra-pulmonary tuberculosis, tuberculous lymphadenitis is the most common one, and its most common site is the neck [1]. Cervical tuberculous lymphadenitis (CTL) accounts for 4.0–5.1% of all tuberculosis cases, and 20.3–50% of extra-pulmonary tuberculosis [2]. In recent years, Indian scholar Akkara et al. [3] showed that cervical lymph node tuberculosis accounted for 5.36% of all tuberculosis cases, so cervical lymph node tuberculosis is quite common clinically.

Cervical tuberculous lymphadenitis is most commonly caused by the spread of Mycobacterium tuberculosis from pulmonary tuberculosis or mediastinal tuberculosis lymphadenitis to cervical lymph nodes through blood circulation or lymphatic tract, or by Mycobacterium tuberculosis inducing the infection in the mouth or at nasopharynx after traveling through the upper respiratory tract of moving with food, especially the infection at cervical superficial and deep lymph nodes where Mycobacterium tuberculosis arrives at after traveling through lymphatic tract from the primary infection focus that it induces in tonsils. This disease manifests often painless masses growing slowly in lateral cervical region, for which the best opportunity of medical treatment is often missed because of the difficulties in early diagnosis, predisposing the patient to the formation of prolonged fistula

H.-j. Wang (✉)
Department of Thoracic Surgery, The Third People's Hospital of Shenzhen, Shenzhen, Guangdong, China

H.-z. Lu
Infectious Disease, The Third People's Hospital of Shenzhen, Shenzhen, China
e-mail: luhongzhou@shphc.org.cn

Y.-x. Yi
Hepatobiliary Surgery, Nanjing Drum Tower Hospital, Nanjing, China

Z.-h. Luo
Department of Nuclear Medicine, Jingxi Provincial People's Hospital, The First Affiliated Hospital of Nanchang Medical College, Jingxi, China

Y.-l. He
Department of Radiology, The First Affiliated Hospital of Nanchang University, Nanchang, Jiangxi, China

P.-x. Lu et al. (eds.), *Diagnostic Imaging of Drug Resistant Pulmonary Tuberculosis*,
https://doi.org/10.1007/978-981-99-8339-1_12

and ulcers, especially in the drug-resistant or multi-resistant cervical tuberculous lymphadenitis.

Gene Chip is of great value in clinical application in the diagnosis of tuberculous lymphadenitis and analysis of drug resistance, and its efficiency in diagnosis and in detection of drug resistance in MTB is generally identical to the classical Mycobacterium tuberculosis culture [4]. Fine needle aspiration cytology in combination with fluorescence quantitative PCR to detect TB-DNA, as reported by Xiaoqin Yu [5], seems to be able to diagnose tuberculosis lymphadenitis more accurately and more rapidly than acid fast staining. Romdhane et al. [6] reported that Genexpert detection for formalin-fixed and paraffin-embedded tissue showed good sensitivity (74%) and perfect specificity (100%) in diagnosing cervical tuberculosis lymphadenitis. GeneXpertMTB/RIF was shown to have a sensitivity of 82.6% and a specificity of 85.0% in comparison with histopathology in 67 cases of tuberculosis lymphadenitis, as reported by Raja [7], with 2 patients (2.9%) having rifampicin resistance. A research by Tadesse [8] reported that positive MTB/RIF, the rifampicin resistant gene, was revealed in 4.7% (4/86) of all patients positive in genetic detection for cervical tuberculosis lymphadenitis. The multidrug-resistant rate was reported by Chengqing Yang [9] to be 11.0% in 210 cases of cervical tuberculosis lymphadenitis. In a group of 127 patients with cervical tuberculous lymphadenitis undergone surgical treatment, which we analyzed retrospectively, 6 cases (4.7%) had rifampicin resistance based on Gene/XpertMTB/RIF.

Based on various pathological process and clinical manifestations, cervical tuberculous lymphadenitis can be categorized into the following four types [10]: (1) Nodular type: It shows slow onset and manifests localized single or multiple swollen lymph node(s) in hard texture, scattered and movable, with mild tenderness, but without adhesion. Along with the progression of the disease, however, tuberculosis lymphadenitis increases in size with a gradual decrease in the mobility and becomes adhered into clusters. This state may persist for months without any obvious change. (2) Infiltration type: The swollen lymph nodes fuse into masses, with obvious perinodal inflammation, adhesion to surrounding tissues and skin, softening at the center (i.e. caseous necrosis), limited mobility, and aggravated pain and tenderness. (3) Abscess type: It shows the softening at the center of the swollen lymph nodes manifesting a gradual expansion or a sudden enlargement with fluctuation, so as to form an abscess. (4) Ulcerative sinus type: The fluctuation of the abscess becomes gradually mild, which is extremely breakable to discharge watery caseous pus, with a delayed healing of the wound and the formation of sinus or ulcer. This categorization is also applicable to the clinical grouping of drug-resistant cervical tuberculous lymphadenitis.

Image examination for drug-resistant cervical tuberculous lymphadenitis is conducive to define diagnosis, evaluate the disease, guide clinical categorization and the option of surgical modalities, and provide a precise range of lymphadenectomy. The typical CT manifestations of cervical tuberculous lymphadenitis in the early stage include multiple nodular opacities in the density of soft tissue in the lateral cervical region, showing high density along the circumference of the lesion complicated sometimes with punctiform calcification. A circular enhancement at the edge of the lesion can be observed in contrasted CT scans, which can fuse and aggregate, with the maximum diameter of the lesion often less than 2 cm, and proliferative tuberculosis lymphadenitis shows homogeneous enhancement. The further progression of the lesion forms signs of abscess or ulcer, with its image findings featuring a giant necrotic cavity fused by multiple lesions and penetrating capsule to infiltrate surrounding tissues, and network edema in subcutaneous fat. Lee et al. [11] summarized CT findings of cervical tuberculous lymphadenitis into four types, including type I showing the density of the lesions almost identical to that of surrounding normal soft tissue; type II illustrating low density in the center of the lymph node with surrounding circular enhancement without the disappearance of surrounding fat layers; type III featuring multi-cavity low-density opacities, with disappearance of surrounding fat layers (this type is the most common one); and type IV manifesting often nodular low-density opacities with loss of normal morphology of original lymph nodes. Image findings of CT scans in cervical tuberculosis lymphadenitis correlate mainly to its pathological stages, showing homogenous-density lesions with obvious enhancement in contrasted CT scans when it is in proliferative or granulomatous stage, and manifesting circular enhancement with adhered/fused lymph nodes and blurred peripheral fat space when it is in the stage of caseous necrosis. It is of great importance to carry out pre-operative evaluation for this disease using routine imaging methods.

12.2 Treatment Principles of Drug-Resistant Cervical Tuberculous Lymphadenitis with Abscess and Ulcerative Sinus

Cervical lymph node tuberculosis drug treatment effect is poor, mainly because the enlarged lymph nodes have a complete capsule, lymph node formation after an abscess, the blood supply in the abscess cavity is poor, and it is difficult for drugs to enter the lesion. In addition, the increase in drug-resistant tuberculosis strains makes patients manifest as neck lumps, abscesses, or sinus tracts that do not heal for a long time, causing a heavy psychological burden and affecting life and work. Jiang Tao et al. [12] applied a therapy of minimally invasiveness plus wound surface vacuum to cervical tuberculous lymphadenitis, which reduced the healed wound scar, enhanced the expression of VEGF and CD34 over the wound surface, decreased the number of post-operative dressing changes, and accelerated wound healing. In addition, good response was achieved by Haijiang Wang et al. [13] using functional regional lymphadenectomy in treating abscess and ulcerative type of cervical tuberculous lymphadenitis.

Cervical tuberculous lymphadenitis is a benign disease, and the surgery aims to eradicate the abscess and resect the swollen lymph nodes. The functional regional lymphadenectomy is performed simultaneously with the eradication of abscess, and an effective intra-operative protection is provided for internal jugular vein, common carotid artery, sternocleidomastoid muscle, omohyoid muscle, supraclavicular cutaneous nerve, greater auricular nerve, occipital minor nerve, accessory nerve, transverse cervical blood vessels and nerves, phrenic nerve, and vagus nerve. Therefore, post-operative recurrence of tuberculosis lymphadenitis can be prevented from, while cervical function is better protected.

Operative procedure of functional regional lymphadenectomy includes general anesthesia and endotracheal intubation; the patient is kept in a supine position, with the shoulder on the affected side underlaid, the head bent backward, the face turned to the contralateral side, and neck on the affected side exposed.

For a lesion located in region IV or Vb, a 5–6 cm long transverse incision is made at a level of 1–2 cm over supraclavicular fossae along the dermatoglyph at the lateral edge of sternocleidomastoid muscle, while previous fistula or incision scar is resected through a fusiform incision centered at them, so as to eliminate pus and caseous necrotic tissues. The sternocleidomastoid muscle and omohyoid muscle are dissociated with simultaneous protection of the accessory nerve and suprascapular nerve, so as to expose carotid sheath and transverse cervical vessels, and remove all swollen lymph nodes, abscesses, fistulae, and scars in regions IV and V. Lymph nodes in region III can be removed through dissociating internal jugular vein upward along the posterior edge of the sternocleidomastoid muscle. When clearing the lymph nodes in region IV, attention should be paid to the protection of the internal jugular vein and thoracic duct or the right lymphatic duct, lest chylous fistula occurs due to incidental damage to it. A grooved drainage tube is indwelt in the wound that has been washed with hydrogen peroxide and iodophor, followed by continuous negative-pressure aspiration and primary suture for the incision.

Pus is removed for patients with cervical tuberculosis lymphadenitis in region I, II, III, or VA, using a 4–8 cm long longitudinal incision at the anterior edge of the sternocleidomastoid muscle. A skin flap is dissociated from the superficial surface of the deep layer of platysma, while attention is paid to the protection of the external jugular vein, the greater auricular nerve, marginal mandibular branch of the facial nerve, and occipital minor nerve. The medial edge of the sternocleidomastoid muscle is dissociated to expose the internal jugular vein with simultaneous protection of accessory nerve and marginal mandibular branch of the facial nerve, so as to clear surrounding swollen lymph nodes and necrotic tissues, followed by dissociation and clearance of lymphatic tissues downward into regions II and III surrounding the internal jugular vein and backward into regions IV and Va surrounding the accessory nerve, with the primary suture for the wound.

The primary suture of the wound with dissociated flap under the platysma or a vacuum sealing drainage (VSD) is required before the wound is sutured, if a patient has a large skin defect post to debridement, with incomplete clearance of lesions and severe inflammatory reaction in local tissues.

Using these surgical modalities, Haijiang Wang et al. [13] treated 68 patients with cervical tuberculous lymphadenitis including 50 in abscess type and 18 in ulcerative sinus type, and post-operative follow-up for 1 year showed accessory nerve injury ($n = 1$), residue of lesion ($n = 2$), post-operative recurrence ($n = 2$), and healed scar post to surgery or delayed healing ($n = 12$), with the incidence of 25% (17/68) for post-operative adverse complications and of 12.0% (6/50) for complications in abscess type patients, which seemed obviously lower than the incidence of 61.1% (11/18) for complications in patients in ulcerative fistula type. The general primary healing rate of wounds was 82.4% (56/68), wherein the primary healing rate for abscess type was 92.0% (46/50), obviously higher than 55.6% (10/18) for the ulcerative sinus type.

A 100% positiveness rate for tuberculous lymphadenitis was observed, based on pathology of post-operative specimen. Bacteriological tests were performed for resected specimens, showing the positiveness rates of 5.9%, 16.2%, 33.8%, 55.9%, and 88.2%, respectively, for acid fast bacilli smear, culture, TB-RNA, TB-DNA, and GeneXpert.

Primary suture of surgical wound can be performed for abscess type and ulcerative sinus type of cervical tuberculosis lymphadenitis post to functional regional cervical lymphadenectomy, and the abscess type showed higher healing rate of primary healing than ulcerative sinus type, with better prognosis in patients receiving surgery earlier. The research by Zhi Wang et al. [14] showed that surgical effectiveness for cervical tuberculosis lymphadenitis correlated to multidrug resistance (MDR), wherein the recurrence was observed in 2 out of 173 patients having received surgery, and both of them were MDR patients.

The peri-operative anti-tuberculosis regimen against cervical tuberculosis lymphadenitis: a post-operative anti-tuberculosis treatment is recommended, which lasts 6 months for a patient without drug resistance and 9 months for a patient complicated tuberculosis at any other site, and the treatment should be based on the drug resistance regimens for a drug-resistant patient.

Two regimens are optional for multidrug-resistant patients [15]. The first is 6LfxBdqLzdCfzCs/12LfxLzdCfzCs (the number represents duration in month) with the total therapeutic course of 18 months and a strengthening period of 6 months. The second regimen, the regimen containing injections, is 6Lfx (Mfx) Bdq (Lzd) Cfz (Cs) PtoZ(E) Am(Cm)/12Lfx (Mfx) CfzCs) Ptoz (E) (the number represents duration in month).

Operation for cervical tuberculous lymphadenitis not only eliminates abscess lesion of tuberculosis but also achieves a functional regional lymphadenectomy eradicating generally the environment where cervical tubercle bacillus inhabits and minimizing bacterial load in vivo. The microenvironment of local residue tubercle bacilli post to clearance of cervical lymph node abscess has good blood supply with high local blood drug concentration, which is more conducive to eradicating bacteria [3].

12.3 Introduction of Typical Cases of Drug-Resistant Cervical Tuberculous Lymphadenitis

12.3.1 Abscess and Ulceration Type of Cervical Tuberculous Lymphadenitis

The patient Ma, a 31-year-old female, complained a mass found on the right neck 2 years before. She noticed a mass on her right neck in May 2018 and received voluntarily TCM treatment for cervical lymphadenitis for half a year, but there was no amelioration. Fine needle aspiration biopsy done in December 2018 in a hospital in Sichuan Province suggested a pathological diagnosis of an observable granulomatous inflammation with necrosis, and the presence of a small amount of acid fast bacilli found in acid fast staining, with positiveness in Mycobacterium tuberculosis DNA. She was diagnosed as cervical tuberculous lymphadenitis and started an anti-tuberculosis treatment with HERZ regimen, followed by regular medication and follow-up. The mass in the right neck ruptured and discharged pus in March 2019, then she underwent surgery in a local hospital, followed by regular dressing changes, but she still had repeated discharge of purulence. She visited again the local hospital in September 2019 and underwent resection for the sinus of the right cervical lymph node. Her wound recovered well after surgery and she continued the previous anti-tuberculosis treatment. Half a year after this resection, however, pyogenesis took place again at the original incision at the right neck. In April 2020, the patient underwent surgery again, dissection and drainage of the cold abscess in the right neck, but there was still recurrent purulence.

Detection was performed for gene mutation for drug resistance in Mycobacterium tuberculosis, showing resistance to ethambutol, and susceptible to fluoroquinolone and the second-line injection drug. Therefore, the regimen was switched to linezolid, cycloserine, moxifloxacin hydrochloride, isoniazid propionate, and amikacin sulfate in April 2020, and linezolid was discontinued because of numbness of both lower extremities. In September 2020, she came to the hospital for re-consultancy.

Physical examination at admission: a transverse scar of a surgical incision anterior to the sternocleidomastoid muscle is observed on the right neck at 1 cm above the right supraclavicular fossa, and measures about 3.0 × 0.5 cm, with an abscess measuring about 2 × 1 cm observed at the incision, which touched soft with fluctuation but without tenderness, showing a ruptured skin with discharge of reddish exudation (Fig. 12.1a). Contrasted cervical CT scans showed multiple lymphadenectasis in bilateral neck and supraclavicular fossa, with thickening of hypodermic soft tissue at the root of the right neck, which involved with skin (Fig. 12.1b, c). Clearance of lesions in cervical tuberculosis lymphadenitis and functional cervical lymphadenectomy was performed under general anesthesia on September 15, 2020, and an anti-tuberculosis treatment was continued, consisting of cycloserine, moxifloxacin hydrochloride, protionamide, and amikacin sulfate, with a total course of half a year for amikacin sulfate. Post-operative follow-up for the patient showed good healing of the incision without recurrence (Fig. 12.1d).

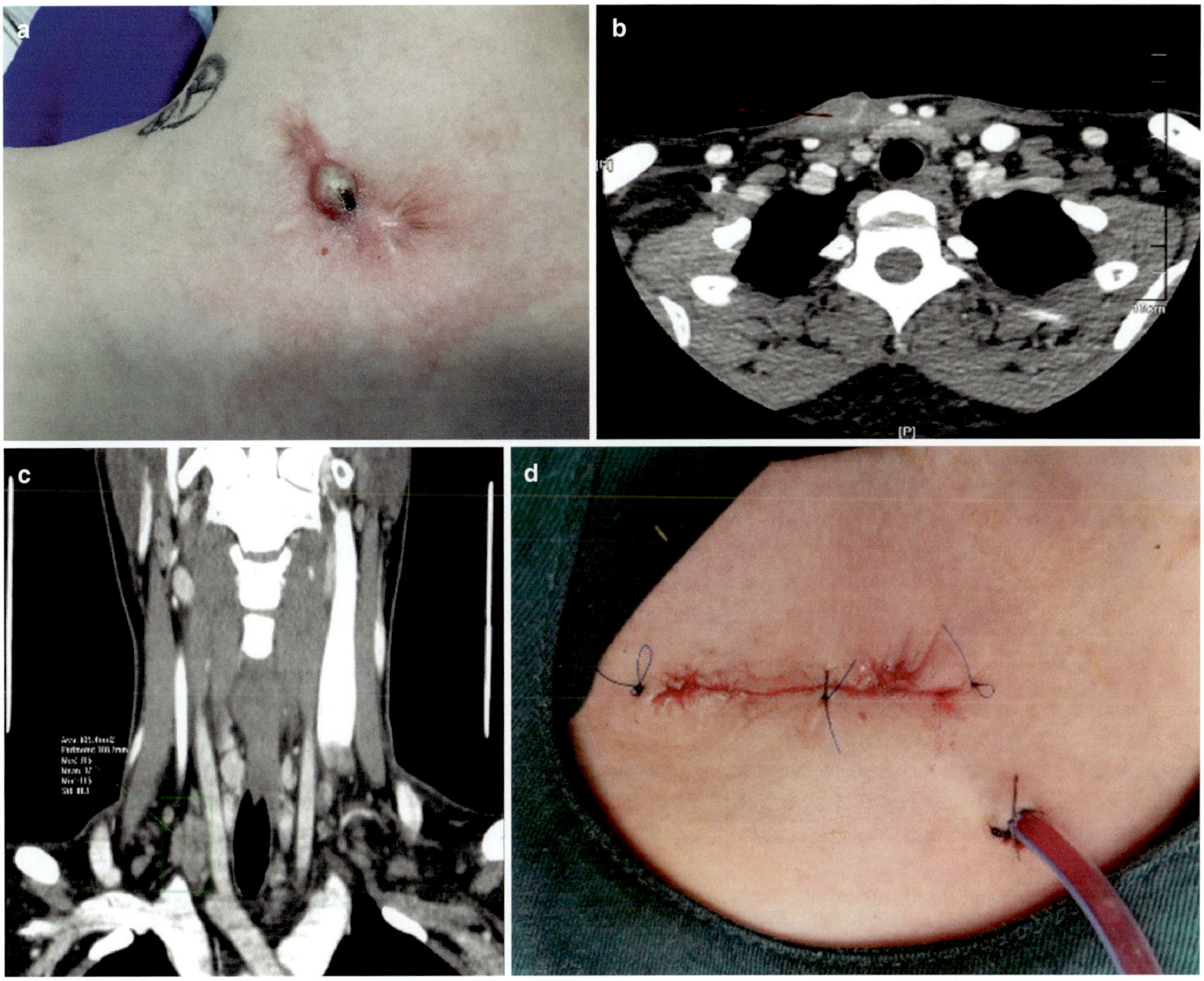

Fig. 12.1 (**a**–**d**) Gross observation and CT image findings of the abscess and ulcerative type of the right cervical drug-resistant tuberculous lymphadenitis prior and post to operation. (**a**) A transverse scar of the surgical incision anterior to the sternocleidomastoid muscle is observed on the right neck 1 cm above the supraclavicular fossa and measures about 3.0 × 0.5 cm, with an abscess at the incision with a size of about 2 × 1 cm. (**b**) Transverse view of contrasted CT scans of the abscess and ulcerative type of the right cervical drug-resistant tuberculosis lymphadenitis shows thickening of hypodermic muscles and soft tissues at the right neck root, which has heterogenous density and enhancement. Lesions extend to dermal surface with irregular adjacent skin. Punctiform calcified foci are observed in swollen lymph nodes, with moderate enhancement in contrasted scans. (**c**) The coronal view of CT scans shows a shadow of an enlarged lymph node measuring about 2.1 × 0.7 cm at the root of the right neck and located at the lateral side of common carotid artery and at the posterior medial side of internal jugular vein, with mild enhancement on contrasted scans. (**d**) The primary suture of the incision is achieved post to the clearance of tuberculosis lesions and functional regional cervical lymphadenectomy

12.3.2 Ulcerative Sinus Type of Multidrug-Resistant Cervical Tuberculous Lymphadenitis

Patient Liu, a 30-year-old female, complained swollen lymph nodes noticed at the right neck for 1 year with rupture and purulence for 3 months and referred to a specialty hospital on March 12, 2020, for in-hospital treatment. Swollen lymph nodes were found in the right neck 1 year before, but she neglected them. Pathology based on fine needle aspiration performed 7 months before in another hospital showed granulomatous inflammation; with concurrent right knee pain and the right axillary lymphadenectasis 5 months before, when she was clinically diagnosed as the right cervical tuberculosis lymphadenitis and pulmonary tuberculosis. She received HREZ quadruple anti-tuberculosis treatment, but her symptoms were not relieved. The skin ruptured with purulence 3 months before, and GeneXpert for Mycobacterium tuberculosis in purulent excretion was positive, which was shown resistant to rifampicin. The anti-tuberculosis, therefore, was switched to a regimen consisting of moxifloxacin, linezolid, clofazimine, cycloserine, ethambutol, and pyrazinamide. Results drug susceptibility test for the culture of Mycobacterium tuberculosis showed resistance to HREMfx, based on which moxifloxacin, pyrazinamide, and ethambutol were withdrawn, and beta-quinoline and isonicotinamide were added to continue the anti-tuberculosis treatment.

Physical examination: Skin rupture and scabs with purulent secretions was observed, with necrotic tuberculous lymphadenitis in the supraclavicular region of the right neck. The size of the rupture with necrosis was about 15 cm*4 cm, with a ruptured sinus of lymph node tuberculosis observable under the muscular layer (Fig. 12.2a). A swollen lymph node in a diameter of about 5 cm was touched in the right axilla, and the skin was thinned with pigmentation and fluctuation. The right knee was swollen with movement disorder.

Adjuvant examination: It was considered probably to be the right cervical tuberculous lymphadenitis, as shown by neck contrasted CT scans on March 17, 2020, which manifested the enlargement of some of the nodules with a newly formed sinus (Fig. 12.2b–d) in comparison with the previous CT finding (February 3, 2020). Chest plain CT scans on November 9, 2019, showed multiple lesions in both lungs, which seemed consistent with secondary pulmonary tuberculosis, with a slight enlargement of the right axillary lymph nodes.

Pre-operative diagnosis: (1) Secondary pulmonary tuberculosis with treatment-naïve multidrug resistance; (2) Multidrug-resistant cervical tuberculous lymphadenitis, in ulcerative sinus type; (3) Axillary tuberculosis lymphadenitis, in abscess type; and (4) tuberculosis of the right knee joint.

The patient received the right cervical functional lymphadenectomy with dissection of lymphadenitis lesions and primary suture with reconstruction for large area skin defect in cervical and thoracic infected wound plus the right axillary lymphadenectomy with dissection of lymphadenitis lesions, under general anesthesia. Caseous necrotic tissues in the swollen lymph nodes were removed intra-operatively, together with cervical subcutaneous purulent excretions, and necrotic and inflammatory skin were trimmed. It was hard to perform primary suture, as shown intra-operatively, due to the large size of the skin defect.

The primary suture was confronted with two puzzles: the reduction of the skin defect and the impossibility of cross-border suture between cervical and thoracic skin.

The former could be solved through dissociating cervical skin distally in the deep layer of platysma, and dissociating chest skin circumferentially in the deep fascia layer, while the latter through suturing the deep fascia of subcutaneous tissue at chest incision onto the deep fascia anterior to the clavicle, and suturing cervical subcutaneous tissue of platysma onto the deep fascia anterior to the clavicle, so as to reduce the skin defect. The cervical skin was shifted laterally by about 2 cm and then sutured, based on the size and location of the skin defect. Then subcutaneous tissue with a large area of skin defects was sutured onto the clavicle bone musculofascia of sternocleidomastoid muscle to reduce the suture tension, before the skin was sutured.

There was a small amount of exudation in the wound after operation, which resulted in a delayed healing. In 1 month post to surgery, a good healing was achieved (Fig. 12.2e). A regimen against multidrug resistance was continued post-operatively, which was discontinued when the medication with bedaquiline was completed, while an anti-tuberculosis treatment was continued, using isonicotinamide propionate, linezolid, clofazimine, and cycloserine.

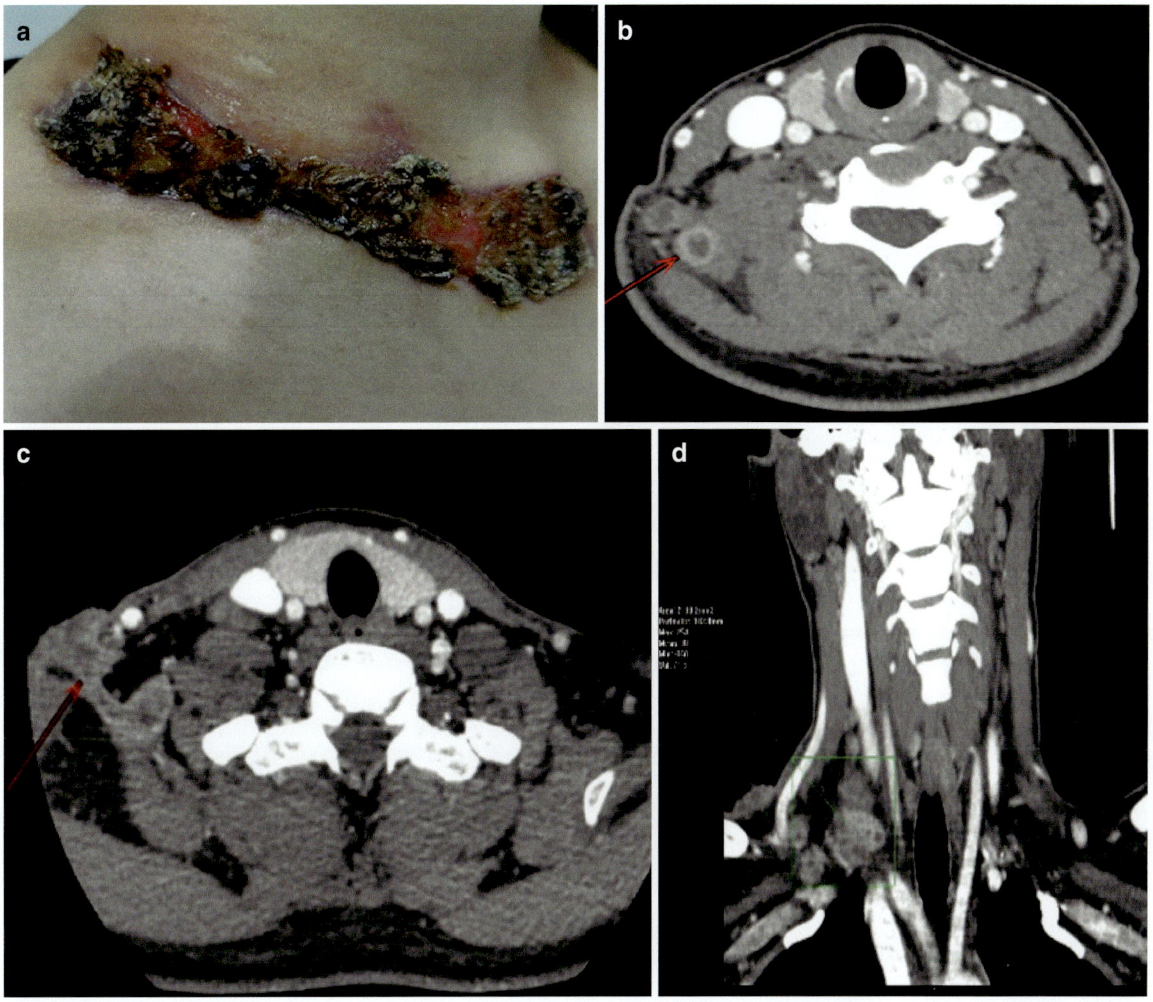

Fig. 12.2 (**a**–**e**) Gross observation and image findings of large area of ulceration caused by multidrug-resistant cervical tuberculous lymphadenitis prior and post to operation. (**a**) A skin ulcer measuring 15 mm × (3–4) cm in the right supraclavicular and subclavicular regions. (**b**) Contrasted neck CT scans show multiple subcutaneous nodular shadows in the density of soft tissues in the right neck (at the level of the fifth cervical vertebrae) and at the root of the neck, with larger ones among them measuring about 10 mm × 12 mm with turbidity in peripheral fat space. (**c**, **d**) Multiple nodular and irregular shadows in density of soft tissue are observed at the root of the neck, with larger ones among them measuring about 23 mm × 15 mm, with the center CT value of about 21HU and turbidity in peripheral fat space. The contrasted scans show the lesions in the circular enhancement, and multiple sinuses are formed inside the lesions, with the rupture of adjacent skin. Shadows of multiple small lymph nodes are observed in regions II–V of the neck. Multiple lymphadenectasis are observed in region V, and enhancement is shown in the center in the contrasted scans, with a small number of necrotic foci at the center. (**e**) The removal of tuberculosis lesions and functional regional cervical lymphadenectomy, followed by the primary suture for the wound and the good healing of the incision in 12 week post to the operation

12.3.3 Abscess Type of Cervical Multidrug-Resistant Tuberculous Lymphadenitis

Patient Li, a female aged 26 years, was admitted on August 13, 2021, with a chief complaint of masses on bilateral neck for 2 years, with the obvious enlargement for 1 month. Masses were found on her bilateral neck 2 years before, and she visited a hospital in Guangzhou City. Neck ultrasound showed multiple swollen lymph nodes on both sides of the neck, considered probably to be tuberculosis, and biopsy of the lymph node on her right neck was performed, with the pathology suggesting tuberculosis lymphadenitis, and an anti-tuberculosis treatment was launched using HREZ regimen. Her cervical masses became larger obviously and neck CT scans showed two circular low-density nodules, with one located in the right cervical region V and the other in the left

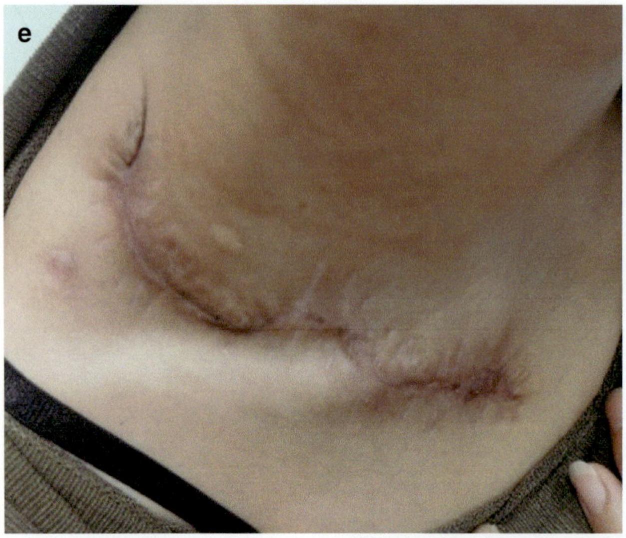

Fig. 12.2 (contiuned)

cervical region II, and both showed irregular low-density area inside and circular enhancement in the contrasted CT scans with even thickness of their wall, illustrating the size of 19 mm × 12 mm (the right) and 25 mm × 17 mm (the left), with a partition shadow within the lesion on the left (Fig. 12.3a–c). The patient underwent bilateral cervical functional lymphadenectomy plus clearance of lesions of tuberculosis abscess, and showed positiveness in GeneXpert detection for Mycobacterium tuberculosis, in segment E of gene rpoB of rifampicin susceptibility, and in genetic mutation for isoniazid resistance in the resected tissue, as well as in GeneXpertMTB nucleic acid (moderate) and in segment E of gene rpoB of rifampicin susceptibility in bronchoalveolar lavage fluid. An anti-tuberculosis treatment based on a regimen against multidrug resistance was given, consisting of bedaquiline, cycloserine, clofazimine, moxifloxacin, and linezolid. The right supraclavicular incision and the left ante-

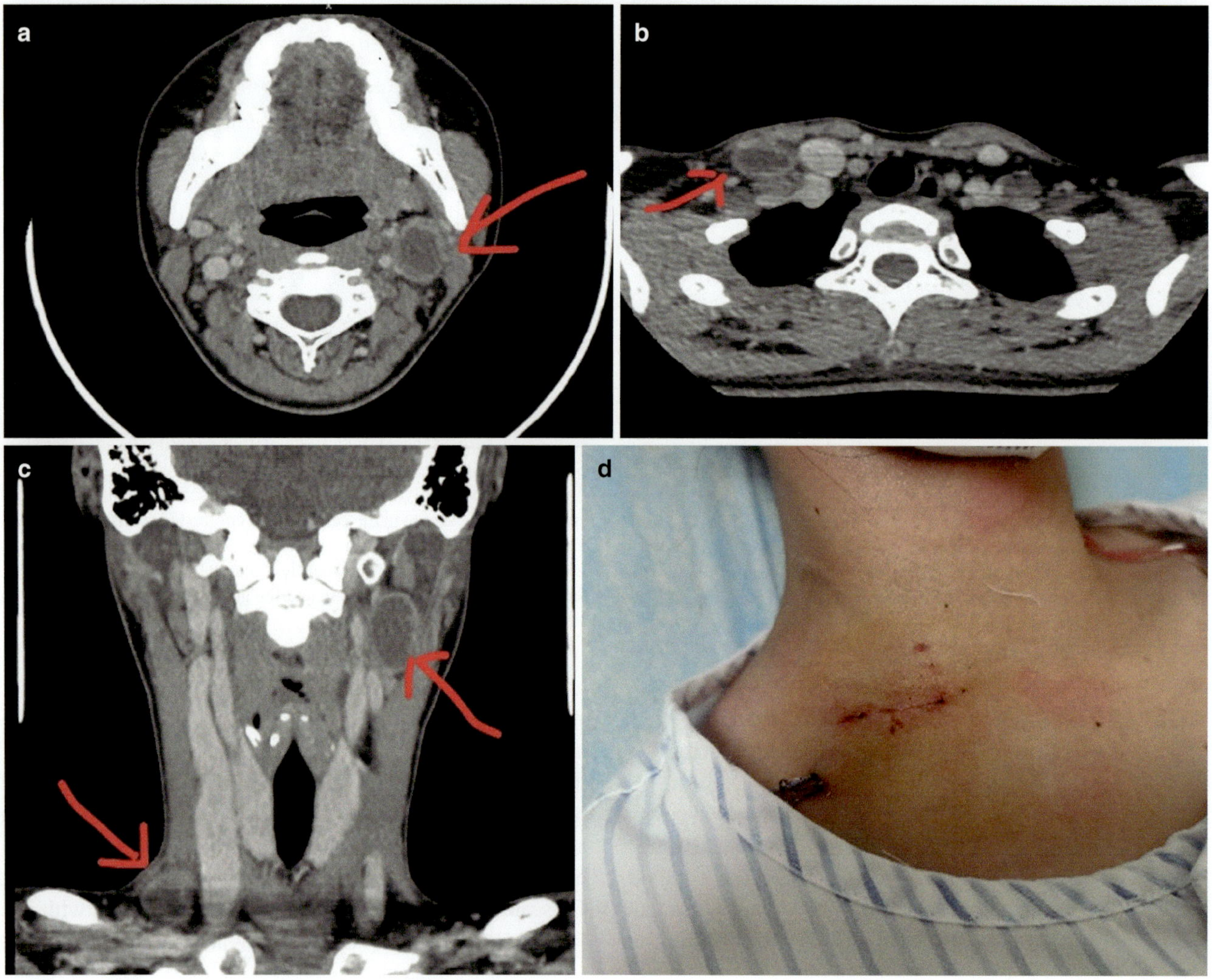

Fig. 12.3 (**a**–**e**) Abscess type of multidrug-resistant cervical tuberculous lymphadenitis. (**a**–**c**) Neck CT scans show two circular low-density nodules, with one located in the right cervical region V and the other in the left cervical region II, and both show irregular low-density area inside and circular enhancement in the contrasted CT scans with even thickness of their wall, illustrating the size of 19 mm × 12 mm (the right) and 25 mm × 17 mm (the left). (**d**, **e**) The right supraclavicular incision and the left anterior sternocleidomastoid muscle incision post to primary cosmetic suture

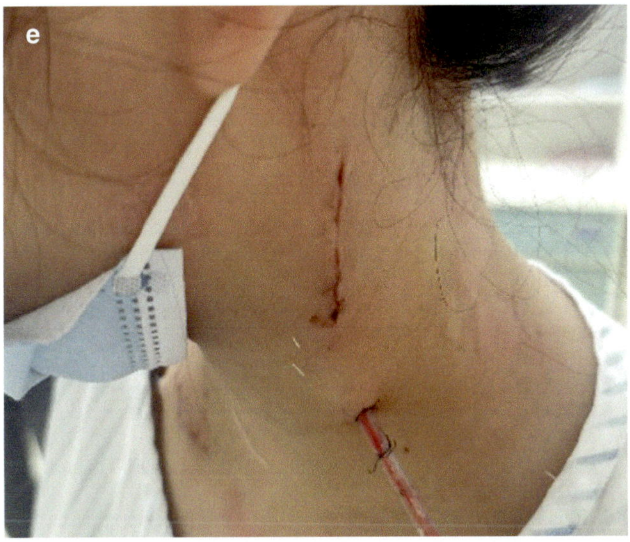

Fig. 12.3 (contiuned)

rior sternocleidomastoid muscle incision were made intra-operatively, which underwent the primary cosmetic suture (Fig. 12.3d, e).

12.3.4 Discussion

Tuberculous lymphadenitis, a common extra-pulmonary tuberculosis, is characterized in the manifestation of painless masses usually seen in the lateral cervical region, slow growth, difficulties in diagnosis in the early stage resulting usually the loss of the best opportunity for medical treatment, and the easy formation of abscess predisposing the disease to an ulcerative sinus with protracted course. Sayaka et al. [16] believed that patients with cervical lymph node tuberculosis who did not respond well to drug therapy, Surgical treatment is feasible and effective, especially for patients with monodrug-resistant or multidrug-resistant.

Ultrasonic diagnosis of cervical tuberculous lymphadenitis is the most convenient and relatively accurate examination [17, 18], based on which this disease can be categorized into four clinical types, including nodule type, infiltration type, abscess type, and ulcerative sinus type. In contrast to the former two types which are curative by anti-tuberculosis medication, the latter two types respond poorly to medication, and the surgical modality adopted previously, such as incision and drainage of abscess and clearance of lesions, have often some defects, including the impossibility of primary suture for the wound, the drain placed in the wound that necessitates prolonged dressing changes and results in protracted course of wound healing, and high recurrence rate. Post-operative recurrence rate for functional regional lymphadenectomy in treating cervical tuberculosis lymphadenitis is lower than that for clearance of tuberculosis foci [19]. Risk factors influencing post-operative responses to surgery for cervical tuberculous lymphadenitis, as considered by Zhi Wang et al. [14], include the largest diameter no less than 3 cm, infiltration of lymph nodes no less than 2 groups, and multidrug resistance.

Surgical indications for cervical tuberculous lymphadenitis include the spreading of the disease along the lymphatic tract, tuberculosis-induced infection, formation of abscess and sinus with protracted disease, the probably hard achievability of the effective concentration at local foci, single or multidrug-resistant tuberculosis, the inability of complete absorption of the therapeutic drugs by lesions, and the intolerability in patients to toxicity and side effects of drugs. Dissection of cervical tuberculosis lymphadenitis lesions plus functional cervical lymphadenectomy has an obvious advantage in reducing post-operative recurrence, and the operation necessitates general anesthesia and achieves the complete removal of the foci.

In case 1, a patient had a cervical lymphadenectasis found for 2 years and was diagnosed as cervical tuberculous lymphadenitis, based on fine needle aspiration biopsy at cervical lymph nodes, and an anti-tuberculosis treatment was launched instantly.

An abscess was formed with rupture, however, in cervical lymph nodes in 3 month post to the biopsy, and an incision with drainage was performed for the abscess followed by dressing changes. No healing was achieved for the wound for half a year, so the second operation (sinus resection) was done, followed by the continuation of anti-tuberculosis treatment. An abscess formed again at the previous incision half a year post to the second operation, and the third operation was performed, the dissection of cold abscess with drainage. Purulence was still discharged post-operatively, and a diagnosis of ethambutol resistance was confirmed based on the genetic detection for drug resistance in the pus. The anti-tuberculosis regimen, therefore, was switched to MfxLzdCsPtoAm, which was continued for 5 months but there was still protracted purulent discharge. Thereafter the fourth operation was performed, and a right cervical subcutaneous abscess was found intra-operatively, with swollen lymph nodes at the root of the right neck on the lateral side of the common carotid artery and on the posterior medial side of the internal jugular vein, which formed caseous necrosis. Therefore, dissection of cervical tuberculosis lymphadenitis plus functional cervical lymphadenectomy was performed again to remove foci thoroughly, followed by a primary suture for the wound and a nearly 18-month follow-up. The patient had discontinued the medication so far, with good healing of the wound without any recurrence.

In case 2, a patient had the right cervical lymphadenectasis found for 1 year with ulcerative purulent discharge for 3 months, showing multidrug resistance in culture of acid fast bacilli in pus, based on which the anti-tuberculosis treatment was switched to the regimen of BdqLzdCsPtoCfz. Cervical tuberculous lymphadenitis resulted in dermal rupture in the right supra- and infra- clavicular regions, measuring 15 cm × (3–4) cm. An enlarged dermal deficit crossing neck and chest was anticipated, making it hard to suture the skin between them, if lymphadenopathy and ruptured skin were removed. An innovative surgical modality, therefore, was adopted to dissociate a skin flap beneath cervical platysma and dissociate thoracic skin beneath thoracic superficial fascia, and the wound was sutured after tension reduction. The primary suture was achieved, with good healing of the wound.

In case 3, the patient had bilateral cervical lymphadenectasis for 2 years, with formation of cervical abscess post to biopsy of cervical lymph nodes, and positiveness in segment E of gene rpoB of rifampicin susceptibility and in isoniazid resistant mutation of Mycobacterium tuberculosis, suggesting the presence of multidrug-resistant tuberculosis, based on which an anti-tuberculosis treatment was given, using the regimen of BdqLzd CsMfxCfz. Thereafter resection of lesions of bilateral cervical tuberculosis lymphadenitis plus functional cervical lymphadenectomy was performed, which achieved the primary cosmetic suture, with good healing shown by follow-up for half a year.

These three cases all had the course of 1–2 year(s) before they sought medical service, which suggested the difficulties in diagnosing definitely cervical tuberculous lymphadenitis in its early stage. Biopsy of fine needle aspiration was performed for cervical lymph nodes in all these cases preoperatively, before abscess of cervical tuberculous lymphadenitis was formed or ulceration with prolonged discharge of pus occurred in these patients. Extreme caution, therefore, should be exercised in choosing this biopsy, if tuberculosis is suspected of. Meanwhile, the presence of drug resistance in cervical tuberculosis lymphadenitis in these cases also confirms the difficulties in diagnosing this disease in its early stage, and timely surgery post to formation of cervical abscess or ulcerative sinus due to progression of the disease is conducive to controlling the disease, especially the drug-resistant diseases, for which the clearance of lesions plus functional regional cervical lymphadenectomy may remove thoroughly cervical tuberculosis lesions, reduce the risk of recurrence and achieve primary or cosmetic suture of the wound. Standardized post-operative anti-tuberculosis treatment may raise cure rate and shorten the course of anti-tuberculosis treatment, which is worth clinical generalizing.

References

1. Gautam H, Agrawal SK, Verma SK, et al. Cervical tuberculous lymphadenitis: clinical profile and diagnostic modalities [J]. Int J Mycobacter. 2018;7(3):212–6.
2. Technical Guidance Group of the Fifth National Epidemiological Sampling Survey of tuberculosis, and Office of the Fifth National Epidemiological Sampling Survey of Tuberculosis. Report on the fifth national epidemiological sampling survey of tuberculosis in 2010. Chin J Antituberc. 2012;34(8):485–508.
3. Akkara SA, Singhania A, Akkara AG, et al. A study of manifestations of extrapulmonary tuberculosis in the ENT region [J]. Indian J Otolaryngol Head Neck Surg. 2014;66(1):46–50.
4. Zeng Z, Zhou J, Tao J, et al. Application of gene chip to the diagnosis of tuberculosis lymphadenitis and analysis on its drug resistance [J/OL]. Chin J Clin (Electr Ed). 2020;14(11):890–4.
5. Yu X, Fang X. The role of fine needle aspiration cytology in combination with fluorescence quantify polymerase chain reaction in diagnosing tuberculosis lymphadenitis [J]. Chin J Tuberc Resp Dis. 2009;32(1):51–4.
6. Romdhane E, Arfaoui A, Benabdessalem C, et al. Performance of GeneXpert ultra in the diagnosis of tuberculous cervical lymphadenitis in formalin fixed paraffin embedded tissues [J]. Tuberculosis. 2020;125:102–12.
7. Raja R, Sreeramulu PN, Dave P, et al. GeneXpert Assay—a cutting-edge tool for rapid tissue diagnosis of tuberculous lymphadenitis [J]. J Clin Tuberc Other Mycobact Dis. 2020;21:100204.
8. Tadesse M, Abebe G, Abdissa K, Aragaw D, Abdella K, Bekele A, et al. GeneXpert MTB/ RIF assay for the diagnosis of tuberculous lymphadenitis on concentrated fine needle aspirates in high tuberculosis burden settings. PLoS One. 2015;10(9):e0137471.
9. Yang C, Dai X, Li Q, et al. A clinical analysis on 210 cases of cervical tuberculosis lymphadenitis [J]. Chin J Antituberc. 2017;39(02):169–73.
10. Guo B, Liu W, Shao B, et al. The role of cervical lymphadenectomy in treating cervical tuberculosis lymphadenitis [J]. Chin J Tuberc Resp Dis. 1998;21(6):352–4.
11. Lee Y, Park KS, Chung SY. Cervical tuberculous lymphadenitis: CT findings [J]. J Comput Assist Tomogr. 1994;18(3):370075.
12. Jiang T, Xue L, Lian G, et al. A research on clinical application of micro-invasiveness in combination with negative pressure wound therapy to surgery of cervical tuberculosis lymphadenitis [J]. Chin J Biomed Eng. 2021;27(01):47–52.
13. Wang H, Zheng S, Huang P, et al. Retrospective analysis of functional regional cervical lymph node dissection in the treatment of abscess and ulcerated cervical lymphatic tuberculosis [J/CD]. Electr J Emerg Infect Dis. 2021;6(4):275–9.
14. Wang Z, Liu J, Li J, et al. Analysis of factors related to responses in 173 cases of cervical tuberculosis lymphadenitis to surgical treatment [J]. Chin J Antituberc. 2016;38(7):559–63.
15. Tuberculosis Branch of Chinese Medical Association. Expert consensus on the treatment of multidrug resistant and rifampicin resistant tuberculosis in China (2019 edition). Chin J Tuberc Resp Dis. 2019;42(10):733–40.
16. Sayaka O, Muneo N, Ayumi M, et al. A clinical review of 38 cases of cervical tuberculous lymphadenitis in Japan—the role of neck dissection [J]. Auris Nasus Larynx. 2017;120(3):276–7.
17. Zheng Q-t, Dong C-f, Lu P-x, et al. The comparative analysis of color doppler ultrasonography and multi-slice CT scan in the diagnosis of cervical lymph node tuberculosis[J].Electronic journal of. Emerg Infect Dis. 2017;2(3):218–22.
18. Xiuling H, Changfeng D. The application value of new ultrasound technique in cervical lymph node tuberculosis[J].Electronic journal of. Emerg Infect Dis. 2021;6(3):255–9.
19. Zhao D, Wang M, Liu J, et al. An observation of effectiveness of functional cervical lymphadenectomy in treating cervical tuberculosis lymphadenitis [J]. Chin J Difficult Complicated Cases. 2019;18(1):60–4.

Investigations on Artificial Intelligence with Its Application to Diagnosis of Drug-Resistant Pulmonary Tuberculosis

13

Qiu-ting Zheng, Lin Guo, Fleming Lure, Ying-yu Huo, Yong Zhong, Wen-feng Wu, and Stefan Jaeger

13.1 Investigations on Automatic Detection of Drug-Resistant Tuberculosis Bacteria with Its Application

Drug resistance in tuberculosis bacteria has always been one of the puzzles to be solved in the treatment of pulmonary tuberculosis. Clinically, methods for detecting drug resistance of tubercle bacillus include mainly the phenotypic drug susceptibility test and drug-resistance gene mutation detection. Among them, phenotypic methods include traditional drug susceptibility detection, microscopic observation of drug susceptibility, and the detection based on the metabolic reaction of tubercle bacillus. The traditional drug susceptibility test is the gold standard for detecting drug-resistant tubercle bacillus, but it is usually time-consuming with high cost, and the operation requires accurate bacterial quantification to match the drug concentration of the medium. The use of this method in hospitals either domestic or abroad is limited by its availability, reliability, accuracy, repeatability, and standardization, and its results have limited guidance on clinical diagnosis and treatment. Therefore, further improvement is required for it. The determination of susceptibility of Mycobacterium tuberculosis to drugs based on its characteristic microscopic observation is characterized by high sensitivity and high specificity. However, the high requirements on personnel engaged in the detection limit the generalized clinical application of the microscopic method. Metabolic reaction of Mycobacterium tuberculosis is a commonly used method for cultivating rapidly Mycobacterium tuberculosis and identifying drug susceptibility. Due to its high automation and low pollution rate, it has been approved by WHO as a recommended method for determining drug resistance in Mycobacterium tuberculosis.

The key point of diagnosis and control of tuberculosis is the fast identification of resistant genotypes of Mycobacteria tuberculosis, based on which the formulation of clinical chemotherapeutic regimens is guided. Theoretically, cultivation of Mycobacteria tuberculosis is not required by the analysis of resistant genotypes based on molecular biology technique, which has advantages including higher expedience and higher safety in comparison with traditional drug susceptibility tests and has become the main direction in research on drug resistances in Mycobacteria tuberculosis. Gene sequencing is to sequence directly drug-resistant genes of Mycobacteria tuberculosis and then compare it with the unified DNA fragments of standard drug-sensitive strain to analyze the distribution of base mutations. The methodology based on drug-resistant genes of Mycobacteria tuberculosis both detects and predicts its drug resistance. Now achievements have been made in artificial intelligence (AI) technology applied to automatic detection of drug-resistant Mycobacteria tuberculosis, e.g., a research by California University suggested the feasibility of using machine learning to identify and predict genes making pathogenic bacteria generate antibiotic resistance [1]. In this research, a detection on Mycobacteria tuberculosis was performed, and antibiotics resistance genes, including 33 known ones and 24 new ones, were identified. The knowledge about which genes are capa-

Q.-t.Zheng (✉)
Department of Medical Imaging, Shenzhen Center for Chronic Disease Control, Shenzhen, Guangdong, China

L. Guo · F. Lure
Shenzhen Zhiying Medical Co., Ltd., Shenzhen, Guangdong, China

Y.-y. Huo · Y. Zhong
School of Electronic Information Engineering, Foshan University, Foshan, Guangdong, China

W.-f. Wu
Jiangxi JF Healthcare Limited Company, Nanchang, Jiangxi, China

S. Jaeger
National Institutes of Health/National Library of Medicine, Bethesda, MD, USA

P.-x. Lu et al. (eds.), *Diagnostic Imaging of Drug Resistant Pulmonary Tuberculosis*, https://doi.org/10.1007/978-981-99-8339-1_13

ble of conferring antibiotic resistance may change therapeutic modalities for contagious diseases in the future. The team engaged in this research, therefore, used a large number of genome sequences and corresponding phenotypes for training, so as to predict whether a group of genes may result in antibiotic resistance. Moreover, this team analyzed further the results predicted based on this algorithm and confirmed the allelic combinations capable of bestowing on strains the antibiotic resistances, thereby exploiting potential mechanism of the evolution of antibiotic resistance through combining genomic model of metabolic network and its machine-learning algorithms. Using the support vector machine (SVM) and artificial neural networks, Salma Jamal et al. [2] established a gene mutation model capable of predicting gene rpoB, inhA, katG, pncA, gyrA, and gyrB in patients with drug-resistant tuberculosis, which was a disaggregated model with a mean accuracy of 85% for all genes detected. Moreover, this research also performed molecular docking and molecular dynamics simulation to investigate the influence of genetic mutations on protein conformation and finally confirmed the observed phenotypes.

13.2 Research Related to Artificial Intelligence in Imaging Diagnosis of Pulmonary Tuberculosis and Their Achievements

The present speed of physician training and their working efficiency around the world cannot catch up with the fast-increasing requirements on imaging data, and the huge working pressure imposed by imaging diagnosis and the lack of clinical experience among doctors engaged in imaging diagnosis in basic level hospitals may easily lead to misdiagnosis and/or missed diagnosis. Artificial intelligence, however, depends upon strong ability in image recognition and profound studying, to solve well puzzles and problems existing in manual processing of big data in medical imaging. Now the application of artificial intelligence to pulmonary medical imaging has become more generalized, and automatic diagnosis has been realized by many studies targeting at diseases such as pulmonary nodules, pulmonary malignancies, and drug-sensitive pulmonary tuberculosis [3, 4]. Some authors, moreover, realized the quantitative analysis on lesions such as pulmonary tumors and corona virus disease 2019 (COVID-19) based on images of CT scans, providing evidences for the diagnosis established by physicians [5]. A certain progress has been made particularly in computer aided diagnostic (CAD) System based on artificial intelligence for pulmonary TB. It has been approved by some large clinical trials [6, 7] that the automatic chest X-ray pulmonary TB detection system utilizing artificial intelligence and machine learning may improve the accuracy of screening diagnosis of pulmonary tuberculosis, and digital image screening system for pulmonary tuberculosis can reduce the time consumed for imaging doctors reviewing images, thereby improving greatly the work efficiency and the accuracy of their diagnosis of pulmonary tuberculosis, which is of great importance in the control of tuberculosis.

Now mature chest X-ray screening systems for pulmonary tuberculosis based on artificial intelligence are available in China and abroad, and those developed by research institutions represented by Delft Imaging Systems (Delft) Netherlands [8–10] and National Library of Medicine (NLM) of National Institute of Health (NIH), USA, have been applied preliminarily to clinical practice with good results achieved [11–13]. Let us take chest X-ray screening system for pulmonary tuberculosis based on artificial intelligence by NLM as an instance. The main structure of the system is a group of modules connectable with the chest imaging system, which are capable of automatically detecting pulmonary regions to extract features of pulmonary images at first, and then using a new automatic algorithm for detecting pulmonary boundaries and making a dichotomous decision to categorize the images into the normal and abnormal ones, with a precision attainable up to 92–95%. Utilizing features such as multi-resolution image texture and edge curvature, the system achieves its categorization via a neural network classifier based on artificial intelligence, and the classifier may achieve an overall precision up to 99.3% and a false positive rate lower than 7%. Given its reliable performance, the chest X-ray automatic detection system for tuberculosis can be used as a mass screening and diagnosis method to categorize patients into "tuberculosis suspected," "slight abnormality," or "recommended for re-examination."

Analytical cloud platforms for pulmonary TB chest X-ray applied to big data of medical imaging have been designed and developed in China, and the installation or cloud interface docking has been completed in nearly 100 hospitals in China, covering Beijing City, Shanghai City, Guangdong Province, Qinghai Province, Shandong Province, Xinjiang Uygur Autonomous Region, Inner Mongolia Autonomous Region, etc., which have significantly improved the detection rate of tuberculosis [2, 14–16] (Fig. 13.1).

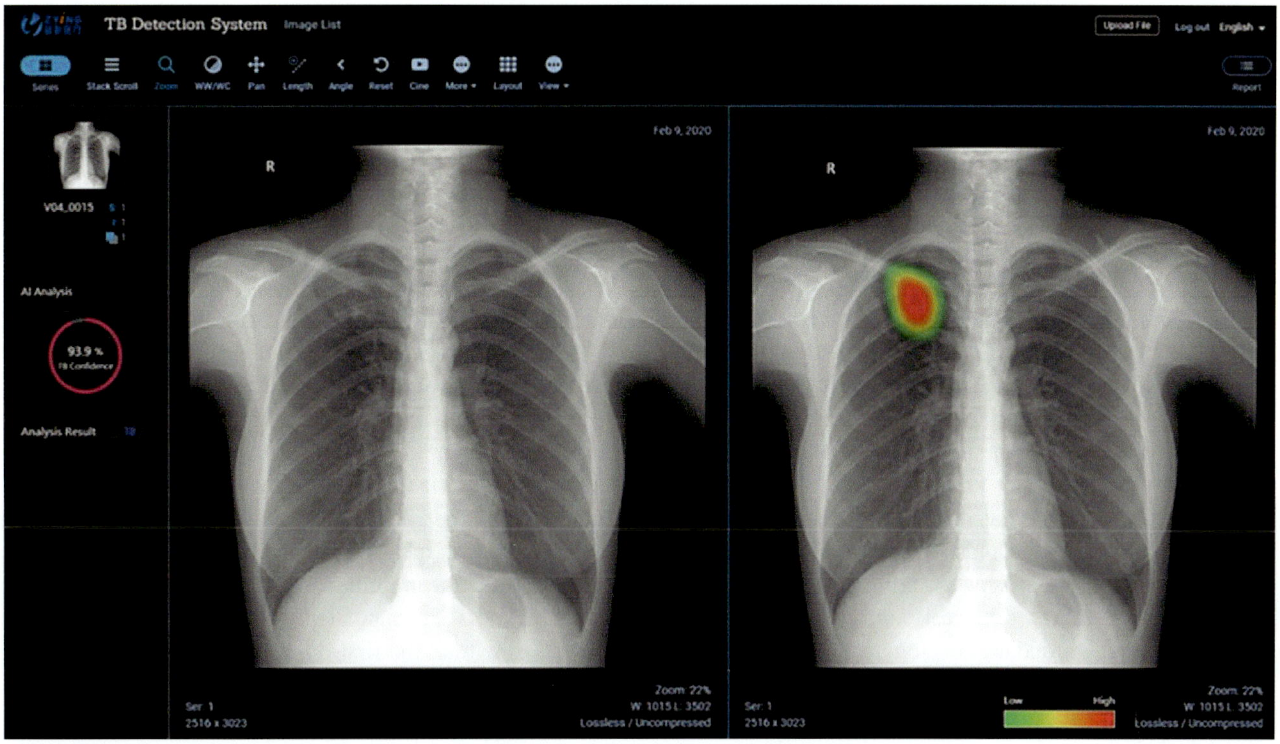

Fig. 13.1 Graphic user interface of the AI-based detection system for pulmonary abnormalities

13.3 Exploitation on Artificial Intelligence in Drug-Resistant Pulmonary Tuberculosis

Though the great progress has been made in image diagnosis of pulmonary TB based on artificial intelligence, most of AI technologies in the domain of medical imaging in China remain in the stage of lesion detection, the typing of image signs and proposal of tentative diagnosis, while the further categorization of pulmonary TB is still in the exploration stage. Despite the availability of the algorithm designed by Blavatnik Institute of Harvard Medical College and capable of detecting resistances to commonly used anti-tuberculosis drugs prior to treatment and the availability of prediction of resistance/susceptibility mutations in Mycobacteria tuberculosis based on artificial intelligence and machine learning, there is still a great gap to realize a real clinical application of artificial intelligence to the diagnosis of drug-resistant tuberculosis.

Accurate clinical categorization and typing of drug-resistant pulmonary tuberculosis facilitate the guidance of clinical diagnosis, treatment, and evaluation of efficacy. Clinically, drug resistance can be categorized into mono-, poly-, multiple-, extensive-, and rifampicin-resistance, based on the number and the categorization of drugs to which a strain is shown resistant in a patient. Among them, rifampicin-resistant, multi-resistant, and extensive-resistant pulmonary tuberculosis are the three main types, having, respectively, their own imaging features shown by chest X-ray and CT scans, manifesting mainly multiple thick-walled intrapulmonary cavities, nodules of different sizes, patchy consolidations and fibrous strips, and some patients show hilar or mediastinal lymphadenectasis and pleural effusion, extensive involvement by lesions, protracted course and possible occurrence of the destroyed lung. Imaging features of drug-resistant pulmonary TB have laid a theoretical foundation for the artificial intelligence system applied to automatic determination of drug-resistant/sensitive pulmonary tuberculosis. Stefan Jaeger et al. [17] developed an artificial intelligence model, which was based on chest X-ray and capable of distinguishing between drug-resistant and drug-sensitive pulmonary tuberculosis, and its results showed that the area under the ROC curve (AUC) was up to 66%, indicating that chest X-ray examination included information about the possibility of the infection with drug-resistant pulmonary tuberculosis. However, due to less information provided by chest X-ray and the smaller sample size included in the research, a bigger data set is required by a further research to increase the accuracy in automatically detecting drug-resistant pulmonary tuberculosis. Gao et al. [18] used artificial intelligence technology based on CT images to predict drug-resistant pulmonary tuberculosis from patients with drug-sensitive pulmonary TB, and the results showed that the best model was a deep convolution neural network based on support vector classifier (SVC), which could achieve a classification accuracy up to 91.11%.

Shenzhen Center for Chronic Disease Control and Shenzhen Zhiying Medical Imaging Co., Ltd. in China applied AI technology to the exploration of the image findings of drug-resistant pulmonary tuberculosis and developed an AI discrimination system for drug-resistant/sensitive pulmonary tuberculosis patients. This system, endowed with a highly complicated pattern recognition, can assist physicians to make accurate determination of drug-resistant pulmonary tuberculosis in early stage and will play a vital role in formulating and modifying clinical treatment plans, observing and evaluating responses, and predicting the prognosis (Figs. 13.2 and 13.3).

Fully automatic artificial intelligence analysis for drug-resistant pulmonary tuberculosis based on characteristics of chest CT imaging is used by the artificial intelligence discrimination system for drug-resistant/sensitive pulmonary tuberculosis patients, and the development is launched on the basis that the developed auxiliary CT detection software for pulmonary tuberculosis is capable of detecting pulmonary tuberculosis lesions. The investigational methods are as follows: (1) segmentation of cavity wall: multi-person parallel marking is performed by three clinical imaging doctors using the online scientific research platform provided by Shenzhen Zhiying Medical Imaging Co., Ltd. to label the cavity's outer wall displayed by chest CT scans as training data. The labeled data sets are divided into a training set, a verification set, and a test set, and a gradient descending method is used to train the target detection network based on convolution (Fig. 13.4), in order to obtain a network model that segments automatically the outer wall of the cavity. The model is used to automatically segment the outer wall of the cavity for the residue data in the experiment. In the limited cavity lesions, the adaptive threshold segmentation is used to extract the inner wall of the cavity, which clearly shows the segmented cavity wall (Fig. 13.5). (2) Extraction of iconographic characteristics of cavity wall: Considering the irregular shape of the cavity, the minimum bounding rectangle is used to obtain the long and short diameters (Fig. 13.6). In respect of the measurement of the thickness of the cavity wall, an outward radiation from the geometric center of the inner wall of the cavity is used to measure the thickness in various angles (Fig. 13.7), and the minimum, maximum, and average values of the thickness are calculated. Image processing operators are used to extract the first-order properties such as energy and average density, calculate the second-order properties such as area and Euclidean distance, and extract the high-order properties such as gray scale co-occurrence matrix and gray scale dependency matrix. (3) Training with classification model: classifiers such as decision tree, support vector machine, and random forests are used to classify features and predict the possibility of drug resistance (Fig. 13.8).

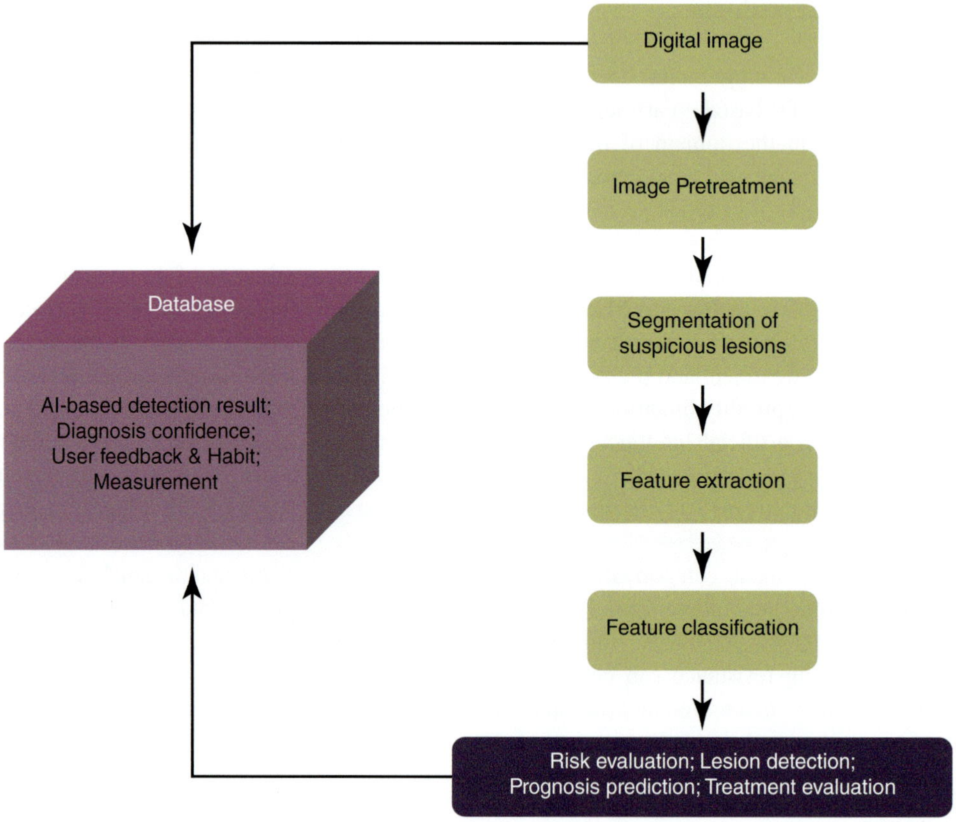

Fig. 13.2 The overall scheme for AI-based automatic detection of drug-resistant tuberculosis

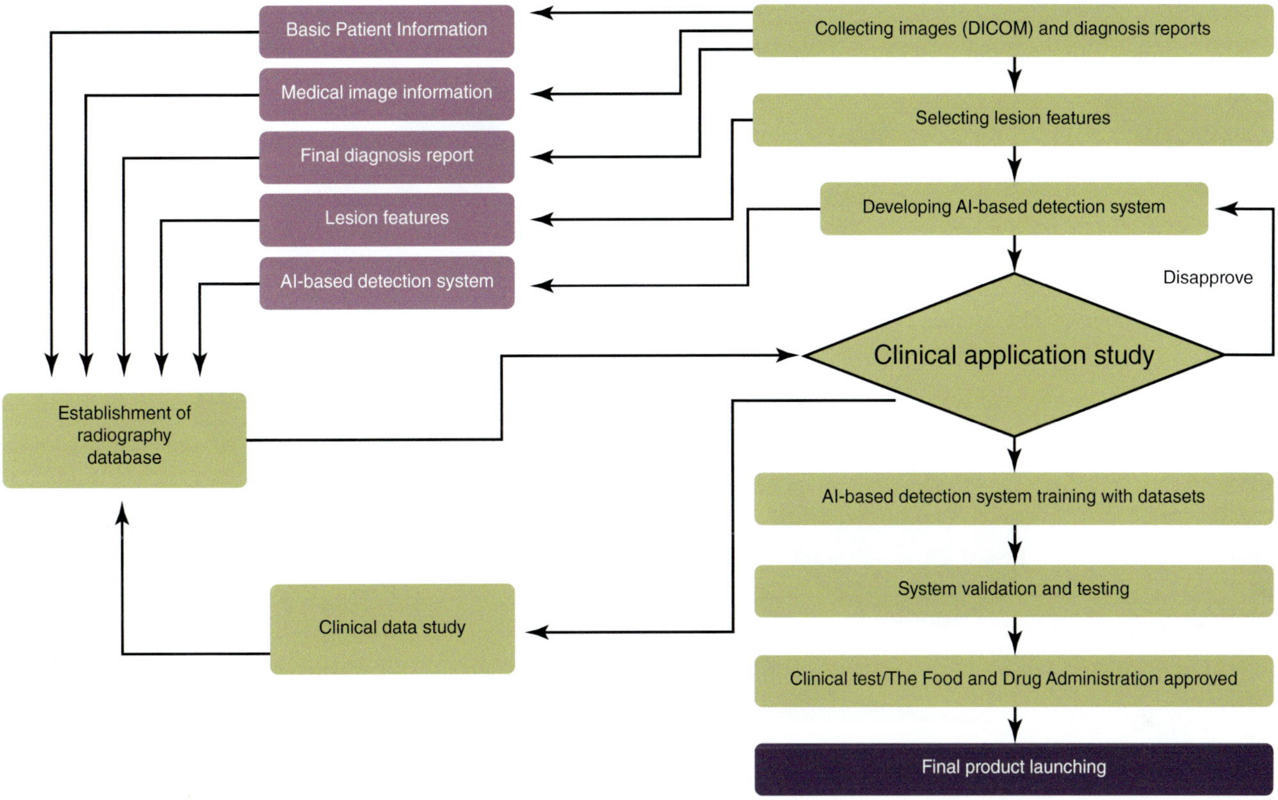

Fig. 13.3 The development process and technical roadmap of AI-based detection system for drug-resistant tuberculosis

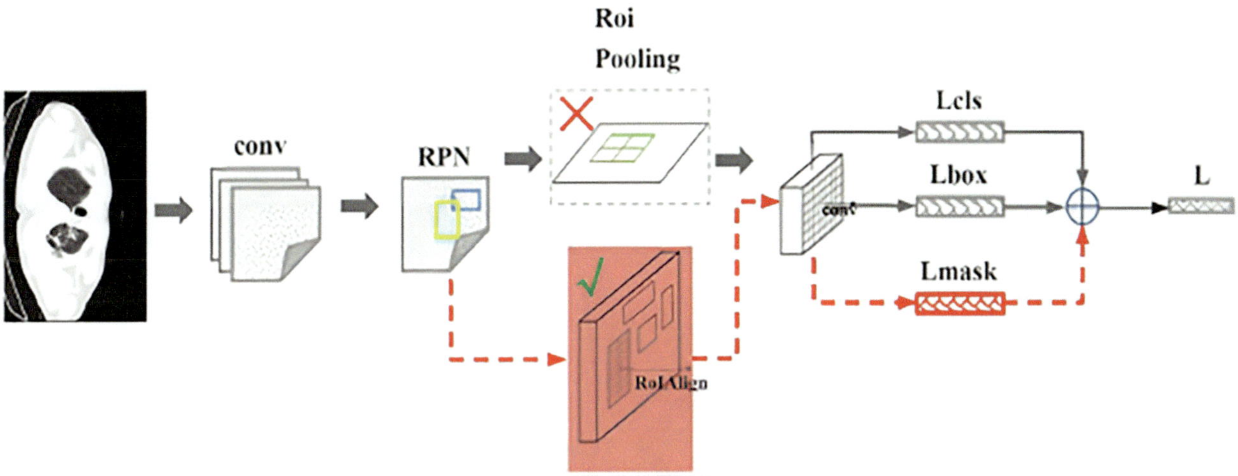

Fig. 13.4 Architecture of the target detection network Mask RCNN

We believe that the artificial intelligence algorithm of diagnostic software will be improved in the future through the joint efforts of medical experts and computer software/hardware research experts, so as to minimize the false positive rate and improve the detection sensitivity. Meanwhile, we also look forward to strengthening the training of both biomedical engineering personnel and imaging physicians, so as to make doctors totally understand the functions and properties of the artificial intelligence diagnosis software system, establish cooperation and mutual trust with the system, and apply it correctly.

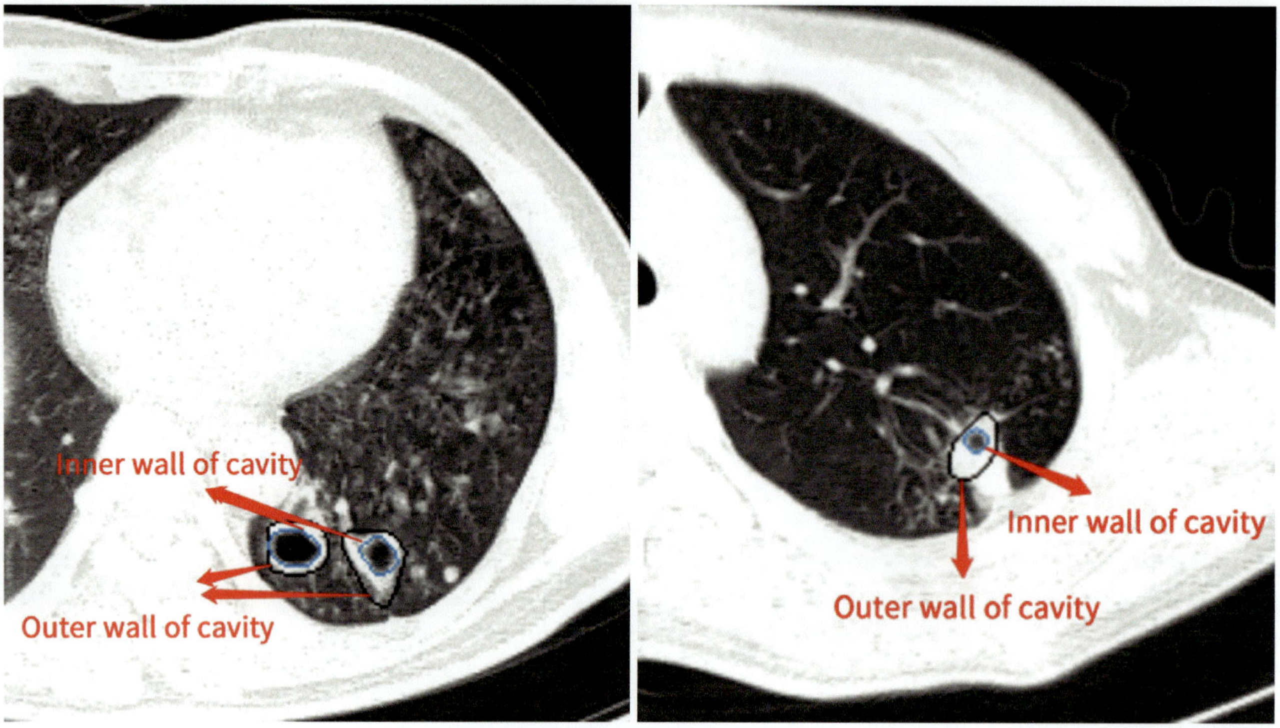

Fig. 13.5 Two examples of automatically segmented cavities by using self-adaptive threshold method: Male, 48 years old, drug-resistant tuberculosis (left); Female, 25 years old, drug-sensitive tuberculosis (right). Black circles represent the outer wall of cavity, and blue circles represent the inner wall of cavity

Fig. 13.6 The minimum bounding rectangle

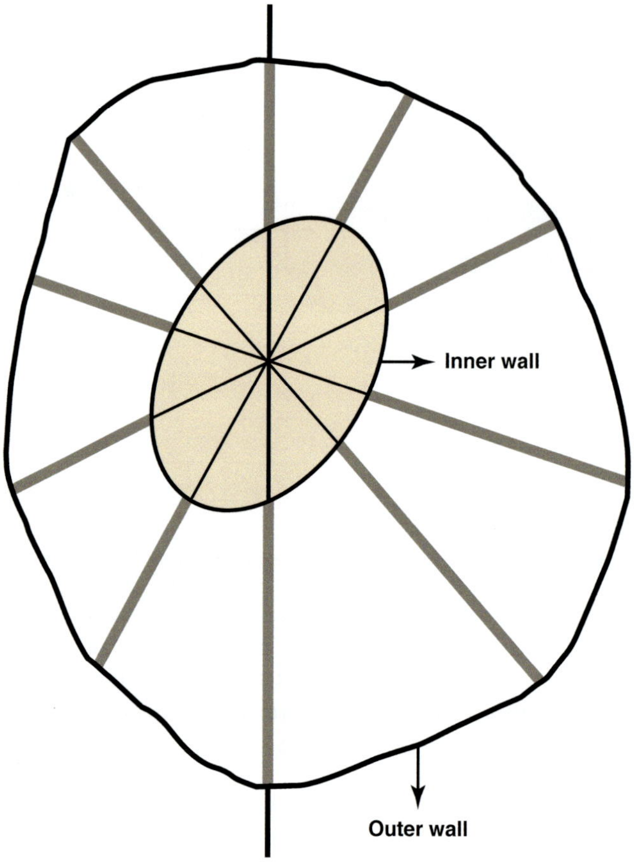

Fig. 13.7 The cavity wall thickness at various angles

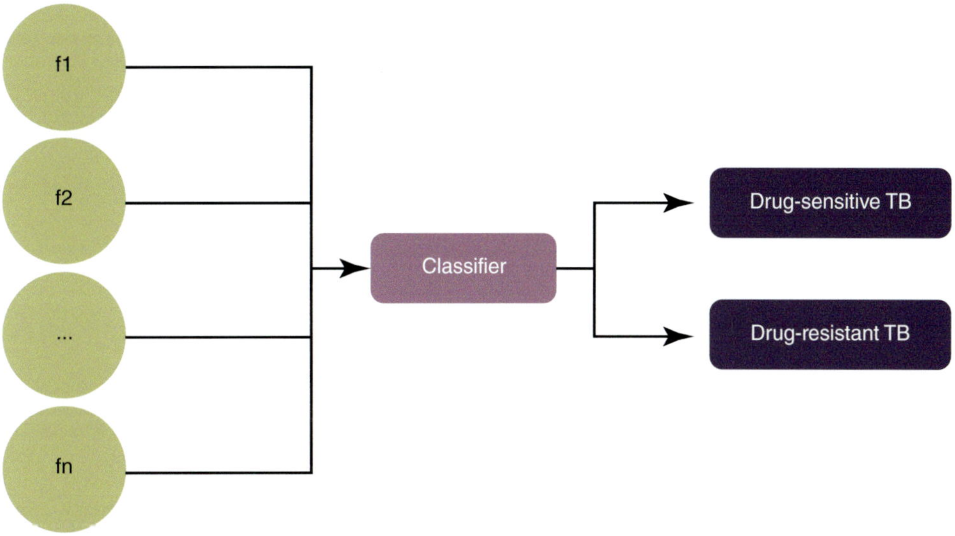

Fig. 13.8 Feature classifier for distinguishing drug-sensitive and drug-resistant tuberculosis

References

1. Chen ML, Doddi A, Royer J, et al. Beyond multidrug resistance: leveraging rare variants with machine and statistical learning models in mycobacterium tuberculosis resistance prediction. EBioMedicine. 2019;43:356–69.
2. Jamal S, Khubaib M, Gangwar R, et al. Artificial intelligence and machine learning based prediction of resistant and susceptible mutations in mycobacterium tuberculosis. Sci Rep. 2020;10(1):5487.
3. Ardila D, Kiraly AP, Bharadwaj S, et al. End-to-end lung cancer screening with three-dimensional deep learning on low-dose chest computed tomography [J]. Nat Med. 2019;25(5):1.
4. Lure FYM, Jaeger S, Antani S. Automated systems for microscopic and radiographic tuberculosis screening [J]. Electr J Emerg Infect Dis. 2017;2(1):5.
5. Zhang K, Liu XH, Shen J, et al. Clinically applicable AI system for accurate diagnosis, quantitative measurements, and prognosis of COVID-19 pneumonia using computed tomography [J]. Cell. 2020;181(5):1423–33.
6. Zhou W, Cheng G, Zhang Z, et al. Deep learning-based pulmonary tuberculosis automated detection on chest radiography: large scale independent testing [J]. Quant Imaging Med Surg. 2022;12(4):2344–55.
7. Fehr J, Konigorski S, Olivier S, et al. Computer-aided interpretation of chest radiography reveals the spectrum of tuberculosis in rural South Africa [J]. NPJ Digit Med. 2021;4(1):106–15.
8. Maduskar P, Muyoyeta M, Ayles H, et al. Detection of tuberculosis using digital chest radiography: automated reading vs. interpretation by clinical officers [J]. Int J Tuberc Lung Dis. 2013;17(12):1613–20.
9. Hogeweg L, Sanchez C, Maduskar P, et al. Automatic detection of tuberculosis in chest radiographs using a combination of textural, focal, and shape abnormality analysis [J]. IEEE Trans Med Imaging. 2015;34(12):2429.
10. Muyoyeta M, Maduskar P, Moyo M, et al. The sensitivity and specificity of using a computer aided diagnosis program for automatically scoring chest X-rays of presumptive TB patients compared with Xpert MTB/RIF in Lusaka Zambia [J]. PloS One. 2014;9(4):e93757.
11. Folio L, Sigelman J, Wang Y, et al. Automatic identification and classification of tuberculosis findings on chest radiographs for global surveillance programs, annual meeting of the American Roentgen Ray Society (ARRS) [J]. J Med Imaging Radiat Oncol. 1974;18(2):174.
12. Jaeger S, Karargyris A, Candemir S, et al. Automatic tuberculosis screening using chest radiographs [J]. IEEE Trans Med Imaging. 2014;33(2):233–45.
13. Karargyris A, Folio L, Siegelman J, et al. Comparing the performance of man and machine for TB screening in chest radiographs [J]. NIH Intramural Res Festival. 2013;12(6):6–8.
14. Yan M-y, Chen G-m, Lai C, et al. Clinical value of artificial intelligence in detecting and analyzing lesions in patients with pulmonary tuberculosis [J]. Electr J Emerg Infect Dis. 2018;3(4):214–7.
15. Nijiati M, Abudukaiyoumu A, Damaola M, et al. Application of artificial intelligence for tuberculosis screening in primary hospital [J/CD]. Electr J Emerg Infect Dis. 2021;6(2):137–41.
16. Xu J, Wang X, Xia L, et al. Application research of remote image aided diagnosis of pulmonary tuberculosis based on artificial intelligence [J]. China Digit Med. 2021;16(8):98–100.
17. Jaeger S, Juarez-Espinosa OH, Candemir S, et al. Detecting drug-resistant tuberculosis in chest radiographs [J]. Int J Comput Assist Radiol Surg. 2018;13(12):1915.
18. Gao XW, Qian Y. Prediction of multidrug-resistant TB from CT pulmonary images based on deep learning techniques. Mol Pharm. 2018;15(10):4326–35.

Differential Diagnosis of Drug-Resistant Pulmonary Tuberculosis

14

Yu-feng Xu, Chuan-jun Xu, Ru-ming Xie, Yan Lv, Wei He, Feng-li Jiang, Hui Zhang, Wei Ma, Guan-qiao Jin, and Pu-Xuan Lu

14.1 Differential Diagnosis of Non-tuberculous Mycobacteria (NTM)[1]

Chuan-jun Xu and Feng-li Jiang

Tuberculosis is a respiratory infectious disease caused by infection of Mycobacterium tuberculosis. The emergence of drug-resistant pulmonary tuberculosis (DR-TB), bringing new challenges to the whole world, is one of the greatest barriers for human beings to conquer tuberculosis and has become a major public health problem endangering human health. Non-tuberculous mycobacteria (NTM), referring to mycobacteria other than Mycobacterium tuberculosis complex and Mycobacterium leprae, invades mainly the lungs and has certain similarities with DR-TB concerning clinical and imaging manifestations, despite their particular traits making them distinguishable to each other [1–9]. Imaging examination, especially chest CT scans expediting and facilitating diagnosis, is of great significance for the diagnosis of both diseases and capable of providing certain evidences for early clinical diagnosis and treatment prior to the confirmation of diagnosis based on the sputum culture results.

14.1.1 Common Points Between Non-Tuberculous Mycobacteria (NTM) and Mycobacteria Tuberculosis

Non-tuberculous Mycobacterium and Mycobacterium tuberculosis share a commonality in cell composition and antigen. Moreover, multiple commonalities also exist in clinical symptoms and pathologies of pulmonary infections that they both induce, with lots of similar features in chest image findings for both, which show usually extensive pulmonary lesions involving multiple lobes [7] with coexistence of multiple lesions.

Lesions induced by Mycobacterium tuberculosis manifest often as inflammatory exudation. In case of progression of lesions, the cavity formed after liquefaction of the central caseous necrotic substance and its discharging through the bronchi leads to the coexistence of the cavity and the consolidation, both of which are tissues lacking blood supply and not easily accessible to antituberculosis drugs, making a large number of latent Mycobacterium tuberculosis survive and resulting in the emergence of multi-drug resistant Mycobacterium tuberculosis. The liquefied necrotic substance can spread to other pulmonary lobes and segments due to causative factors such as coughing and gravity, thereby resulting in bilateral, multi-segmental, and multi-lobar distri-

[1]Chuan-jun Xu is the corresponding author for the Sect. 14.1.

Y.-f. Xu (✉)
Department of Radiology, Peking University First Hospital, Beijing, China

C.-j. Xu
Department of Radiology, The Second Hospital of Nanjing, Nanjing University of Chinese Medicine, Nanjing, China

R.-m. Xie
Department of Radiology, Beijing Ditan Hospital, Capital Medical University, Beijing, China

Y. Lv · W. He
Department of Medical Imaging, Beijing Chest Hospital, Capital Medical University, Beijing, China

F.-l. Jiang
Department of Radiology, Zhongda Hospital, Medical School, Southeast University, Nanjing, China

H. Zhang
Department of Radiology, The Third People's Hospital of Shenzhen, Shenzhen, Guangdong, China

W. Ma
Department of Radiology, The Third People's Hospital of Longgang, Shenzhen, Guangdong, China

G.-q. Jin
The Affiliated Cancer Hospital of Guangxi Medical University, Guangxi, China

P.-X. Lu
Diagnostic Imaging, Shenzhen Center for Chronic Disease Control, Shenzhen, China

P.-x. Lu et al. (eds.), *Diagnostic Imaging of Drug Resistant Pulmonary Tuberculosis*,
https://doi.org/10.1007/978-981-99-8339-1_14

bution of lesions, or even the whole lung distribution. However, the extensive distribution of lesions induced by non-tuberculous mycobacteria is related possibly to protracted course of NTM pulmonary diseases and concurrent underlying pulmonary diseases. Image findings of infections caused by mycobacteria tuberculosis or non-tuberculous mycobacteria manifest often as coexistence of a variety of changes including cavities, bronchiectasis, nodules, and infiltrations [6, 9].

14.1.2 Differences Between Non-tuberculous Mycobacteria and Mycobacteria Tuberculosis

There is no obvious difference between non-tuberculous mycobacteria and mycobacteria tuberculosis concerning either clinical symptoms including cough, hemoptysis, fever, night sweat, etc., or gender [4, 5]. However, NTM pulmonary lesions are often secondary to underlying diseases, and one of the risk factors of NTM pulmonary diseases is the destructed biological structure of pulmonary tissues. Moreover, the course is shorter in multi-drug resistant pulmonary tuberculosis than in NTM, due to virulence being weaker in non-tuberculous mycobacteria than in mycobacteria tuberculosis. Also, NTM has different image findings of chest CT scans comparison with DR-TB.

14.1.2.1 NTM Pulmonary Disease Is More Prone to Thin-Walled Cavities

NTM infection will first induce the formation of granuloma in the terminal bronchioles and then spread through the bronchi while destroying muscular layers of the air tract, which will be narrowed or even blocked, resulting in increased pressure within the bronchial lumen, followed by emergence of thin-walled cavities [1] (Fig. 14.1).

Patients with pulmonary tuberculosis who experience liquefaction and discharge of caseous necrotic substances are more likely to develop thick-walled cavities, and most of which are fibrotic in patients with drug-resistant TB due to prolonged existence of these cavities. Consolidations are commonly observed along the periphery of thick-walled cavities in MDR-TB, in contrast to satellite foci often found surrounding thin-walled cavities in NTM lung disease [10]. Sometimes it is difficult to distinguish them based on the thickness of the cavities, and 33% of NTM patients manifest thin-walled cavities, which may be related to the thinning process of the cavity wall at a certain stage during the progression of the disease [11].

14.1.2.2 NTM Pulmonary Disease Is More Prone to Bronchiectasis

Pulmonary infection induced by NTM manifests mainly as pulmonary granulomatous lesions, but rarely as caseous necrosis. The former involves easily bronchioles and large airways, thereby causing bronchiectasis [2], which is commonly observed in the left lingual segment and the right middle lobe [5] (Fig. 14.2). Bronchiectasis has been pointed out by some studies to be a susceptible factor to NTM infection [8]. There is no significant difference in terms of bronchiectasis and thickening of bronchiole wall between these two diseases, except that MDR-TB more frequently involves the upper lobes, while NTM more frequently involves middle and lower lobes [10].

14.1.2.3 NTM Pulmonary Disease Manifests Usually as Centrilobular Nodules

Centrilobular nodules may be formed by granulomas or necrotic substances scattered in bronchial lumen [1]. Image findings in CT scans show clustered micronodules, most of which are less than 5 mm, with parenchyma infiltration rarely observed around the bronchus and bronchioles (Fig. 14.3). Nodules and bronchiectasis are typical image findings of NTM [5]. Due to liquefaction and discharging of caseous necrotic tissues, drug-resistant pulmonary tuberculosis manifests as disseminations along bronchial periphery and in other pulmonary fields and seems more prone to the emergence of acinar nodules.

14.1.2.4 Drug-Resistant Tuberculosis Is More Likely to Involve Adjacent Pleura

Mycobacterium tuberculosis may invade the visceral pleura of patients and cause pleurisy in the early stage, which subsequently results in pleural thickening and pleural effusion. Due to its protracted course, drug-resistant pulmonary tuberculosis is more prone to pleural adhesion and calcification. Pleural effusion occurs in 4.3% of NTM patients and in 21% of MDR-TB patients [5].

14.1.2.5 Drug-Resistant Pulmonary Tuberculosis Is More Destructive to Lung Tissue

The strains inducing drug-resistant pulmonary tuberculosis have stronger pathogenicity and cause significant damage to pulmonary tissues, especially in multi-drug resistant pulmonary tuberculosis, which is characterized in longer course, emergence of new lesions in the background of previous local lesion without amelioration, unceasing progression of lesions with enlargement of their scope, and final emergence of pulmonary consolidation, destructive pneumonophthisis, atelectasis and reduction of pulmonary volume [5]. In NTM

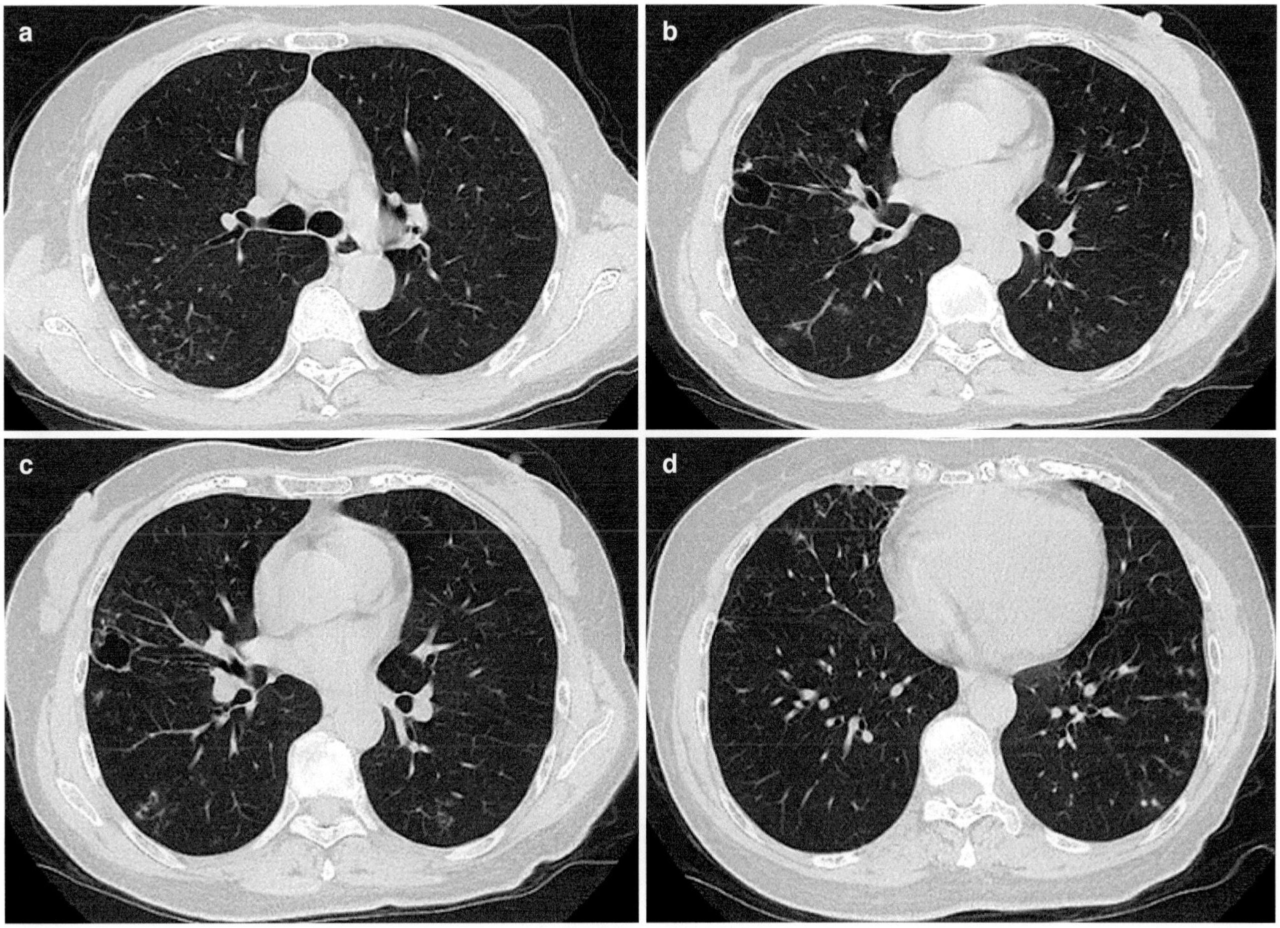

Fig. 14.1 (**a**–**d**) A 65-year-old female with NTM pulmonary disease. (**a**) Multiple tree-in-bud signs are observed in the upper and middle lobes of the right lung; (**b**) mild bronchiectasis is seen in the right upper lobe, and a thin-walled cavity can be seen in the right middle lobe; (**c**, **d**) mild bronchiectasis is observed in the right middle lobe with multiple tree-in-bud signs around the bronchiectasis, and scattered subpleural nodular shadows are present in the left lower lobe

lung diseases, however, pulmonary consolidations and atelectasis occur only when the large air tracts are involved, and this risk is lower [12].

14.1.2.6 Main Predisposing Sites for NTM Lung Diseases are the Right Middle Lobe and the Lingual Segment of the Left Upper Lobe

The percentage of bronchiectasis and cavitation involving the lingual segment of the left lobe and the right middle lobe is higher in patients with NTM pulmonary diseases than in those with multi-drug resistant pulmonary tuberculosis [4, 5], but there is no significant difference in the scope involved by nodules between these two groups of patients.

Though it is very hard to distinguish clinically drug-resistant pulmonary tuberculosis from NTM pulmonary diseases, a differentiation can be made for these two diseases according to clinical and laboratory examinations and image findings [13]. In case of a difficult differentiation, it is very important to seek assistance from immunological detection results, sputum culture bacteriology, and drug susceptibility test to confirm the diagnosis, based on which a targeted regimen can be provided.

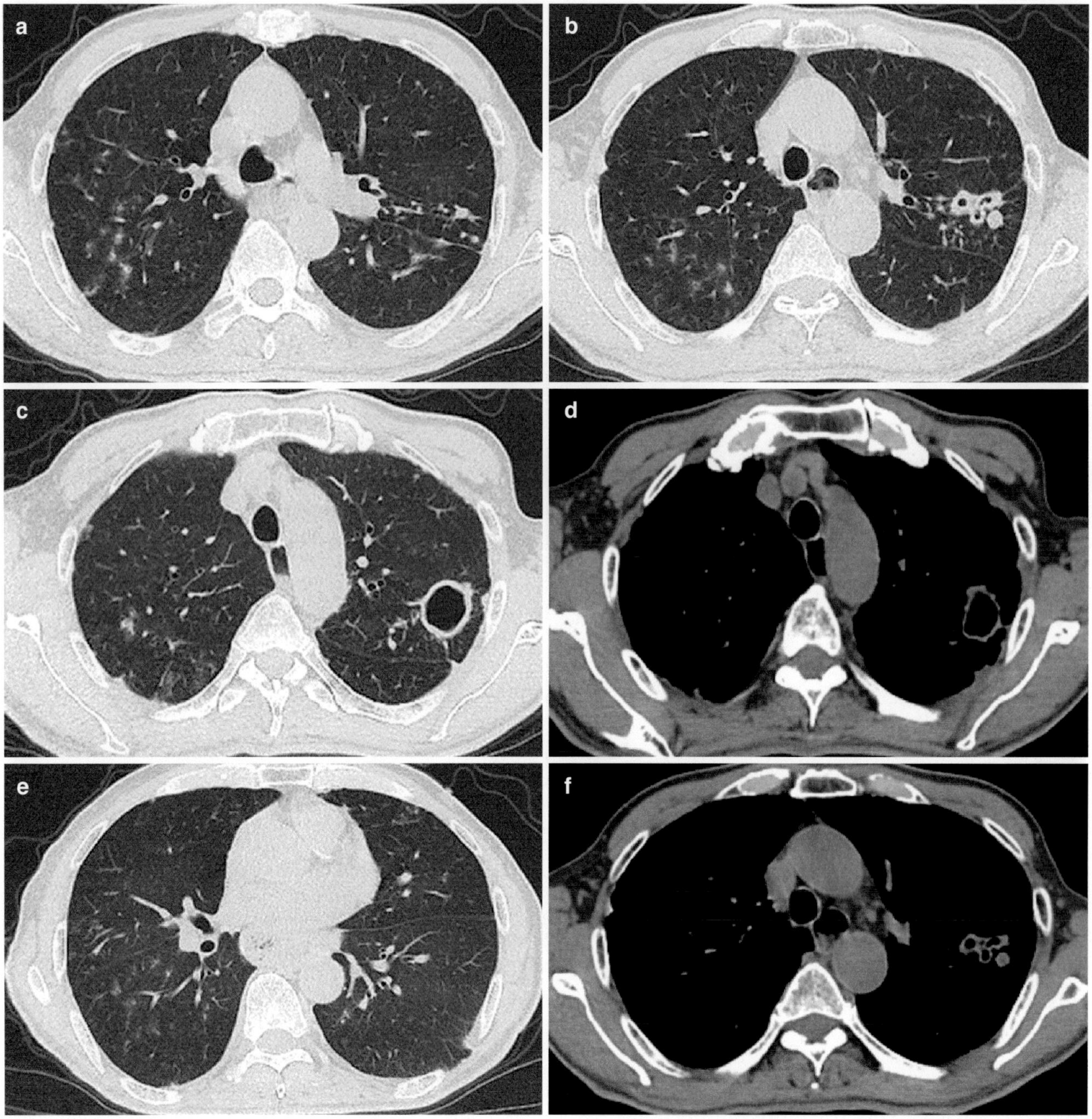

Fig. 14.2 (**a**–**f**) A 71-year-old male post to operation of esophageal cancer, suffering from NTM pulmonary disease. (**a**) Lung window of chest CT scans shows a small patchy opacity in the right upper lobe, and a patchy-strip high-density opacity in the left upper lobe; (**b**) a small patchy opacity is observed in the right upper lobe, and clustered bronchiectasis with small nodular opacities is noticed in the left upper lobe; (**c**) mediastinal window of CT scans shows thickened bronchial wall of clustered bronchiectasis and high-density nodular opacities in the left upper lobe; (**d**) small patchy opacities are noticed in the right upper lobe, which are distributed mainly in subpleural regions; a cavity with smooth interior wall is observed in the subpleural region of the left upper lobe, and there are thickened bronchial wall, bronchiectasis, and cords adjacent to the cavity; (**e**) mediastinal window of CT scans shows the wall of the cavity in the left upper lobe seems complete; and (**f**) lung window of CT scans shows scattered small patchy opacities in the right lower lobe and the lingual segment of the left upper lobe

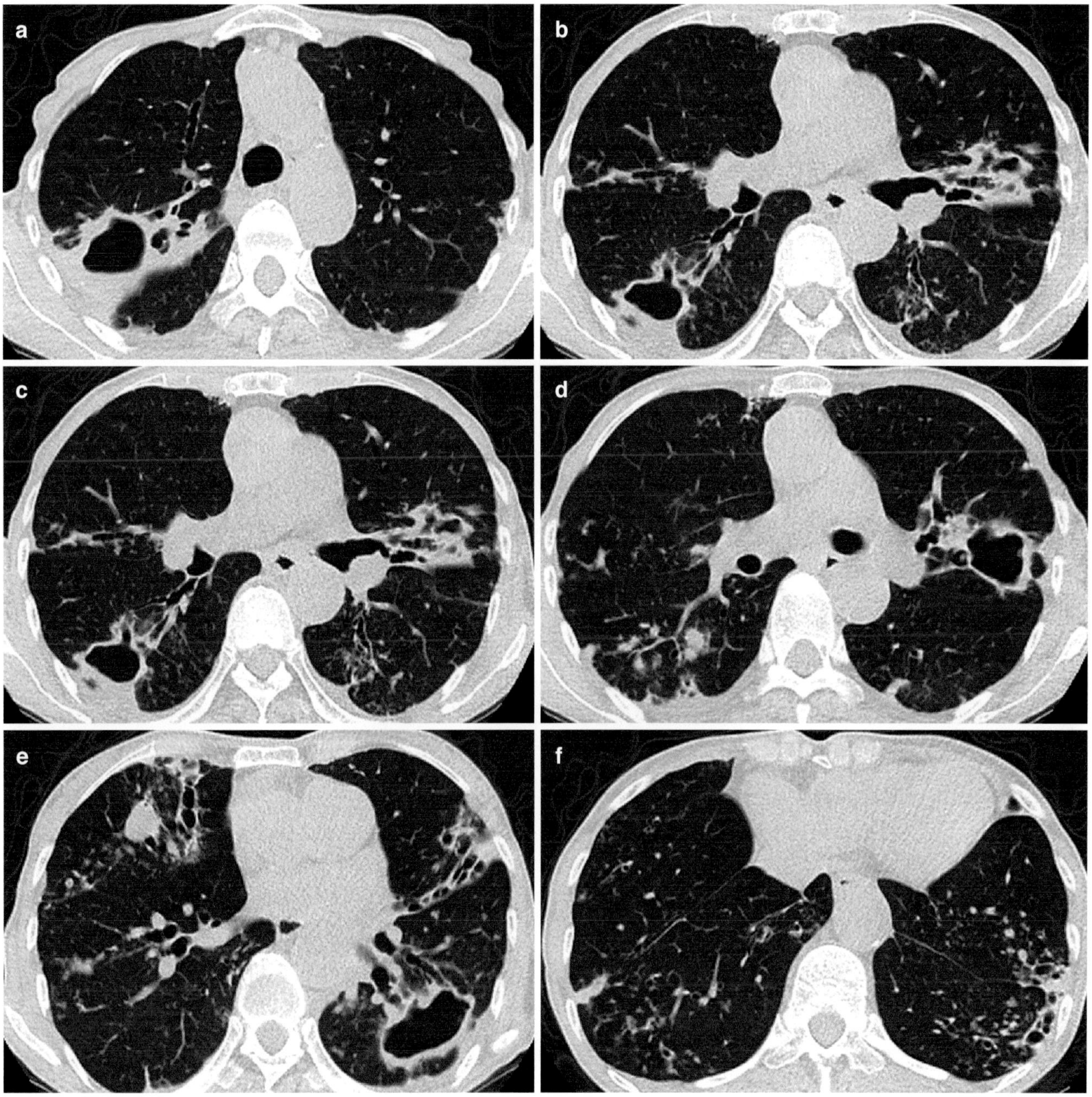

Fig. 14.3 (**a**–**f**) A 68-year-old male with NTM pulmonary disease. (**a**–**c**) Lung window of chest CT scans shows cavities in the right middle lobe (**a**, **b**) and in the lingual segment of the left upper lobe (**c**) with smooth interior wall, and clustered bronchiectasis in the lingual segment of the left upper lobe (**b**); (**d**) multiple bronchiectasis are observed in the right middle lobe and the lingual segment of the left upper lobe, with thickened bronchial wall and multiple nodular opacities around the bronchiectasis; (**e**) bronchiole expansions and small nodular opacities are observed in both lower lungs, which are mainly distributed in subpleural region

14.2 Differential Diagnosis of AIDS Complicated with Pulmonary Tuberculosis[2]

Ru-ming Xie and Pu-Xuan Lu

The incidence rate of drug-resistant TB has been increasing during recent years in both HIV-negative pulmonary TB patients and HIV infected/AIDS patients complicated with pulmonary TB [14, 15]. In 2015, WHO defined three categories of tuberculosis occurring from 2016 to 2020: tuberculosis, multi-drug resistant tuberculosis, and tuberculosis complicated with AIDS, while China was in the list of countries with high burden related to all these three categories [16, 17]. Besides the differentiation between drug-susceptible and drug-resistant pulmonary tuberculosis in daily work, importance should also be attached to the differential diagnosis between drug-resistant pulmonary tuberculosis and AIDS complicated pulmonary tuberculosis. As for the latter two diseases, chest imaging is an important adjunctive diagnostic method, in addition to those required by confirmation of diagnosis including laboratory bacteriology, molecular biology, and immunology. Chest imaging, a simple and rapid examination characterized by distinct features supported by a large amount of literature data, may achieve the improvement of prognosis through realizing the early-stage targeted treatment launched in time based on imaging diagnosis in most of patients.

14.2.1 Pathological Basis for AIDS Complicated with Pulmonary Tuberculosis

The atypical pathological changes in patients with AIDS complicated with pulmonary tuberculosis result in the diversity in imaging manifestations. Wenke Zhu et al. [18] analyzed pathological data from biopsy in correlation to CT image findings in 13 AIDS patients complicated with pulmonary tuberculosis and found that these patients manifested nodules, masses, or patchy consolidations, but cavities rarely observed in pulmonary lesions. Patients who present with patches and consolidation have the pathology lacking typical tuberculous nodules and Langhans giant cells, but show caseous necrosis, inflammatory cell infiltration, or inflammatory granuloma instead. In patients manifesting pulmonary nodules or masses, the pathology shows lymphocytes, proliferation of fibrous tissue or infiltration with epithelioid cells, with infiltration of inflammatory cells and a small amount of necrotic pulmonary tissues observed in some of the lesions, while there were no typical tuberculous nodules or Langhans giant cells, with caseous necrosis rarely observed in pathological changes. The ability of macrophages to inhibit the growth of Mycobacterium tuberculosis is reduced when the immunity of AIDS patients is extremely low, as some authors have noted, and the low level of allergic reaction cannot cause caseous necrosis in lung tissue, which is also one reason why cavities rarely form in AIDS patients complicated with tuberculosis [19].

Patients with drug-resistant pulmonary tuberculosis and those with normal immunity share common features in pathological manifestations, which are mainly characterized by exudations, proliferation, and necrosis. Tuberculous nodules, consisting of epithelial cells, Langhans giant cells, lymphocytes gathered locally in the periphery and the small number of reactively proliferating fibroblasts, are prone to caseous necrosis inside. Characteristic tuberculous nodules, therefore, are of great importance for the pathological diagnosis of tuberculosis. Secondary caseous necrosis, moreover, may occur in case of the presence of a great amount of Mycobacteria tuberculosis, strong virulence, low systemic resistance, or strong allergic reaction in the host, which is also one of vital reasons for the emergence of cavities, proliferative lesions, and caseous pneumonia in patients with pulmonary tuberculosis.

14.2.2 Image Findings in AIDS Patients Complicated with Pulmonary Tuberculosis

14.2.2.1 Image Findings in AIDS Complicated with Pulmonary Tuberculosis and Its Correlation to Count of $CD^{+}4$ T lymphocytes

Image findings of pulmonary tuberculosis lesions are almost the same in pulmonary TB patients with normal immunity and those in the early stage of HIV infection when immune mediation is absent and count of $CD4^{+}T$ lymphocytes cell is more than 200 cells/μL. The lesions, often located in the posterior apical segment of the upper lobs and/or the dorsal segment of the lower lobes, manifest mainly as multiple morphologic lesions including infiltrative patchy consolidations, nodular masses, cavities, and tree-in-bud signs in lungs (Fig. 14.4), or miliary pulmonary tuberculosis characterized in "homogeneity in three aspects" in both lungs. However, tuberculosis lymphadenitis and extra-pulmonary tuberculosis are relatively rarely observed [20]. There is no specific predisposing site for pulmonary tuberculosis, which manifests as exudative lesions distributed in multiple segments and lobes of both lungs, with patchy opacities and consolidations in different sizes and disseminated lesions in the lungs (Fig. 14.5), in case of CD+4 T lymphocytes lower than 200 cells/μL in AIDS patients in middle/advanced stage compli-

[2] Ru-ming Xie is the corresponding author for the Sect. 14.2.

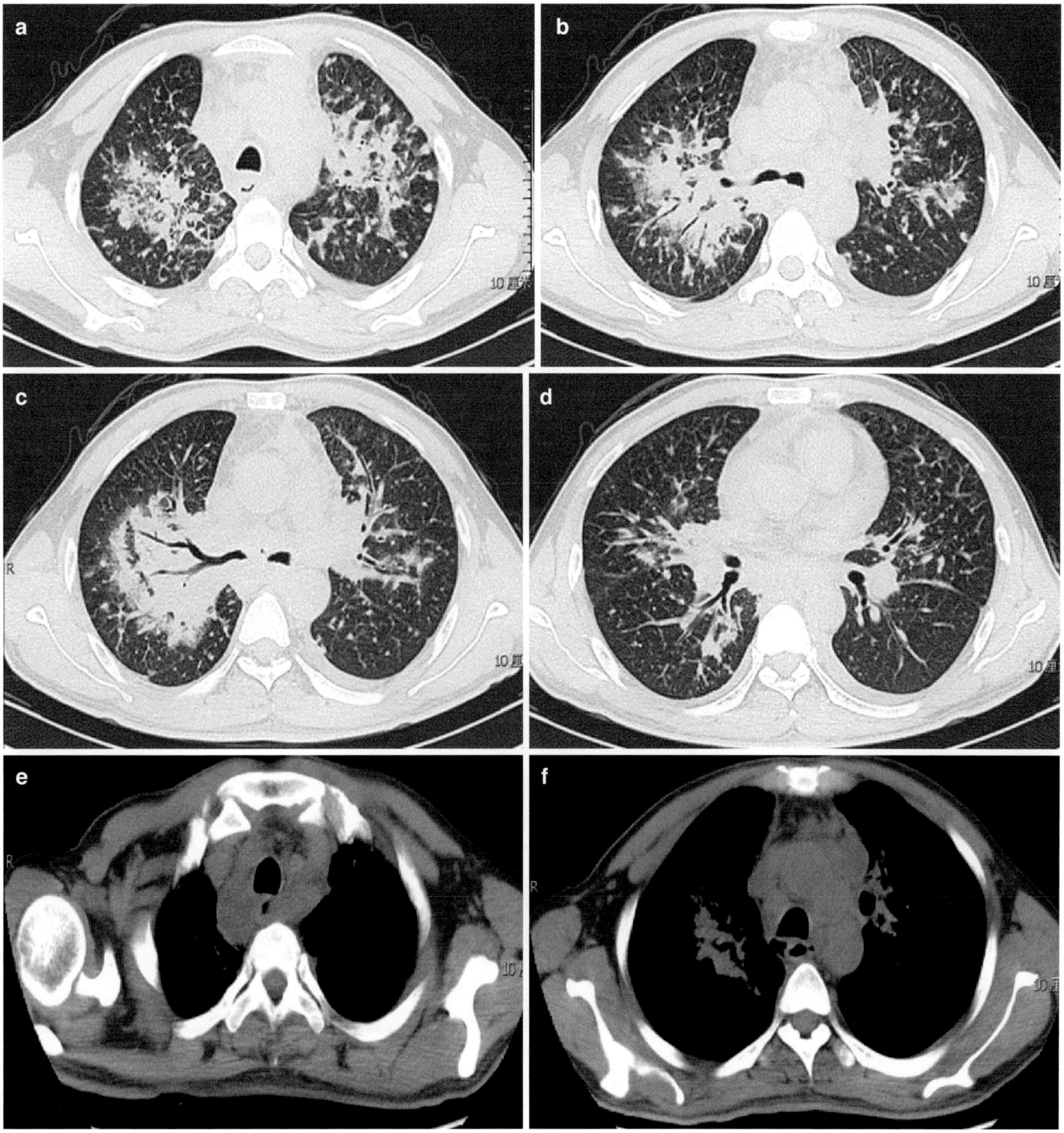

Fig. 14.4 (**a**–**f**) A 34-year-old male, with CD4+T lymphocytes of 20 cells/μL. AIDS complicated with pulmonary tuberculosis. (**a**–**d**) Lung window of chest CT scans shows large patches of consolidations distributed diffusively in both lungs, with disseminated nodules of various sizes. (**e**, **f**) Mediastinal window of chest CT scans shows lymphadenectasis in regions 2R, 4, 5, and 6, and liquefaction of lymph nodes in region 6, which manifests as a low density in CT scans

cated pulmonary tuberculosis. When lesions are dominantly exudative, it is difficult to distinguish them from a general nonspecific inflammation. Hilar and mediastinal tuberculosis lymphadenitis are common complications, and hematogenous dissemination often occurs, which is prone to small patchy fusion. It has been reported by literature [21–24] that the lower the immunity is in patients with pulmonary tuberculosis, the less likely the cavity will occur. The reason for this, based on analysis by researchers, lies in the reduced ability of macrophages to inhibit the growth of Mycobacterium

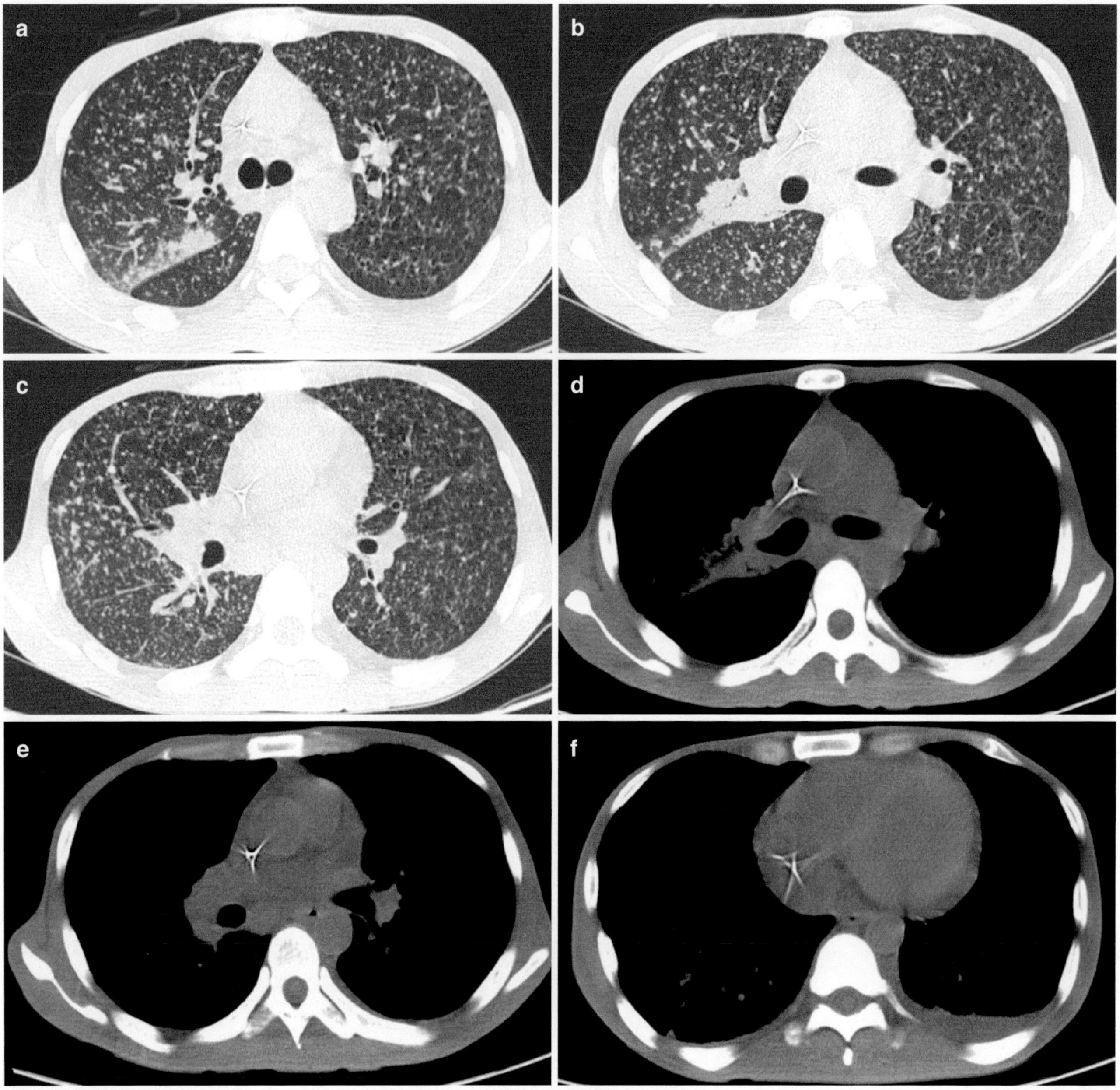

Fig. 14.5 (**a**–**f**) A 25-year-old male, with CD4+ T lymphocytes of 20 cells/μL. AIDS complicated with pulmonary tuberculosis. (**a**–**c**) Lung window of chest CT scans shows that both lungs are diffused with miliary opacities in uneven distribution and various sizes, and some lesions fuse into small patches. A sub-segmental consolidation is observed in the posterior segment of the upper lobe of the right lung, and a few exudative flocculence is seen at the distal side of the consolidation. (**d**–**f**) Mediastinal window of chest CT scans shows mediastinal and hilar lymphadenectasis, with a small amount of bilateral pleural effusion

tuberculosis and the lowered allergic reaction, which cannot cause caseous necrosis in lung tissue and so less cavities are formed.

14.2.2.2 Characteristic Image Findings in AIDS Complicated with Pulmonary Tuberculosis

In their early study, Leung et al. [25] compared the images of HIV infection/AIDS patients complicated with pulmonary TB to those of HIV-negative patients with pulmonary TB and found that imaging characteristics in HIV infected/AIDS patients were similar to those seen in primary pulmonary tuberculosis. Primary pulmonary tuberculosis, as shown by results of subsequent researches [26–28] on this topic, seems to be more common in AIDS patients. It mainly manifests as intra-thoracic tuberculosis lymphadenitis, and mediastinal and/or hilar lymphadenectasis, which may be single or multiple. The latter has a wider distribution and a higher incidence of mutual fusion. These patients exhibit a lower rate of lymph nodes calcification than tuberculosis patients without AIDS and manifest common central necrosis of lymph nodes, with ulceration observable in hilar lymph nodes invading adjacent pulmonary field. According to the analysis conducted by researchers [23], it has also been found that chest image findings in AIDS patients complicated with pulmonary tuberculosis are commonly characterized by atypical changes. First of all, the atypical location of lesions is commonly observed in both lower pulmonary fields in chest X-ray and in the right middle lobe or both lower lobes on CT scans. These lesions commonly involve multiple segments and lobes, progress rapidly, and are characterized by exudation and consolidation with large patchy consolidations. Signs of bronchial disseminations (such as acinar nodules and tree-in-bud signs) and proliferative and caseous foci in both upper pulmonary fields or apical fields are rare. Lesions complicated with cavities or fibrosis are also infrequent. Moreover, the incidence is significantly higher for miliary pulmonary tuberculosis and extra-pulmonary tuberculosis in AIDS patients, and the miliary lesions are prone to small fragmental fusion. The incidence of tuberculous pleural effusion or pericardial effusion complications is higher in AIDS patients than in non-AIDS patients [23, 29–31].

14.2.2.3 AIDS Complicated with Pulmonary Tuberculosis Is Prone to Concurrent Mixed Infection by Multiple Pathogens

The extremely low cellular immune in AIDS patients makes them more susceptible to mixed pulmonary infections caused by multiple pathogens such as bacteria, viruses, fungi, etc. Image findings of pulmonary lesions can be complicated, which may easily lead to misdiagnosis or delayed diagnosis of pulmonary tuberculosis in cases where it is complicated with an infection induced by another pathogen.

14.2.2.4 Immune Reconstitution Inflammatory Syndrome of Pulmonary Tuberculosis

Immune reconstitution syndrome related to tuberculosis in AIDS patients is defined as the emergence of clinical symptoms in patients with latent infection of tuberculosis in case of the decreased plasma HIV load and the increase in $CD4^{+}T$ lymphocytes cell count in AIDS patients post to the start of HAART treatment, or as the deterioration/progression of tuberculosis post to HAART treatment [32]. Immune reconstitution syndrome may manifest as newly appearing exudative patches, consolidations, and nodules in the lung, and some patients may have cavities with peripheral satellite foci, as well as signs including pleural thickening, pleural effusion, and pericardial effusion [33]. Patients with preexisting pulmonary tuberculosis may manifest as the aggravation of intra-pulmonary tuberculosis lesions post to HAART treatment, showing the increased number of exudative lesions, the enlargement of the lesion range and even the appearance of lumps and consolidations, the emergence of cavities in some of the lesions, and the appearance of extensively disseminated lesions in both lungs. In addition, there will be obvious enlargement of mediastinal tuberculosis lymphadenitis within a short period, with obvious liquefaction necrosis and fusion of lesions. The obvious progression of hematogenous disseminated pulmonary tuberculosis within a short period may manifest as progressive signs of extensive patchy fusion. There will be increase in pleural effusion and pericardial effusion [32, 33].

14.2.3 Differentiation Diagnosis Between Drug-Resistant Pulmonary Tuberculosis and AIDS Complicated with Pulmonary Tuberculosis

Based on a great amount of literatures [15, 34–37] reporting characteristics of image findings of drug-resistant pulmonary tuberculosis (including single-, poly-, multi-, quasi extensive-, extensive- and rifampicin resistances), the overall characteristics of the lesions include common involvement of at least three pulmonary fields, high incidence of cavitation with often more than three, and thick-walled cavities commonly observable, despite the minor difference among different drug-resistant groups. Compared with types of resistance, including single-, poly-, and multi-resistance, extensive drug-resistant tuberculosis (XDR-TB) is more likely to have a larger number of cavities and to cause unilateral destroyed lung and intra-pulmonary dissemination. The unresponsiveness of drug-resistant pulmonary tuberculosis to antituberculosis therapies predisposes the lesions to a protracted course, with an increase in both size and number of lesions, and recurrent dissemination of pathogens in the lungs. Other image findings commonly observed also include centrilobular nodule, tree-in-bud sign, plaque with consolidation, bronchiectasis, and pleural involvement.

Though both drug-resistant pulmonary tuberculosis and AIDS complicated with pulmonary tuberculosis have extensive distribution of lesions in lungs, they have distinct features in their image findings [20, 34–41].

1. Cavities are rarely observed in AIDS complicated with pulmonary tuberculosis. AIDS complicated with pulmonary tuberculosis manifests as nodules, masses, or patchy consolidations with intra-pulmonary disseminations, but cavities are rarely observed. The authors [18] analyzed pathological data from needle biopsy in correlation to CT image findings in AIDS patients complicated with pulmonary tuberculosis and found that patients showing patchy intra-pulmonary consolidations lacked typical tuberculous nodules and Langhans giant cells in their pathology,

but manifested as caseous necrosis and inflammatory cell infiltration or changes of inflammatory granuloma. Proliferation of lymphocytes and fibrous tissue or infiltration of epithelioid cells was shown in patients with nodules and masses, and infiltration of inflammatory cells and a small amount of lung tissue necrosis were also seen in some lesions. The capacity of macrophages capable of inhibiting the growth of Mycobacteria tuberculosis is lowered in case of extremely reduced immunity, such as in AIDS patients. Additionally, decreased levels of anaphylaxis prevent pulmonary tissue from generating caseous necrosis or forming cavities. Therefore, fewer cavities are observed in AIDS patients.

2. Image findings dominated by exudation can make it difficult to differentiate from nonspecific inflammation. In AIDS patients, immunity may lead to pulmonary tuberculosis lesions that are dominated by exudations and appear as cloud floccules, patches, or consolidations in imaging findings. This is in contrast to typical features of pulmonary tuberculosis which show the coexistence of lesions in multiple lobes, multiple segments and multiple forms.
3. Intra-pulmonary bronchiectasis is rarely observed in AIDS patients complicated with pulmonary tuberculosis. AIDS patients, if complicated with infection of tuberculosis, may often exhibit as acute progression, exudation, consolidation, and dissemination due to their extremely low immunity. In comparison, drug-resistant tuberculosis is a chronic disease due to poor response to antituberculosis treatment. Bronchiectasis occurs due to the traction of bronchi caused by contracture of scar tissue resulting from fibrosis post-healing of peri-bronchial lesions or damage to bronchial structures caused by chronic, protracted pulmonary diseases. Bronchiectasis, though not a typical feature in image findings in drug-resistant pulmonary tuberculosis, has a high incidence as reported by literature.
4. The presence of high incidence of primary tuberculosis, a high incidence of hematogenous disseminated pulmonary tuberculosis, and the coexistence of multiple types of pulmonary tuberculosis in one case are characteristics observed in AIDS patients complicated with pulmonary tuberculosis but rarely observed in any type of drug-resistant pulmonary tuberculosis. Only a few literature reports have indicated that lymphadenectasis with circular enhancement in contrasted CT scans may occur in drug-resistant tuberculosis.
5. Mixed infection induced by multiple pathogens is one of the characteristics of AIDS complicated with pulmonary tuberculosis. The reduced immunity predisposes the patients to the complications induced by other pathogens (such as bacteria, viruses, fungi) in addition to pulmonary infection caused by Mycobacterium tuberculosis, thereby complicating the image findings of pulmonary tuberculosis, which has atypical image findings as its intrinsic character. Therefore, it has a distinct difference when compared to drug-resistant pulmonary tuberculosis, which exhibits typical imaging characteristics of pulmonary tuberculosis.
6. Immune reconstitution inflammatory syndrome in AIDS patients complicated with pulmonary tuberculosis differs from drug-resistant pulmonary tuberculosis in their dynamic manifestations of image findings. Immune reconstitution inflammatory syndrome in patients with pulmonary tuberculosis is defined as the deterioration and progression occurring for intra-pulmonary tuberculosis lesions in some of the AIDS patients complicated with pulmonary tuberculosis in week 1–4 of HAART treatment, most commonly observed in week 2. If antituberculosis treatment is continued, amelioration with absorption of lesion may occur. Drug-resistant pulmonary tuberculosis, however, has poor or even no response to antituberculosis treatment, with persistent presence and progression of cavities, repeated bronchial dissemination and even destroyed lungs, which has the intrinsic difference compared with immune reconstitution inflammatory syndrome in AIDS patients complicated with pulmonary tuberculosis.

14.3 Differentiation Diagnosis with Drug-Sensitive Tuberculosis[3]

Yan Lv and Wei Ma

Drug-resistant pulmonary tuberculosis (DR-TB) and drug-sensitive pulmonary tuberculosis (DS-TB) differ in etiology, pathogenesis, treatment regimen, prognosis, and harms to public health. Therefore, it is extremely important to find out features and differences in clinical symptoms, laboratory examinations, and imaging findings. Among them, the chest imaging examination is simple and intuitive, providing objective value for diagnosis and response evaluation. Therefore, DR-TB should be timely differentiated in the chest imaging examination for patients with pulmonary tuberculosis, so that early treatment can be initiated and prognosis improved.

[3] Yan Lv is the corresponding author for the Sect. 14.3.

14.3.1 Both DS-TB and DR-TB Have Pathological Basis of Pulmonary Tuberculosis, and the Same Characteristics in Their Image Findings

1. Location of lesions: According to the literature both domestic and abroad concerning researches on pulmonary tuberculosis, a consensus has been reached. The predisposing locations for pulmonary tuberculosis, based on the relationship between anatomical characteristics and hemodynamic characteristics such as blood flow and ventilation, typically include the posterior apical segment of the upper lobes and the dorsal segment of the lower lobe, particularly in the subclavian region. Lesions can be solitary or multiple, distributed within one or multiple segments, or appear in a multi-lobar distribution.
2. Intra-pulmonary lesions and related intra-thoracic lesions: The basic pathological features of pulmonary tuberculosis include exudative, proliferative, and degenerative lesions, all of which are typical changes of tuberculosis. Multiple lesions may coexist simultaneously, or one certain type of lesion may dominate. Image findings of CT scans manifest as different signs, based on the different nature of lesions.
   (a) Patchy or spherical opacities: Pathologically, patches or consolidations represent exudative alveolitis or caseous pneumonia, which is the most common sign in the early stage of pulmonary tuberculosis. The image shows blurred edges of the lesion and the complications of ground glass opacities in some of the lesions, indicating an active disease. Yan Lu et al. [42] studied the image findings of 323 patients with active pulmonary tuberculosis, and the results showed that lobar and sub-segmental consolidation accounted for 90.7%, and the enlarged lesion range might show segmental or lobar high-density opacities. Particularly, it was emphasized that caseous foci are more likely to occur in focal, segmental, or lobar consolidation and manifest as punctiform and patchy low-density opacities prone to cavitation after communicating with the bronchus and to bronchial dissemination, which could better represent the activity of the lesions. Spherical lesions and masses are other manifestations, and it is easier to diagnose them when they are complicated by cavitation. If there is no cavity, an enhanced scan is necessary, which is characterized by mildly to moderately contrasted small patchy low-density opacities that appear capsule-like or scattered with blurred edges.
   (b) Bronchial disseminated lesions: It manifests mainly as centrilobular nodules, including "tree-in- bud sign" and branch linear opacities, air-cavity nodules or acinar nodules. Tree-in-bud sign in pulmonary tuberculosis is a characteristic imaging finding of bronchial dissemination caused by Mycobacterium tuberculosis. The efficiency of high-resolution CT (HRCT) or thin-layer CT scan appears to be optimal. The pathological basis of "dendritic" image is caseous necrotic substances filled in the lumen of terminal bronchioles, while the "tree-in-bud" sign is the image of caseous substances filled in the respiratory bronchioles and alveolar ducts [43–46]. The incidence of "tree-in-bud" sign, as reported by literature, was 45–67% in active pulmonary tuberculosis. It is noteworthy that this sign represents a lesion of bronchioles, which are small airway. This sign may occur not only in the bronchial disseminated lesions of pulmonary tuberculosis, but also in corresponding infectious lesions such as bronchiolitis and diffuse pan-bronchiolitis. Both of which are inflammation of bronchiole wall, often manifested as blurred edges and gradual narrowing of lumen due to exudation or hyperplasia. "Tree-in-bud sign" of pulmonary tuberculosis, however, is the caseous substance filling in the bronchioles, often appearing as smaller branches and larger buds with clearer edges. It is important to differentiate between these two signs. The pathological basis of the airspace nodule is the consolidation of the air cavity around the bronchioles. This nodule is located at the center of the pulmonary lobules, as shown by HRCT examination or thin-layer CT images. It is more commonly observed in peripheral regions of the lung with uniform density and a CT value often lower than that of the adjacent blood vessels. The airspace nodule appears as a nodular lesion with fuzzy edges, which can also take on a "fascicular" or "plum petal" shape. It is also known as acinar nodules because their size is similar to an acinus [47]. The nodules always have lobar, sub-segmental or segmental distribution, or appear as satellite foci around the main focus. All these signs are manifestations of bronchial dissemination at different stages, and the difference in their appearance is just because of the different locations of the disseminated lesions in different sizes and shapes.
   (c) Miliary nodule opacities: The focus on chest CT is shown as multiple clustered miliary nodules and is called as dense miliary shadow by some scholars [48]. Its pathological basis is tuberculous granulomatous nodule in bronchial submucosa and pulmonary interstitial structure. Image findings in CT scans manifest as nodules ranging from 1 to 3 mm with the relatively clear border in intensive or clustered distribution and in coexistence with exudative inflammatory patches [49]. The lesions are limited in segments or lobes or distributed in multiple lobes and segments

in both lungs, which are observed in the acute inflammatory stage of pulmonary tuberculosis. This sign is also called "sarcoid galaxy sign" by some researchers, and the lesion may also manifest as "reversed halo sign" based on the different distribution of nodules and their presentations [49]. Recently, some scholars [50] call them "fireworks sign," which may describe this sign more concretely and vividly as a whole. According to the amount of local nodules accumulated in the lesion, different morphological manifestations are formed, which can be categorized in three groups: halo sign, anti-halo sign and the uniform, based on the morphological characteristics. The halo sign is defined as having more lesions at the center compared to fewer lesions at the peripheral, anti-halo sign as having the fewer lesion at the center compared to more lesions at the peripheral, and the uniform as having an even distribution of lesions both at the center and peripheral. Multiple forms of fireworks signs may appear in the same patient, and small nodules forming fireworks signs correspond to caseous necrotic granuloma in bronchioles and alveoli, which are considered a type of bronchial dissemination. Despite subtle differences between researches or their descriptions, their common point is that all these signs suggest the presence of active pulmonary tuberculosis.

(d) Cavity: Cavitation is the common image finding of pulmonary tuberculosis and one of the manifestations of active tuberculosis. Most patients with cavities have positive sputum bacteria. The pathology of a cavity can be categorized into following groups based on its origin, shape of its wall and its peripheral location: (1) mouth-eaten cavity, also called non-wall cavity, is observed in caseous pneumonia and has different sizes and irregular shapes. (2) Thin-walled cavity, which has a thickness of wall less than 3 mm and is observed commonly in the early stage of cavitation. (3) Caseous cavity, refers to a cavity formed in a tuberculoma by central or eccentric dissolution of a caseous focus, with a thicker layer of caseous material and thinner layers of granulation tissue and fibrous tissue. (4) Fiber cavity, which evolves through protracted courses from lesions above, has a three-layer structure consisting of a caseous necrotic layer, a granulation layer and a fibrous tissue layer (the thickest layer), and the cavity has a rigid appearance. Cavities in pulmonary tuberculosis are typically classified into mouth-eaten, thin-walled, and thick-walled cavities on image findings, based on pathological manifestations. This categorization based solely on image findings, however, is deemed by some researchers not enough to fully reflect the etiology of the cavity and its response to treatment. Therefore, the cavity of pulmonary tuberculosis can be categorized into two groups: the infiltrative cavity and the fibrous cavities, based on their morphology. The infiltrating cavity, mainly surrounded by exudative lesions, is a solitary thick-walled cavity in most cases, with a liquid-gas plane observable inside. The fibrous cavitation, which is observed in multiple thin-walled cavities in most cases, is characterized by a periphery dominated by fibrosis and the presence of calcification on the interior wall in some cases. Cavities in different categories respond differently to treatment. Infiltrative cavities are more prone to dynamic changes during treatment, while no obvious changes are observed in fibrous cavities [51].

(e) Bronchial change: It consists of thickening of bronchial wall and bronchiectasis. The thickening of the bronchial wall manifests as cuff sign and track sign, with its thickness greater than that of the bronchi at the same level. The bronchi at all levels can be affected, especially the thickening of drainage bronchi wall in proximity to the cavity, which is relative specific. Bronchiectasis in pulmonary tuberculosis, previously deemed as a sequel of lesions, is actually a sign of non-active pulmonary tuberculosis [52, 53]. Recent researches, however, suggest that signs of reversible bronchiectasis may occur in active pulmonary tuberculosis within the consolidation or in the drainage bronchi near the consolidation or cavity. The wall of the enlarged bronchi may appear even or manifest as tumor-like or varicose expansion, especially in case of bronchiectasis within consolidations or nodules complicated with focal erosion-like changes. This can be one of the signs used to differentiate between active pulmonary tuberculosis and other infections [54].

(f) Interstitial changes: Pulmonary tuberculosis is a disease transmitting and disseminating through air tract, but interstitial changes as a secondary sign have received great attention from scholars in recent years. Based on results of domestic research, interstitial changes mainly manifest as intra-lobular fine reticuloid opacities, micronodules, tree-in-bud sign, ground glass opacities, thickening of interlobular septum and airway walls, with a detection rate of 100.0% (43/43), 100.0% (43/43), 76.7% (33/43), 62.8% (27/43), 53.5% (23/43), and 55.8% (24/43), respectively. Various degrees of absorption can be achieved after antituberculosis treatment, and the rate is higher than 93% for any one of the four signs at the end of consolidated treatment (6 months) [55].

(g) Changes of mediastinal lymph nodes: Along with the progression of lesions, mediastinal lymphadenopathy may show a blurred fat space in the periphery of lymph nodes or even the fusion of lymph nodes, which is of specificity shown on enhanced scans. Enhancement may appear in lymph nodes during the proliferative stage, and small focal low-density regions may emerge along with the development of caseous foci within the lesions. Most of these regions exhibit typical circular enhancement, and in case of fused lesions, they display compartmentalized or honeycomb enhancement. Calcification may occur in lymph nodes as the disease progresses.

(h) Pleural changes: It presents as pleural thickening, and nodular or flat nodular protrusions may occur, with smooth surface, heterogeneously reduced density inside, and enhanced edge in contrasted scans. Its pathology is granulomatous inflammatory necrosis showing a tuberculoma-like manifestation. Extrapleural fat hyperplasia or pleural calcification may occur in patients with prolonged course of disease, and most of them are complicated with pleural effusion and prone to partition or wrapping formed within a short period, which is caused by the components contained in the pleural effusion. Fibrous strips and bands with blurred edges are commonly observed in subpleural regions in lungs, due to reasons such as lymphatic drainage and inflammatory exudation [56]. Pleural effusion may be absorbed gradually during antituberculosis treatment, but changes of pleural tuberculoma-like changes may not be synchronous, but manifest as shrinkage, enlargement, or emergence of new lesions instead. The overall tendency, however, seems good along with the progress of treatment cycles.

14.3.2 Differentiation of Image Findings Between DR-TB and DS-TB

Results from numerous literature show that DR-TB has identical lesion nature and morphology in image findings when compared to DS-TB, but has a certain difference except for image findings of general pulmonary tuberculosis or DS-TB, due to different innate molecular biological behavior of DR-TB.

1. DR-TB has severe lesions with extensive distribution. Image findings in HIV(-) adult pulmonary pt DMR-TB are prone to multiple lesions in large sizes with significant involvement of both lungs [34], as concluded by A Literature Review of Radiological Signs Related to Multi-Drug Resistant Pulmonary Tuberculosis, which analyzed 17 articles identified fully relevant to the analytical aim out of 427 articles retrieved in PubMed (https://www.ncbi.nlm.nih.gov/pubmed) with their titles and abstracts screened and only literature in English retained. It was shown by results of a comparative study on CT Imaging in 127 cases of multi-drug resistant pulmonary tuberculosis and drug-sensitive tuberculosis that chest image findings of MDR-TB patients were complicated, who had a higher incidence of pulmonary parenchyma damages and involvement of a larger number of pulmonary segments as compared with drug-sensitive pulmonary tuberculosis, and the number of patients with lesions infiltrating at least three pulmonary lobes was higher in the observational group than in the control [57]. A similar conclusion was also obtained by Chenghai Li et al. [58] in an analysis of CT signs in patients with different types of drug-resistant and drug-sensitive pulmonary tuberculosis. They found that those with drug-resistant pulmonary tuberculosis had wider distribution of lesions, with more cases of involvement of at least three pulmonary lobes when compared with DS-TPB and was more prone to involvement of atypical sits of pulmonary tuberculosis. The results show that multi-drug resistant tuberculosis is involved with more commonly at least three pulmonary fields with concurrent destroyed lungs, as observed in the research by Dejie Gao et al. [59]. This is considered to be related to the innate nature of multi-drug resistant pulmonary tuberculosis as an acquired resistance, which resulted in the emergence of resistant bacteria induced by reduced drug concentration within lesions due to difficulties in drug penetration caused by severely destroyed lungs with extensive fibrous hyperplasia resulting from protracted courses, recurrent diseases, and repeated intra-pulmonary dissemination. Results of the research by Baoyun Cai et al. [60] showed that destroyed lungs may occur within a short period (within 1 year) for patients with drug-resistant pulmonary tuberculosis, with the lesions in the contra-lateral lung involving with at least two sites. The distribution of lesions is extensive not only in patients with MDR-TB but also in those with initial mono-resistant tuberculosis exhibiting active signs as its dominant CT manifestations [36]. Results from a research with 102 patients of acquired drug-resistant pulmonary tuberculosis and 36 patients susceptible to antituberculosis drugs showed that number of tuberculosis lesions exceeding 4 was one of the main risk factors of acquired resistance [61], which proved conversely that drug-resistant pulmonary tuberculosis had multiple lesions with extensive involvement.
2. DR-TB has multiple nodules and multiple cavities. Multiple lesions are commonly observed in DR-TB, which is prone to the development of nodules and cavities, with thick-walled cavities as its feature. The number

of tuberculosis lesions more than 3 complicated with cavitation is the risk of developing drug-resistant pulmonary tuberculosis [23]. The possibility of MDR-TB is high in case of multiple punctiform nodules appearing in multiple pulmonary fields [62]. Yixiang Wang et al. [34] concluded in their literature review that the maximum diameter of pulmonary cavity ≥30 mm with cavity number ≥3 and regions containing cavity ≥2 pulmonary fields in HIV (-) adults correlated to pulmonary MDR-TB, though nMDR-TB and ptMDR-TB did not differ greatly in incidence of cavitation. A comparative analysis on image findings between DMR-TB and XDR-TB showed that XDR-TB seemed probably more aggressive, with larger and more cavities, and thicker wall than MDR-TB, showing the mean thickness of 8.0 mm for the cavity wall in MDR-TB cohort in comparison with 11.5 mm in XDR-TB cohort, and the mean size of cavity of 21 mm in MDR-TB cohort in comparison with 36 mm in XDR-TB cohort. Compared with DS tuberculosis patients, those with primary MDR tuberculosis have higher incidence of multiple cavities. Early detection and timely treatment can be achieved based on the finding of multiple cavities in imaging [63].

3. Bronchial involvement is commonly observed in DR-TB patients. Except for multiple cavities and nodules in drug-resistant tuberculosis patients, image findings of CT scans, such as the frequency of bronchiectasis, correlate with drug-sensitive tuberculosis patients [39, 64] and are commonly observed in MDR and XDR tuberculosis patients [39], which is possibly related to chronic disease history of many ptMDR patients. In the research on single-resistant patients, the incidence of either bronchial wall thickening or lumen stenosis is higher in the observational cohort than in the drug-sensitive cohort [36]. The research by Chenghai Li et al. [58] showed that the incidence of bronchial wall thickening is higher in MDR-TB and XDR-TB, as well as in single-resistant pulmonary tuberculosis, compared to drug-sensitive cohort, but without significant difference among all drug-resistant types. The incidence of bronchial wall thickening or stenosis is positively correlated with the load of Mycobacterium tuberculosis, and the greater the bacterial load, the easier the airway is damaged. Conversely, Mycobacteria tuberculosis is prone to natural resistance to drugs due to the increasing bacterial load caused by airway stenosis and obstructed drainage, as well as the multiplication of this bacteria into a great amount when caseous necrosis occurs during the process from onset to development of TB.
4. Calcification of mediastinal and hilar lymph nodes is rarely observed in DR-TB patients. Observation of chest CT scans for nMDR-TB patients shows rarely calcification of mediastinal and hilar lymph nodes, and calcification of either intra-pulmonary lesions or lymph nodes is more common in DS-TB than in nMDR-TB, suggesting DS-TB patients may have a chronic disease course, while nMDR-TB has a relatively more acute onset and greater severity [39]. Same results were also obtained by the research [36] conducted by Genming Chen et al. showing CT manifestations of treatment-naïve single-resistant pulmonary tuberculosis were dominantly active signs, with incidence of calcification of either hilar or mediastinal lymph nodes lower than that in the cohort of drug-sensitive patients.

The onset age of DR-TB is considered younger, as suggested by other literature concerning comparative researches on DR-TB and DS-TB. Genming Chen et al. [36] concluded in the research on CT Imaging of Treatment-Naïve Single-Resistant Pulmonary Tuberculosis that the mean age was (38 ± 18.6) years in the single-resistance cohort, which was younger than that in DS-TB cohort with statistical difference. Similar results were observed by Jihoon Cha et al. [64], suggesting younger age in MDR-TB and XDR-TB patients than in DS-TB patients ($p < 0.001$), the absence of difference between MDR-TB and XDR-TB patients, the median age of 38 years in either MDR-TB patients or XDR-TB patients. Although having not achieved consistent results based on all literature studies, the data of age may provide some possible

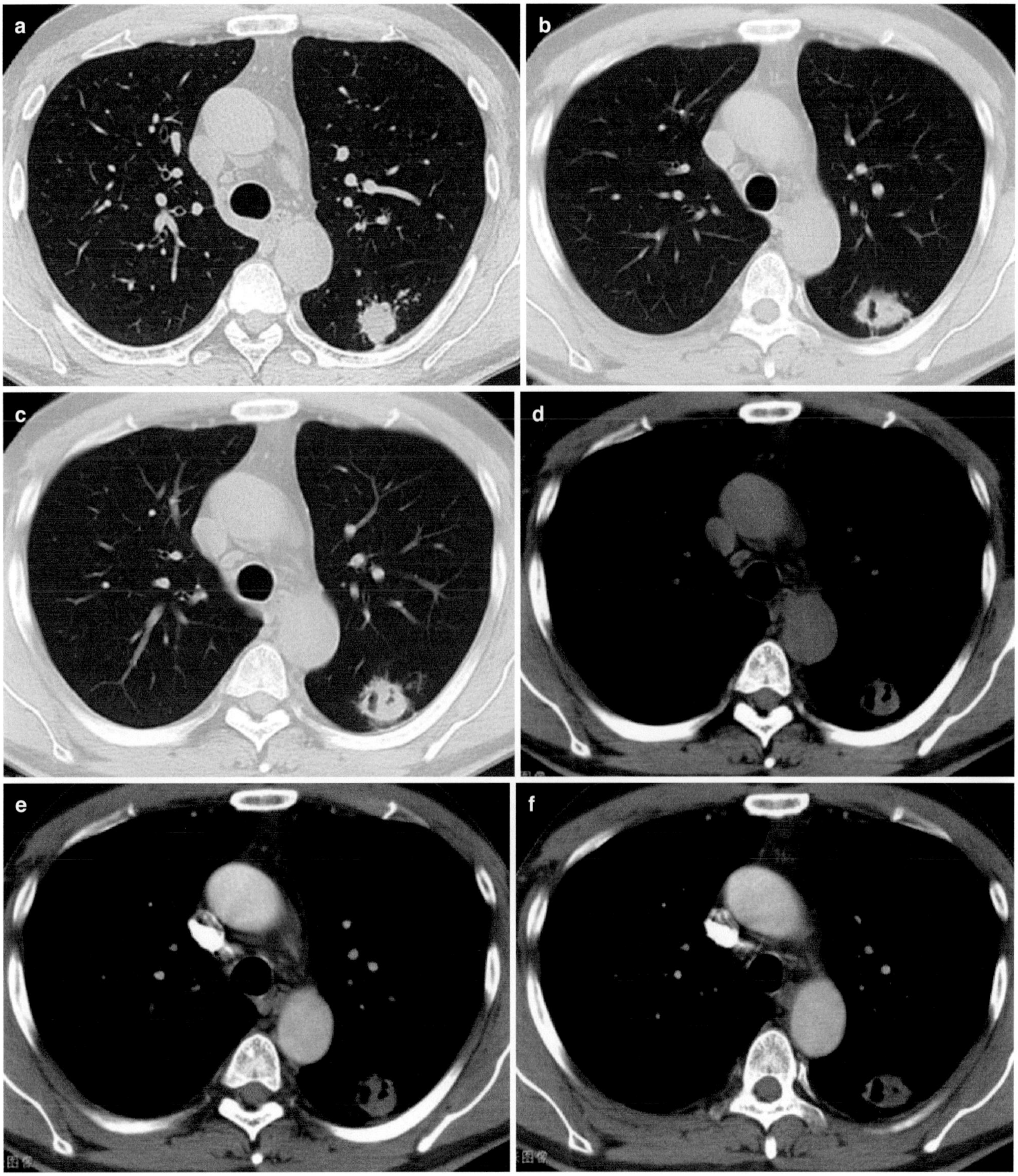

Fig. 14.6 (**a**–**f**) A 43-year-old patient, with drug-sensitive pulmonary tuberculosis. (**a**–**c**) Lung window of chest CT scans shows a nodule with clear edge in the dorsal segment of the left lower lobe, with a cord observable adhered to adjacent pleura. Small cavities are seen within parenchyma with their peripheries distributed with satellite lesions, some of which appear in "tree-in-bud sign." (**d**–**f**) Mediastinal window of chest CT scans shows high-density nodules with clear edges in the dorsal segment of the left lower lobe, without enhancement shown by contrasted scans

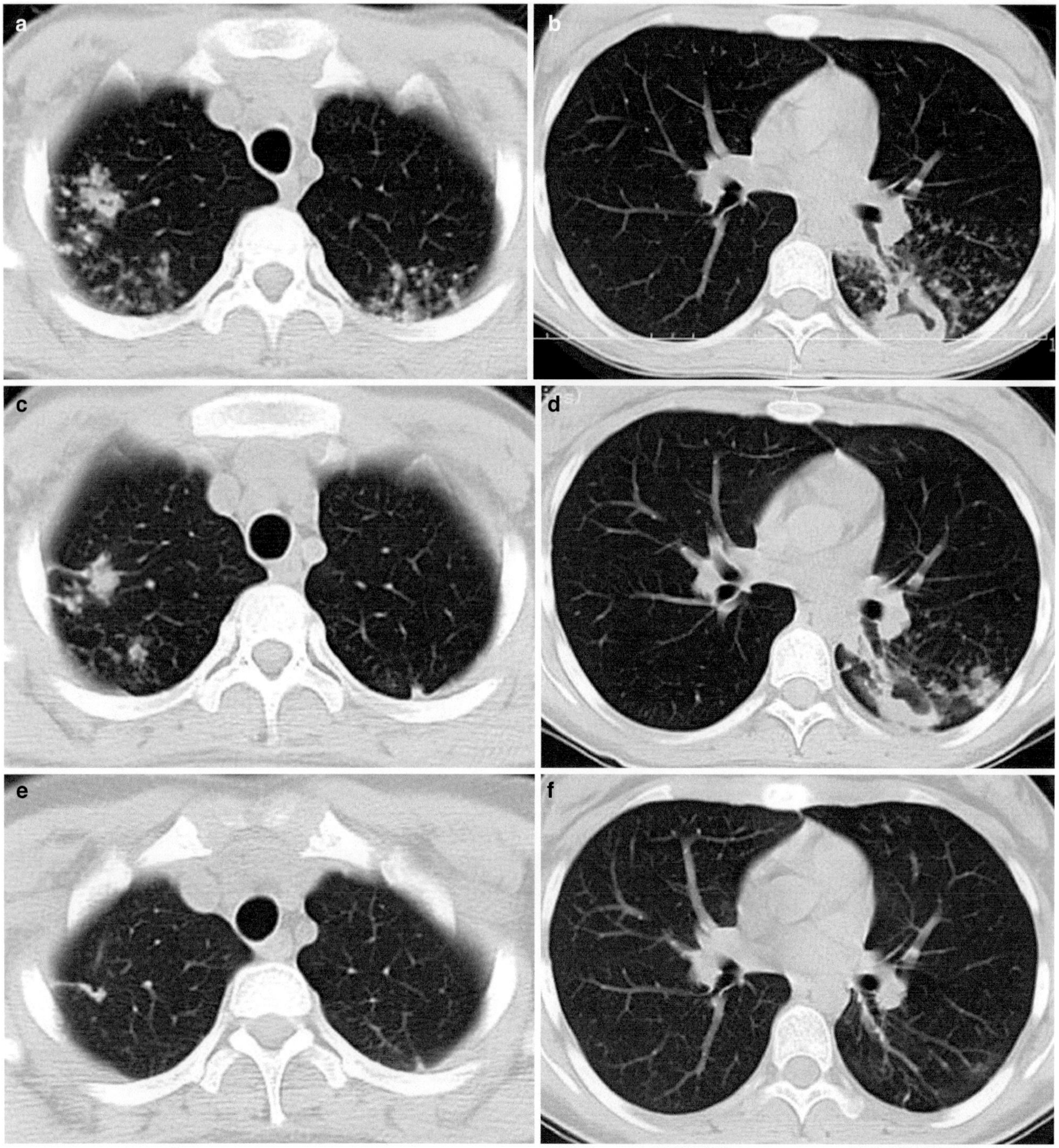

Fig. 14.7 (**a–f**) A female patient aged 13 years, with drug-sensitive pulmonary tuberculosis. (**a**, **b**) Lung window of chest CT scans shows thick-walled cavities with smooth interior wall in the apical segment of the right upper lobe and in the dorsal segment of the left lower lobe prior to treatment. Lesions in the left lower lobe seem larger in size, with a drainage bronchus nearby. Multiple "tree-in-bud signs" with blurred edges are observed surrounding the lesions and in the posterior apical segment of the left upper lobe. (**c**, **d**) Lung window of chest CT scans at re-examination after 3 months of antituberculosis treatment shows obvious decrease in size and number of the lesions, with the closure of cavities in the right upper lobe. (**e**, **f**) Re-examination 1.5 years after discontinuation of antituberculosis treatment shows overall absorption of lesions in both lungs, with residue of small amount of fibrous lesions

differences, thus providing a hint for the diagnosis of DR-TB (Figs. 14.6 and 14.7).

14.4 Differentiation Diagnosis with Pulmonary Fungal Infection[4]

Wei He and Hui Zhang

China not only ranks among countries with the highest incidence of drug-resistant tuberculosis, but also witnesses the gradual increase in fungal infections due to widely use of broad-spectrum antibiotics, immunosuppressants, adrenocortical hormones and cytotoxic drugs as well as more and more popularization of organ transplantation and instrument placement during recent years. There are similarities in some respect of clinical and imaging manifestations between pulmonary tuberculosis and fungal infection, predisposing them to misdiagnosis. Moreover, pulmonary fungal infection is also one of the common complications of pulmonary tuberculosis. Suzhen Peng et al. analyzed Mycobacterium tuberculosis detected in 77 patients with multi-drug resistant pulmonary tuberculosis and found that Mycobacterium tuberculosis could not be cultured in sputum of 71.43% (55/77) of the patients after 6-month antituberculosis treatment, which was significantly lowered compared with the 100% positive rate at their enrollment, indicating that satisfactory results were achieved by the treatment. Mycobacteria tuberculosis, however, was cultured again in sputum of 11 patients in month 12 of the treatment. The overall fungal infection rate was 36.36% (28/77) in 77 patients with multi-drug resistant pulmonary tuberculosis, compared with 12.98% observed at their first hospitalization, showing a significant increase in the detection rate of fungi when antituberculosis treatment was prolonged to month 6 and 12. This suggests that a great importance should be attached by physicians to the culture of fungi when they are performing antituberculosis treatment and modify the regimens timely based on results of drug susceptibility test, so as to achieve individualized treatment.

Radiology is of great importance on diagnosis of pulmonary infections, and chest X-ray is a diagnostic tool used for screening, but it has a limited sensitivity. Lung magnetic resonance imaging is a new diagnostic tool that has been introduced into the assessment of pulmonary parenchyma and has the great advantage of not using ionizing radiation. In a latest research, Yan et al. [65, 66] found the sensitivity of 3.0 TMRI was superior to that of HRCT (90.5% vs. 86.9%) when detecting infiltrating pulmonary fungal infections. However, other researches have reported lower sensitivity of MRI compared to HRCT in detecting primary signs (i.e., the halo sign) of vascular invasive pulmonary aspergillosis. It is considered in some researches that imaging examination can serve as an approach to identify pulmonary fungal infection [65], and CT plays an important role in early detection, diagnosis, and differentiation diagnosis of pulmonary infection, as well as evaluating their responses to treatment.

14.4.1 Pulmonary Mycosis

Categorization of pulmonary mycosis: Pulmonary mycosis is defined as pulmonary diseases caused by fungi, referring mainly to fungal inflammation of lungs and bronchi or related diseases. Clinically, fungi are usually divided into pathogenic fungi (causing primary and exogenous fungal infections) and conditional pathogenic fungi (opportunistic pathogenic fungi). The most common fungi causing pulmonary mycosis at present include Candida, Aspergillus, and Cryptococcus neoformans, followed by Coccidioides, mucor, histoplasma, and Talaromyces marneffei.

Main pathogenic fungi in lower respiratory tract are categorized into: (1) Saccharomycetes: Candida (Candida albicans), non-Candida (Cryptococcus, Trichosporum, and Saccharomyces); (2) Mycetes: Aspergillus or non-Aspergillus; (3) Dimorphic fungi: Coccidioides, Paracoccidioides, Histoplasma, sporothrix, Blastomyces, and Geotrichum; and (4) Eumycetes: Pneumocystis jiroveci, Nocardia, Actinomycetes, and Botryomyces [67].

Invasive pulmonary mycosis is defined usually as acute/chronic pathological changes and pathophysiological processes of tissue damage, pulmonary dysfunction and inflammatory reaction caused by fungi invading directly into pulmonary tissue or bronchi and growing and proliferating there. Generally, it does not include bronchial/pulmonary fungal infection induced by parasitic fungi and allergy to it and can be categorized into two groups: the primary and the secondary.

14.4.2 Image Findings for Pulmonary Mycosis

Pulmonary mycosis can be caused by multiple pathogenic bacteria, and they either differ or are identical in various respects of image findings with overlaps often observed among them but without specific signs, which predisposes its diagnosis to the great difficulties, thereby resulting in the potential delay in treatment due to the misdiagnosis to be tuberculosis or infections induced by other stains or missed diagnosis, or potential overtreatment due to the misdiagnosis to be malignancies such as lung cancer [68].

Features of image finding of fungal infection include: (1) acute phase: pneumonia shadow (possibly segmental or non-segmental, or patchy); or miliary (hematogenous) nodules,

[4]Wei He is the corresponding author for the Sect. 14.4.

which are found in patients with immunosuppression; (2) recovery phase: the nodular lesion containing or not containing cavity and crescent sign; (3) chronic phase: calcification may appear in chest image findings in some of the fungal infection (such as histoplasmosis); and (4) disseminating diseases (spreading to other organs), which occurs mainly in patients with immunosuppression [69].

Image finding of CT scans of pulmonary mycosis, based on morphology of lesions, can be categorized into mass- or nodule-predominant type, aspergilloma type, cavity type, and pneumonia type (manifesting dominantly as pulmonary consolidations and ground glass opacities) [68–70]. Now, shadows of nodules or masses with its halo sign are considered to be manifestations with specificity in early phase for pulmonary mycosis. The halo sign, however, may also occur in other lesions, such as bacterial infection, granulomatous lesions, and even some malignant lesions, due to their potential peripheral vascular exudation or hemorrhage, or local infiltration by malignant cells. Therefore, the diagnostic value of this sign should be differentiated by closely combining clinical history and relevant examinations [71]. Image findings of CT scans for pulmonary inflammation manifest as irregular patchy and wedge-shaped consolidations differing in size and morphology with blurred or clear border, which are commonly observed in sub-pleura region. The lesions may fuse into honeycomb-shaped or geographic consolidations, which can involve multiple pulmonary segments or lobes, seeming like the manifestations of segmental or lobar pneumonia and may can coexist with nodules or masses and their "halo sign." The pathological basis for the formation of wedge-shaped consolidation is the hemorrhagic pulmonary infarction of small segments caused by invasion of pulmonary arterioles by fungi [72]. Wedge-shaped consolidation, as reported by literature, is a characteristic change in the early phase of invasive pulmonary aspergillosis and has an incidence as high as 80%, higher than that of "halo sign." Aspergilloma is a relatively characteristic change in pulmonary fungal infection.

Thin-layer CT scans with its image finding combined with MPR images are superior to ordinary CT scans in displaying CT signs such as halo signs, ground glass opacities, grids, linear shadows, and small nodules ($P < 0.05$) and conducive to diagnosis of pulmonary fungal infections [70]. Halo sign, crescent sign, and cavitation inside the consolidation, though considered as characteristic manifestations of pulmonary fungal infection based on diagnostic criteria formulated by European Organization for Research on Treatment of Cancer and Mycology Study Group (EORTC/MSG) [73], are not frequently observed in clinical practice, while pulmonary nodules and ground glass opacities are also common manifestations in CT scans [74].

Finding in chest CT scans seems complicated in AIDS patients with concurrent pulmonary mycosis, and their common manifestations include multiple nodules, cavities, consolidations, and ground glass opacities in both lungs [75].

14.4.3 Main Image Findings in Fungal Infections [68]

1. Pulmonary infections induced by different fungi, such as Aspergillus, Candida, Cryptococcus, mucor, Pneumocystis jiroveci, and Actinomycetes, differ in the image findings.
   (a) Pulmonary aspergillosis: It is a group of acute/chronic pulmonary diseases induced by Aspergillus infection or by Aspergillus antigen inhaled and includes allergic aspergillosis, parasitic aspergillosis, and invasive pulmonary aspergillosis (IPA). Aspergillus fumigatus is the most common one that causes pulmonary aspergillus infection, while aspergillus flavus and mucor are uncommon. Aspergillus is distributed extensively in nature and exists in necrosis of organic substances, moldy grains, forages, water, soil, cloths, and furniture. Aspergillus is a conditional pathogenic fungus.

   Pathological changes mainly include acute extensive necrotic pneumonia, eccyesis, and formation of granuloma consisting of epithelial cells and macrophages. Aspergillus hypha proliferating in pulmonary tissue and invading into blood vessels may cause necrotizing vasculitis and bacterial thrombotic hemorrhage, thereby resulting in hematogenous dissemination of Aspergillus. Other histopathological reactions include parenchyma nodular damages, bronchial granulomatous damages, and invasive tracheobronchial inflammation. Image findings include multiple pulmonary nodules (40%) which have the halo shadow (representing pulmonary hemorrhage) with the specificity. Fifty percent of the nodules may form cavities within two weeks and the air crescent sign may appear, which means the advent of the recovery phase of the disease, implying the raised reactivity of granulocytes. It is noteworthy that air crescent sign may also occur in pulmonary tuberculosis, infections induced by actinomycetes or mucor, infectious embolus and tumor. Other signs, meanwhile, should be paid attention to, such as parabronchial shadows and focal pulmonary consolidations [70].

   Acute invasive pulmonary aspergillosis: Chest X-ray shows wedge-shaped shadows, patchy infiltrating shadows, solitary or multiple nodules, etc., with cavities formed inside the lesions, while pleural effusion is rare. Characteristic changes can be found by chest CT, including halo sign in the early phase of the disease (about within one week). This refers to a circular ground glass opacity surrounding the lesions, which is induced by edema or hemorrhage at the circumference of the lesions, followed by the wedge-shaped shadow occurring later (about one week later) with its bottom side adjacent to the pleura and its tip directing toward hila, seeming similar to pulmonary infarction induced by pulmonary vascular embolism. Air crescent sign occurs later (in week 2 or 3), manifesting as a crescent transparent area emerging within the pre-existing lesion, which is commonly observed in neutrophil recovery phase in patients with immunosuppression and induced by the contraction of the infarct focus. Aspergillus can be formed in the lesion in the advanced phase. Acute invasive pulmonary aspergillosis progresses rapidly and usually shows an obvious increase in size of the lesions within a few days, which is also one of characteristic imaging findings.

Chronic necrotic pulmonary aspergillosis, observed commonly in the middle-aged and old people, shows unilateral or bilateral pulmonary infiltrative lesions or nodules on its chest image findings, which have irregular borders and emerge in most cases in dorsal segments of the lower lobes and the upper lobes, complicated with or without cavitation. Fifty percent of patients with cavities have aspergilloma and often exhibit thickening at the adjacent pleura.

Airway invasive pulmonary aspergillosis, commonly observed in patients with neutropenia and AIDS patients, has the following clinical manifestations and image findings:

(1) Acute tracheobronchitis: Findings in chest X-ray are normal in most cases, with increased lung markings occasionally observable. (2) Bronchiolitis, which manifests as centrilobular nodule and "tree-in-bud sign" in HRCT. (3) Bronchopneumonia: small patchy consolidation is observable in pulmonary peripheral regions distributed with bronchioles. (4) Obstructive bronchopulmonary aspergillosis, which shows a cloddy growth of aspergillus in the lumen, with other manifestations similar to ABPA, including its predilection sites in the lower lobes and complications such as bilateral bronchiectasis, a large amount of mucoid impaction, and atelectasis caused by bronchial obstruction.

(b) Parasitic pulmonary aspergillosis: Aspergillus can invade pulmonary lesions with cavities inside and cystic bronchodilation, while the hyphae proliferates to form clumps, which become characteristic aspergillomas. The pulmonary parenchyma surrounding the cavity is rich in blood vessels and may form hemangioma. There is hyperplasia of granulation on the cavity wall, accompanied by infiltration with chronic inflammatory cells and inflammatory reactions in pulmonary parenchyma around the cavity. Additionally, there is obvious thickening commonly seen at the adjacent pleura. Image findings of chest X-ray of pulmonary aspergilloma are characterized by uniform opacity, with a circular or semi-circular transparent region in its upper part, indicating the presence of air crescent sign (Monod Sign). The appearance of the image may vary depending on changes in body posture. The typical lesion occurs in upper lobes [70]. Chest CT scans not only show the typical aspergilloma, but also manifest as a spongy structure composed of cavities and lumens without an air crescent sign. At this time, the aspergilloma is fixed. CT scans can also identify the aspergilloma which is immature or forming, so it can show the rough and disordered network structure of irregular air chamber, which will subsequently fuse gradually to form the mature typical aspergilloma or remain in the stage of network structure without further development.

(c) Allergic bronchopulmonary aspergillosis (ABPA): ABPA is characterized by immune response to Aspergillus fumigatus antigen existing in bronchial branches, which results in pulmonary infiltration and proximal bronchiectasis. Allergic bronchopulmonary aspergillosis, a relatively common type of eosinophilic pneumonia, has an allergic pathogenesis rather than an infectious one, with its lesions located in bronchi and lungs. The main allergen is Aspergillus, with Aspergillus fumigatus being the most common one. ABPA involves type-I and type-III hypersensitivities. Lung infiltration, tissue damage, or central bronchiectasis is caused by damages induced by IgG antibody against Aspergillus fumigatus produced through chronic and continuous stimulation by Aspergillus fumigatus and its antigen, as well as damages induced by protease secreted by Aspergillus fumigatus.

Nonspecific image findings include pulmonary infiltration, atelectasis, emphysema, fibrosis, pulmonary lobar contraction with pulmonary vacuoles, and pneumothorax. Pulmonary infiltrations commonly observed or with the earliest occurrence shown by chest X-ray are distributed in homogeneous patches, which are usually temporary, recurrent, transitional, more common in the upper lobes, and occasionally extending the whole lungs, with variable size of their infiltration. Their dissipation is promotable by oral corticosteroids. Other potential diseases should be considered, if the infiltration never dissipates at the same site, or even expands. The presence of infiltration indicates the activity of the disease. The recurrent infiltration at the same site suggests the potential central bronchiectasis might have occurred there. Atelectasis is also more common and may involve any one of the pulmonary lobes. Specific changes in image findings of central bronchiectasis include central bronchiectasis at the proximity and the normal distal end, which is different from peripheral bronchiectasis caused by infection. Central bronchiectasis exists in ABPA and cystic fibrosis, but has not been observed in any other diseases. Cystic fibrosis, however, is extremely rare in China. Therefore, it should generally be considered as ABPA, once central bronchiectasis occurs. Image findings of Chest X-ray shows characteristic parallel lines, circular shadows, bands or toothpaste like-shadows and fingerstall shadow. HRCT is a sensitive and specific method for diagnosing bronchiectasis.

2. Bronchopulmonary candidiasis: The pathogenic bacteria are mainly Candida albicans, followed by Candida tropicalis and Candida chrysotile. In case of the primary or secondary reduction or dysregulation of immunity occurs or in the background of pre-existing lesions of bronchi and lungs, the Candida in the cavity and upper respiratory tract can invade the respiratory system and cause infection, without specificity in image findings [75]. Bronchopulmonary candidiasis can be divided clinically into three types: bronchitis type, which shows increase in bilateral lung markings in middle and lower lung fields in image findings of chest X-ray; bronchopneumonia type, which shows diffusive punctiforms, small or large patches in middle and lower fields of both lung; and pneumonia type including primary Candida pneumonia and secondary Candida pneumonia, which manifests as punctiform shadows, irregular patches, and fused extensive consolidations in middle and lower parts of both lungs in its image findings with lesions rarely observable in apical part of lungs, but with occasionally cavities or pleural effusion and possibly hilar lymphadenectasis. Image findings in chest X-ray for secondary Candida pneumonia may be negative, especially in patients receiving immunosuppressant treatment, while the imaging findings in a few patients show pulmonary interstitial lesions, as well as miliary shadows or and a tendency of fusion. G test is conducive to the diagnosis, though it is not capable of differentiating invasive Candida from Aspergillus infection [68].

3. Pulmonary cryptococcosis: Cryptococcus neoformans invades mainly the central nervous system and lungs, often occurring in patients with low immune function such as those suffering from malignant tumors, leukemia or lymphoma, or those exposed to high-dose glucocorticoids or chemotherapy. Cryptococcus neoformans is round or oval in the tissue, with a diameter of 4–6 um. The cell is surrounded by a broad and thick capsule and does not form hyphae or spores. It exists mainly in soil and pigeon dung and can also be found in air, fruits, and vegetables.

   Pulmonary cryptococcosis mainly occurs in young and middle-aged male [76] and tends to affect individuals with impaired immune function. However, it is not uncommon in people with normal immunity and exists alone or simultaneously with cryptococcosis in other parts. 1/3 to 1/2 of the patients having pulmonary lesions manifest pulmonary nodules without any symptom, which are often identified in chest X-ray examination. Solitary large spherical lesions or nodular lesions are commonly observed and sometimes misdiagnosed as pulmonary tuberculosis or lung cancer. Moreover, most of the lesions are located in the peripheric zone of the pulmonary fields, and the edges of the lesions are not smooth, with long spicules and ground glass opacities. Some of the lesions have straight edges, seeming like "knife cut sign," and some of the nodules have limited thickening of blood vessel texture penetrating deeply into the lesions [14]. A few cases manifest as acute pneumonia. Imaging findings show that lesions on chest X-ray may manifest commonly as the distribution in bilateral lungs or in unilateral lung or are confined to a certain pulmonary lobe with various appearances [68, 77, 78]: (1) solitary mass, measuring 2–7 cm in diameter. (2) Solitary or multiple nodules. (3) Solitary or multiple patches, about 10% of these patients have cavitation, which is often the secondary pulmonary cryptococcosis. (4) Diffuse miliary shadows. (5) Acute interstitial pneumonia, which is rare. A mixture of various manifestations may coexist. Calcification and caseous necrosis are rare among all types, while cavity, pleural effusion, and lymphadenectasis are rare as well. The lesions are mostly located in the sub-pleura region, accompanied by halo sign, proximal air bronchogram, thin-walled cavity and the septum inside the cavity, with a relatively homogenous moderate enhancement, without significant necrosis [76].

4. Pulmonary mucormycosis: It rarely occurs with nonspecific symptoms. Chest image finding may show solitary or multiple infiltrations or nodules, sometimes with wedge-shaped changes. The predisposing sites are mostly the upper lobes, and both lungs can be involved simultaneously. Lesions rarely occur in lower lobes [79]. Interstitial pneumonia or tumor-like changes, either sin-

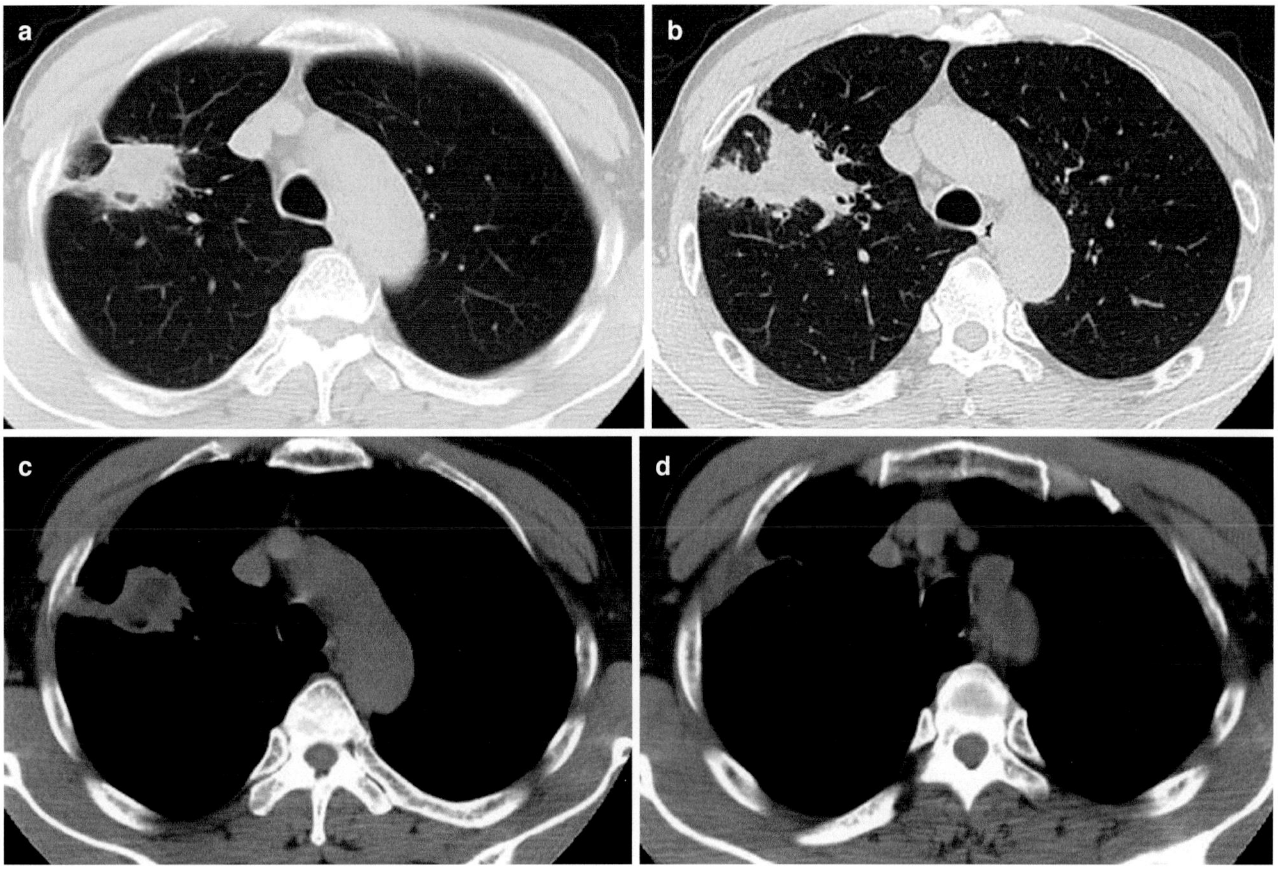

Fig. 14.8 (**a**–**d**) A 55-year-old male, with actinomycete infection confirmed by puncture pathology. (**a**, **b**) The lung window of chest CT scans shows irregular patchy shadows in the upper lobe of the right lung. There are nodular lesions linearly connected with the adjacent pleura and surrounded by patchy, cord-like and punctiform high-density opacities. (**c**, **d**) The mediastinal window of chest CT shows the heterogeneous density of nodules, with the shadows observable in liquefaction density and the formation of small cavities, and the adjacent pleura is thickened

gle or multiple, can be observed in some of the patients, while halo sign, crescent sign, and cavity may also occur. Lesions exhibit blurred edge after contrast enhancement, with occasional pleural effusion observed. Hypoxemia may occur clinically, in case of a large thoracic lesion.

5. Pneumocystis jiroveci pneumonia (PJP): It is an opportunistic fungal infectious disease in respiratory system caused by Pneumocystis jirovecii. This bacteria can parasitize in the alveoli of healthy human being, usually in the form of cysts and trophozoites, and can be removed out of body through the combined action of cellular immunity and activated phagocytes. Only when the immune function is low and the ability to remove this bacteria is reduced, its proliferation in large amount in alveoli may occur, and inflammatory reaction in the host will damage alveoli-capillary surface, thereby causing inflammatory exudation in the alveoli. Typical image findings shown by chest X-ray include ground glass opacities or grid shadows distributed diffusively in both lungs or near hila, which can progress into consolidations. Lesions shown by CT or HRCT manifest as scattered or diffusely distributed ground glass opacities or consolidations, with interlobular septal thickening [80]. About 1/3 of the patients may have solitary or multiple shadow(s) of thin-walled cysts, which can appear in any lobe or segment of the lungs with upper lobes as the predisposing sites, and pneumothorax may occur concurrently. Atypical manifestations include segmental or lobar consolidations, focal nodules with or without cavitation. Pleural effusion and hilar/mediastinal lymphadenectasis are extremely rare.
6. Pulmonary actinomycosis: Its CT manifestations vary along with the progression of the lesions, with a great diversity. Lesions are commonly located near the peripheral lobar zone adjacent to the pleura (Fig. 14.8) and often manifest as patchy pulmonary inflammatory infiltration, multiple nodular irregular dense opacities (but solitary nodule is extremely rare), shadows of tumors, and even cavitation [81], in the initial and progressing stages. Pulmonary actinomycosis has the manifestation similar

to that of bacterial pneumonia, pulmonary abscess, pulmonary tuberculosis or peripheral lung cancer, so its misdiagnosis rate is extremely high. The disease progressing to the advanced stage may invade the pleura to cause pleurisy or empyema and also invades mediastinum and chest wall, resulting in abscess and rib osteomyelitis. The manifestation has a certain specificity, based on which the possibility of actinomycete infection in lungs should be considered, when there is complication of rib destruction and formation of fistula in chest wall, especially when sulfur particles are found in the fistula. In addition, sulfur granules may also be found in the sputum of patients, but histological and microbiological examinations are required to confirm the diagnosis.

14.4.4 Differential Diagnosis Based on Image Findings Between Drug-Resistant Pulmonary Tuberculosis and Fungal Pneumonia

1. The differential diagnosis for lesions manifesting as solitary nodules or masses: Tuberculomas are often located in the dorsal segments of the upper and lower lobes, with surrounding satellite foci and calcifications. Nodules or masses in fungal pneumonia are mostly located in subpleura regions, with cavities and halo signs observable, but pleural depression sign is extremely rare, generally without hilar or mediastinal lymphadenectasis [70].
2. Differential diagnosis of diffuse pulmonary fungal infection and pulmonary tuberculosis: Pulmonary tuberculosis, located bilaterally in upper lobes and the dorsal segments of the lower lobes in most cases, is positive in sputum tubercle bacillus. Image findings manifest dominantly as patchy and punctiform disseminating foci, and commonly as cavities, calcifications, and fibrous cords, which show responsiveness to antituberculosis treatment. Diffuse fungal infection, however, often has concurrent underlying diseases and manifests dominantly as nodules, masses, and consolidations, which do not respond to antituberculosis treatment.

   Pulmonary cryptococcosis (PC) is easily misdiagnosed as bacterial negative pulmonary tuberculosis if there is the coexistence of multiple patches, nodules, and masses. Cryptococcosis has larger number of cases identified during health examination, less cases with symptoms including cough, expectoration, fever and fatigue, and no great difference in cases with symptoms including hemoptysis, chest pain, night sweat, and weight loss, as compared with pulmonary tuberculosis. The sites where lesions occur, as shown by image findings, are significant in differentiating pulmonary tuberculosis from PC. The predisposing sites of PTB are still the posterior segment of the upper lobes and the dorsal segment of the lower lobes, and the multiple lesions diffusively and bilaterally distributed are dominantly observed in both upper lungs, compared to PC which shows no such rule in lesions distribution. Ground glass opacity (halo sign) surrounding lesions or in neighboring pulmonary fields occurs in 40% of PC lesions, as reported by literature, though sometimes it is difficult to distinguish it from the intra-pulmonary congestion post to hemoptysis. In addition, cryptococcal antigen latex agglutination test is a highly specific method for diagnosing cryptococcus infection and also an effective approach for differentiating PC from other diseases. Given the low positive rate of sputum culture, however, suspected cases should undergo latex agglutination test as early as possible, and sputum test and fiberoptic bronchoscopy should be repeated, with pathological examination necessitated to confirm the diagnosis [78].
3. Differential diagnosis of cavity: Cavities of tuberculoma are mostly located in the hilum, with "satellite foci" often observed surrounding the lesions. The predisposing sites include pulmonary apex and the dorsal segment of the lower lobes. The shadow of movable nodules seen in the cavity is not a unique sign of pulmonary aspergillosis, and it is observable sometimes in case of necrotic substances in lung abscess, fissure-like cancerous cavities, and accumulation of tuberculoma lysate with cavities. However, when the "halo sign" appears in its peripheries, potential fungal infection is first considered [82].

   The incidence rate of cavity morphology, including honeycomb or air crescent sign, partitions inside the cavity, smooth interior wall and morphological consistency in case of multiple cavitations, is higher in fungal infection than in tuberculosis. On the contrary, the incidence of classic distribution of cavities, eccentric cavity, bronchial involvement around the cavity, and time for cavity absorption or closure >6 months is higher in pulmonary tuberculosis than in pulmonary fungal infection. There is no obvious difference between fungal infection and pulmonary tuberculosis concerning data of cavities, such as their size, number, thickness of its wall, morphology, and enhancement [82].

   Based on results of logistic regression analysis on signs of pulmonary fungal cavity and pulmonary tuberculosis cavity, three indexes including bronchial involvement, consistent cavity morphology, and the duration >6 months for absorption of the cavity favor the diagnosis of the cavity in pulmonary mycosis, while bronchial involvement with absorption time >6 months favors the diagnosis of tuberculosis cavity [82].

Small cavities or vacuoles and residual bronchial shadows can be observed in lesions induced by actinomycetes, and the vacuoles are often suspended inside lesions without the formation of a liquid level. This is due to the presence of immovable necrotic tissues, actinomycetes and sulfur particles around the vacuoles, which can be distinguished from other lesions with cavitation [81].

4. Differentiation between pulmonary fungal infection and pulmonary tuberculosis based on main signs: Differentiation was performed, as shown by literatures [82], in 36 patients with pulmonary fungal infection from lung cancer and pulmonary tuberculosis based on main signs including superficial/deep lobulation, air bronchogram, short/long spurs, vacuoles and halo sign, all of which except for vacuoles showed that the incidence obviously is lower in tuberculosis cohort than in fungal infection cohort, while there are higher incidence of satellite foci, calcification, and obvious lymphadenectasis observed in the tuberculosis cohort compared to the fungal infection cohort ($P < 0.05$). The added value of enhanced CT scans demonstrated a statistically significant difference ($P < 0.05$) between the cohort with pulmonary fungal infection and the tuberculosis cohort.

   Image findings show a great diversity in fungal infection, and the diagnosis of pulmonary mycosis can be confirmed based on "crescent sign" typical of aspergilloma, while ground glass opacity and "halo sign," if present, are characteristic manifestations of fungal infection. Moreover, multiple lesions in both lungs with greatly diverse signs and rapid evolution suggest the possibility of fungal infection.

5. Differentiation diagnosis of patients manifesting diffusive miliary nodules: An analysis by Jinxin Liu et al. [31] of 112 AIDS patients with single pathogenicity with concurrent diffusive miliary pulmonary nodules showed that Mycobacteria tuberculosis and fungi were the most common, suggesting that a certain difficulty existed in the differentiation diagnosis for these nodules if based solely on morphology and size, and considering accompanying signs may offer help to differentiation diagnosis. The types of distribution of diffusive miliary nodules in infections with Mycobacteria tuberculosis included random distribution (n = 47) and centrilobular distribution (n = 18), with 8 cases exhibiting coexisting random-centrilobular distribution. The types of distribution of diffusive miliary nodules in fungal infection included random distribution (n = 36) and centrilobular distribution (n = 16) which included 7 cases of coexisting random-centrilobular distribution. The types of distribution of diffusive miliary nodules in bacterial infection included 10 cases of centrilobular distribution. χ^2 test on image findings about accompanying signs shown by chest and abdomen CT scans between Talaromyces marneffei infection and pulmonary tuberculosis suggested diffusive miliary pulmonary nodules with pleural effusion correlated closely to AIDS complicated with infection of Mycobacteria tuberculosis ($n = 31$) and was also observed in 5 cases with Talaromyces marneffei infection (χ^2 = 14.024, $P < 0.01$). Diffusive miliary nodules with mesenteric lymphadenectasis correlated closely to Talaromyces marneffei infection (n = 5) and were also observed in 5 cases with Mycobacteria tuberculosis infection (χ^2 = 23.015, $P < 0.01$).

6. Differentiation diagnosis between pulmonary aspergilloma and tuberculoma. Both pulmonary aspergilloma and tuberculoma shown by chest X-ray are more common in the upper pulmonary fields. Pulmonary aspergilloma is spheroidal or oval, while tuberculoma is round or ellipse (Fig. 14.9). Pulmonary aspergilloma usually has a crescent transparency over its uniform-density sphere, but the sphere may change along with posture change. Tuberculoma are commonly uneven with calcification and cavitation. The border of pulmonary aspergilloma is clear or slightly rough, while the border of tuberculoma is generally clear [83].

In conclusion, drug-resistant pulmonary tuberculosis and fungal infections often occur concurrently, with certain similarities in their clinical features and image findings, despite having specific features in their own image findings. The

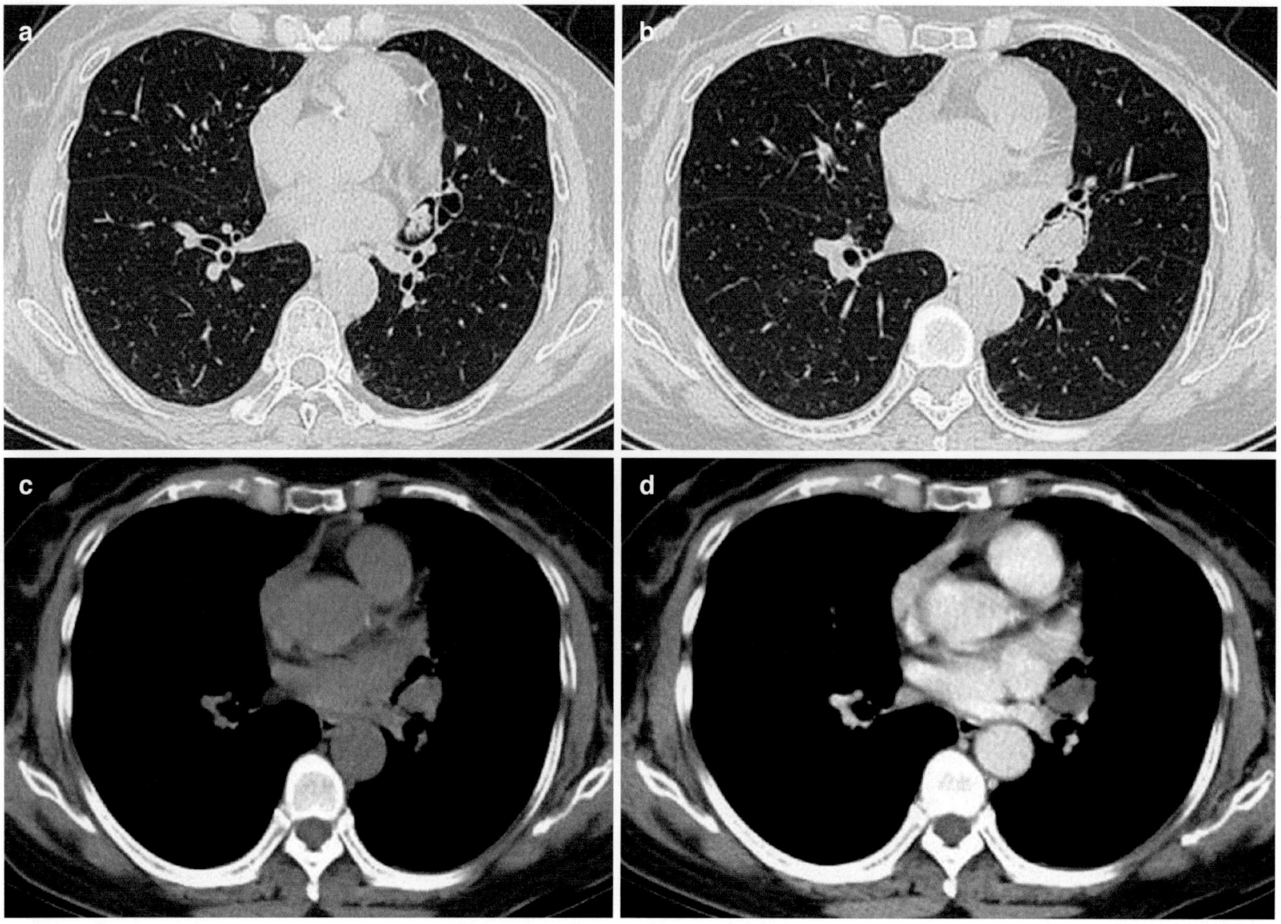

Fig. 14.9 (**a**–**d**) A 70-year-old female with pulmonary aspergilloma. (**a**, **b**) Lung window of chest CT scans shows multiple shadows of pneumatocele, with nodular high-density shadows inside. (**c**) Mediastinal window of chest CT scans shows the mean CT value of nodules inside pneumatocele is about 31 HU, (**d**) No obvious enhancement is shown by contrasted scans, without obvious mediastinal lymphadenectasis. Post-operative pathology: consistent with bronchiectasis complicated with Aspergillus infection

possibility of concurrent fungal infection should be considered, when drug-resistant pulmonary tuberculosis responds poorly to treatment or image findings evolve rapidly. A correct diagnosis can be made by combining the results of other laboratory tests or etiological examinations, and a pathological test may be necessary to confirm the diagnosis.

References

1. Xie Z, Li H, Song M, et al. A comparative analysis of CT image findings of non-tuberculous mycobacterial pulmonary disease, active pulmonary tuberculosis and multi-drug resistant pulmonary tuberculosis [J]. J Med Imaging. 2020;30(12):2224–7.
2. Wang D, Li Y, Wei Y, et al. A meta analysis of clinical features and image findings of non-tuberculous mycobacterial pulmonary diseases and pulmonary tuberculosis [J]. Pract Clin J Integr Trad Chin Western Med. 2021;21(16):1–4.
3. Lin A, Yang X, Liu G, et al. A discussion on misdiagnosis of non-tuberculous mycobacteria pulmonary diseases [J]. Clin Misdiagn Misther. 2016;29(9):8–10.
4. Tingshan Y, Shen X, Long X, et al. A comparative analysis on CT image findings between non-tuberculous mycobacteria pulmonary diseases and multi-drug resistant pulmonary tuberculosis [J]. Tianjin Med J. 2017;45(6):628–31.
5. Li C, Sun C, Jin W. A comparative analysis of image findings of chest CGT scans between non-tuberculous mycobacteria pulmonary diseases and multi-drug resistant pulmonary tuberculosis [J]. Clin Focus. 2021;36(6):530–4.
6. Qin Z, Ma G. More attention should be paid to non-tuberculous mycobacteria pulmonary diseases [J]. Chin J N Clin Med. 2021;14(1):13–8.
7. Dong X, Chen H, Hong J, et al. Characteristics of thin-layer CT scans of multi-drug resistant secondary pulmonary tuberculosis [J]. Chin J Clin. 2013;7(21):9494–7.
8. Tian J, Bang X, Li Y, et al. A comparative study on CT image findings between non-tuberculous mycobacteria pulmonary diseases and active pulmonary tuberculosis [J]. J Youjiang Med Univ Natl. 2020;42(3):294–8.

9. Chen B, Chen H, Yanni D, et al. Expert consensus on imaging diagnosis of non-tuberculous mycobacterial pulmonary disease [J]. J Chin Res Hosp. 2021;8(3):1–6.
10. Kahkouee S, Esmi E, Moghadam A, et al. Multidrug resistant tuberculosis versus non-tuberculous mycobacterial infections: a CT-scan challenge[J]. Braz J Infect Dis. 2013;17(2):137–42.
11. Ellis SM, Hansell DM. Imaging of non-tuberculous (atypical) mycobacterial pulmonary infection[J]. Clin Radiol. 2002;57(8):661–9.
12. Anjos LRBD, Parreira PL, Torres PPTS, et al. Non-tuberculous mycobacterial lung disease: a brief review focusing on radiological findings[J]. Rev Soc Bras Med Trop. 2020;53:e20200241.
13. Jinwei X, Xin Z, Zhen C. Comparative analysis of CT findings between non-tuberculous mycobacterial pulmonary disease and secondary pulmonary tuberculosis[J/CD]. Electron J Emerg Inf Dis. 2020;5(2):113–7.
14. Friedland G. Tuberculosis, drug resistance, and HIV/AIDs: a triple threat[J]. Curr Infect Dis Rep. 2007;9(3):252–61.
15. Zhu Y, Zhang Z, Shi Y. Progress of imaging diagnosis of AIDS complicated with drug-susceptible, drug-resistant and extensive-resistant tuberculosis [J]. Radiol Pract. 2011;26(9):941–3.
16. Wei-ye Y, Wei-guo T, Luo Y-t, et al. 2018 WHO tuberculosis report: key data analysis for global and China[J/CD]. Electron J Emerg Inf Dis. 2018;3(4):229–34.
17. World Health Organization. Global tuberculosis report 2018[EB/OL][2018-09-18]. http://www.who.int/tb/publications/global_report/en/.
18. Zhu W, Puxian L, Yue X, et al. A comparative analysis on CT image findings and pathology in AIDS patients complicated with pulmonary tuberculosis [J]. Radiol Pract. 2011;26(9):931–3.
19. Li Y, Xia L, Jingru Z, et al. Comparative analysis of pulmonary CT findings between AIDS patients with MDR-TB and non AIDS patients with MDR-TB[J/CD]. Electron J Emerg Inf Dis. 2021;6(1):27–30.
20. Puxuan L, Weiye Y, Zhu W, et al. Image findings of AIDS and its correlation to CD4+T lymphocytes in AIDS patients complicated with pulmonary tuberculosis [J]. Chin J Tuberculosis Respir Dis. 2005;28(1):16–9.
21. Fang-jun W, Li-fei W, Guang-ping Z, et al. Imaging features of pulmonary tuberculosis in low CD4+T cell count HIV infected patients[J/CD]. Electron J Emerg Inf Dis. 2017;2(3):237–9.
22. Zhu W, Puxuan L, Weiye Y, et al. Manifestations of CT scans and its correlation to $CD4^{+}T$ lymphocytes in AIDS patients complicated with pulmonary tuberculosis [J]. J Med Imaging. 2007;15(4):256–9.
23. Ru-ming X. Imaging findings of AIDS complicated with thoracic tuberculosis[J/CD]. Electron J Emerg Inf Dis. 2017;2(3):192.
24. Kim JY, Jeong YJ, Kim KI, et al. Miliary tuberculosis: a comparison of CT findings in HIV-seropositive and HIV-seronegative patients[J]. Br J Radiol. 2010;83(987):206–11.
25. Leung AN, Brauner MW, Gamsu G, et al. Pulmonary tuberculosis: comparison of CT findings in HIV-seropositive and HIV-seronegative patients[J]. Radiology. 1996;198(3):687–91.
26. De-Chun L, Hong-Jun L. Clinical-imaging-pathological analysis of 48 cases of AIDS patients and HIV infected persons[J/CD]. Electron J Emerg Inf Dis. 2019;4(3):152–5.
27. Song Shulin L, Yibo PR, et al. Curative effect observation on anti-tuberculosis therapy for AIDS patients complicated with mediastinal lymph node tuberculosis[J/CD]. Electron J Emerg Inf Dis. 2020;5(4):253–7.
28. Zhao D, Ma D. Imaging diagnosis of AIDS complicated with pulmonary tuberculosis [J]. Chin J Med Imag Technol. 2002;18(2):147–8.
29. Xie Z, Dai F. An analysis on HRCT image findings and its correlation to CD4+T lymphocytes in AIDS patients complicated with miliary pulmonary tuberculosis [J]. Radiol Pract. 2013;28(2):150–3.
30. Song W, Zhao Z, Zhao D, et al. Image findings of AIDS complicated with disseminating pulmonary tuberculosis [J]. Chin J Radiol. 2013;47(1):13–7.
31. Liu J, Li J, Guan Y, et al. Image findings of high-resolution CT scans for AIDS complicated diffusive miliary pulmonary tuberculosis [J]. Chin J Radiol. 2013;47(11):993–6.
32. Deng Y, Liu Y. A study on tuberculosis-associated immune reconstitution inflammatory syndrome (IRIS) occurring in AIDS patients during antiviral therapy. Indian J Med Res. 2015;33(11):700–4.
33. Huang H, Puxuan L, Liu S, et al. Manifestations of chest CT scans in AIDS patients with concurrent immune reconstitution inflammatory syndrome (IRIS) [J]. Radiol Pract. 2009;24(9):955–8.
34. Yi-xiang W, Chung MJ, Skrahin A, et al. Literature analysis of radiological signs related to multidrug-resistant tuberculosis[J/CD]. Electron J Emerg Inf Dis. 2018;3(2):244–53.
35. Luyao M, Qiuting Z, Punxuan L, et al. Pulmonary multi-drug resistant tuberculosis: a radiological review [J/CD]. Electron J Emerg Inf Dis. 2021;6(1):58–65.
36. Genming C, Guan-xun C, Shao-qian Z, et al. CT scanning of mono-resistant pulmonary tuberculosis during initial treatment[J/CD]. Electron J Emerg Inf Dis. 2018;3(2):111–4.
37. Sun H, Tang S, Jin G. Image findings of chest CT scans for extensive-resistance pulmonary tuberculosis [J]. Chin J Antituberculosis. 2011;33(2):123–5.
38. Weiye Y, Tan Wei-guo L, Pu-xuan. Classification and imaging manifestations of drug-resistant pulmonary tuberculosis[J/CD]. Electron J Emerg Inf Dis. 2019;4(1):42–7.
39. Li D, He W, Chen B, et al. Primary multidrug-resistant tuberculosis versus drug-sensitive tuberculosis in nonHIV-infected patients: comparisons of CT findings [J]. PLoS One. 2017;12(6):e0176354.
40. Kim W, Lee KS, Kim HS, et al. CT and microbiologic follow-up in primary multidrug-resistant pulmonary tuberculosis[J]. Acta Radiol. 2016;57(2):197–204.
41. Chuchottaworn C, Thanachartwet V, Sangsayunh P, et al. Risk factors for multidrug-resistant tuberculosis among patients with pulmonary tuberculosis at the Central Chest Institute of Thailand[J]. PLoS One. 2015;10(10):e0139986.
42. Yan L, Li C, Xie R, et al. A study on image findings of HRCT in treatment-naïve secondary active pulmonary tuberculosis [J/CD]. Chin J Exp Clin Inf Dis. 2015;9(5):643–8.
43. Hong SH, Im JG, Lee JS, et al. High resolution CT findings of military tuberculosis[J]. J Comput Assist Tomogr. 1998;22(2):220–4.
44. Nakanishi M, Demura Y, Ameshima S, et al. Utility of high-resolution computed tomography for predicting risk of sputum smear-negative pulmonary tuberculosis[J]. Eur J Radiol. 2010;73(3):545–50.
45. Xiwei L, Wang M, Shen J. Application of tree-in-bud sign to radiological diagnosis of pulmonary tuberculosis [J]. Chin J Antituberculosis. 2004;26(5):275–9.
46. Zhao C, Zhang J, He Y. The value of thin slice scanning of multi-slice spiral CT in diagnosing active pulmonary tuberculosis [J]. Chin J Antituberculosis. 2011;33(10):671–4.
47. Ma D. Differentiation diagnosis of multiple pulmonary nodules based on high resolution CT scans [J]. Chin J Radiol. 2001;35(9):647–50.
48. Zhou X. The importance attached to analysis of CT signs in pulmonary tuberculosis [J]. Chin J Antituberculosis. 2016;38(5):339–41.
49. Heo JN, Choi YW, Jeon SC, et al. Pulmonary tuberculosis: another disease showing clusters of small nodules [J]. AJR Am J Roentgenol. 2005;184(2):639–42.
50. Fang R, Zhongzhong W, Jian W, et al. Firework sign manifested in CT scans of active pulmonary tuberculosis [J]. Chin J Radiol. 2019;53(3):196–9.
51. Junyang HZ, Zhou X, et al. CT manifestations and their pathological basis of cavitation in pulmonary tuberculosis [J]. Chin J Med Imag Technol. 2007;23(12):1831–3.

52. Im JG, Itoh H, Shim YS, et al. Pulmonary tuberculosis: CT findings–early active disease and sequential change with antituberculous therapy[J]. Radiology. 1993;186(3):653–60.
53. Beigelman C, Sellami D, Brauner M. CT of parenchymal and bronchial tuberculosis[J]. Eur Radiol. 2000;10(5):699–709.
54. Ko JM, Kim KJ, Park SH, et al. Bronchiectasis in active tuberculosis[J]. Acta Radiol. 2013;54(4):412–7.
55. Jianlin W, Shen J, Kai X, et al. Value of CT scans in diagnosing secondary pulmonary tuberculosis dominated by interstitial changes and in evaluating its responses to treatment [J]. Chin J Antituberculosis. 2012;34(4):207–11.
56. Wang D, Yang X, Yan L, et al. An analysis of characteristic dynamic mechanical changes of CT signs in early-phase of onset in tuberculous pleurisy [J]. Chin J Antituberculosis. 2018;40(7):677–81.
57. Li C, Zhao P, Shengxiu L, et al. CT image findings and its clinical correlation in 127 cases of multi-drug resistant pulmonary tuberculosis [J]. Chongqing Med. 2014;43(23):3078–80.
58. Li C, Zhou X, Yan L, et al. An analysis on CT signs in patients with various types of drug-resistant and drug-susceptible pulmonary tuberculosis [J]. Chin J Antituberculosis. 2018;40(7):707–12.
59. Gao D, Wang S, Qiu L. An analysis on image findings of chest CT scans in 86 multi-drug resistant pulmonary tuberculosis [J]. J Clin Pulm Med. 2012;17(7):1265–6.
60. Cai B, Chu N, Kang W, et al. Drug-resistance analysis and clinical characteristics in 115 cases of tuberculous destroyed lung [J]. Chin J Antituberculosis. 2012;34(6):380–3.
61. Daling Z, Yang S, Chen L. An analysis on risk factors of acquired drug-resistant tuberculosis and interventions [J]. J Bengbu Med Coll. 2018;43(8):1109–11.
62. Cheon H. Comparison of CT findings of between MDR-TB and XDR-TB: a propensity score matching study[J]. Imaging Med. 2017;9(5):125–9.
63. Kim SH, Min JH, Lee JY. Radiological findings of primary multidrug-resistant pulmonary tuberculosis in HIV-seronegative patients[J]. Hong Kong J Radiol. 2014;17(1):4–8.
64. Cha J, Lee HY, Lee KS, et al. Radiological findings of extensively drug-resistant pulmonary tuberculosis in non-AIDS adults: comparisons with findings of multidrug-resistant and drug-sensitive tuberculosis[J]. Korean J Radiol. 2009;10(3):207–16.
65. Peng S, Hou Y, Cheng S, et al. Clinical significance of mycological examinations in patients with multi-drug resistant pulmonary tuberculosis [J]. J Clin Pulm Med. 2013;18(11):2049–50.
66. Yan C, Tan X, Wei Q, et al. Lung MRI of invasive fungal infection at 3 Tesla: evaluation of five different pulse sequences and comparison with multidetector computed tomography (MDCT)[J]. Eur Radiol. 2015;25(2):550–7.
67. Cai B, Li L, et al. PUMC respirology. 2nd ed. Beijing: Peking Union Medical College Press; 2011. p. 918–39.
68. Wang G, Mao H, He H, et al. A discussion of CT radiological manifestations in pulmonary mycosis [J]. J Med Imaging. 2010;20(4):585–7.
69. Weissleder R, Wettenberg J, Mukesh G, Arisinghani, et al. Primer of diagnostic imaging. 5th ed. Beijing: Peking University Publishing House; 2016.
70. Li L, He L, Li S, et al. The value of MSCT post-processing technology in diagnosis and differential diagnosis of fungal pneumonia [J]. Radiol Pract. 2014;29(3):292–5.
71. Yan C, Yue Y, Jianbin F, et al. Diagnostic value of MSCT for pulmonary fungal diseases [J]. Radiol Pract. 2010;25(11):1228–30.
72. Leung AN, Gosselin MV, Napper CH, et al. Pulmonary infections after bone marrow transplantation: clinical and radiographic findings[J]. Radiology. 1999;210(3):699–710.
73. De Pauw B, Walsh TJ, Donnelly JP, et al. Revised definitions of invasive fungal disease from the European Organization for Research and Treatment of Cancer/Invasive Fungal Infections Cooperative Group and the National Institute of Allergy and Infectious Diseases Mycoses Study Group (EORTC/MSG) Consensus Group[J]. Clin Infect Dis. 2008;46(12):1813–21.
74. Park SY, Kim SH, Choi SH, et al. Clinical and radiological features of invasive pulmonary aspergillosis in transplant recipients and neutropenic patients[J]. Transpl Infect Dis. 2010;12(4):309–15.
75. He W, Chen W, Chen N, et al. An analysis on diagnostic value of radiology for Pulmonary candidiasis [J]. Chin J Inf Control. 2011;10(2):116–9.
76. Lan C, Weng H, Li H, et al. A retrospective analysis on 117 cases of pulmonary cryptococcosis [J]. Chin J Tuberculosis Respir Dis. 2016;39(11):862–5.
77. Lan L, Shu J, Tang G, et al. Manifestations of multi-slice spiral CT in pulmonary fungal infection [J]. J Luzhou Med College. 2015;38(6):588–92.
78. Fan L. A clinical analysis on 31 cases of cryptococcal pulmonary disease with image findings suspected of pulmonary tuberculosis [J]. J Clin Pulm Med. 2009;14(8):1049–51.
79. Pu-Xuan L, Zhou B-P. Diagnostic imaging of emerging infectious diseases[M]. Cham: Springer; 2015.
80. Jin-ming Q, Ren-hua WU. The imaging manifestations of pneumocystis jiroveci pneumonia[J]. Electron J Emerg Inf Dis. 2019;4(4):235–9.
81. Wang Z, Haixia G, Zhang H. CT manifestations in pulmonary actinomycosis [J]. Med Rec. 2014;20(9):1716–8.
82. Wang X. A study on HRCT in differentiation diagnosis for cavitation in pulmonary fungal infection and in tuberculosis and their dynamic comparison [D]. Guangzhou Med Coll. 2016;2016:1–78.
83. Qiu C, Lu P-X, Wu S-P. Pulmonary aspergillosis: diagnosis and Cases[M]. Cham: Springer; 2019. p. 27–79.

15 Treatment of Drug-Resistant Pulmonary Tuberculosis

Guo-fang Deng, Miao-na Liu, Liang Fu, Nu Zhang, Jian Zheng, Qiu-qi Chen, Chao Chen, Tong-xia Li, Shui-hua Lu, and Hong-zhou Lu

Drug-resistant tuberculosis (DR-TB) comprises mainly multidrug- or rifampicin-resistant tuberculosis (MDR/RR-TB), rifampicin-susceptible isoniazid-resistant tuberculosis (Hr-TB), and extensively drug-resistant TB (XDR-TB). Compared with drug-susceptible tuberculosis, DR-TB has more incredible treatment difficulty and challenges patients, medical practitioners, and the medical service system. The increasing burden of DR-TB is substantially threatening the global realization of WHO's strategic goal of "terminating tuberculosis." Taking Shenzhen, China, as an example, both the ratio of resistance to any drug (34.78%) and multidrug resistance rate (12.06%) in Mycobacterium tuberculosis are high there, as revealed by studies [1]. In order to further prevent DR-TB, WHO issued the first edition of the Integrated Guideline on DR-TB Treatment based on the latest and the most comprehensive evidence-based data and put forward proposals concerning treatment, administration, and care for DR-TB patients. Related policies and guidelines were renewed in June 2020, i.e., Module 4 of Integrated Guideline on Tuberculosis: Treatment of Drug-Resistant Tuberculosis, after this referred to as the Guidance [2].

G.-f. Deng (✉) · L. Fu · Q.-q. Chen · C. Chen · S.-h. Lu
Department of Tuberculosis, The Third People's Hospital of Shenzhen, Shenzhen, Guangdong, China

M.-n. Liu · J. Zheng
Department of Pharmacy, The Third People's Hospital of Shenzhen, Shenzhen, Guangdong, China

N. Zhang
Department of Pharmacy, Shenzhen Center for Chronic Disease Control, Shenzhen, Guangdong, China

T.-x. Li
Department of Tuberculosis, Qingdao Chest Hospital, Qingdao, Shandong, China

H.-z. Lu
Infectious Disease, The Third People's Hospital of Shenzhen, Shenzhen, China

15.1 Treatment of Isoniazid-Resistant Pulmonary Tuberculosis[1]

Guo-fang DengLiang Fu, Shui-hua Lu and Hong-zhou Lu

Hr-TB is defined as tuberculosis induced by a strain of Mycobacterium tuberculosis proven in vitro resistant to isoniazid and susceptible to rifampicin. Newly diagnosed Hr-TB patients undergoing standardized regimens recommended by WHO in comparison with drug-susceptible tuberculosis patients, as shown by the latest systematic review, have a higher level of treatment failure rate (11% vs. 1%), recurrence rate (10% vs. 5%), and acquired resistance rate (8% vs. 0.3%) [3], the higher likelihood for lost to follow-up (70%) and transition of drug resistances, and a higher percentage of patients with concurrent resistance to rifampicin [4]. Targeting this actuality, WHO established a Guidelines Development Group (GDG) in April 2017, which reviewed strictly the best evidence for the treatment of Hr-TB, through using for the first time the Grading of Recommendations Assessment, Developmental and Evaluation (GRADE) based on a methodology of evidence quality and recommended intensity grading, according to procedures specified by the WHO Guidelines Development Committee, provided recommendations for proper regimens in the treatment of Hr-TB and its cycles, and issued these recommendations on March 16, 2018 [5]. These recommendations supplement the WHO Guidelines on Drug-Resistant Tuberculosis Treatment 2016 and replace the previous WHO recommendations on Hr-TB treatment.

[1] Guo-fang Deng is the corresponding author for the Sect. 15.1.

P.-x. Lu et al. (eds.), *Diagnostic Imaging of Drug Resistant Pulmonary Tuberculosis*,
https://doi.org/10.1007/978-981-99-8339-1_15

15.1.1 Treatment Regimens

As for tuberculosis patients diagnosed susceptible to rifampicin (R) and resistant isoniazid (H), a treatment consisting of R, ethambutol (E), pyrazinamide (Z), and levofloxacin (Lfx) for six months is recommended (a recommendation under a specific condition, with a very low quality of evidence) [2, 6].

Remark: A fixed-dose combination (FDC) consisting of four drugs (HREZ) may be used when the approved "REZ" FDC regimen is not available to limit the use of bulk drugs, thus making the regimen HREZ-Lfx. The patient's susceptibility to fuoroquinolones should be determined before starting treatment.

15.1.2 Guidelines Implemented

1. Streptomycin or any other injection is not recommended to be added to the treatment regimen for tuberculosis patients diagnosed as susceptible to R and resistant to H [2, 7–9] (a recommendation under a specific condition, with a very low quality of evidence).
2. The regimen alternative to Lfx if it does not apply to a patient.

   6(H)REZ should be a regimen alternative to Lfx if it is not tolerable or the resistance to it occurs [10, 11].
3. A consideration of the dosage of H

   There is no clear evidence of whether the increased H dosage will benefit patients. The limited data makes it impossible to evaluate responses to high dosage of H (10–15 mg/kg/day). However, GDG discusses the modification of the dosage of H based on molecular mutation types for H resistance. Evidence from experiments in vitro suggests that the disease responses are likely to H with increased dosage in case of a specific mutation of inhA and the absence of any katG mutation. Therefore, the dosage of H can be increased up to 15 mg/kg/day. KatG mutation usually results in high resistance to H when there is no response to H despite its increased dosage [12].
4. Dosage of Lfx

   Although individual patient data (IPD) failed to obtain clear evidence to guide the dosing frequency of 6(H)REZ-Lfx regimen, intermittent or fractioned dosing should be avoided [5, 13, 14]. The dosage of Lfx is recommended to be based on body weight in case of insufficient information concerning the best dosage (remark 4).

   Remark 4: Studies that were covered by this IPD analysis related to Lfx with a usual dosage of 750–1000 mg/day, moxifloxacin (400 mg/day) or galtixacin (400 mg/day), as well as fluoroquinolones, the antiquities deemed no longer as a recommended component in a regimen for DR-TB, such as ciprofloxacin and ofloxacin. Please refer to the "WHO Frequently Asked Questions (FAQs) on Hr-TB Treatment Guidelines" for more information on dosing regimens.
5. A consideration about the prolongation of the treatment course beyond 6 months

   A prolongation of the treatment course is considered for Hr-TB patients with extensive cavitation or those with slowed-down negative conversion in sputum smear/culture. Among the latter, those with rifampicin resistance must be excluded, and those resistant to fluoroquinolones and pyrazinamide should also be excluded as well if possible, who need close monitoring and follow-up [5].
6. Monitoring and evaluation of the treatment

   Patients undergoing (H)REZ-Lfx must monitor their clinical and laboratory indicators during treatment [15]. Results of drug-susceptibility testing (DST) for rifampicin, fluoroquinolones, and pyrazinamide should be tracked in case of no response or treatment failure [16]. In order to lower the risk of acquired drug resistance, adding a single anti-tuberculosis drug should be avoided for patients with persistent positive sputum smear or culture at the end of 2 months of treatment, those responding poorly to clinical treatment, and those without recent DST results.

   Hr-TB regimen, just like any other anti-tuberculosis regimen, needs safety precautions to ensure rapid identification and correct handling of any serious adverse event. Since prolonged exposure to pyrazinamide may increase hepatotoxicity, close clinical monitoring, especially liver function tests, should be performed for all patients receiving this regimen. If applicable, the level of glutamic oxaloacetic transaminase should be monitored in all patients. Suppose it is not possible to monitor all patients undergoing Hr-TB regimen due to limited resources. In that case, it is strongly recommended to monitor high-risk patients monthly, such as those with concurrent viral hepatitis or those with a history of severe alcoholism. In addition, the correct dosage recommended for pediatric patients must be followed to prevent and treat potential toxicities of ethambutol (such as retrobulbar neuritis) in them. Early signs of ethambutol toxicity in older children can be detected by red-green discrimination tests and retrobulbar neuritis should be monitored as early as possible when appropriate in the pediatric population [17].

15.1.3 Consideration of Hr-TB Applied to Specific Populations

1. Only 2% of patients undergoing the Hr-TB regimen are children, as revealed by IPD evaluation for this population. Therefore, the response to this regimen is yet to

be evaluated in the pediatric population alone. However, because components of this regimen have always been standard drugs available for treating pediatric tuberculosis, it is plausible to apply this adult regimen to the pediatric population, in whom a guiding recommendation is formulated based on an evaluation of responses [2].

2. Although IPD analysis provides no evidence supporting the prolongation of treatment courses in patients with extensive lesions, 6(H) REZ-Lfx regimen should be extended beyond six months as appropriate for cavitary pulmonary tuberculosis and those positive persistently in sputum bacteria (culture or smear under microscopy) at the end of 3-month treatment or later based on their situation [18]. The extended courses may increase the risks of adverse events in some of the patients (please refer to "Monitoring and Evaluation" mentioned above for more information) [2].
3. Studies on responses to an extended course of anti-tuberculosis treatment have been carried out, irrespective of whether antiretroviral therapy (ART) is used, in HIV patients with concurrent drug-susceptible pulmonary tuberculosis [19]. The recurrence rate was 2.4 times higher in patients exposed to 6-month anti-tuberculosis treatment without ART than those exposed to 9-month anti-tuberculosis treatment. An extension of the regimen containing rifampicin beyond 6 months in drug-susceptible pulmonary tuberculosis patients receiving ART did not show obvious benefit [13]. Present studies available now showed that only a few patients received ART. Based on WHO guidelines, nevertheless, the first task in treating pulmonary tuberculosis patients with concurrent HIV infection is to ensure that ART should be initiated within eight weeks after the start of anti-tuberculosis treatment (regardless of $CD4^{+}T$ lymphocyte cell count) [20]. Therefore, HIV-positive patients are recommended to undergo a treatment using (H)REZ-Lfx regimen for 6 months.
4. Patients with extrapulmonary TB have no data concerning how to perform standardized treatment specific to patients with extrapulmonary Hr-TB, and regimens recommended by WHO may also be effective in these patients. The treatment for extrapulmonary TB patients should be communicated closer to infectious physicians and related specialists, and treatment duration with caring measures should be defined according to individual differences among patients [2].

15.2 Treatment of Multidrug-/Rifampicin-Resistant Pulmonary Tuberculosis[2]

Guo-fang DengQiu-qi Chen, and Tong-xia Li

Expanded indications for new full-oral regimens and new anti-tuberculosis drugs are proposed by "Module 4 of Integrated Guideline on Tuberculosis: Treatment of Drug-Resistant Tuberculosis" [2], including short-course regimens against MDR/RR-TB, the course exceeding six months using bedaquiline (BDQ), BDP used in pregnant period and BDP in combination with delamanid (DLM). The guideline focuses specifically on the initiation of effective anti-tuberculosis regimens from the point of view of public health, offering recommendations concerning full-oral short-course regimens against MDR/RR-TB, long-course regimens against MDR/RR-TB, monitoring of responses in patients with MDR/RR-TB, the initiation of ART for HIV-infected patients receiving the second-line anti-tuberculosis treatment, surgery options for MDR-TB patients during their medication, and caring and supporting measures for MDR/RR-TB patients.

15.2.1 The Short-Course Full-Oral BDQ Regimen During Treatment for MDR/RR-TB

15.2.1.1 Treatment Regimen

A 9-12-month full-oral regimen containing BDQ is recommended for patients with a confirmed diagnosis of MDR/RR-TB who meet certain conditions, i.e., previous exposure to the second-line anti-TB drugs included in this regimen of no more than one month; patients with fluoroquinolone (FQ) resistance that can be excluded; the absence of disseminated tuberculosis; and the absence of severe extrapulmonary tuberculosis [2] (conditional recommendation, with very low quality of evidence).

Based on the standardized short-course anti-tuberculosis regimens recommended by WHO, this regimen has its injection substituted for bedaquiline. It uses a combination of levofloxacin/moxifloxacin (Mfx), ethionamide (Eto), ethambutol, isoniazid (high dosage), pyrazinamide, and clofazimine (Cfz) for four months which can be extended to month 6 in case of persistent positive sputum smear at the end of month 4, followed by a 5-month treatment combining levofloxacin/moxifloxacin, clofazimine, ethambutol, and pyrazinamide. This renewal recommends conditionally a short-course treatment regimen, i.e., the regimen consists of

[2]Guo-fang Deng is the corresponding author for the Sect. 15.2.

4-6 Bdq(6m)-Lfx(Mfx)-Cfz-Z-E-Hh-Eto/5Lfx (Mfx)-Cfz-Z-E, and this new short-course regimen is recommended as the standard regimen [2].

15.2.1.2 Guidelines Implemented

1. Application to subgroups: (1) HIV-positive patients: They are suitable for this full-oral short-course regimen, but adverse reactions and drug interactions should be considered [21–24]. (2) Children: Data for children younger than 14 years are extremely limited, so it is unevaluable. However, there is no reason to reject the application of full-oral short-course protocol to the pediatric population, just as the long-course full-oral protocol applies to children over 6 years old [25]. (3) Pregnant and breastfeeding women: Adverse influences by ethionamide on embryos have been confirmed in animal experiments, so it is recommended to formulate individualized long-course regimens to treat MDR/RR-TB in pregnant and breastfeeding women [2]. (4) Extrapulmonary tuberculosis: The only available data is the data of full-oral short-course regimen in treating pulmonary TB patients complicated with mild extrapulmonary tuberculosis, which is still unevaluable in patients with disseminated tuberculosis and severe extrapulmonary tuberculosis.
2. Precautions for using full-oral short-course regimens: (1) no resistance or highly suspected resistance to any drug contained in the regimen is permitted; the full-oral short-course regimen is indicated to treat a patient with either inhA or katG mutation site as shown by genetic detection, but not to treat a patient with both; it is unevaluable because of the absence of data concerning the resistance to pyrazinamide [10]; (2) the previous exposure to any second-line drug contained in this regimen should not exceed one month, except for patients with bacteria proven susceptible to this second-line drug; (3) absence of either disseminated tuberculosis or severe extrapulmonary tuberculosis; (4) no pregnancy; (5) the age should be no younger than 6 years for children. The full-oral long-course regimens are recommended in case of any inconsistency with these conditions [2].
3. Selection of fluoroquinolones: Data provided by South Africa showed that 83% of patients used levofloxacin, and the rest used moxifloxacin. Both have similar efficacy in treating MDR, but moxifloxacin in the short-course regimen containing the injection shows a slightly higher cumulative cardiac toxicity compared with levofloxacin in the full-oral short-course regimen. Therefore, levofloxacin is prioritized by the full-oral short-course regimen. Notably, levofloxacin's musculoskeletal toxicity in children is slightly higher than that of moxifloxacin. No matter which drug is chosen, therefore, it is essential to monitor adverse drug reactions [2, 26, 27].
4. Treatment cycles: 4 months of intensive phase (sometimes extendable to month 6), followed by 5 months of continuation phase, for a total course of 9 months. The course of bedaquiline is strictly limited to six months [2].
5. Monitoring and evaluation: Monthly sputum smear microscopy and sputum culture should be done, ideally at the same time, to monitor the response to treatment. Attention should be paid to monitor the emergence of acquired drug resistance. Appropriate actions and quick reactions should be done in responding to adverse events, and recurrence should be monitored after the withdrawal of the drug.

15.2.2 Long-Course Regimens in Treating MDR/RR-TB (Table 15.1)

15.2.2.1 Treatment Regimens

The WHO Integrated Guideline on Treatment of Drug-Resistant Tuberculosis 2020 recommends standardized long-course regimens, i.e., 6 Lfx (Mfx)-Bdq-Lzd-Cfz-Cs (Trd)/12 Lfx (Mfx)-Lzd-Cfz-Cs (Trd). For an MDR/RR-TB patient requiring a long-course regimen, the regimen should contain all three drugs in Group A and at least one drug in Group B to ensure the presence of at least 4 and 3 potentially effective drugs, respectively, at the initiation of anti-tuberculosis treatment and in the subsequent treatment period post to the end of BDQ cycles. Both drugs in Group B should be contained

Table 15.1 Categorization of drugs recommended for long-course regimen against MDR-TB

Group	Drug	Abbreviation
Group A: Inclusion of all three drugs in group A (except for the drug that cannot be used)	Levofloxacin or Moxifloxacin	Lfx Mfx
	Bedaquiline	Bdq
	Linezolid	Lzd
Group B: Addition of one or two drug(s) in group B (except for the drug that cannot be used)	Clofazimine	Cfz
	Cycloserine or Terizidone	Cs Trd
Group C: Drugs in group C should be added, when drugs in group A and B cannot form a complete regimen	Ethambutol	E
	Delamanid	Dlm
	Pyrazinamide	Z
	Imipenem/ cilastatin or Meropenem	Ipm-Cl n Mpm
	Amikacin or streptomycin	Am (S)
	Ethionamide or protionamide	Eto Pto
	Para-aminosalicylic acid	PAS

in the regimen if only 1 or 2 drugs in Group A can be included. If drugs in Group A and B cannot constitute an effective regimen, drugs in Group C should be chosen for compensation [2] (conditional recommendation, with a very low quality of evidence).

15.2.2.2 Application to Subgroups

1. Isoniazid susceptible but rifampicin resistant: for TB patients with rifampicin resistance but without isoniazid resistance, an individualized long-course regimen (supplemented with isoniazid) or standardized short-course regimen can be an option, with the latter requiring the consistency with certain conditions. High-dosage isoniazid is still intended to treat isoniazid-susceptible patients or those resistant to low-dosage isoniazid but susceptible to high dosages. However, high-dosage isoniazid is not included in Group A, B, and C (unevaluable due to limited data) [2, 28]. The WHO Guideline on Multidrug-resistant Tuberculosis 2016 shows good responses in the pediatric population to high-dosage isoniazid, which can improve the treatment success rate [29].
2. Despite the fewer pediatric cases included by the meta-analysis on individual patients in 2018, WHO recommends the same treatment principle in pediatric patients as that in adults. Years of practical experience also show that the categories of drugs and their combinations are roughly the same in children as in adults. Bedaquiline is indicated for the treatment in children no younger than 5 years, and delamanid in children no younger than 3 years, as recommended by GDG. However, only 50 mg tablets are available for delamanid, and separating tablets from children may reduce efficacy [25]. Injections should be avoided as much as possible in pediatric patients, especially young children with mild diseases. It is necessary to monitor the hearing change if an injection is needed because hearing impairment will permanently affect children's linguistic ability and learning abilities. Similarly, in pediatric patients and adults, the anti-tuberculosis treatment course usually lasts 18–20 months and should be determined in also considering responses to treatment. As for pediatric patients with fewer pulmonary lesions, the course may be shortened to below 18 months.
3. Extrapulmonary tuberculosis and tuberculous meningitis: Individualized long-course regimen is also indicated for the treatment of extrapulmonary tuberculosis. The regimens can be modified as appropriate based on specific sites of lesions. Regimens against MDR/RR-TB meningitis should be formulated according to the results of strain DST and characteristics of drugs penetrating the blood–brain barrier. Levofloxacin and moxifloxacin can penetrate well the blood–brain barrier [30], while ethionamide/protionamide, cycloserine/terizidone, linezolid, imipenem-cilastatin can penetrate it as well [31, 32]. Exposure to imipenem-cilastatin predisposes pediatric patients to epilepsy, so meropenem is prioritized. High-dosage isoniazid and pyrazinamide may achieve effective therapeutic concentration in cerebrospinal fluid, and of course, the resistance to them should be determined first. Para-aminosalicylic acid and ethambutol, which can hardly penetrate the blood–brain barrier, are not considered effective drugs. Amikacin and streptomycin penetrate only the meninges in the inflammatory state. The meningeal permeability of clofazimine, bedaquiline, and delamanid remains unclear, lacking relevant investigational data [33–35]. In addition, it should be noted that the drug concentration in cerebrospinal fluid is not equal to that in the meninges or brain.
4. Pregnancy: Amikacin, streptomycin, protionamide, and ethionamide are generally contraindicated in pregnant women, for they may be teratogenetic. Based on WHO Guideline 2018 [5], the use of these drugs in long-course regimens has been decreasing. The safety of bedaquiline and delamanid applied to pregnant women still lacks data. GDG evaluated observational data in studies from South Africa on 58 pregnant patients exposed to bedaquiline in 2019 and concluded the possible correlation between bedaquiline to low birth weight without findings of any other adverse outcome [36]. Generally speaking, more research on drug safety during pregnancy is needed due to the lack of data.
5. HIV infection: Attention may be paid to the interaction between drugs, such as between bedaquiline and efavirenz [2].
6. Extensive-foci tuberculosis: The treatment courses should be determined according to responses to treatment (such as negative conversion at the end of month 2) and other risk factors influencing potentially the efficacy [2].
7. Injection: The intensifying and the consolidating periods are no longer distinguished if no injection is contained in the regimen. Even if bedaquiline, linezolid, and delamanid are only used at the beginning of the treatment, this period is no longer called the intensifying period.

15.2.2.3 Guidelines Implemented

1. Kanamycin and capreomycin are not recommended in the long-course regimen for MDR/RR-TB patients (conditional recommendation, with a very low quality of evidence).
2. LFX and MFX should be included in the long-course regimen for MDR/RR-TB patients (strong recommendation, with a moderate quality of evidence).
3. BDQ should be included in the long-course regimen for MDR-TB patients younger than 18. (strong recommendation, with a moderate quality of evidence); BDQ can be used in the long-course regimen for MDR-TB patients aged between 6 and 17 years (condi-

tional recommendation, with a very low quality of evidence).

4. Linezolid (LZD) should be included in the long-course regimen for MDR-TB patients (strong recommendation, with a moderate quality of evidence).
5. Clofazimine and cycloserine/terizidone can be included in the long-course regimen for MDR/RR-TB patients (conditional recommendation, with a very low quality of evidence).
6. Ethambutol can be included in the long-course regimen for MDR-TB patients (conditional recommendation, with a very low quality of evidence).
7. Delamanid can be included in the long-course regimen for MDR/RR-TB patients younger than three years (conditional recommendation, with a moderate quality of evidence).
8. Pyrazinamide can be included in the long-course regimen for MDR-TB patients (conditional recommendation, with a very low quality of evidence).
9. Imipenem or meropenem can be included in the long-course regimen for MDR-TB patients (conditional recommendation, with a very low quality of evidence).
10. Amikacin can be included in the long-course regimen for MDR/RR-TB patients no younger than 18 years in case of proven susceptibility to it with appropriate approaches for monitoring its adverse reactions. If unavailable, amikacin can be substituted for streptomycin under the same premise (conditional recommendation, with a very low quality of evidence).
11. Ethionamide and protionamide cannot be added to the long-course regimen for MDR/RR-TB unless bedaquiline, linezolid, clofazimine, or delamanid is not used, or there are no other better optional drugs to constitute the regimen (conditional no-recommendation, with a very low quality of evidence).
12. PAS cannot be added to the long-course regimen against MDR/RR-TB unless bedaquiline, linezolid, clofazimine, or delamanid is not used or there are no other better optional drugs to constitute the regimen (conditional no-recommendation, with a very low quality of evidence).
13. Clavulanic acid should not be included in the long-course regimen for MDR/RR-TB patients (conditional objection, with a very low quality of evidence).
14. The course, recommended to be 18–20 months for most MDR/RR-TB patients receiving the long-course regimen, can be modified according to responses in patients to the treatment (conditional recommendation, with a very low quality of evidence).
15. A continued treatment for 15–17 months post to negative conversion is recommended for most MDR/RR-TB patients receiving the long-course regimen. The course can be modified according to responses in patients to the treatment (conditional recommendation, with a very low quality of evidence).
16. The intensifying period is recommended to be 6–7 months for the majority of MDR/RR-TB patients receiving the long-course regimen containing AMK or SM, and the course can be modified according to responses in patients to the treatment (conditional recommendation, with a very low predicted efficacy reliability).

The safety-related guidance on extended exposure of BDQ (beyond 6 months), the combination of BDQ and DLM, and BDQ exposure during pregnancy are provided in the part of individualized long-course regimens against MDR/RR-TB in this guideline.

15.2.3 Using Tubercle Bacillus Culture to Monitor the Responses of MDR-TB

Simultaneous usage of sputum smear and sputum culture is recommended to monitor responses to the treatment in MDR/RR-TB patients receiving the long-course regimen (strong recommendation, with moderate quality of evidence). The monthly culture is prioritized during the treatment [2, 37–39].

A persistent bacteriological conversion achieved from the positive to the negative is widely used to evaluate responses to treatment. Culture, a bacteriological tuberculosis diagnostic test more sensitive than a direct microscopic smear, also facilitates phenotypic DST. However, many logistical organizations and well-equipped laboratories are required. At the same time, culture is performed to reduce cross-contamination, ensure proper conditions for bacterial growth, and make them meet other quality standards [40]. Besides the greater requirement on resources, the attainability of its results post to a delay for weeks or months is an obvious contrast to the relative immediacy of direct microscope results. However, the latter cannot confirm the survival of Mycobacteria tuberculosis. Though capable of providing rapid and reliable diagnosis, molecular technology cannot replace culture or microscopy to monitor the condition of bacteria during treatment.

15.2.4 Initiation of Antiretroviral Therapy (ART) in Patients Receiving Treatment with the Second-Line Anti-tuberculosis Regimen

The initiation of ART as soon as possible (within 8 weeks) post to the start of the anti-tuberculosis course is recommended for HIV positives requiring the second-line regimen for treating multidrug-resistant tuberculosis, irrespective of CD4^{+} T lymphocyte cell count of them [2] (strong commendation, with a very low quality of evidence).

The strong recommendation of ART is based on the indirect evidence in active tuberculosis patients exposed to ART. Irrespective of CD4^{+}T lymphocyte cell count, ART should be initiated as soon as possible once the anti-tuberculosis treatment proceeds smoothly, preferably after 2 weeks of anti-tuberculosis treatment and no later than eight weeks of it. ART should be initiated during the first 2 weeks of anti-tuberculosis treatment [20].

15.2.5 Recommendation of Surgery for MDR-TB Patients

15.2.5.1 Recommendations

Selective pneumectomy (lobectomy or wedge excision) is recommended to be performed simultaneously, while the recommended MDR-TB regimen is used for MDR/RR-TB patients [2] (conditional recommendation, with a very low quality of evidence).

15.2.5.2 Rules of the Implementation

Pneumectomy for MDR-TB patients can only be considered on the prerequisite of good surgical facilities, well-trained and experienced surgeons, and careful patient screening.

15.2.5.3 Monitoring and Evaluation

IPD meta-analysis showed no significant difference in mortality between patients with and without surgery. There is no sufficient data from the American Epidemiological Society (AES) concerning surgical complications or long-term sequela (some may be fatal), as required by a significant analysis. Despite the unknown situation of perioperative complications, GDG believes that surgical treatment is generally beneficial.

15.3 Treatment of Extensive Drug-Resistant Pulmonary Tuberculosis[3]

Liang Fu and Guo-fang Deng

Anti-tuberculosis injection has been gradually losing its status as the center in the treatment of MDR-TB during the past decade and has been replaced by other oral drugs with better efficacy and fewer adverse reactions. In consideration of the emergence of resistance to bedaquiline and linezolid, moreover WHO organized an online expert seminar on the XDR-TB definition in October 2020 [41], reviewing the epidemiological data of XDR-TB and recommendations on its diagnosis and treatment by WHO, and offering essential modifications for the definition and treatment regimens of XDR-TB and Pre-XDR-TB.

15.3.1 Definition

WHO redefined XDR-TB due to the substitution of anti-tuberculosis injection for oral drugs and the emergence of drug resistance to bedaquiline and linezolid. The updated definition of XDR-TB is tuberculosis induced by a Mycobacterium tuberculosis strain that conforms to the MDR/RR-TB definition and is resistant simultaneously to fluoroquinolones and at least one of the other drugs in Group A (levofloxacin or moxifloxacin, bedaquiline, and linezolid). Pre-XDR-TB is defined as tuberculosis induced by a Mycobacterium tuberculosis strain that conforms to the MDR/RR-TB definition and is simultaneously resistant to any fluoroquinolones [41].

15.3.2 Treatment Regimens

The regimen consisting of bedaquiline, pretomanid, and linezolid (BPaL), also known as the BPaL (6~9BDQ+PA-824+LZD), is used for 6–9 months if conditions permit the study [2, 41] (conditional recommendation, with a very low quality of evidence).

BPaL is based on the results of the clinical trial Nix-TB conducted in South Africa [42]. This trial showed a treatment success rate close to 90% in XDR-TB patients and the MDR-TB cohort with intolerance or poor response to the treatment. The trial had a generally good safety, with advantages including fewer drugs in a combination of only three, a short course reduced from 2 years down to 6–9 months for MDR/XDR-TB treatment, full-oral administration without any injection, and convenient management for patients [2]. However, Nix-TB has deemed as a trial of a very low level of evidence by WHO and recommended to be used conditionally under conditions for implementable studies, given its nature of a single-arm, open-label, and observatory cohort trial conducted in one country (South Africa) without control.

[3]Liang Fu is the corresponding author for the Sect. 15.3.

15.3.3 BPaL Regimen Is Intended to Treat Patients Who Must Meet the Following Conditions

1. Bacteriological diagnosis of pulmonary tuberculosis, which is confirmed resistant to rifampicin and fluoroquinolones based on laboratory evidence;
2. Aged no younger than 14 years;
3. Body weight no less than 35 kg;
4. Informed consent is obtained from the patient;
5. The patient is not in the period of pregnancy or lactation and is willing to take effective contraceptive measures;
6. Not allergic to any drug contained in BPaL regimen;
7. No resistance to any drug contained in the regimen is shown by susceptibility test, or the previous exposure to these drugs lasts less than 2 weeks;
8. There is no extrapulmonary tuberculosis, including meningitis, other types of central nervous system tuberculosis, or tuberculous osteomyelitis [2, 41].

15.4 Mechanism and Clinical Application of Important New Drugs and the Recommended Drugs Against Drug-Resistant Pulmonary Tuberculosis[4]

Nu Zhang, Miao-na Liu, Jian Zheng and Chao Chen

Since the discovery of streptomycin (S) by Waksmanin in 1944 and its application to the treatment of tuberculosis [43], various types of anti-tuberculosis drugs have emerged successively and promoted greatly anti-tuberculosis medication. However, the rapid growth of DR-TB has become the biggest challenge to curbing tuberculosis [44]. The significant progress in the development of new anti-tuberculosis drugs such as BDQ, Dlm, and pretomanid (PA-824) [45, 46] boosted WHO to perfect the guideline again in 2020 and to renew DR-TB treatment regimen, which would reverse the current passive situation of DR-TB treatment dramatically and promote the implementation of the tuberculosis termination strategy quickly [47].

[4]Nu Zhang is the corresponding author for the Sect. 15.4.

15.4.1 Summary of Important New Drugs and the Recommended Drugs Against Drug-Resistant Pulmonary Tuberculosis

15.4.1.1 Summary of the Recommended Drugs Against Drug-Resistant Tuberculosis

Because of their high efficacy and good tolerance, traditional anti-tuberculosis drugs, such as rifamycins, pyrazinamide, and ethambutol, are still the first-line treatment drugs for rifampicin-susceptible drug-resistant tuberculosis when they have laboratory and clinical evidence suggesting their efficacy. However, anti-tuberculosis injections are no longer used as the first option in marketing oral drugs. At the same time, fluoroquinolones, especially levofloxacin, and moxifloxacin, have become the recommended drugs against MDR-TB because of their significant effects in treating MDR-TB. Other oral anti-tuberculosis drugs, such as linezolid, clofazimine, cycloserine, and terizidone, are still the core drugs for treating MDR-TB or XDR-TB [2].

15.4.1.2 Summary of New Drugs against Pulmonary Tuberculosis

1. **Post-market new drugs:** Since 2012, three new anti-tuberculosis drugs have been approved for marketing, including BDQ developed by Johnson & Johnson Pharmaceutical Company in the USA approved for marketing in 2012, recommended in 2013 by WHO with a limited application to a long-course regimen for MDR-TB [48], and used in more than 50 countries and regions; Dlm developed by Otsuka Pharmaceutical Co., Ltd Japan and approved for marketing in 2014 as a component in the long-course regimen against multidrug-resistant tuberculosis, with an expansion of its applicable age rang in 2016 [49]; and pretomanid (PA-824) developed by Global Alliance for TB Drug Development and approved for marketing by FDA in 2019, showing an excellent inhibitory effect on Mycobacterium tuberculosis strain in both replication and non-replication periods [50].
2. **New drugs in clinical trials:** Now there are 23 new chemical entity drugs in clinical trials, and 4 of them have their development participated by China [51]. The focus of these chemicals in present clinical trials is the exploration of new mechanisms or new targets, particularly targets of mycobacterium tuberculosis (MTB), which is conducive to a great extent to reducing potential adverse reactions of drugs in hosts. Moreover, the mechanism of immune regulation also manifests great potential advantages in addition to classical targets, becoming a critical investigation direction.

15.4.2 Main Mechanisms of Important New Drugs and the Recommended Drugs Against Drug-Resistant Pulmonary Tuberculosis

TB is a disease caused by the complex of Mycobacterium tuberculosis, among which the most common and important human pathogenic bacteria is Mycobacterium tuberculosis (MTB), and the acid resistance of its cellular wall is the main distinguishable feature. MTB cell wall is mainly composed of the core, lipopolysaccharide, and lipoarabinomannan (LAM). The core is linked covalently by mucin, arabinogalactan, and mycolic acid, which is the main component of the cellular wall and accounts for more than 50% of the total weight [52].

15.4.2.1 Drugs Influencing the Formation of Cellular Wall

1. The unique characteristics of the MTB cellular wall make it the main target in the early exploitation of anti-tuberculosis drugs. Isoniazid is the first drug discovered to act upon the cell wall of MTB. As a prodrug, it inhibits inhA (the enoyl carrier protein reductase) after being activated by the peroxidase katG. It influences the synthesis of mycotic acid, the cell wall component, to damage the cellular wall of bacteria and cause it to die due to the loss of acid resistance and hydrophobicity. KatG and inhA are the main mutated genes causing isoniazid resistance [53]. Ethionamide is a derivative of isoniazid and has a mechanism of action similar to isoniazid. Ethambutol, a drug introduced later, is an analog of arabinose acting upon arabinoglycosyltransferase (AftA) and hindering the synthesis of arabinogalactan and arabinoglycan to achieve the bactericidal effect. The common mutation point of ethambutol-resistant strain is mainly codon 306 of gene embB in the AftA coding gene [53]. Cycloserine, a derivative of D-alanine, causes cell wall defects, weakens its acid resistance, and achieves the effect of sterilization and bacteriostasis through inhibiting competitively the racemase (Ar) and synthetase (Dd) of D-alanine, which acts as biological synthetases of cell wall mucin [53]. Terizidone and cycloserine belong to phenazine derivatives with a similar mechanism of action.
2. Dlm is a nitroimidazole derivative and a prodrug. Once activated by nitroreductase Ddn, it inhibits the synthesis of methoxy mycotic acid and ketone mycotic acid, thereby affecting the formation of the cellular wall [54]. Pretomanid (PA-824) has a mechanism similar to that of Dlm, but it is shown by some studies to target also at the pentose phosphorylation pathway to result in the accumulation of pentose phosphate, thereby leading to the toxic accumulation of methyl-glyoxal and the stagnation of cell growth [55].
3. Recent years have witnessed abundant drugs in clinical trials acting to block the synthesis mechanism of the cellular wall, especially the decahydronaphthalene ribose phosphate epimerase (DprE1) that affects the synthesis of arabinan. Now four new chemical entities have entered the phase-II clinical studies, namely BTZ-04, PBTZ-169, TBA-7371, and OPC-167832 [56–59]. SQ109, one of the new ethylenediamine obtained through screening structural modifications of ethambutol [60], affects the synthesis of the cellular wall by acting upon the membrane protein 3 (MmpL3) target [61] and is superior to ethambutol concerning safety, efficacy, and tolerance.

15.4.2.2 Drugs Influencing Synthesis of Proteins

1. Drugs influencing the synthesis of proteins have a long history and include aminoglycosides applied first and linezolid which has become a hot spot in recent years. Aminoglycosides combine mainly the 30S subgroup of the ribosome, and linezolid inhibits mainly its 50S subgroup, both of which achieve bacteriostat by interfering with the synthesis of MTB proteins [53].
2. The investigation on inhibition of targets of protein synthesis is another investigational focus of anti-tuberculosis drugs, e.g., GSK3036656, one of the new boron-containing heterocyclic compounds developed by GlaxoSmithKline Pharmaceuticals having leucyl-tRNA synthetase (LeuRS) as its target, which is an aminoacyl-tRNA synthase (aaRS), a family of enzymes necessary for protein synthesis in all cells [62]. Now this compound is in a phase-II clinical trial. Meanwhile, new oxazolidinones, including PNU100480 [63] and LCB01-0371 [64], inhibit the synthesis of proteins via 23SrRNA acting upon 50S subunit and have stronger inhibition on Mycobacterium tuberculosis in comparison with linezolid. Now they are also in phase-II clinical trials.

15.4.2.3 Drugs Affecting Synthesis of Nucleic Acids

Drugs that act on nucleic acids can be categorized into two groups. One group acts on DNA and is represented by fluoroquinolones. It acts on DNA cyclooxygenase (topoisomerase II) and causes breakage of DNA strands on bacterial chromosomes, thereby inhibiting DNA replication and transcription and achieving sterilization; wherein mutation of gyrA, the encoding gene of DNA cyclooxygenase, means the occurrence of moderate or high resistance to fluoroquinolone, while the mutation of gyrB means the occurrence of a slight resistance to fluoroquinolones. The other group acting upon RNA, however, is represented by rifamycins and intervenes synthesis of DNA and proteins RNA to cause the death of bacteria through inhibiting activities of DNA-dependent RNA polymerase and therefore inhibiting transcription of mRNA. The mutation of rpoB, the polymerase-dependent encoding gene, makes MTB generate resistance to rifamycin [53].

15.4.2.4 Drugs Affecting Energy Metabolism

1. Pyrazinamide, a derivative of nicotinamide, can be converted into pyrazines acid by amidase (PZA enzyme) in MTB bacteria. At the same time, it interferes with the actions of dehydrogenase by replacing nicotinamide in MTB bacteria, hinders the use of oxygen by MTB, and affects its normal metabolism. The resistance to it is induced in case of mutation of pncA (the gene encoding PZA), which inactivates the PZA enzyme and inhibits the conversion of pyrazines acid [53].
2. **Bedaquiline** (BDQ), a diarylquinoline, kills MTB by affecting ATP synthesis of MTB by inhibiting the activity of the proton pump of the ATP synthase of MTB [65]. This new mechanism of action of **bedaquiline** (BDQ) provides a reference for developing a new generation of anti-tuberculosis drugs. BAJ-876 belongs to the analogs of **bedaquiline**, and its mechanism of action is the same as that of **bedaquiline**, except that the substitution of the naphthalene ring of **bedaquiline** for 3,5 dimethoxy-4-pyridine ring reduces the cardiotoxicity of **bedaquiline** significantly [66]. This drug is currently in a phase-I clinical trial.
3. An imidazopyridine drug Q203 developed by Qurient Company can act on the subunit QcrB of cytochrome bc1 complex and interrupt electron transmission in the respiratory chain of Mycobacteria tuberculosis, thereby affecting ATP synthesis of Mycobacteria tuberculosis and exerting its effectiveness [67]. Now this drug is in a phase-II clinical trial. At the same time, it obtained the qualification of FDA-approved orphan drug fast track for the treatment of Mycobacterium tuberculosis infection in 2015 because of its new mechanism of action.

15.4.2.5 Drugs with Other Mechanisms

AMG-634, an inhibitor of phosphodiesterase IV (PDE4), inhibits the production of tumor necrosis factor- α (TNF- α) and interleukin-12 (IL-12), manifests an inhibitory effect on interleukin-1β (IL-1β) induced by bacterial lipopolysaccharide (LPS), reduces significantly the subsequent human inflammatory reactions caused by bacterial infection. It can also achieve good clinical responses, although it does not directly kill the bacteria [68, 69]. Now a phase-II clinical trial is ongoing. The immunoregulatory mechanism of oral inhibitors is of great potential advantage in resolving drug resistance of tuberculosis, which may become an important subsequent research direction.

15.4.3 Values in Clinical Application and Precautions of Important New Drugs and the Recommended Drugs Against Drug-Resistant Pulmonary Tuberculosis

15.4.3.1 Rifamycins

Rifamycins characterized by good oral absorption, wide tissue distribution, broad antibacterial spectrum, and strong killing effect on MTB in either the reproductive or quiescent periods are still the cornerstone of treatment regimens for drug-resistant drugs rifampicin-susceptible tuberculosis.

1. A certain induction effect on liver drug enzymes can be observed in all rifamycins, among which rifampicin has the strongest induction. A weaker induction effect, however, can be exerted on liver drug enzymes by rifabutin than by rifampicin, so the latter should be selected when a combination is necessary for a drug-resistant tuberculosis patient complicated with AIDS [70].
2. Only about 17% of rifapentine is excreted through the kidneys, and there is no need to modify the dose for patients with renal failure and/or on hemodialysis.
3. The exposure to rifamycins alone generally does not induce the elevation of transaminases. However, they may cause liver injury when used for a prolonged period with the fixed-dose combination (FDC) of pyrazinamide, ethambutol, and isoniazid. Anti-tuberculosis drugs might not be suspended, and liver-protection treatment be performed under close observation if aminotransferase is less than three times the upper limit of normal value (ULN) without obvious symptoms or jaundice. However, these drugs should be discontinued and therapy of liver protection performed with close observation if aminotransferase is no less than three times the upper limit of normal value (ULN), the patient has symptom or hemobilirubin is no less than three times [71].

15.4.3.2 Ethambutol

Ethambutol has a synergistic effect with other drugs and may delay the development of resistance to other drugs. No cross-resistance is found between this product and other anti-tuberculosis drugs, and it is still the first-line drug optioned by regimens for MDR-T.

Ethambutol may cause optic nerve damage, with clinical manifestations including eye discomfort, foreign body sensation, vision abnormality, and vision loss. It should be discontinued in time if the optic nerve damage is found clinically. Additional treatment should be performed, which consists of large doses of vitamin B, nicotinic acid, compound Danshen, and zinc sulfate [71]. Moreover, the occurrence of retrobulbar optic neuritis is related to its dosage. Therefore, it should be used with caution in those with reduced renal function or renal failure because of the cumulative poisoning that it might induce in them. Attention should be paid to the check of the visual field, vision, and red-green discernibility.

15.4.3.3 Pyrazinamide

Most MDR-TB patients are complicated with chronic pulmonary inflammation. Pyrazinamide has strong antibacterial activity in the acidic environment induced by inflammation. It also has a synergistic effect with fluoroquinolones but without any cross-resistance with any other anti-tuberculosis drug. It is still the first-line drug for the treatment of MDR-TB.

Pyrazinoic acid, the metabolite of pyrazinamide, is capable of inhibiting the excretion of uric acid by renal tubules (promoting the reabsorption of uric acid), thereby causing hyperuricemia with probable manifestations including gout arthralgia and/or dysfunction. The patient's diet should be modified, food-increasing uric acid be avoided, and symptomatic treatment be given. The medication should be discontinued if necessary.

15.4.3.4 Fluoroquinolones

High generations of fluoroquinolones, the most effective drugs against MTB, can achieve satisfactory clinical responses and occupy an absolute predominance in treatment regimens for MDR-TB. Fluoroquinolones commonly used to treat drug-resistant tuberculosis include levofloxacin, moxifloxacin, and gatifloxacin. However, galtixacin may induce hypoglycemia, hyperglycemia, or new-onset diabetes, so it is not recommended as the prioritized choice [53].

1. Fluoroquinolones are concentration-dependent antibacterial drugs, and administration once a day is preferred.
2. Fluoroquinolones may cause the prolongation of QT interval, and levofloxacin has fewer cardiac toxicities than moxifloxacin [26]. Levofloxacin, therefore, is preferred in the full-oral short-course regimens.
3. Moxifloxacin is excreted less through the kidney, and a reduction of the dosage of moxifloxacin is not needed in patients with impaired renal function, including those on dialysis.

15.4.3.5 Linezolid

Linezolid has nearly 100% oral bioavailability and good permeability in tissues and body fluids. It may achieve good clinical responses in treating MDR-TB and XDR-TB, thereby becoming the first-line drug for treating MDR-TB and XDR-TB.

1. This product can cause thrombocytopenia. The blood routine should be monitored weekly within one month of exposure, followed by a re-examination once every 2 weeks, for patients prone to bleeding, having thrombocytopenia, or exposed to this product in combination with platelet-reducing drugs or exposed to this product alone for more than 2 weeks. If anemia and thrombocytopenia worsen progressively, the dosage should be reduced, or the drug should be discontinued, with blood routine closely monitored.
2. The product, having the effect of monoamine oxidase inhibitor, may raise blood pressure if it is used in combination with adrenergic drugs and may induce 5-hydroxytryptamine syndrome if it is used in combination with the 5-hydroxytryptamine inhibitor, an antidepressant.
3. This product can cause peripheral neuritis and optic neuritis and requires routine visual examination prior to treatment with monthly monitoring of visual changes during treatment when it is used in combination with anti-tuberculotic drugs having the same adverse reactions (such as ethambutol). The dosage should be reduced, or the drug should be discontinued in case of the occurrence of hypoplasia [72, 73].

15.4.3.6 Bedaquiline

Bedaquiline (BDQ) has replaced anti-tuberculosis injections and become the first-line drug in oral regimens for MDR-TB and XDR-TB because of its unique mechanism, good pharmacokinetics characteristics, and significant clinical efficacy.

1. Phase-II clinical study [74] showed that BDQ had a higher risk of death than the placebo group, and concerning it, FDA issued a "black box" warning.
2. It is contraindicated in ventricular arrhythmia patients with Q-T interval >500 ms. Monitoring of ECG should be performed during treatment with the Product while avoiding combination with any other drug prolonging Q-T interval. Manifestations of adverse heart events should be observed closely with ECG monitored when it is really necessary to use it in combination with drugs that may increase cardiac toxicity, such as moxifloxacin and clofazimine. After the syncope occurs, a clinical evaluation and electrocardiogram should be performed immediately to understand the prolongation of the QT interval.
3. The combination with CYP3A4 inducer with potent effects (such as rifamycins) or moderate effects (such as efavirenz) may weaken the therapeutic effect of the product, so this combination should be avoided during the treatment. The advantages and disadvantages should be weighed when it is combined with potent CYP3A4 inhibitors (such as protease inhibitors), and the continuous application should be at most 14 days [73].

15.4.3.7 Delamanid (Dlm)

Although its clinical experience is limited, delamanid (Dlm) as a new drug has a therapeutic effect on drug-resistant tuberculosis, which is still worthy of recognition, especially considering its advantages, including fewer drug interactions and a wide age range, which make it included in the long-term regimen for MDR/RR-TB patients [2].

More attention should be paid to cardiac toxicity during treatment, and ECG monitoring in high frequency should be performed throughout treatment, particularly for patients with risk factors and when it is combined with any other drug that may increase cardiac toxicity (such as moxifloxacin). If a prolongation >500ms of Q-T interval is observed before the first administration or during treatment, the drug should not be administered, or it should be discontinued [75].

15.4.3.8 Pretomanid (PA-824)

Despite the short duration on the market for pretomanid (PA-824), the BPaL regimen centering on pretomanid achieved good responses in South Africa [42], with good safety and advantages including exposure to fewer drugs, shorter course, full oral, and convenience for patients, making it highly anticipated in the future treatment of XDR-TB.

Regimen BPaL consisting of this product, **bedaquiline (BDQ), and linezolid may induce adverse reactions, including liver injuries, bone marrow suppression, and peripheral nerve and optic neuropathy, so attention should be paid to the monitoring of indicators such as liver function and whole blood cell count, as well as symptoms such as visual impairment** [76].

References

1. Liang F, Zhang P, Deng G, et al. An analysis of drug resistance in 3309 strains of Mycobacterium tuberculosis [J/CD]. Electron J Emerg Inf Dis. 2017;2(1):31–4.
2. WHO. WHO consolidated guidelines on tuberculosis. Module 4: treatment - drug-resistant tuberculosis treatment[M]. Geneva: World Health Organization; 2020.
3. Gegia M, Winters N, Benedetti A, et al. Treatment of isoniazid-resistant tuberculosis with first-line drugs: a systematic review and meta-analysis[J]. Lancet Infect Dis. 2017;17(2):223–34.
4. Liang F, Weiming L, Huihua Z, et al. A retrospective cohort study of clinical characteristics and treatment regimens of drug-resistant tuberculosis containing isoniazid-resistance[J/CD]. Electron J Emerg Inf Dis. 2021;6(4):306–10.
5. World Health Organization. WHO treatment guidelines for isoniazid-resistant tuberculosis: supplement to the WHO treatment guidelines for drug-resistant tuberculosis[R]. Geneva: World Health Organization; 2018. p. 1–31.
6. Fregonese F, Ahuja SD, Akkerman OW, et al. Comparison of different treatments for isoniazid-resistant tuberculosis: an individual patient data meta-analysis[J]. Lancet Respir Med. 2018;6(4):265–75.
7. Voogt GR, Schoeman HS. Ototoxicity of aminoglycoside drugs in tuberculosis treatment[J]. S Afr J Commun Disord. 1996;43:3–6.
8. Gülbay BE, Gürkan OU, Yildiz OA, et al. Side effects due to primary antituberculosis drugs during the initial phase of therapy in 1149 hospitalized patients for tuberculosis[J]. Respir Med. 2006;100(10):1834–42.
9. Bloss E, Kuksa L, Holtz TH, et al. Adverse events related to multidrug-resistant tuberculosis treatment, Latvia, 2000-2004[J]. Int J Tuberc Lung Dis. 2010;14(3):275–81.
10. World Health Organization. The use of molecular line probe assays for the detection of resistance to second-line anti-tuberculosis drugs: policy guidance[R]. Geneva: World Health Organization; 2016. https://apps.who.int/iris/bitstream/handle/10665/246131/9789241510561-eng.pdf?sequence=1.
11. World Health Organization. Rapid communication: molecular assays as initial tests for the diagnosis of tuberculosis and rifampicin resistance[R]. Geneva: World Health Organization; 2020. https://apps.who.int/iris/bitstream/handle/10665/330395/9789240000339-eng.pdf.
12. Lempens P, Meehan CJ, Vandelannoote K, et al. Isoniazid resistance levels of Mycobacterium tuberculosis can largely be predicted by high-confidence resistance-conferring mutations[J]. Sci Rep. 2018;8(1):3246.
13. World Health Organization. Guidelines for treatment of drug-susceptible tuberculosis and patient care, 2017 update[R]. Geneva: World Health Organization; 2017. https://apps.who.int/iris/bitstream/handle/10665/255052/9789241550000-eng.pdf?sequence=1.
14. Nahid P, Dorman SE, Alipanah N, et al. Official American Thoracic Society/Centers for Disease Control and Prevention/Infectious Diseases Society of America Clinical Practice Guidelines: treatment of drug-susceptible tuberculosis[J]. Clin Infect Dis. 2016;63(7):e147–95.
15. Hornik CP, Herring AH, Benjamin DK Jr, et al. Adverse events associated with meropenem versus imipenem/cilastatin therapy in a large retrospective cohort of hospitalized infants[J]. Pediatr Infect Dis J. 2013;32(7):748–53.
16. Oxlade O, Falzon D, Menzies D. The impact and cost-effectiveness of strategies to detect drug-resistant tuberculosis[J]. Eur Respir J. 2012;39(3):626–34.
17. World Health Organization. Guidance for national tuberculosis programmes on the management of tuberculosis in children[R]. Geneva: World Health Organization; 2014. https://apps.who.int/iris/bitstream/handle/10665/112360/9789241548748_eng.pdf?sequence=1.
18. Zha BS, Nahid P. Treatment of drug-susceptible tuberculosis[J]. Clin Chest Med. 2019;40(4):763–74.
19. Ahmad Khan F, Minion J, Al-Motairi A, et al. An updated systematic review and meta-analysis on the treatment of active tuberculosis in patients with HIV infection[J]. Clin Infect Dis. 2012;55(8):1154–63.
20. World Health Organization. Consolidated guidelines on the use of antiretroviral drugs for treating and preventing HIV infection: recommendations for a public health approach. 2nd ed. Geneva: World Health Organization; 2016. https://apps.who.int/iris/bitstream/handle/10665/208825/9789241549684_eng.pdf?sequence=1.
21. Brill MJ, Svensson EM, Pandie M, et al. Confirming model-predicted pharmacokinetic interactions between Bedaquiline and lopinavir/ritonavir or nevirapine in patients with HIV and drug-resistant tuberculosis[J]. Int J Antimicrob Agents. 2017;49(2):212–7.
22. Svensson EM, Dooley KE, Karlsson MO. Impact of lopinavir-ritonavir or nevirapine on Bedaquiline exposures and potential implications for patients with tuberculosis-HIV coinfection[J]. Antimicrob Agents Chemother. 2014;58(11):6406–12.
23. Svensson EM, Aweeka F, Park JG, et al. Model-based estimates of the effects of efavirenz on Bedaquiline pharmacokinetics and suggested dose adjustments for patients coinfected

with HIV and tuberculosis[J]. Antimicrob Agents Chemother. 2013;57(6):2780–7.
24. Cerrone M, Bracchi M, Wasserman S, et al. Safety implications of combined antiretroviral and anti-tuberculosis drugs[J]. Expert Opin Drug Saf. 2020;19(1):23–41.
25. World Health Organization. WHO consolidated guidelines on drug resistant tuberculosis treatment[R]. Geneva: World Health Organization; 2019. https://apps.who.int/iris/bitstream/handle/10665/311389/9789241550529-eng.pdf?ua=1.
26. Borisov S, Danila E, Maryandyshev A, et al. Surveillance of adverse events in the treatment of drug-resistant tuberculosis: first global report[J]. Eur Respir J. 2019;54(6):1901522.
27. World Health Organization. Active tuberculosis drug-safety monitoring and management (aDSM). Framework for implementation[R]. Geneva: World Health Organization; 2015. https://apps.who.int/iris/bitstream/handle/10665/204465/WHO_HTM_TB_20.15.28_eng.pdf?sequence=1.
28. Dooley KE, Miyahara S, von Groote-Bidlingmaier F, et al. Early bactericidal activity of different isoniazid doses for drug resistant TB (INHindsight): a randomized open-label clinical trial[J]. Am J Respir Crit Care Med. 2020;201(11):1416–24.
29. Harausz EP, Garcia-Prats AJ, Law S. Treatment and outcomes in children with multidrug-resistant tuberculosis: a systematic review and individual patient data meta-analysis[J]. PLoS Med. 2018;15(7):e1002591.
30. Thwaites GE, Bhavnani SM, Chau TT, et al. Randomized pharmacokinetic and pharmacodynamic comparison of fluoroquinolone for tuberculous meningitis[J]. Antimicrob Agents Chemother. 2011;55(7):3244–53.
31. Donald PR. The chemotherapy of tuberculous meningitis in children and adults[J]. Tuberculosis. 2010;90(6):375–92.
32. Sun F, Ruan Q, Wang J, et al. Linezolid manifests a rapid and dramatic therapeutic effect for patients with life-threatening tuberculous meningitis[J]. Antimicrob Agents Chemother. 2014;58(10):6297–301.
33. Akkerman OW, Odish OF, Bolhuis MS, et al. Pharmacokinetics of bedaquiline in cerebrospinal fluid and serum in multi-drug-resistant tuberculous meningitis[J]. Clin Infect Dis. 2016;62(4):523–4.
34. Tucker EW, Pieterse L, Zimmerman MD, et al. Delamanid central nervous system pharmacokinetics in tuberculous meningitis in rabbits and humans[J]. Antimicrob Agents Chemother. 2019;63(10):e00913–9.
35. Holdiness MR. Cerebrospinal fluid pharmacokinetics of the antituberculosis drugs[J]. Clin Pharmacokinet. 1985;10(6):532–4.
36. Loveday M, Hughes J, Sunkari B, et al. Maternal and infant outcomes among pregnant women treated for multidrug/rifampicin-resistant tuberculosis in South Africa[J]. Clin Infect Dis. 2021;72(7):1158–68.
37. World Health Organization. Guidelines for the programmatic management of drug-resistant tuberculosis, 2011 update[R]. Geneva: World Health Organization; 2011. https://www.who.int.
38. Kurbatova EV, Gammino VM, Bayona J, et al. Frequency and type of microbiological monitoring of multidrug-resistant tuberculosis treatment[J]. Int J Tuberc Lung Dis. 2011;15(11):1553–5.
39. Mitnick CD, White RA, Lu C, et al. Multidrug-resistant tuberculosis treatment failure detection depends on monitoring interval and microbiological method[J]. Eur Respir J. 2016;48(4):1160–70.
40. World Health Organization. Tuberculosis laboratory biosafety manual[R]. Geneva: World Health Organization; 2012. https://apps.who.int/iris/bitstream/handle/10665/77949/9789241504638_eng.pdf.
41. World Health Organization. Meeting report of the WHO expert consultation on the definition of extensively drug-resistant tuberculosis, 27-29 October 2020[R]. Geneva: World Health Organization; 2021.
42. Conradie F, Diacon AH, Ngubane N, et al. Treatment of highly drug-resistant pulmonary tuberculosis[J]. N Engl J Med. 2020;382(10):893–902.
43. Sakula A. Selman Waksman (1888-1973), discoverer of streptomycin: a centenary review[J]. Br J Dis Chest. 1988;82(1):23–31.
44. World Health Organization. Global tuberculosis report 2020 [R]. Geneva: WHO; 2020.
45. Liangzi Y, Ren Tantan F, Dong X, et al. Bedaquiline in the treatment of pulmonary drug-resistant tuberculosis: safety and efficacy[J/CD]. Electron J Emerg Inf Dis. 2021;6(4):302–5.
46. Zhao-jing Z, Wei J, Feng-min H, et al. Resistance analysis of extensively drug-resistant Mycobacterium tuberculosis isolates against linezolid[J]. Electron J Emerg Inf Dis. 2017;2(3):160–3.
47. WHO. The end TB strategy global strategy and targets for tuberculosis prevention, care and control after 2015 [EB/OL]. Geneva: World Health Organization; 2015. https://apps.who.Int/Iris/handle/10665/162760.
48. World Health Organization. The use of bedaquiline in the treatment of multidrug-resistant tuberculosis: interim policy guidance[M]. Geneva: WHO; 2013.
49. World Health Organization. The use of delamanid in the treatment of multidrug-resistant tuberculosis in children and adolescents: interim policy guidance [M]. Geneva: WHO; 2016.
50. Lenaerts AJ, Gruppo V, Marietta KS, et al. Preclinical testing of the nitroimidazopyran PA-824 for activity against Mycobacterium tuberculosis in a series of in vitro and in vivo models [J]. Antimicrob Agents Chemother. 2005;49(6):2294–301.
51. Zi-hao Z, Zhang W-x, Tian-lei L, et al. Research progress in anti-tuberculosis drugs[J/OL]. J Pharm. 2022;57(4):892–902.
52. McNeil MR, Brennan PJ. Structure, function and biogenesis of the cell envelope of mycobacteria in relation to bacterial physiology, pathogenesis and drug resistance; some thoughts and possibilities arising from recent structural information[J]. Res Microbiol. 1991;142(4):451.
53. Journal of Pharmacy. Drug-resistant tuberculosis chemotherapy guidelines (2019)[J]. China Issue Magaz. 2019;41(10):1025–73.
54. Sotgiu G, Pontali E, Centis R, et al. Delamanid (OPC-67683) for treatment of multi-drug-resistant tuberculosis[J]. Exp Rev Anti-Inf. 2015;13(3):305–15.
55. Baptista R, Fazakerley DM, Beckmann M, et al. Untargeted metabolomics reveals a new mode of action of Dretomanid (PA-824)[J]. Sci Rep. 2018;8(1):5084.
56. Makarov V, Manina G, Mikusova K, et al. Benzothiazinones kill Mycobacterium tuberculosis by blocking arabinan synthesis [J]. Science. 2009;324(5928):801–4.
57. Tiwari R, Miller PA, Cho S, et al. Syntheses and antituberculosis activity of 1,3-benzothiazinone sulfoxide and sulfone derived from BTZ043[J]. ACS Med Chem Lett. 2015;6(2):128–33.
58. Shirude PS, Shandil R, Sadler C, et al. Azaindoles: noncovalent DprE1 inhibitors from scaffold morphing efforts, kill Mycobacterium tuberculosis and are efficacious in vivo [J]. J Med Chem. 2013;56(23):9701–8.
59. Hariguchi N, Chen X, Hayashi Y, et al. OPC-167832, a novel carbostyril derivative with potent anti-tuberculosis activity as a DprE1 inhibitor [J]. Antimicrob Agents Chemother. 2020;64(6):e02020.
60. Sacksteder KA, Protopopova M, Barry CE, et al. Discovery and development of SQ109: a new antitubercular drug with a novel mechanism of action[J]. Future Microbiol. 2012;7(7):823–37.
61. Tahlan K, Wilson R, Kastrinsky DB, et al. SQ109 targets MmpL3, a membrane transporter of trehalose monomycolate involved in mycolic acid donation to the cell wall core of Mycobacterium tuberculosis [J]. Antimicrob Agents Chemother. 2012;56(4):1797–809.
62. Palencia A, Li X, Bu W, et al. Discovery of novel oral protein synthesis inhibitors of Mycobacterium tuberculosis that target leucyl-tRNA synthetase [J]. Antimicrob Agents Chemother. 2016;60(10):6271–80.

63. Barbachyn MR, Hutchinson DK, Brickner SJ, et al. Identification of a novel oxazolidinone (U-100480) with potent antimycobacterial activity [J]. J Med Chem. 1996;39(3):680–5.
64. Jeong JW, Jung SJ, Lee HH, et al. In vitro and in vivo activities of LCB01-0371, a new oxazolidinone [J]. Antimicrob Agents Chemother. 2010;54(12):5359–62.
65. Andries K, Verhasselt P, Guillemont J, et al. A diarylquinoline drug active on the ATP synthase of Mycobacterium tuberculosis [J]. Science. 2005;307(5707):223–7.
66. Sutherland HS, Tong AST, Choi PJ, et al. 3,5-Dialkoxypyridine analogues of Bedaquiline are potent antituberculosis agents with minimal inhibition of the hERG channel [J]. Bioorg Med Chem. 2019;27(7):1292–307.
67. Abrahams KA, Cox JA, Spivey VL, et al. Identification of novel imidazo[1,2-a]pyridine inhibitors targeting M. tuberculosis QcrB [J]. PLoS One. 2012;7(12):e52951.
68. Houslay MD. Underpinning compartmentalised cAMP signalling through targeted cAMP breakdown [J]. Trends Biochem Sci. 2010;35(2):91–100.
69. Guo J, Lin P, Zhao X, et al. Etazolate abrogates the lipopolysaccharide (LPS)-induced downregulation of the cAMP/pCREB/BDNF signaling, neuroinflammatory response and depressive-like behavior in mice [J]. Neuroscience. 2014;263:1–14.
70. The Treatment Committee of the Japanese Society for Tuberculosis. Clinical use of rifabutin, a rifamycin-class antibiotic, for the treatment of tuberculosis. Kekkaku. 2011;86(1):43.
71. Academic Work Committee of China Anti TB Association. Expert consensus on the clinical use of fixed dose compound of anti-tuberculosis drugs [M]. Chin J Anti-tuberculosis. 2020;42(9):885–93.
72. Tuberculosis Branch of Chinese Medical Association, Preparation Group of Expert Consensus on Linezolid in Anti-tuberculosis Treatment. Expert consensus on linezolid in anti-tuberculosis treatment [J]. Chin J Tuberculosis Respir Dis. 2018;41(1):14–9.
73. Tuberculosis Branch of Chinese Medical Association. Expert consensus on the clinical application of bedaquiline, a new anti-tuberculosis drug (2020) [J]. Chin J Tuberculosis Respir Dis. 2021;44(2):81–7.
74. Diacon AH, Pym A, Grobusch MP, et al. Multidrug-resistant tuberculosis and culture conversion with Bedaquiline[J]. N Engl J Med. 2014;371(8):723–32.
75. World Health Organization. Interim policy guidance for the use of Delamanid in the treatment of MDR-TB[R]. WHO/HTM/TB/2014.23. Geneva: World Health Organization; 2014.
76. National Association for the Prevention of Tuberculosis, Tuberculosis Prevention and Control Center under Chinese Center for Disease Control and Prevention. Recommendation of application of Pretomanid (PA-824) to the treatment of multidrug resistant tuberculosis [J]. Chin J Antituberculosis. 2022;44(1):38–43.

An Analysis of Dynamic Changes in Image Findings During Treatment of Drug-Resistant Pulmonary Tuberculosis

16

Pu-Xuan Lu, Fang-jun Wei, Dai-lun Hou, Guan-qiao Jin, Lin Li, Pei-ying Liu, Ji-li Wu, and Ming-yuan Yuan

Drug-resistant pulmonary tuberculosis has become a major challenge to public health endangering seriously the health of both patients and healthy population, due to its high infectivity, prolonged treatment cycle, low cure rate, and high mortality [1, 2]. Early diagnosis and early application of appropriate combined chemotherapy may improve effectively the cure rate and curb the transmission of this disease. The present detection of drug-resistant strains of pulmonary tuberculosis is mainly based on the isolation and cultivation of sputum Mycobacterium tuberculosis by laboratory examination, followed by the confirmed by drug sensitivity test. Also, it can be confirmed by TB polymerase chain reaction (TB-PCR) in sputum samples, by identification of strains of Mycobacterium tuberculosis, or by detection of drug resistance mutation gene of Mycobacterium tuberculosis [3]. Clinically, the diagnosis of patients can be delayed because of the prolonged cycle required by some laboratory technologies for detecting mycobacterium tuberculosis, and the negative results in both smear and culture of sputum Mycobacteria tuberculosis in some patients. Imaging examination, especially CT scans, has the great significance in the diagnosis and differential diagnosis of drug-resistant pulmonary tuberculosis, its dynamic follow-up and evaluation of responses to treatment during the process of diagnosis and treatment of this disease, because of its fast scanning and clear imaging [4]. Guidance can be offered, particularly for the clinical diagnosis of drug-resistant pulmonary tuberculosis and the formulation of precise therapeutic regimens. This involves understanding the first image findings, determining the potential advent of a new drug-resistant strain during the treatment, and appraising image findings concerning whether it occurs the immune inflammatory reaction reconstruction syndrome during the treatment against drug-resistant pulmonary tuberculosis with concurrent AIDS.

P.-X. Lu (✉)
Diagnostic Imaging, Shenzhen Center for Chronic Disease Control, Shenzhen, China

F.-j. Wei
Department of Radiology, The Third People's Hospital of Shenzhen, Shenzhen, Guangdong, China

D.-l. Hou
Department of Radiology, Beijing Chest Hospital, Capital Medical University, Beijing, China

G.-q. Jin
The Affiliated Cancer Hospital of Guangxi Medical University, Guangxi, China

L. Li · P.-y. Liu
Department of Radiology, Lin Yi People's Hospital, Shandong, China

J.-l. Wu
Department of Medical Imaging, The Fourth People's Hospital of Taiyuan, Taiyuan, Shanxi, China

M.-y. Yuan
Department of Radiology, Affiliated Zhoupu Hospital, Shanghai University of Health and Medicine Science, Shanghai, China

16.1 Analysis of the First CT Imaging Findings of Drug-Resistant Pulmonary Tuberculosis

16.1.1 Drug-Resistant and Drug-Susceptible Pulmonary Tuberculosis Share the Similar Image Findings

Drug-resistant and drug-susceptible pulmonary tuberculosis are generally similar, as far as the findings of the first CT scans are concerned [5–7]. Both of them share the main manifestations of the active pulmonary tuberculosis, including lobular-central nodules, tree-in-bud signs, ground-glass opacities, lobular/massive consolidations, nodules or masses, solitary or multiple cavities, bronchial wall thickening, and stenosis and dilation of bronchial lumen. The reason for the first pulmonary CT scan is usually a respiratory symptom such as cough and expectoration for which a patient seeks medical service in a hospital, and the image findings in lungs are similar to that of the drug-susceptible pulmonary tuberculosis (Fig. 16.1). Based on the literature [8], the presence of the extensive lesions suggestive of the initial treatment single drug-resistant pulmonary

P.-x. Lu et al. (eds.), *Diagnostic Imaging of Drug Resistant Pulmonary Tuberculosis*,
https://doi.org/10.1007/978-981-99-8339-1_16

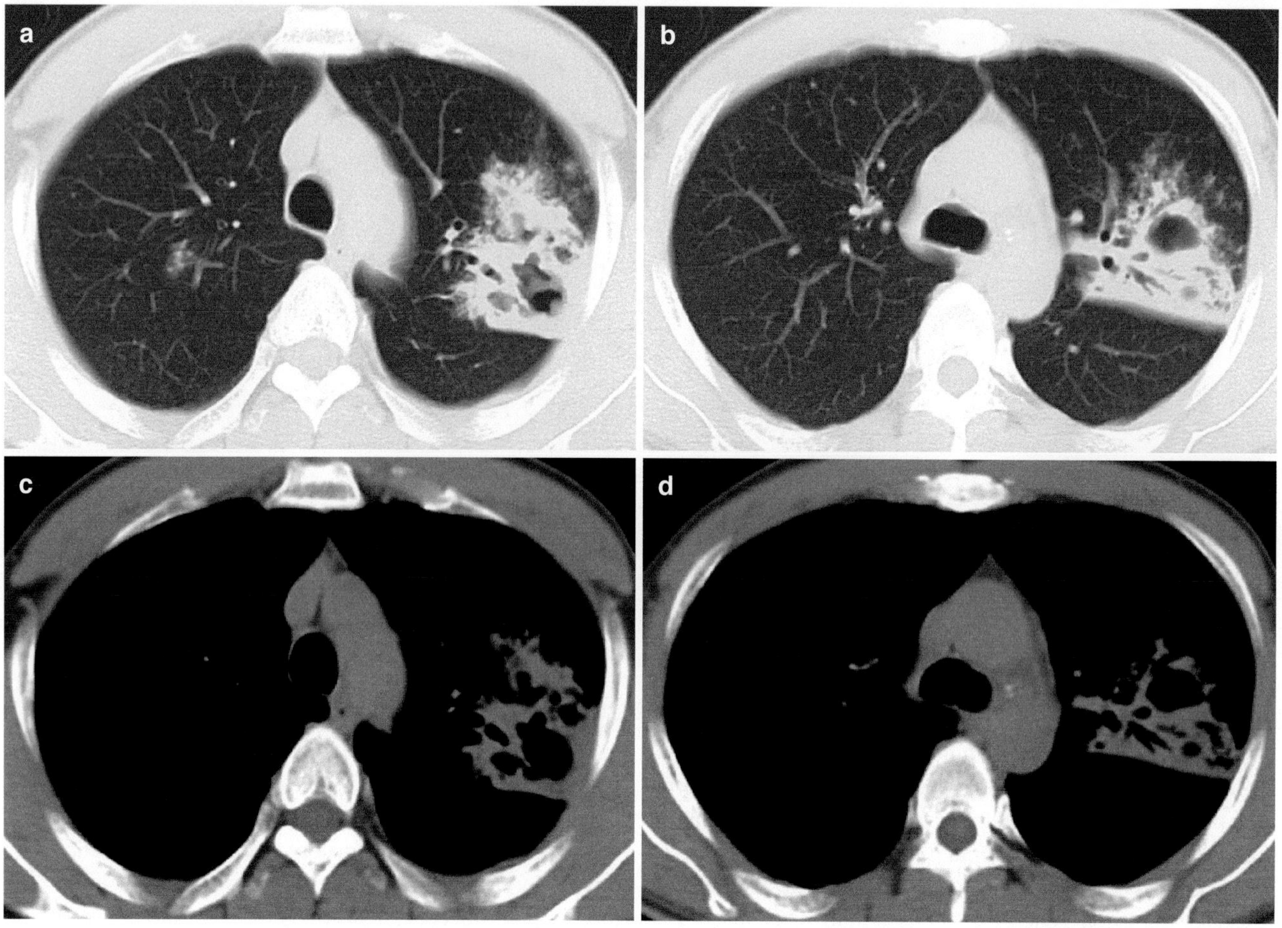

Fig. 16.1 (**a–d**) A 37-year-old male, complaining cough and expectoration for one month, is diagnosed with initial treatment single drug-resistant pulmonary tuberculosis. (**a**, **b**) Lung windows show a large consolidation in the apical-posterior segment of the left upper lobe, and multiple mouth-eaten cavities and air bronchogram are observed inside the consolidation. A small patch is shown in the posterior segment of the right upper lobe; (**c**, **d**) mediastinal windows show the co-existence of a large consolidation, a mouth-eaten cavity, and the image of a bronchiectasis in posterior apical segment of the left upper lobe, and the lesions adhere to the thickened lateral pleura on the left side, without any calcification among the lesions

tuberculosis, including large lobar or segmental consolidations, mouth-eaten cavity, thickening of bronchial wall, and the absence of hilar lymphatic calcification, is conducive to the imaging diagnosis of this disease.

16.1.2 Image Findings of Pediatric Drug-Resistant Pulmonary Tuberculosis Manifest Small Patches and Small Nodules

Atypical clinical symptoms are observed in some of pediatric patients with drug-resistant pulmonary tuberculosis, who manifest mainly the fever or mild cough but show only small patches and small nodules (Fig. 16.2). Besides considering the possibility of pulmonary tuberculosis, therefore, the evidences supporting the diagnosis of pulmonary tuberculosis shall be searched positively, such as sputum smear and culture of Mycobacteria tuberculosis, molecular biological detection, laboratory detection of Mycobacterium tuberculosis in bronchoscopic alveolar lavage fluid, and detection of genetic mutation of Mycobacterium tuberculosis, so as to determine the potential presence of drug-resistant pulmonary tuberculosis, as for an initial treatment patient with atypical clinical symptoms manifesting patchy or nodular opacities in findings of his/or CT scans [9].

16.1.3 Image Findings of the Drug-Resistant Pulmonary Tuberculosis Identified by CT Scans in an Asymptomatic Person or During Health Examination

Active pulmonary tuberculosis is defined as a disease manifesting corresponding clinical symptoms and signs of tuber-

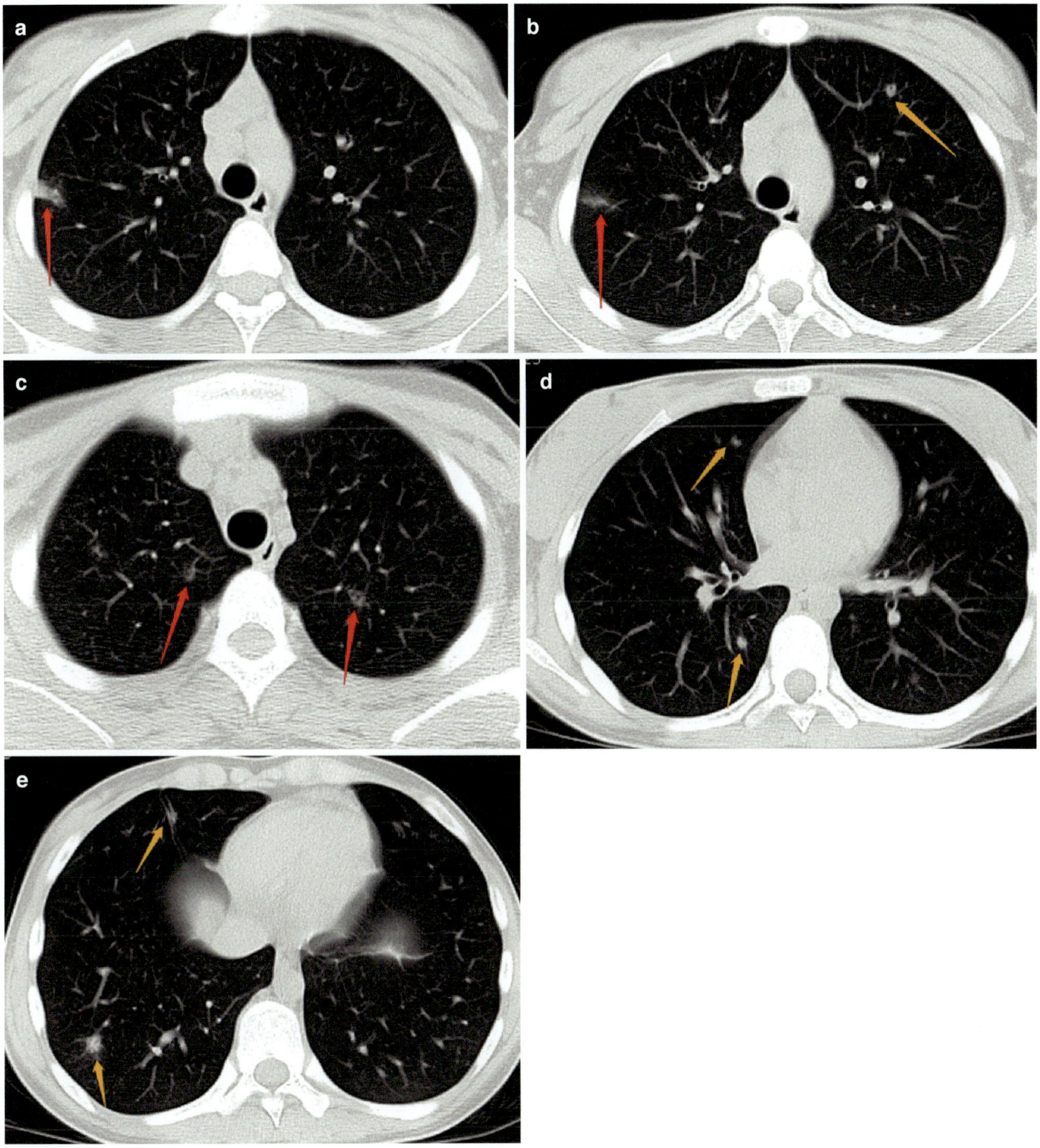

Fig. 16.2 (**a**–**e**) An 11-year-old girl complaining fever, headache, and stomachache with vomiting for 14 days, and lassitude of the extremities with wordless for 3 days. Sputum culture (+) and result of drug susceptibility show the resistance to levofloxacin. ** The diagnosis is initial treatment single-resistant pulmonary tuberculosis: levofloxacin. A CT scan shows patchy shadows of the upper lobe of both lungs (red arrow) and the left upper lung and right lower lung (yellow arrow)

culosis, with evidences supporting its diagnosis, including results of etiological, pathological, and radiological examinations for Mycobacterium tuberculosis [5, 10]. Meanwhile, cases are seen in clinical practice, which have no symptoms or signs but show the pulmonary abnormality in CT scans during health examination. Manifestations of CT scans can be relied on to carry out the initial determination of whether it is pulmonary tuberculosis, in case of the absence of clinical symptoms, signs, and laboratory etiological evidence. If it is suspected to be pulmonary tuberculosis, we should also determine whether it is active or non-active pulmonary tuberculosis based on the image findings. Non-active pulmonary tuberculosis is defined as a disease having no clinical symptoms and signs related to active tuberculosis, showing negative result in bacteriological test, and conforming to at least one out of the five radiological manifestations while excluding any other factors that might induce changes of pulmonary image findings. The five radiological manifestations include (1) calcified lesion (solitary or multiple); (2) strips, with clear border; (3) sclerotic lesion; (4) clean cavity; and (5) thickened and adhered pleura with calcification [11].

Case Report (Figs. 16.3 and 16.4)

The patient, a 28-year-old male, had no fever or cough. Chest CT scans for his health examination on November 7, 2019, revealed nodules, patches, and strips in both upper lungs, manifesting a co-existence of exudative, proliferative, fibrotic, and calcified lesions as its characteristic image find-

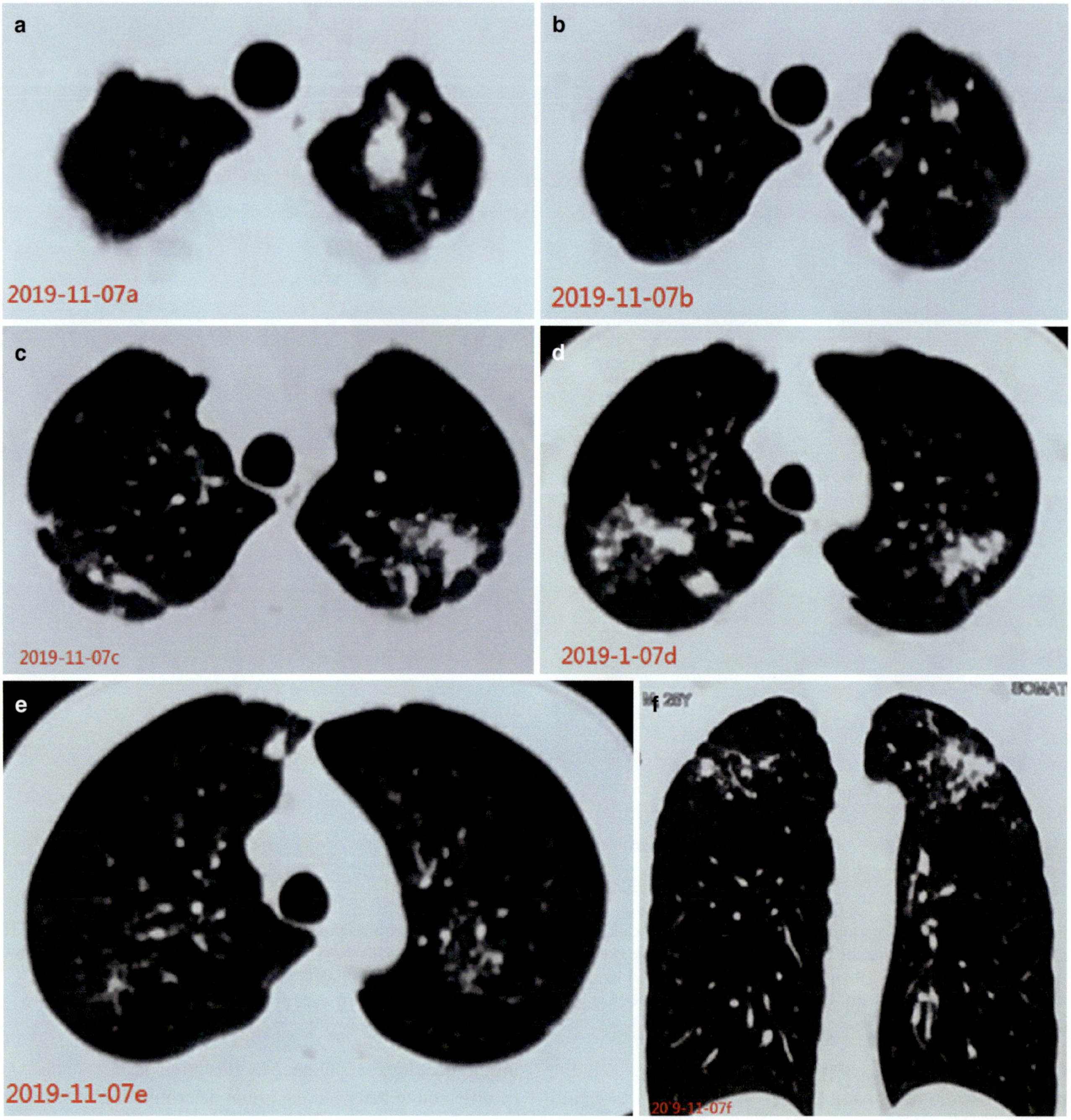

Fig. 16.3 (November 7, 2019), a male aged 28 years had no symptoms such as fever or cough, but pulmonary abnormality was revealed during health examination. (**a**–**e**) Nodules with blurred boundaries as well as patches and strips with increased density are shown in both upper lobes in cross sections of lung windows of CT scans, which are more significant in the left upper lung. (**f**) Nodules and irregular patches are displayed in posterior apical segments of both lungs by coronal section of three-dimensional reconstruction images

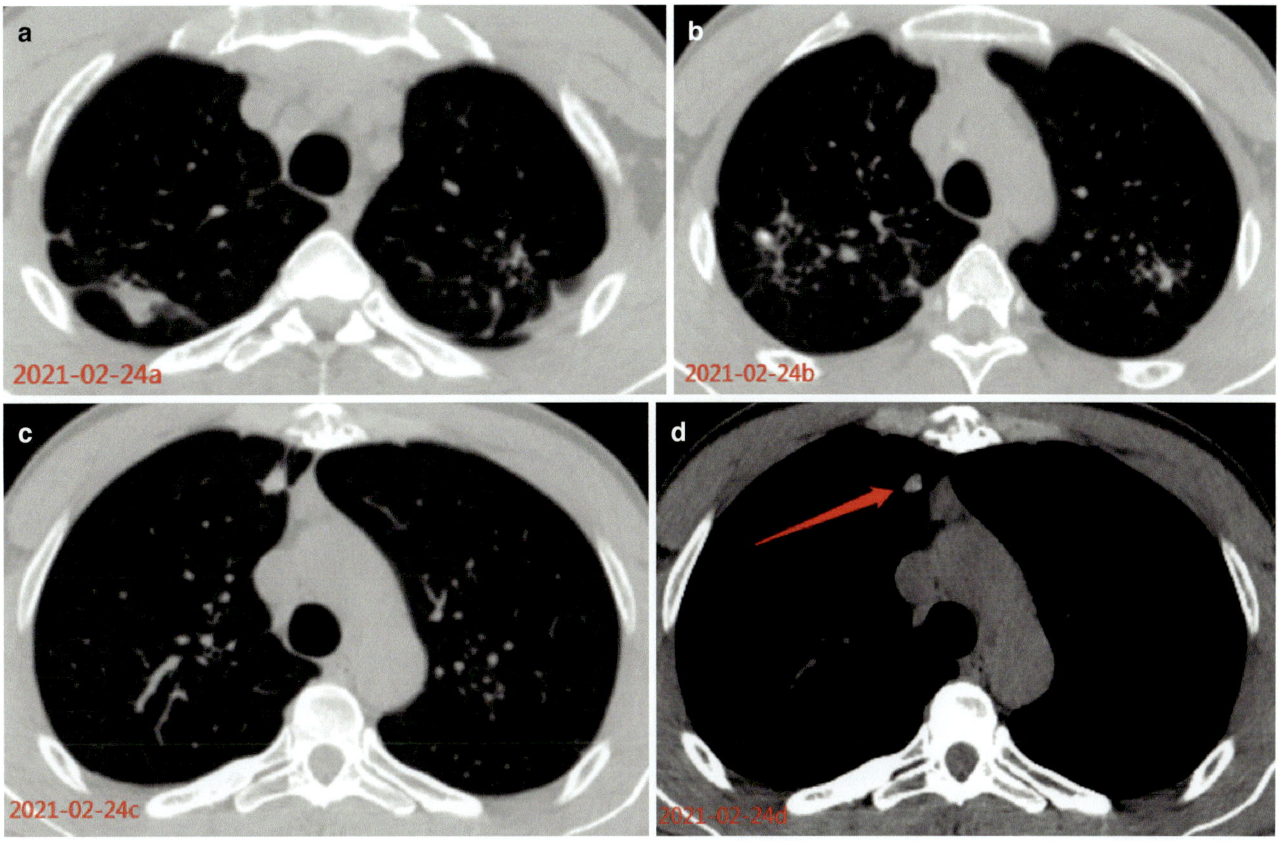

Fig. 16.4 (February 24, 2021): Re-examination of chest CT scans post to 15-month anti-tuberculosis treatment. (**a–c**) Lung windows show high-density nodules and patches in both upper lungs, and most of these lesions have clear boundary. (**d**) High-density patches with punctiform calcifications (indicated by the red arrow) among them are shown in the right upper lobe by the mediastinal window

ings. It was considered probably the pulmonary tuberculosis, based on the location and pathological characteristics of the lesions. The non-active pulmonary tuberculosis could be excluded, because of the presence of blurred ground-glass opacities in both lungs with exudative lesions.

Laboratory detection of Mycobacterium tuberculosis and drug-resistant gene in bronchoalveolar lavage fluid on November 23, 2019, suggested positiveness result in Mycobacteria tuberculosis and mutation of KatG gene (probably resistant to isoniazid). The anti-tuberculosis treatment was launched instantly based on results of radiological and laboratory examinations, and an obvious absorption and amelioration of the lesions were shown after 15-month treatment.

16.2 CT Evaluation of New Drug-Resistant Strains Potentially Appearing During the Treatment Against Drug-Resistant Pulmonary Tuberculosis

Satisfactory responses are shown to most of regimens tailored to the drug-resistant diagnosis and its category confirmed by culture of Mycobacteria tuberculosis, drug susceptibility test, and related genetic detection. Treatment failure and re-treatment, however, can be caused by multiple factors such as the side effects of anti-tuberculosis drugs and the compliance of patients, which are witnessed by the prolonged treatment course for anti-drug resistant pulmonary tuberculosis. Chest image findings manifest the increase in both number and scope of lesions, or the appearance of solitary or multiple cavities [12, 13]. A great importance should be attached, therefore, to regular follow-up of chest imaging in addition to regular detection of renal and hepatic functions of patients, sputum culture and smear of Mycobacteria tuberculosis aiming to understand the negative conversion of Mycobacteria tuberculosis, and drug susceptibility test, during the process of anti-tuberculosis treatment. Potential causality should be screened in case of the absence of absorption or the presence of progression is identified for the pulmonary tuberculosis, and whether there is an infection by a new drug-resistant strain should be considered. Image findings of a newly occurring drug-resistant stain during the treatment against a drug-resistant pulmonary tuberculosis manifest mainly the continuous enlargement of the previous pulmonary lesions, such as pulmonary consolidation, cavitation, nodules, and patches, on the basis of their partial or whole absorption post to the previous anti-tuberculosis treatment.

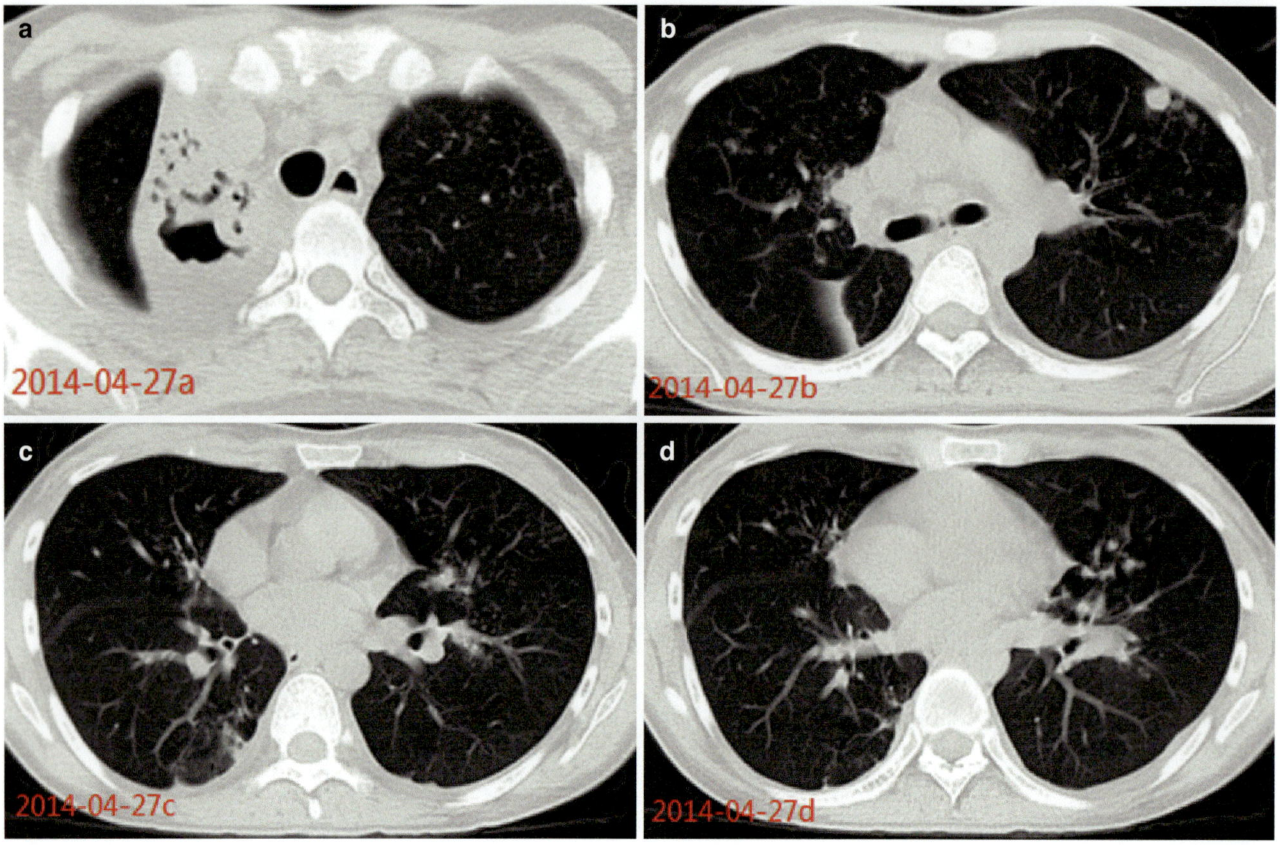

Fig. 16.5 (April 27, 2014 **a**–**d**) Drug-resistant pulmonary tuberculosis. The first chest CT scans on April 27, 2014, post to admission. (**a**) Pulmonary windows show atelectasis of the right upper lobe, with a mouth-eaten cavity and bronchiectasis. (**b**–**d**) Lung windows show nodules of the pleura of the right upper lung (**b**); high-density patches are observed in the dorsal segment of the right lower lobe, and some of them are adhered to the pleura (**c**); the lingual segment of the left lung is scattered with multiple patches, small nodules, and tree-in-bud signs (**d**)

Case 1 (Figs. 16.5, 16.6, 16.7, and 16.8)

The patient, a female aged 26 years, had the onset of cough in November 2012, with an expectoration of a little clear sputum without any obvious inducement, when she visited a local disease control institute and was diagnosed with pulmonary tuberculosis positive in sputum smear. She received anti-tuberculosis treatment using 2HRZ/4HR for 7 months until a somewhat recovery, when she voluntarily discontinued the treatment. The recurrence of symptoms was witnessed between August 26 and September 5, 2013, and she sought medical service in an outpatient department in a specialty hospital, where she was diagnosed with pulmonary tuberculosis negative in sputum smear requiring re-treatment and the right tuberculous pleurisy. She underwent a therapy consisting of rifampicin, pyrazinamide, streptomycin, ethambutol, and levofloxacin. After 2-month treatment, streptomycin was discontinued and the rest of drugs in this regimen was continued up to now. Re-examination of CT scans during this period showed the absorption and shrinkage of the lesions, and multiple sputum smear revealed negative results.

She was admitted to hospital on April 20, 2014, for further diagnosis and treatment. The result of laboratory detection showed the infection of acid-fast bacillus, based on which she was diagnosed with drug-resistant pulmonary tuberculosis.

Case 2 (Figs. 16.9, 16.10, 16.11, and 16.12)

Patient Liu, a 52-year-old male, had no fever or cough. A pulmonary shadow was noticed in his health examination in January 2018, which was considered to be pulmonary tuber-

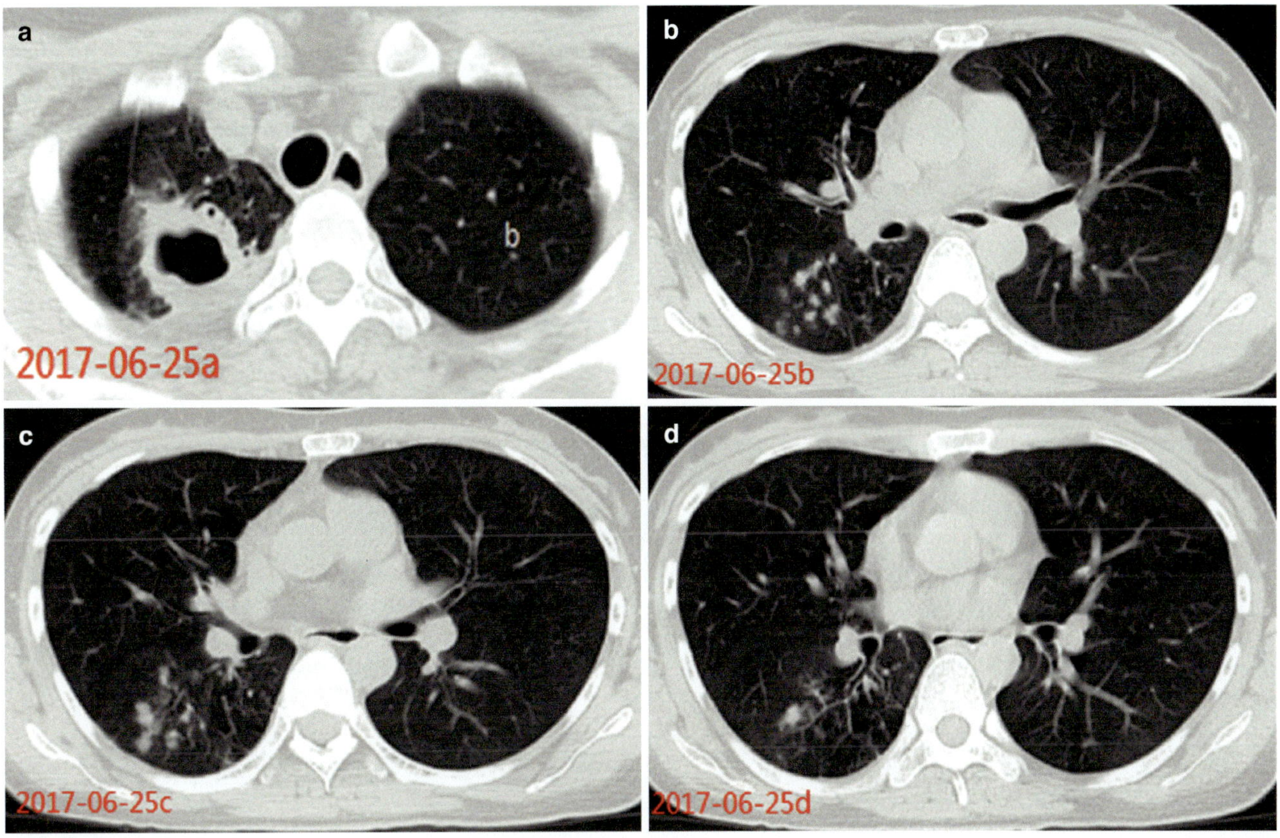

Fig. 16.6 (June 25, 2017 **a**–**d**). Drug-resistant pulmonary tuberculosis and CT re-examination on June 25, 2017. (**a**) Lung windows show a certain absorption and recovery of the previous caseous pneumonia in the right upper lobe, but a large thick-walled cavity is still observed in the right upper lung with the smooth interior wall and its posterior–interior wall adhered locally with the pleura. Patches and small nodules are observed in the dorsal segment of the right lower lobe, which increase in number compared with lesions shown by the previous CT scans. Image findings show an overall absorption and amelioration of the lesions, but active tuberculosis lesions still exist

culosis. He visited a specialty hospital, and chest CT scans on February 13, 2018, revealed patches and nodules in both upper lungs, suggesting bilateral pulmonary tuberculosis. Bronchoscopic alveolar lavage fluid was shown positive in acid-fast staining of tuberculosis, and he was diagnosed with bilateral pulmonary tuberculosis. CT re-examination performed on April 9, 2018, post to two-month anti-tuberculosis treatment showed an absorption and amelioration of lesions in both upper lobes, and the treatment was continued. During this period, CT re-examination on September 7, 2018, showed an absorption of lesions in both lungs. CT re-examination on February 2, 2019, showed the increase in both size and number of tuberculosis lesions in both upper lungs, and the image findings suggested the likeliness of drug-resistant pulmonary tuberculosis. He visited a specialty hospital, where laboratory culture of Mycobacteria tuberculosis was done together with drug susceptibility test, showing resistance to isoniazid, streptomycin, rifampicin, and ethambutol. Based on these results, therefore, a regimen against the drug-resistant pulmonary tuberculosis was switched to and continued for 6 months. After that chest CT scans were re-examined on August 13, 2019, which showed patches and nodules in the right lung with a little amount of small nodules in the left upper lobe, suggesting an obvious absorption and amelioration of tuberculosis lesions in both upper lobes compared with those shown by CT scans on February 2, 2019.

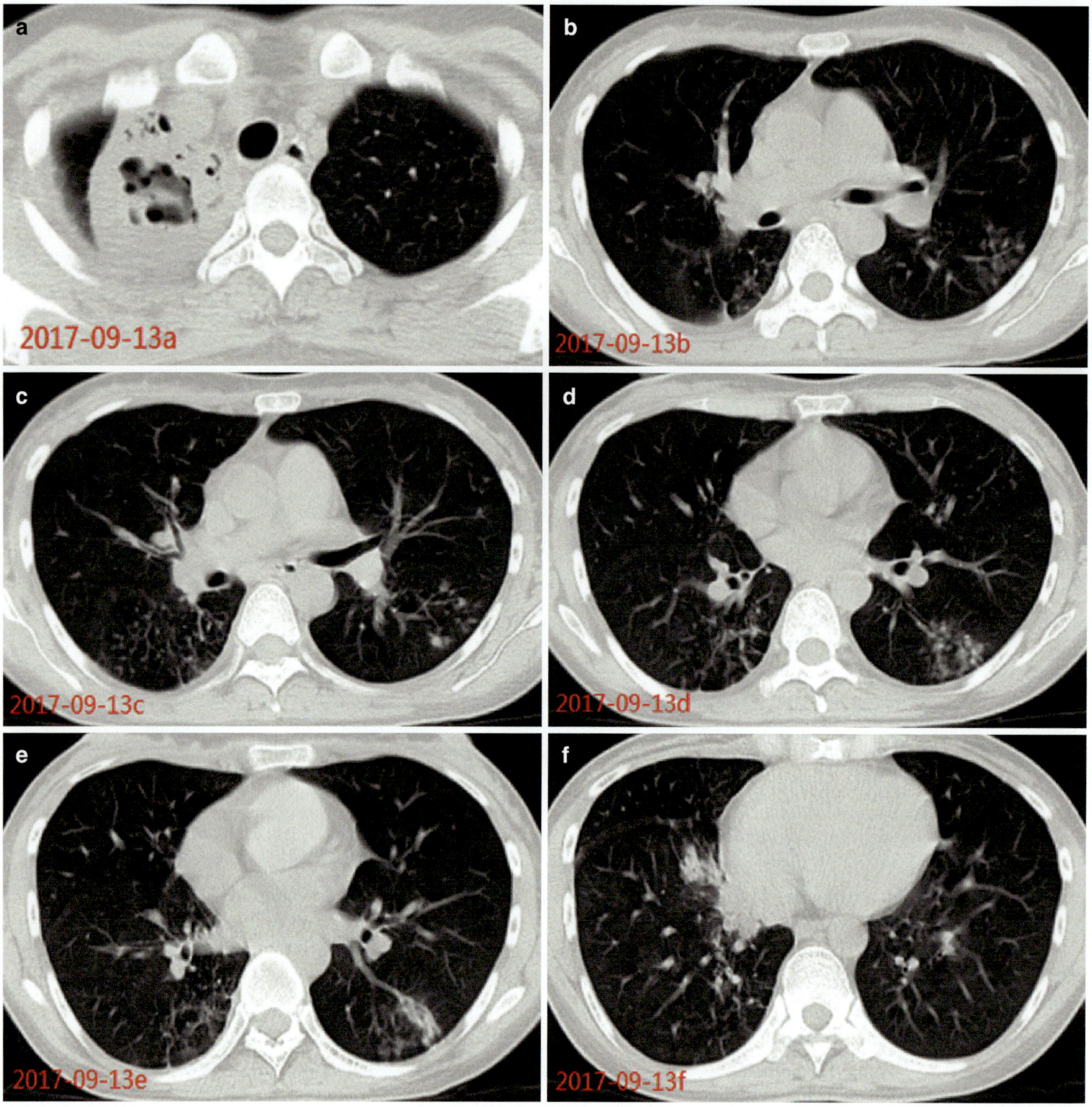

Fig. 16.7 (September 13, 2017 **a**–**f**). CT re-examination on September 13, 2017, shows a progression of tuberculosis lesions, suggesting not so good a response to the treatment and the likely presence of drug-resistant strains. Laboratory tests post to admission confirmed the recurrent atelectasis and caseous pneumonia in the right upper lobe as shown by the previous lung windows a., showing a progression of lesions compared with chest CT scans on June 25, 2017. (**b**–**f**) Lung window shows a certain absorption and decreased number of lesions in the dorsal segment of the right lower lobe, and patches, small nodules, and tree-in-bud signs are observed in the anterior basal segment of the right lower lobe and the left lower lobe, and these lesions show a progression compared with the previous CT scans

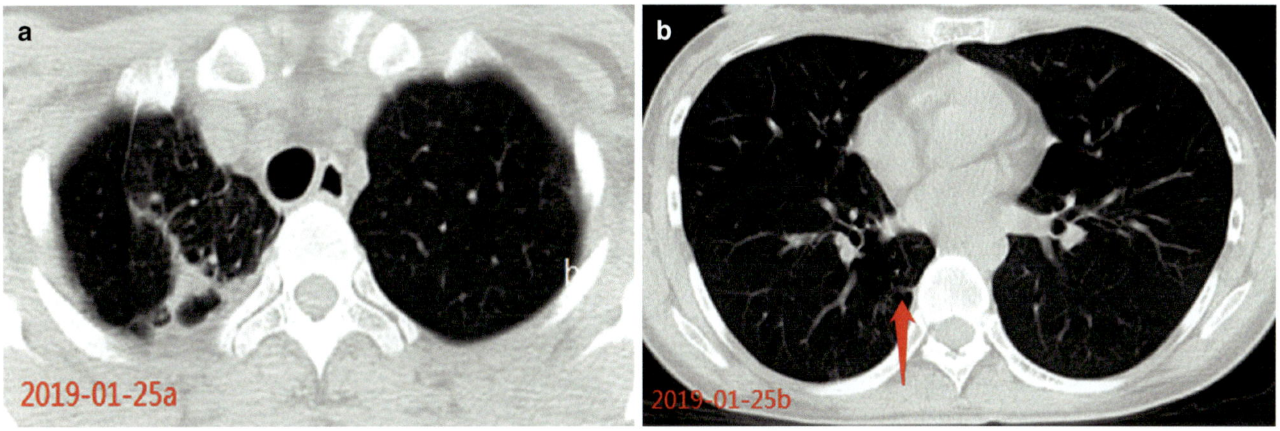

Fig. 16.8 (January 25, 2019 **a**, **b**). Treatment was continued for 16 months after the regimen against drug-resistant pulmonary tuberculosis was modified. CT re-examination performed on January 25, 2019, shows the obvious amelioration in both lungs. (**a**) Pulmonary windows show the obvious post-treatment absorption and amelioration of lesions of caseous pneumonia in the right upper lobe, and only strips, high-density patches, and local pleural thickening are observable. (**b**) Lung windows show a little amount of fibroproliferative lesions in the right lower lobe (indicated by the red arrow)

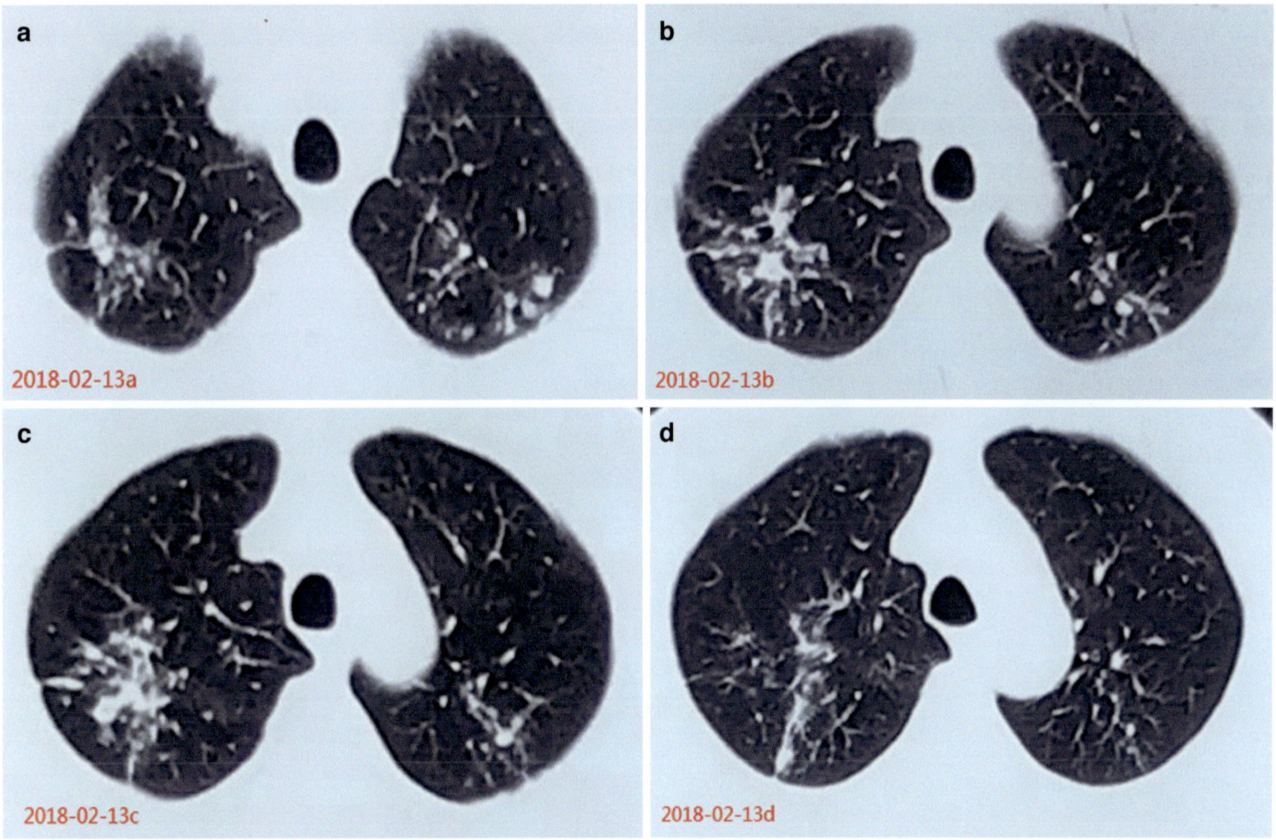

Fig. 16.9 (February 13, 2018 **a**–**d**). The patient had no discomfort, and a pulmonary shadow was revealed during health examination. (**a**–**d**) Patches and nodules are shown in both upper lobes and some of them are integrated, which seemed significant in the right upper lung

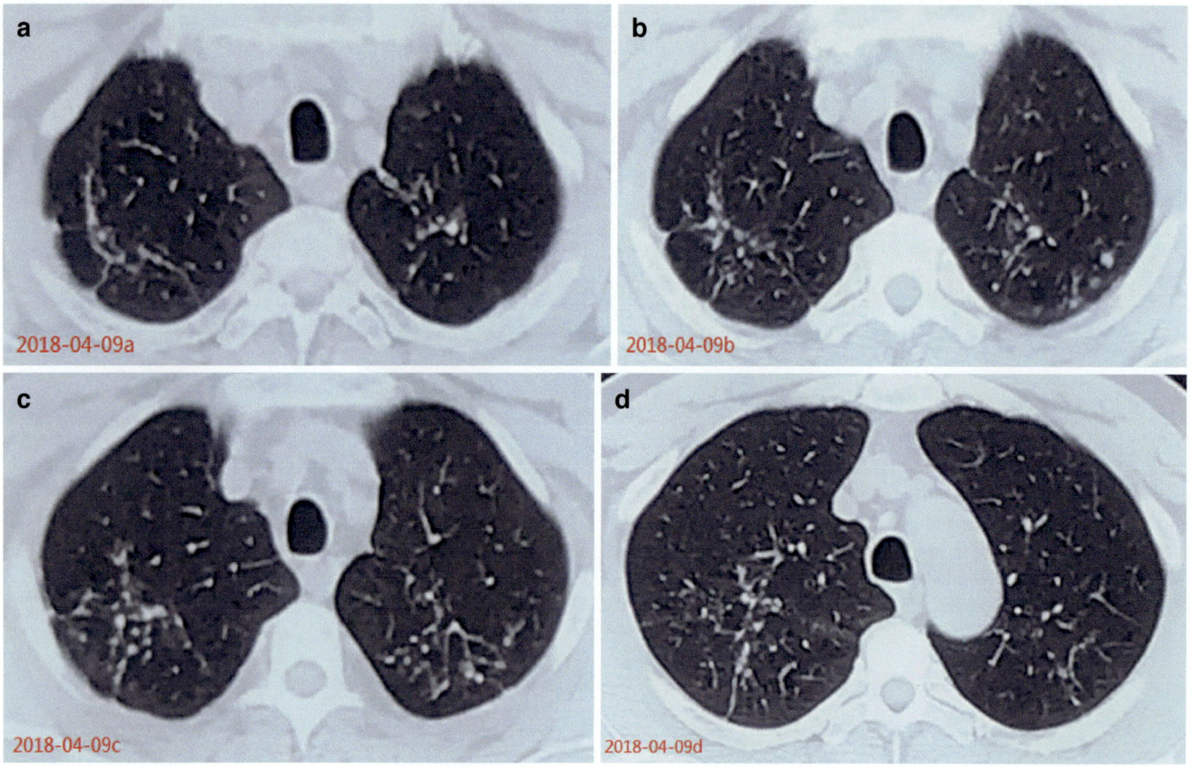

Fig. 16.10 (April 9, 2018 **a–d**). Re-examination of chest CT scans on April 9, 2018, post to anti-tuberculosis treatment. (**a–d**) Pulmonary windows of CT scans show strips and small nodules in both lungs, suggesting an absorption and amelioration of tuberculosis lesions in both lungs compared with chest CT scans on February 13, 2018

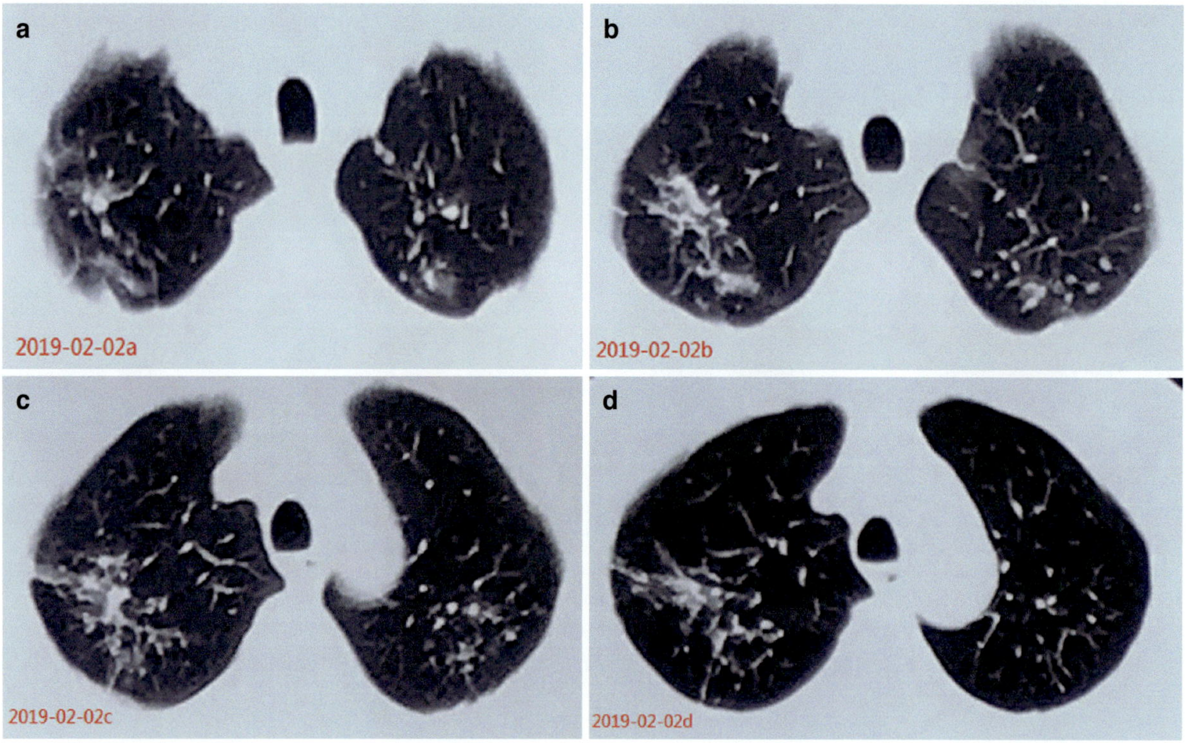

Fig. 16.11 (February 2, 2019 **a–d**). Re-examination of chest CT scans on February 2, 2019, shows the increased size of tuberculosis lesions in both upper lungs, and revealed a progression of them compared with chest CT scans on April 9, 2018, suggesting not so good a response to the treatment and the presence of a drug-resistant pulmonary tuberculosis

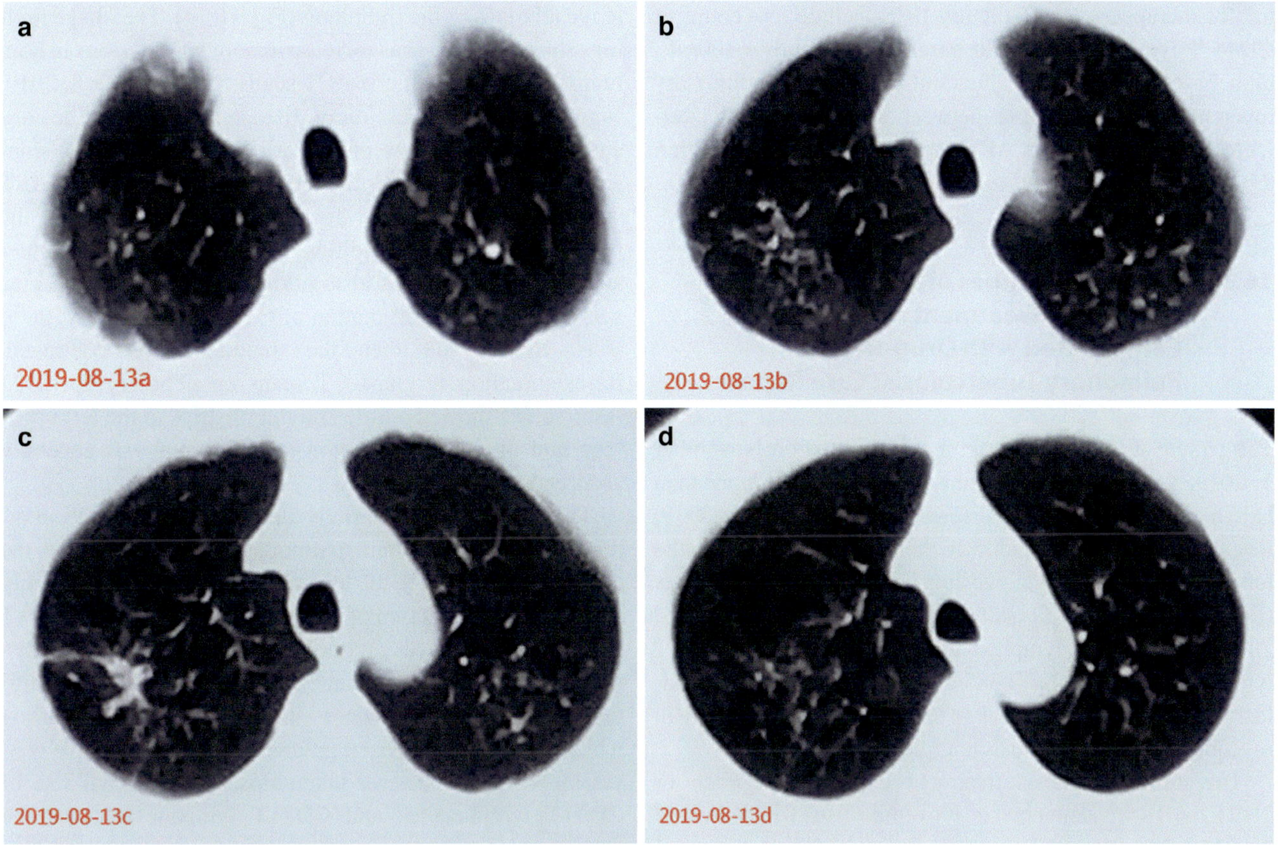

Fig. 16.12 (August 13, 2019 **a**–**d**). Re-examination of chest CT scans on August 13, 2019, post to 6-month treatment against drug-resistant pulmonary tuberculosis. (**a**–**d**) Patches and nodules are shown in the right upper lung, and a little amount of nodules in the left upper lung, showing an obvious absorption and amelioration of these lesions compared with those shown by chest CT scans on February 2, 2019

16.3 CT Appraisal of Immune Reconstitution Inflammatory Syndrome (IRIS) Occurring During the Treatment Against AIDS Complicated with Drug-Resistant Pulmonary Tuberculosis

16.3.1 Summary of Immune Reconstitution Inflammatory Syndrome (IRIS)

Immune reconstitution inflammatory syndrome (IRIS) is defined as a group of clinical syndromes occurring during immunity recovery post to highly active anti-retroviral therapy (HAART) in AIDS patients and manifesting mainly as fever, the occurrence of hidden infection or aggravation or deterioration of pre-existing infection. A variety of latent or active opportunistic infections can cause IRIS after HAART, such as tuberculosis and nontuberculosis mycobacterium infection, pneumocystis pneumonia, etc. IRIS usually occurs within 3 months post to antiviral treatment and needs to be differentiated from primary or newly occurring opportunistic infections. (1) Reduction of HIV load and/or increase in $CD4^+$ T lymphocytes appears after AIDS patients receive HAART and anti-tuberculosis treatment, and clinical symptoms of opportunistic infections such as tuberculosis deteriorate. While AIDS patients complicated with tuberculosis respond to HARRT and anti-tuberculosis treatment, there are still concurrent inflammations, aggravation of tuberculosis and increased size of lesions or occurrence of new lesions. This aggravation of clinical symptoms is not related to new opportunistic infections, adverse drug reactions, drug resistance or treatment failure. (2) Therapeutic contradictory IRIS commonly observed in clinical practice is defined as the potential re-aggravation of tuberculosis symptoms due to the enhanced immunity in responding to inflammation post to anti-tuberculosis and ART treatment given to AIDS patients complicated with tuberculosis. In addition to fever, patients may have pleural infiltration or occurrence of new tubercle nodules, as well as mediastinal or peripheral lymphadenectasis, cutaneous or visceral tuberculous abscesses, tuberculous arthritis, or osteomyelitis. A meta-analysis showed that the incidence of IRIS in HIV/AIDS patients with concurrent tuberculosis was 18%, and TB-IRIS related deaths seemed uncommon, accounting for 2% [14]. Risk factors of therapeutic contradictory IRIS include low count of CD4+ T lymphocytes cell at baseline, especially <100/μL; high baseline viral load; disseminated or extrapulmonary tuberculosis; lower interval between anti-tuberculosis treatment and the initiation of ART, especially its initiation within 2 months prior to the anti-tuberculosis treatment [15].

16.3.2 Dynamic Changes of Image Findings During the Treatment Against AIDS Complicated with Drug-Resistant Pulmonary Tuberculosis: Case Report

The patient was a 43-year-old male admitted on November 5, 2019, with a chief complaint of coughing for more than half a month. His first CT scans on November 8, 2019, revealed a large patch shadow in the left upper lobe, with the left pleural effusion, suggesting pulmonary tuberculosis (Fig. 16.13). HIV test result was positive on November 19, 2019, with CD4+ T lymphocyte count of n = 16/ul, CD8+T lymphocytes count of n = 385/ul, the positive result in acid-fast bacilli in sputum smear (4+) and the positive result in mycobacterium tuberculosis complex (+).

The anti-tuberculosis treatment using the regimen of 2HREZ/4HR was launched on November 19, 2019, followed by HAART. Rifampicin resistance was found by rpoB genetic and mutation detection (Xpert MTB/RIF) for Mycobacteria tuberculosis on December 1, 2019, based on which the regimen against tuberculosis was switched to 6Am-Mfx-Cs-Pto-E-Z/18Mfx-Cs-Pto-E-Z. Chest CT scans on December 27, 2019, showed an obvious enlargement of the large patchy consolidation with the obvious increased number of lesions in the left lung, and high-density patches in the all lobes of the right lung (Fig. 16.14). The image findings showed an obvious increase in number of lesions in both lungs compared with chest CT scans on November 8, 2019, suggesting the progression of disease with enlarged lesions and occurrence of new pulmonary lesions, which was considered to be IRIS. Anti-tuberculosis treatment and HAART were continued clinically for 3 months, and after that the patient was in good condition without cough or any other symptoms. An obvious absorption of lesions in both lungs was shown by re-examination of CT scans on April 1, 2020 (Fig. 16.15), and then the treatment was continued. Re-examination of chest CT scans on February 23, 2021 (Fig. 16.16) showed a little amount of strips in the left upper lung and the exudative lesion in both lungs was generally absorbed.

This patient was definitely diagnosed with AIDS combined with drug-resistant pulmonary tuberculosis, and the double infection led to the low immunity, manifesting mainly as the obvious reduction of CD4+T lymphocytes and CD8+T lymphocytes, with the reduced defensive response to disease, and the atypical image findings. HAART and anti-tuberculosis treatment were carried out clinically, during which HIV load decreased gradually with the negative conversion of Mycobacteria tuberculosis, the gradual rise of CD4+T lymphocytes and CD8+T lymphocytes, and the enhancement of systemic immunity of the patient. Generally, IRIS occurs within 1–3 months of treatment, with the image findings showing the worsening of the disease, the enlarged lesions, and the occurrence of new pulmonary lesions. At this time point, we shall not doubt or deny our previous diagnosis on the basis of non-responsiveness to treatment and the disease progression, but continue HAART and anti-tuberculosis treatment, and carry out imaging follow-up syn-

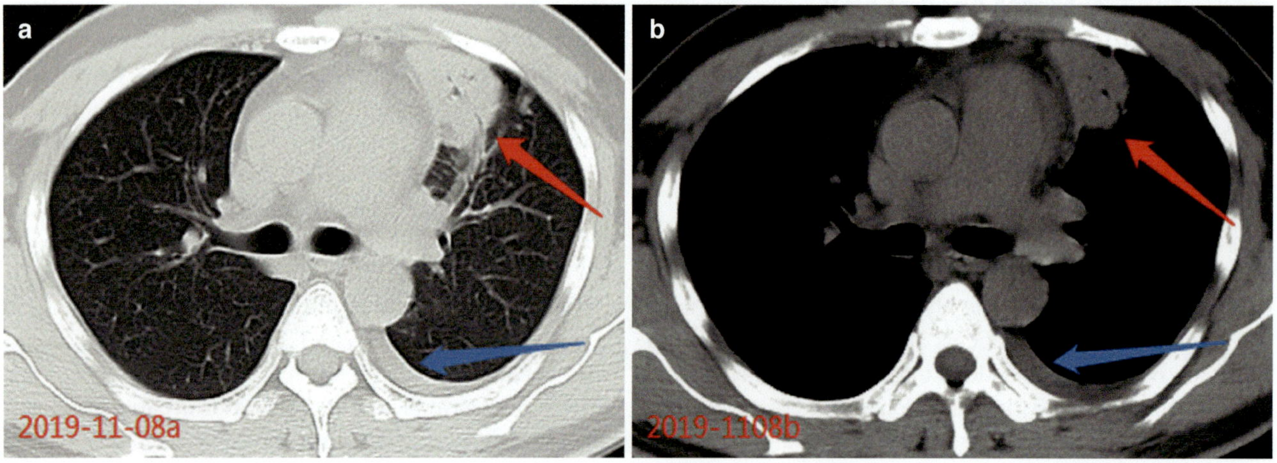

Fig. 16.13 (November 8, 2019 **a**, **b**). Re-examination of chest CT scans on November 8, 2019. Lung windows of CT scans show a large patchy consolidation in the left upper lung, and a bronchogram (indicated by a red arrow) is observed inside the consolidation, which is adhered with the anterior chest wall and the pericardium. A small patch is observed at the outer front of consolidation, and an arch high-density shadow (indicated by the blue arrow) is seen in the left thoracic cavity. (**b**) Mediastinal windows of CT scans show a consolidation in the left upper lung with a high density similar that to chest wall muscles (indicated by the red arrow)

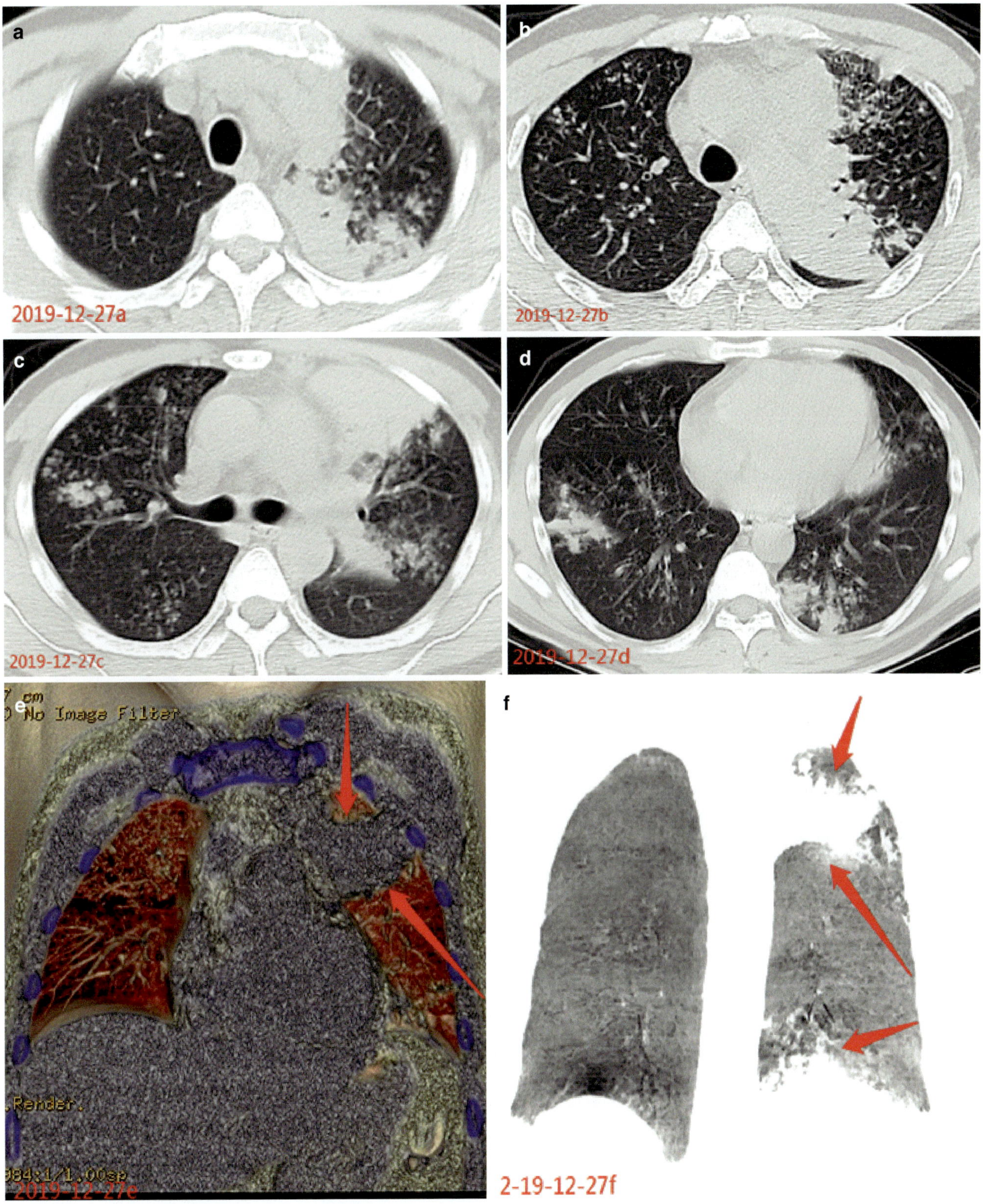

Fig. 16.14 (December 27, 2019 **a–h**) CD4+T lymphocyte count was 75/ul and CD8+T lymphocyte count 413/ul post to the 40-day anti-tuberculosis treatment synchronized with HAART, and the re-examination was done on December 27, 2019. (**a–d**) Lung windows of chest CT show multiple patchy consolidations in both lungs, and multiple large patchy high-density consolidations in the left lung, manifesting an obviously increased number and progression of lesions in both lungs in comparison with chest CT scans on November 8, 2019, and suggesting the presence of IRIS. (**e**, **f**) Colorful images of three-dimensional CT reconstruction show the consolidation in the left lung. (**g**, **h**) Mediastinal windows of CT scans show the large patchy consolidation in the left upper lung and patchy high-density shadows in the left lower lobe and the right upper lobe

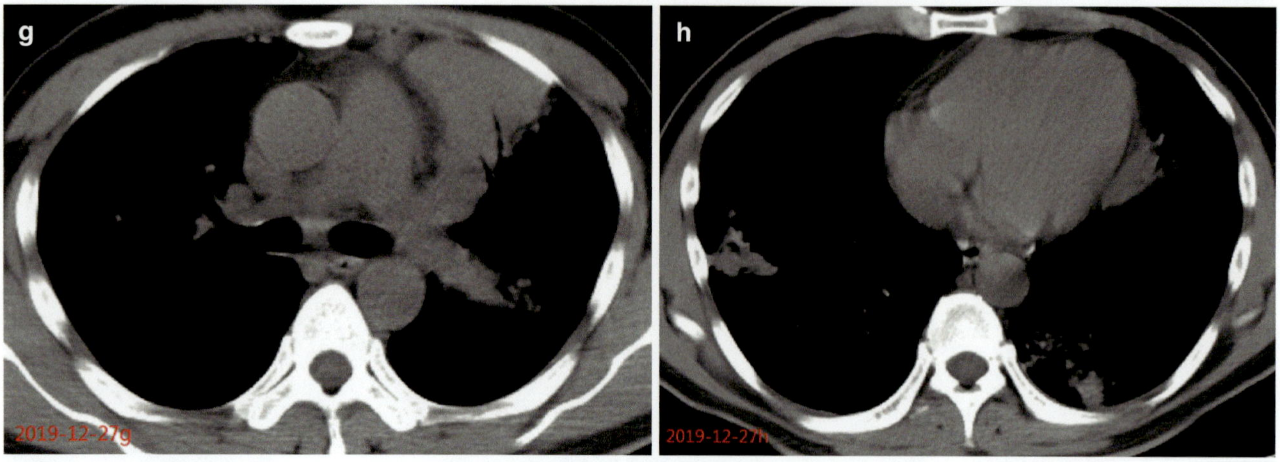

Fig. 16.14 (continued)

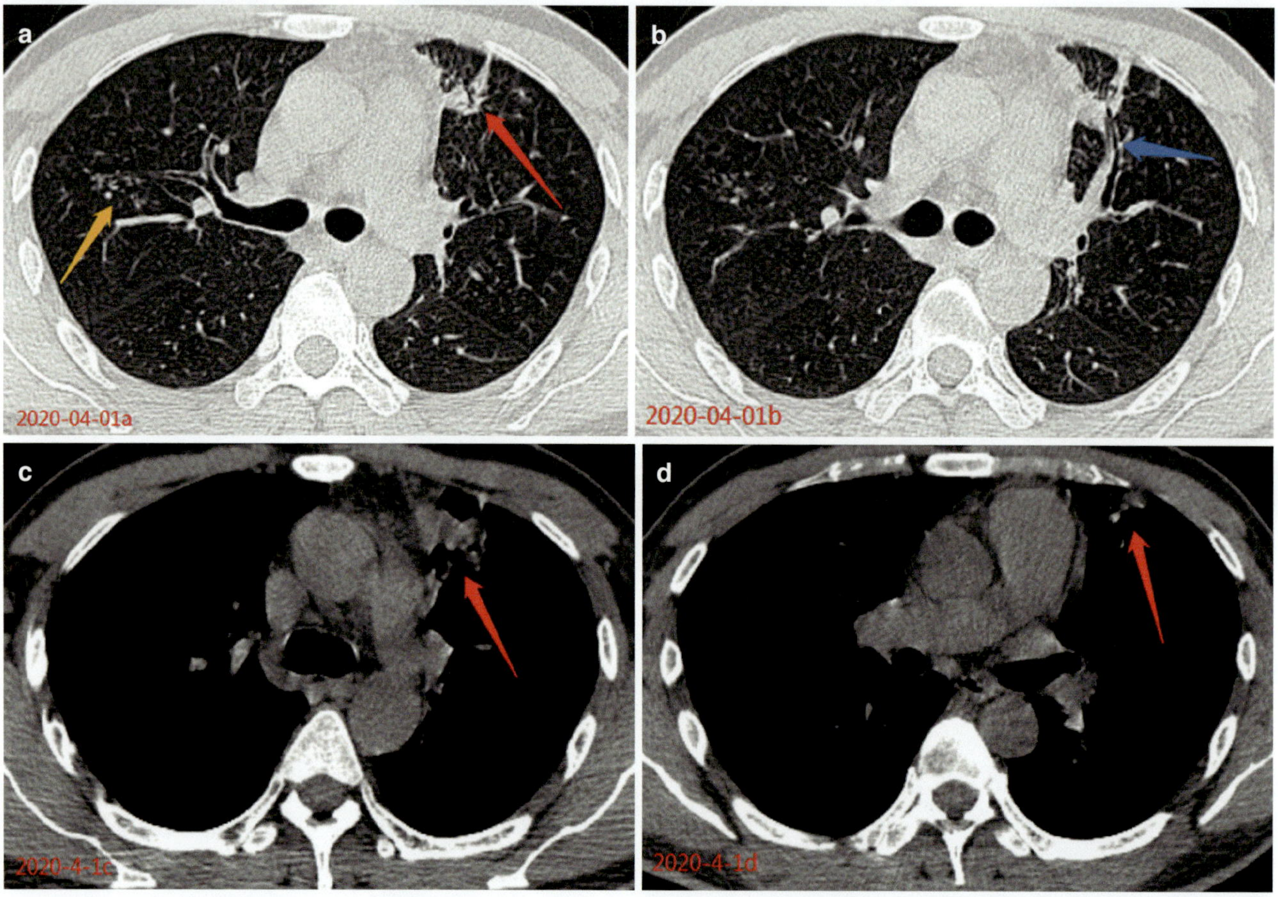

Fig. 16.15 (April 1, 2020 **a**–**d**). Re-examination of chest CT scans was done on April 1, 2020, post to the continuation of anti-tuberculosis treatment for 132 days synchronized with HAART. (**a**) Patches and strips (indicated by the red arrow) are shown in the left upper lung by lung windows of CT scans, which also reveal a little amount of punctiform high-density shadows (indicated by the yellow arrow) in the right upper lung. (**b**) Lung windows of CT scans show patches and bronchiectasis (indicated by the blue arrow) in the left upper lobe. (**c**, **d**) Mediastinal windows of CT scans show high-density patches (indicated by the red arrow) in the left upper lung. In comparison with CT scans on December 27, 2019, lesions in both lung show the obvious absorption and amelioration, suggesting the response to the treatment

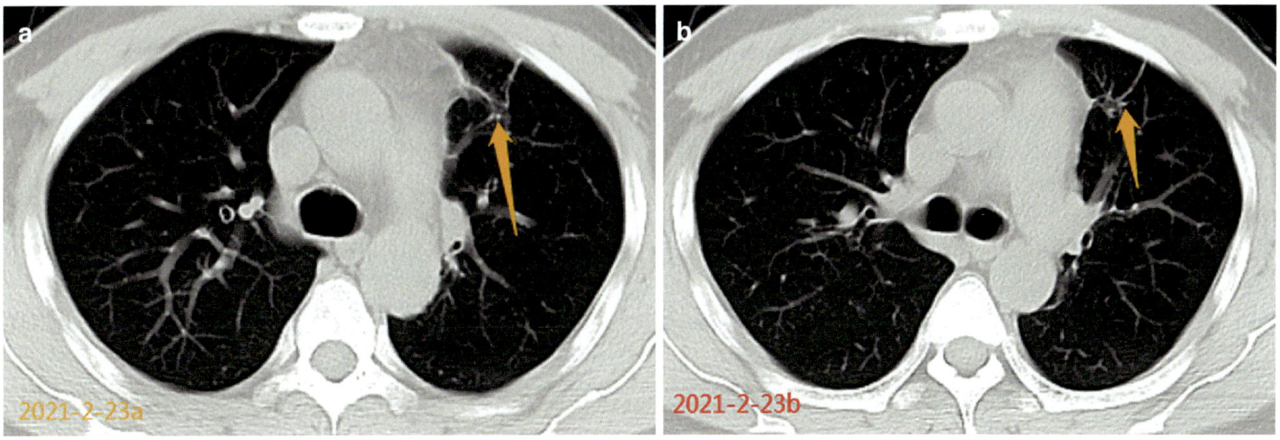

Fig. 16.16 (February 8, 2021 **a**, **b**) CD4+T lymphocyte count was 219/ul and CD8+T lymphocyte count 1429/ul post to the continuation of anti-tuberculosis treatment for 15 months synchronized with HAART, and the re-examination was done on February 23, 2021. (**a**, **b**) Lung windows of CT scans show strips in the left upper lung (indicated by the yellow arrow)

chronized with detection of changes in CD4+T lymphocytes, CD8+T lymphocytes and HIV load, based on which we will find the amelioration of tubercle lesions of the patient, the rise of CD4+ and CD8+ T lymphocytes, and the lowered HIV load. In this case, re-examination of CT scans performed post to the anti-tuberculosis treatment for 40 days showed an obvious increase in the size and number of lesions, suggesting the occurrence of IRIS. A general absorption of lesions, however, was achieved post to the continuation of anti-tuberculosis treatment for another 14 months.

References

1. World Health Organization. Global tuberculosis report 2022[EB/OL]. Geneva: WHO; 2020. https://www.who.int/teams/global-tuberculosis-programme/tb-reports/global-tuberculosis-report-2022.
2. Song Min L, Puxuan FW, et al. The global tuberculosis report 2022: key data analysis for China and the global world[J/CD]. Electron J Emerg Inf Dis. 2023;8(1):1–6.
3. Yumei W, Ziyi L, Jinfu P. Evaluation of Mycobacterium tuberculosis 16Sr RNA+DNA and 23S DNA detection in diagnosis and treatment of pulmonary tuberculosis[J]. Electron J Emerg Inf Dis. 2020;5(2):118–21.
4. Yu W, Tan W-g, Lu P-X. Classification and imaging manifestations of drug-resistant pulmonary tuberculosis[J]. Electron J Emerg Inf Dis. 2019;4(1):42–7.
5. National Health and Family Planning Commission of the People's Republic of China. Diagnostic criteria of pulmonary tuberculosis (WS 288-2017) [J]. Electron J Emerg Inf Dis. 2018;3(1):59–61.
6. Pu-Xuan L. Interpretation of the latest diagnostic criteria for pulmonary tuberculosis in China[J]. Electron J Emerg Inf Dis. 2018;3(1):57–8.
7. Imaging Committee on Infections, Chinese Society of Radiology; Committee on Infectious Disease; Radiology Committee, Chinese Medical Doctor Association. Imaging diagnostic criteria of pulmonary tuberculosis[J]. Electron J Emerg Inf Dis. 2021;6(1):1–6.
8. Chen G, Cheng G-X, Zhu S-q, et al. CT scanning of mono-resistant pulmonary tuberculosis during initial treatment[J]. Electron J Emerg Inf Dis. 2018;3(2):111–4.
9. Fang W-j, Song M, Han Y-y, et al. Characteristic CT images of pulmonary tuberculosis in children under three years of age[J]. Electron J Emerg Inf Dis. 2019;4(4):252–6.
10. Weijun F, He Yulin X, Chuanjun, et al. Interpretation of imaging diagnostic criteria of pulmonary tuberculosis[J]. Electron J Emerg Inf Dis. 2021;6(1):73–8.
11. Puxuan L, Zhou B. Chest radiological clinical diagnosis for AIDS[M]. Beijing: Beijing Science Press; 2012.
12. Li C, Zhou X, Yan L, et al. An analysis of CT manifestations in different types of drug resistant patients and in drug-susceptible patients with pulmonary tuberculosis [J]. Chin J Antituberculosis. 2018;40(7):707–12.
13. Yan X, Xiwei L, Cai C, et al. A retrospective analysis of CT sign evolution in multi-resistant pulmonary tuberculosis patients who failed treatment [J]. Chin J Antituberculosis. 2020;42(6):549–57.
14. AIDS and Hepatitis C Professional Group, Society of Infectious Diseases, Chinese Medical Association Chinese Center for Disease Control and Prevention. Chinese guidelines for diagnosis and treatment of HIV/AIDS (2018 edition)[J]. Electron J Emerg Inf Dis. 2019;4(2):65–84.
15. Professional Committee of HIV Combined with TB, Chinese Association of STD and AIDS Prevention and Control. Expert consensus on diagnosis and treatment of tuberculosis in patients with human immunodeficiency virus/acquired immunodeficiency syndrome[J/CD]. Electron J Emerg Inf Dis. 2022;7(1):73–87.

17 Prevention and Prognosis of Drug-Resistant Tuberculosis

Wei-guo Tan, Yong-yi Lu, Rong Chen, Qi An, and Zhun Yu

17.1 Prevention Strategies

17.1.1 Recognize the Seriousness of the Drug-Resistant Tuberculosis Situation

Drug-resistant tuberculosis (DR-TB) is a major challenge in global tuberculosis control efforts, posing a substantial threat to population health. According to the global tuberculosis report 2021 released by World Health Organization (WHO), there was an estimated 9.9 million cases (95% CI: 8.9 million to 11 million) of TB in 2020, equating to 127 cases per 100,000 (range: 114–140 cases). In 2020, 132,222 cases of MDR/RR-TB were detected and 25, 851 cases of pre-extensively/extensively drug-resistant TB, in a total of 157,903 cases, a decrease of 22% from 201,997 cases in 2019 [1]. In recent years, China has increased its efforts in tuberculosis prevention and control, innovative strategies, multi-sectoral collaboration, and community engagement. Good results have been achieved in different aspects of tuberculosis prevention and treatment. However, there is a rise in drug-resistant tuberculosis and multidrug resistance, which has worsened China's tuberculosis prevention and control situation.

W.-g. Tan (✉) · R. Chen
Tuberculosis Prevention and Control Department, Shenzhen Center for Chronic Disease Control, Shenzhen, Guangdong, China

Y.-y. Lu (✉)
Bloomberg School of Public Health, Johns Hopkins University, Baltimore, MD, USA

Q. An
Urban Planning Department, Faculty of Architecture, Harbin Institute of Technology, Shenzhen, Guangdong, China

Z. Yu
Department of Cardiovascular, Southern University of Science and Technology Hospital, Shenzhen, Guangdong, China

17.1.2 Reduce Resistance-Causing Variables

Drug-resistant tuberculosis is divided into intrinsic drug resistance and acquired drug resistance. Drug resistance generated by particular medication resistance mutation in the non-resistant genome due to some factors such as nonstandard, insufficient and incomplete treatment, poor patient compliance, and poor drug quality during the treatment process is referred to as acquired drug resistance. Intrinsic drug resistance caused by patients infected with drug-resistant mycobacterium tuberculous is known as primary drug resistance and it is also caused by transmission and induced resistance [2].

Drug-resistant tuberculosis was triggered by selection pressure generated by clinical irregular use of anti-tuberculosis medications [3]. In the past, drug resistance acquired due to irregular treatment was always considered a factor contributing to the high frequency of drug-resistant tuberculosis. Therefore, our strategies for prevention and control drug-resistant tuberculosis are primarily focused on reducing acquired drug resistance as a result of non-adherence to anti-TB treatment [4]. However, there is growing evidence that drug-resistant tuberculosis is caused predominantly through transmission rather than insufficient under treatment, which is a primary factor of the drug-resistant tuberculosis epidemic. According to a comprehensive study of XDR-TB genotyping from South Africa, 69% of the XDR-TB patients have never been treated for MDR-TB [4]. Experts analyze the reasons for the MDR-TB epidemic in China and found that 60% of the MDR-TB patients are the newly treated patients, which indicates that 60% of the MDR-TB patients are caused by the transmission of the primary drug resistance [5–7]. Analyzing the reasons for drug resistance among the retreatment patients, the study found that 84% of the retreatment patients were primary drug resistance [8]. Meanwhile, experts also point out that more than 40% of the MDR-TB patients are caused by recent transmission [7]. Under the current DR-TB epidemic situation in

P.-x. Lu et al. (eds.), *Diagnostic Imaging of Drug Resistant Pulmonary Tuberculosis*,
https://doi.org/10.1007/978-981-99-8339-1_17

China, even though acquired drug resistance is relatively low, most of the people may still be infected with drug-resistant mycobacterium tuberculosis. At this point, the most important factors for drug-resistant TB prevention should be early detection and control of the source of infection, as well as strengthening patients' regular treatment and management and reducing the burden of drug-resistant TB at the same time.

17.1.3 Early Detection

Early diagnosis and the prevention of TB transmission are the most strengthened tool to prevent drug-resistant tuberculosis transmission and the foundation of tuberculosis control. According to WHO, early detection of tuberculosis, common drug susceptibility testing, and systematic screening of high-risk populations are the main component of patient-centered care and prevention, which is also the main strategy for eradicating tuberculosis. Researches have shown that even with existing second-line regimens, expanding MDR-TB diagnosis and treatment are predicted to lower MDR-TB incidence rate at the population level [9]. Drug susceptibility testing (DST) method requires longer time to identify mycobacterium tuberculosis growth and drug resistance. During this process, patients may be inappropriately treated and drug-resistant strains may continue to spread, which increases the incidence of drug-resistant tuberculosis. Therefore, early and rapid diagnosis tests of tuberculosis and drug-resistant tuberculosis are important for patients and public health prevention and control. It not only improves patients' prognosis and survival rates but also helps to prevent drug resistance and the spread of drug resistance strains to the community. The development of a rapid tuberculosis culture system and molecular detection system with worldwide implementation has significantly shortened the time it takes to diagnose tuberculosis. However, factors such as technology, economics, and geography limit access to drug-resistant tuberculosis diagnostic testing, including Xpert MTB/RIF, GeneXpert, and whole-genome sequencing, to only a small group of people in most low- and middle-income countries. Only 51% of tuberculosis patients have received the test for rifampicin resistance over the world.

1. BACTEC MGIT 960 detection system: This current detection system is the common automatic culture device for the combination of rapid culture, detection, and DST of MTB. The principle is to use continuous fluorescence detection technology to measure the change in O_2 concentration in the culture tube produced by the growth of MTB to measure whether MTB is drug resistant. Compared with the proportional detection, BACTEC MGIT 960 detection system in detecting INH, RIF, EMB, and SM drug-resistant genes were, respectively, 97.55–97.77%, 91.62–98.78%, 94.97–96.73%, and 93.86–96.73%, which were highly consistent [10]. This detection method has short detection time but is costly. In addition, the culture-based method requires trained faculties and laboratories with stringent biosafety levels to protect technicians and the environment. Therefore, there are some limitations to using this approach to detect resistance, especially in low- and middle- income countries.
2. Sensititre MYCOTB: This susceptibility testing of mycobacterium tuberculosis is widely used and approved by FDA and CFDA and it uses the broth micro-dilution method. The MYCOTB drug susceptibility contains three first-line anti-tuberculosis drug (INH, RIF, and EMB) and nine second-line anti-tuberculosis drugs (aminosalicylate sodium, kanamycin A, amikacin, capreomycin, levofloxacin, moxifloxacin, prothionamide, ethionamide, cycloserine, linezolid, and bedaquiline) including 12 anti-tuberculosis meditations. Meanwhile, it can also detect the minimum inhibitory concentration (MIC) of MTB clinical isolate, which provides more accurate medication resistance data. This method uses an automated sample addition instrument, which accelerates sample addiction while reducing the pollution caught by manual pollution. This ensures the accuracy of the results and MYCOTBI can directly evaluate MIC's drug without the usage of special equipment. Lots of research have proved that MYCOTBI has good consistency with the gold standard ratio of drug susceptibility test results [11–15].
3. Xpert MTB/RIF: Based on semi-quantitative nested real-time fluorescence quantitative PCR, five overlapping probes were designed for the hot spot mutation region of rpoB gene to detect MTB and RR-DR in samples. This method combines automatic sample processing, DNA preparation, nucleic acid amplification, and target sequence into a combined automatic detection method. In 2010, MTB/RIF was first recommended for diagnosis of adult pulmonary tuberculosis from sputum specimens. In 2013, it was recommended for the diagnosis of some extra-pulmonary tuberculosis and pediatric TB. In 2017, WHO recommended it be used in suspected cases to detect MTB complexes and RIF resistance screening. According to meta-analysis results, Xpert MTB/RIF detection was 89% sensitive and 99% specific as a first-line test in smear microscopy. Xpert MTB/RIF detect MTB sensitivity is 67% and the specificity is 99% as additional test of smear negative PTB. The Xpert MTB/RIF has a sensitivity of 98% for tuberculosis regarding smear-positive and culture-positive tuberculosis [16]. Compared with the gold standard, the sensitivity of Xpert MTB/RIF for detecting RFP resistance is 86.8–97.93% and the specific is 95.3–98% [16–18]. In addition, compared to smear microscopy, Xpert MTB/RIF improves the detection rate of

Mycobacterium tuberculosis (MTB) by 23%, thereby reducing the likelihood of misdiagnosis between MTB and non-tuberculous mycobacteria (NTM) [16]. Xpert MTB/RIF directly detects clinical samples, and it is automatically completed in the reaction box during the whole experimental process. This operation is simple and reduces the risk of cross-contamination between the samples and it can significantly reduce the detection time for RIF resistance from 4 to 8 weeks (culture and DST) to 2 h, which helps physicians with quickly identifying MDR-TB patients, giving accurate treatment planning and reducing MDR-TB spreading within the community. WHO recommends Xpert MTB/RIF as initial detection for all tuberculosis patients. However, only 15 out of 29 countries with high TB prevalence rate recommend Xpert for drug resistance testing among tuberculosis patients. According to a report from a large multicenter cohort study in 18 countries, only 4% of HIV/TB receives Xpert detection. The widespread Xpert implementation was prevented by factors such as high-cost and laboratory equipment. In addition, if Xpert finds evidence of rifampicin drug resistance, second-line DST should be started immediately in order to stop the undiscovered XDR-TB from continuing to spread. Research shows that among 1332 patients with rifampicin tuberculosis resistance, only 44% had second-line DST using both a fluoroquinolone and a second-line injectable medication. It is urgent to strengthen the testing of second-line anti-tuberculosis medications.

4. Technology of the whole-genome sequencing: Whole-genome Sequencing (WGS) technology is also based on whole-genome sequence analysis, can quickly and comprehensively analyze drug resistance mutation, and has high sensitivity and specificity [19–21]. Compared with traditional drug susceptibility testing, it has some advantages shown as below. First of all, WGS technology can quickly and comprehensively detect all known resistance-related genes and it can receive DST results for more drugs and provide accurate treatment planning or adjust medicine for MDR patients and reduce the risk of transmission and development of drug resistance mutations. In addition, MGS can identify new drug resistance mutations and DNA as detection objects rather than the risk of exposure to live bacteria and has good biological safety. Besides, MGS technology has become more mature and the cost is decreasing. Compared with other rapid test methods, its price is low and it could be widely used in clinical practice. Research indicates that WGS has an over 85% sensitivity and specificity for the identification of INH, RIF, PZA, Lfx, Am, Km, Cm, SM, and Pto detection. However, the current WGS technology is complicated and subject to stringent conditions. There are many different types of drug resistance-related genes needed to be tested. Meanwhile, the expense of the required testing equipment and detection is high. If we want to achieve large-scale clinical application especially in low-income areas, we might also need to address the issues as below: professional software for analysis, professional experts, database, infrastructure, economic costs, DNA (standardization of acquired procedure, quality requirement), and the identification of new resistance mutations [22–24].

Laboratory capacity and technology play an important role in the early detection among patients, and they are also the greatest limitations of patient detection. The solution to MDR-TB prevention and control lies in enhancing the capacity of grassroots laboratories in disease detection. The grassroots tuberculosis laboratories detection technology results in the delayed diagnosis in the source of infection, which prolong the transmission time. We have to take effective interventions to increase the grassroots laboratories ability and detect MDT-TB patients in a timely manner.

17.1.4 Early Standard Treatment

On a global scale, 61% of tuberculosis patients receive rifampicin resistance detection in 2019. Compared with previous years, only 37% of MDR/TB patients were included. Timely and reasonable anti-tuberculosis treatment can effectively cure drug resistance tuberculosis patients, eradicate infectivity, and stop transmission. Research study has shown that drug susceptibility testing is available for all previously treated patients with active pulmonary tuberculosis and 85% of the MDR-TB patients receive the appropriate MDR-TB treatment. The incidence rate of MDR-TB can be reduced by 26% by 2025.

China's latest "Guidelines for Chemotherapy of Drug-resistant Tuberculosis (2019 Edition)" (also referred as guidelines) points out that [25]:

1. The principle for chemotherapy regimens for rifampicin sensitive and drug resistance patients is to select first-line and anti-tuberculosis medications as much as possible. Fluoroquinolones (FQs) anti-tuberculosis drugs are recommended when first-line anti-tuberculosis drugs cannot be combined into an effective four drug chemotherapy regimen.
2. For rifampicin resistance tuberculosis patients, the long-term chemotherapy regimen's anti-tuberculosis medications were divided into three groups—ABC. Group A was the first-line drug, group B was the subsequent treatment, and group C was the third-line therapy. The group C treatment would be used when both group A and B stop working. In addition, there are some points that should be considered. Oral medications are preferred compared with injectable medications, reliability

of available DST methods, population resistance levels, patients' tolerance and resistance to drugs, and potential drug-drug interaction. A specific plan is recommended as below: (1) Recommended plan 1 for MDR-TB patients: Lfx(Mfx)-Bdq(Lzd)-Cfz-Cs-Z(E, Pto)/12–14Lfx(Mfx)-Cfz-Cs-Z(E, Pto); Recommended plan 2: If Bdq and Lzd are not available, 6Mfx(Lfx)-Cfz-Cs-Am(Cm)-Pto(E, Z)/12–14Mfx(Lfx)-Cfz-Cs-Pto (E, Z). (2) For pre-XDR-TB patients if resistant to fluoroquinolones (FQs), recommended plan 1 is: 6 Bdq-Lzd-Cfz-CS-Z(Pto)/14–18 Lzd-Cfz-Cs-Z(Pto); recommended plan 2 is:6 Lzd(Bdq)-Cfz-CS-Am(Cm)-Z-Pto/14–18 Cfz-CS-Z-Pto. The recommended regimen for resistance to second-line injections is: 6 Lfx(Mfx)-Bdq(Lzd)-Cfz-Cs-Z (Pto)/12–14 Lfx(Mfx)-Cfz-Cs-Z(Pto). (3) A short-course chemotherapy treatment of 9–12 months can be utilized for patients with recently diagnosed tuberculosis who have not received or have not taken second-line anti-tuberculosis medications for less than 1 month. The regimen recommends:4–6Am-Mfx-Pto-Cfz-Z-H^h-E/5Mfx-Cfz-Z-E.

In 2020, WHO released the latest integrated guidelines for the treatment of drug-resistant tuberculosis (referred to as the 2020 guidelines) [26], which recommended for the first time a short-course treatment regimen without injections for the first time recommending a short-course treatment plan without injections: 4–6 months bedaquiline(bdq)-levofloxacin/Mfx-Cfz-Z-E-H^h-ethionamide (Eto)/5Lfx/Mfx-Cfz-Z-E, and recommend it as the first choice for quinolone-susceptible MDR/RR-TB patients. Experts also point out that this planning is added to the new drug Bdq and abandons the injection drug. However, given the situation in China, there are some difficulties in abandoning the use of injection drugs. First of all, the high drug resistance of FQs, short-course therapy regimen is challenging. Linezolid (Lzd), Cfz, and other anti-tuberculosis medications have production and supplies issues, making them unavailable in some group A and group B of the 2020 edition of the guidelines. Some anti-tuberculosis drugs are expensive such as Bdq, the parts that have not been covered by health insurance, high-cost of oral regimens, which is unaffordable for most patients. Currently in China, there are no clinical short-term regimens containing Bdq, and lots of clinical studies have to contain more clinical research on supporting effective and safety data for all-oral short-term regimens in Chinese patients. However, injection has been widely used in China for many years because of the low-cost medical insurance reimbursement, reduced financial burdens on patients, and a rich clinical experience. Thus, most of the physicians and patients would lean toward an injectable regimen [27].

According to the 2020 edition of guideline, for MDR-TB patients with FQs resistance, MDR-TB patients who have not been exposed to Bdq and Lzd or who have been exposed for less than 2 weeks, 6–9 months of Bdq + pratomanib + Lzd (also known as BPaL) may be utilized. Treatment with the BPaL regimen highlights the fact that some of the current medications are ineffective for XDR-TB patients. BpaL can be considered as a last resort. However, patients must be assessed as baseline before treatment, as well as to monitor and manage side effects while undergoing treatment and to be followed up for 24 months after the treatment is completed. Pratomanib has not yet been authorized for marketing in China and further clinical research is needed to verify its safety and effectiveness. Besides, Bdq and Lzd are expensive, which put a heavy financial burden on patients, and the Lzd adverse effect rate is high. Therefore, some scholars believe that the clinical application of BpaL in China is difficult.

17.1.5 Latent Tuberculosis Infection (LTI) Preventive Treatment

17.1.5.1 Prophylaxis in Patients with Isolated LTBI

Currently, there are 4 kinds of medicines commonly used to prevent contacts of pulmonary tuberculosis patients, 6–9 months of once-daily isoniazid, 3 months of twice-weekly isoniazid combined with rifapentine, 3 months of once-daily isoniazid combined with rifampicin (these three regimens are strongly advised by the WHO in the "Guidelines for the Management of Latent Tuberculosis Infection" and "High Confidence Regimen"), and 1 month of once-daily isoniazid plus rifapentine and 4 month of once-daily rifampicin (conditional recommendation). Specific dosing times are shown in Table 17.1.

WHO recommends the 6–9 months INH single-drug regimen as the first-line for preventive treatment for LTBI patients. Numerous studies show that the 6-month INH single-regimen is an effective way to lower the prevalence of active pulmonary tuberculosis in the LBTI population. However, due to the lengthy treatment of INH single-drug regimen is too long, poor patients adherence to medication and risk of hepatotoxicity, its effectiveness in tuberculosis prevention is prevented by insufficient acceptance and low treatment rate. The 3 months isoniazid and rifapentine regimen is a new regimen with fewer adverse reactions and higher completion rate in the LBTI population [28]. In 2010, a multicenter randomized clinical trial tested the effectiveness of 3HP in LBTI patients at a high risk of developing tuberculosis patients. The American CDC recommends direct observation of the 3HP regimen for LTBI, even though this regimen has significant limitations for people with HIV and children between the age of 2 and 11 [29]. Some research has shown that the 3-month isoniazid and rifampicin regi-

Table 17.1 Tuberculosis prevention treatment plan

Treatment plan	Medicine	Dose				Directions	Treatment
		Adults		Children			
		<50 kg	≥50 kg	mg/kg times	Maximum dose (mg/times)		
Isoniazid monotherapy	Isoniazid	300	300	10	300	Once a day	6–9 months
Intermittent rifapentine-isoniazid combination regimen	Isoniazid	500	600	10–15	300	Twice a day	3 months
	Rifapentine	450	600	10 (>5 years old)	340 (>5 years old)		
Isoniazid and rifampicin combination regimen	Isoniazid	300	300	10	300	Once a day	3 months
	Rifampicin	450	600	10	450		
Rifampin monotherapy	Rifampicin	450	600	10	450	Once a day	4 months

men can reduce the development of active pulmonary tuberculosis as well as the incidence of severe pulmonary tuberculosis in the LBTI group. However, the 3-month isoniazid and rifampicin combination regimen and 4-month rifampin monotherapy still need more high-quality clinical research in randomized control trials to explore its efficacy and safety.

17.1.5.2 LTBI Prophylaxis in Close Contact of MDR-TB

It might be ineffective to MDR-TB using the drug susceptible LBTI standard treatment methods for INH and RFP. To prevent the development of MDR-TB, researchers recommend prophylactic treatment for LTBI patients based on the susceptibility results of the primary case. Close contacts of patients with MDR-TB or isoniazid-resistant patients were at higher risk of MTB infection compared with drug susceptible close contacts. However, there was no significant difference in the risk of developing TB. Research has shown that using preventive treatment methods can reduce the incidence rate of MDR-TB by approximately 90%. The 2020 edition guideline recommends close contact of MDR-TB with individualized risk assessment and preventive treatment after their exposure intensity by following clinical evaluation [26]. By using TST or IGRAS, these could confirm patient history, medical resistance, and LBTI. This can prevent the side-effect of LBTI by using a 6-month fluoroquinolones regimen and provide opportunities for fluoroquinolone use in the close contact of MDR-TB.

Studies have shown that prophylactic treatment with fluoroquinolones combined with other first- and second-line anti-tuberculosis drugs can effectively reduce the incidence of active pulmonary tuberculosis in LTBI patients who are in close contact with MDR-TB. After three years of surveillance, a trial of MDR-LTBI therapy revealed that 89 percent of contacts who completed the 12-month fluoroquinolone regimen did not develop MDR-TB. The subjects exhibited great compliance and good tolerance while being observed daily by the professionals, and no significant adverse events were discovered [30]. A systematic review suggests that prophylactic treatment of patients with latent infected MDT-TB could reduce the risk of tuberculosis morbidity. The most effective method is to use the combination between FQ and ethionamide, which is more expensive and less cost-effective compared with other options. FQ and ethambutol were most effective, followed by FQ alone, then pyrazinamide and ethambutol, but pyrazinamide discontinuation rates were higher [31]. Specialist consensus recommends that fluoroquinolones can be used as a prophylactic treatment to high-risk contacts (close contacts of children younger than 5 years and immunocompromised). If the primary patient has proven FQ susceptibility or low FQ resistance, they should use levofloxacin [32]. If DST verifies ofloxacin resistance or high-level of FQ resistance, patients should use moxifloxacin. The European CDC and the American Thoracic Society also recommend the use of fluoroquinolones for prophylactic treatment of LTBI in close contact with MDR-TB. WHO guidelines only recommend preventive treatment for LTBI close contacts with MDR-TB in high-risk groups (children, people receiving immunosuppressive therapy, HIV-positive people, etc.). Nevertheless, regardless of whether they are receiving preventive medication or not, close contacts of MDR-TB should be followed up for 2 years. WHO also recommends levofloxacin for 6-month for tolerant children with MDR-TB. This medicine could be taken with other medications, such as ethambutol and ethionamide, but should be followed up for 2 years with close attention for any signs and suggestive TB symptoms and initiation of treatment if needed [25]. Regarding LBTI for close contact of RR-TB, we could use a similar treatment for LTBI in close contact with MDR-TB. However, if the primary case is sensitive to INH, a regimen of once-daily isoniazid for 6–9 months can be used.

There is a lack of clinical randomized trials of high-quality fluoroquinolones combined with other first- and second-line anti-tuberculosis drug regimens for the treatment of MDR-TB in close contact with LTBI. More research is needed to determine the safety and effectiveness of this combination. At the same time, it should also conduct a clinical trial in adults, children, HIV-infected individuals, which could improve preventive methods, dosage, and treatment for MDR-TB contacts. New drug studies should also be conducted to evaluate the safety and efficacy of prophylactic regimens in MDR-TB close contacts.

17.1.6 Vaccine

BCG is the only TB vaccine that is currently approved, which is effective in preventing both military and pediatric tuberculosis meningitis. Drug resistance tuberculosis remains to be a key priority that cannot be accomplished solely through early diagnosis and adequate treatment. It also requires preventive treatment and effective vaccination. WHO recommends that single-dose BCG vaccine can be provided as soon as after a baby is born in countries with a high TB prevalence. BCG is only offered to newborns and infants or to older children with negative skin tests for TB infection in countries with low TB prevalence.

17.1.7 Infection Control

Tuberculosis infection control is a series of measures to largely reduce the risk of tuberculosis spreading in the population. This includes the development and implementations of infectious control policies at all levels such as public or private clinics, school, community, welfare institution, nursing home, and home setting. Community infectious control focuses on reducing overall tuberculosis exposure and preventing transmission in tuberculosis families. At a societal level, infectious control includes improving standard living and creating an environment that would prevent tuberculosis transmission. Interrupting the transmission of drug-resistant TB is critical to achieving the global goal of ending the TB epidemic. Therefore, interventions are necessary to quickly identify the sources of transmission and then prevent human-to-human transmission by reducing airborne concentration of infectious droplet nuclei and exposure times of susceptible populations.

17.1.7.1 Administrative Control

Administrative control aims at reducing tuberculosis transmission by reducing exposure, and specific interventions include triage and patient isolation systems (i.e., managing patient movement to identify and isolate suspected TB cases in a timely manner), prompt initiation of effective treatment, and respiratory hygiene.

WHO recommends to classify the people with TB symptoms and signs and designated TB medical institutions should develop reasonable medical procedures, strictly adhere to the pre-examination and triage system, and patients are sorted into segregated pathways to care. These could reduce the mycobacteria spread to other persons in high-risk environments, healthcare staff, and patients. However, the implementation of any triage system needs to consider the fast track of TB services and reduce healthcare wait and travel times. Besides, community health workers are crucial for the quick detection of suspected tuberculosis cases, use of referral systems, and rapid tuberculosis diagnosis, and other community-level treatments. Community health workers can help with improving early detection of TB cases and reducing the risk of transmission throughout the community. People with confirmed TB infectious cases should be isolated in designated places, and physicians should give effective treatments for the TB patients to reduce the spread of mycobacterium tuberculosis to health workers, visitors to health-care facilities, or other people in settings with a high risk of transmission.

17.1.7.2 Environmental Control

The purpose of environmental control is to reduce the concentration of air droplet nuclei in the air. In order to avoid nosocomial infection, designated TB medical institutions need to divide TB infection risk areas and have strict regional management. The three principles of dilution, filtration, and disinfection can be used to reduce the infectivity of the air and reduce the risk of tuberculosis transmission. For example, by using special ventilation systems to maximize airflow velocity or filtration, controlling the direction of airflow to reduce the spread of infection; or using UV sterilization systems for air disinfection. Primary medical institutions should also ensure that the area layout is reasonable and well ventilated when suspicious patients are treated, examined, and managed.

UV-air disinfection is one of the most well-studied and cost-effective ways to reduce the spread of TB [33]. In Eastern European or Central Asian countries, there is a high percentage of new cases of MDR-TB because of the low natural ventilation, longer hospital stays. Therefore, widespread use of UV sterilization systems is considered as a particularly useful adjunctive TB transmission control method. Studies have shown that 254 nm UV light fixtures typically installed on the walls or ceilings of patient rooms, along with appropriate air mixing fans, are estimated to reduce TB transmission by 80% [34]. A research study evaluating whether the use of UV sterilization in TB laboratories could substantially reduce TB infection rates among health-care workers showed that implementing UV-air disinfection interventions reduced the absolute risk of LTBI by 14.8% in this population, and 14.8% among health workers. The number of TB cases decreased by 0.29 cases/100 person-years [35]. Studies have shown that mechanical ventilation combined with other environmental control measures, including the use of ultraviolet light for air disinfection in wards and public areas, can reduce the positive rate of tuberculin skin test (TST) for medical staff by 4.1–8.8% [36].

The use of ventilation systems, including natural ventilation, mechanical ventilation, mixed-mode ventilation, high-efficiency recirculation air filters, and room air purification equipment, is an effective intervention to reduce the spread of *M. tuberculosis* to health workers, people visiting health-care facilities, or high-risk settings. Several studies have shown a reduction in the incidence of LTBI among health workers following interventions with mixed-mode ventilation [36, 37]. The decision to use natural ventilation, hybrid ventilation, mechanical ventilation or HEPA filters for a system is largely dependent on the needs of the specific environment, climate, cost-benefit assessment, and resource sustainability to ensure proper design and continued stringent standards and maintenance. The use of poorly designed or poorly maintained ventilation systems results in insufficient airflow, which can lead to the spread of Mycobacterium tuberculosis associated with health-care facilities. Inadequate ventilation also increases the risk of transmission in other non-medical gathering places, such as schools, nursing homes, and welfare homes.

17.1.8 Management of Drug-Resistant Patients

17.1.8.1 Management Method

The whole process of supervision and management is the main management method of drug-resistant tuberculosis. Due to the long-term treatment of drug-resistant tuberculosis patients, most patients need 24 months or even longer. Besides, since the treatment is difficult, it will bring greater social problems once the treatment fails. Effective treatment and management strategies must be implemented throughout the course of treatment to ensure that patients follow the principles of early, combined, moderate, regular, and whole-course medication. Chinese "Guidelines for Chemotherapy of Drug-resistant Tuberculosis (2019 Short Edition)" [25] pointed out that all MDR-TB patients should take full-course supervised chemotherapy. This means each time when the patients took medicines, they would be directly supervised by a specially trained medical staff during the whole process of treatment. However, home-supervised medication is not recommended for MDR-TB patients. Meanwhile, a combination of inpatient treatment and outpatient treatment is suggested to be used to manage MDR-TB patients during treatment. This is because most MDR-TB patients are seriously ill with a long course of treatment and many types of combination drugs. More sensitive TB patients are prone to serious adverse drug reactions. Therefore, MDR-TB patients should be hospitalized first after being diagnosed. After the condition is relatively stable, they can be discharged to continue treatment and management in community or village clinics. For those patients who are unwilling to be hospitalized due to financial difficulties and other reasons, a full-course outpatient treatment can be used. Chemotherapy for DR-TB requires a combination of multiple drugs because the adverse reactions of drugs are difficult to predict, especially second-line anti-tuberculosis drugs. The reason for this often leads to patients discontinuing their medications due to adverse drug reactions, which is detrimental to therapeutic efficacy and even exacerbates drug resistance. Rapid assessment, diagnosis, and management of adverse events are extremely important because adverse drug reactions, such as adverse drug reactions, can affect treatment outcomes, leading to treatment failure and higher mortality. Therefore, when formulating a treatment plan, health education should be given to patients to inform patients of the possible adverse reactions of each drug and the necessity of insisting on completing a full course of treatment, so as to enhance the psychological preparation of patients for possible adverse drug reactions. During the treatment process, the occurrence of adverse events should be closely monitored, recorded, and reported to clinicians in a timely manner. Hence, effective preventive or treatment measures can be taken to deal with possible or already occurred adverse drug reactions and to maximize the guarantee of chemotherapy for drug-resistant tuberculosis. Most adverse events are easily identifiable and are usually reported by patients properly, but some need to be detected through regular inspections and laboratory screening monitoring.

17.1.8.2 Outpatient Management

When a patient is diagnosed and begins outpatient treatment, county-level disease prevention and control institutions or primary medical and health institutions need to implement the treatment and management of the patient, which mainly includes the following four aspects:

1. **The first home visit:** After receiving the notification from the higher-level professional institution, the primary medical and health institution needs to conduct the first follow-up visit to the patient within 72 h. The follow-up should include: jointly determine the personnel who

supervise the administration of medicines with the patients; evaluate the living environment of the patients; carry out publicity and education on the knowledge of tuberculosis prevention and control; If physicians do not see the patient within 72 h in 2 visits, the primary doctor should report to the county (district) level disease prevention and control institution.

2. **Supervise medication administration:** During the period of taking the medicine, the patient can choose to be supervised by the supervisor, or they can use the intelligent tool to record their medicine taking.
3. **Follow-up evaluation**: (1) Follow-up of patients by primary doctors. For patients supervised by medical staff, medical staff should record the results of patient follow-up assessments at least once a month; for patients administered by non-medical staff or by intelligent tools, doctors in primary medical and health institutions should follow-up once every 10 days during the intensive period of the patient, and once a month during the continuous treatment period. Then the physicians record it on the "Tuberculosis Patient Follow-up Service Record Form" Follow-up situation. (2) Follow-up visits of patients to designated TB medical institutions.

   When the patient is followed up, the doctor in the designated medical institution should ask the patient's medication status, verify the patient's remaining medication, evaluate the patient's medication compliance, whether there is any missed or wrong medication. Medical staff can also ask the patient if there is any adverse drug reaction and take appropriate measures according to the situation. Physicians also have to assess the patient's psychological and social support status, complete regular clinical assessments and laboratory tests, and fill in the relevant information in the outpatient medical record. At the same time, adjust the patient's management method according to the number of missed doses: if the patient misses more than 6 doses in a month, physicians have to "strengthen the management" of the patient based on a targeted strengthening management plan according to the specific situation of the patient's missed dose and then notify the grassroots level.
4. **Closing evaluation**: When a patient ends treatment, the designated medical institutions for tuberculosis at the county (district) level shall promptly inform the primary medical and health institutions and disease prevention and control institutions of the relevant information on the cessation of treatment. The designated medical institutions for tuberculosis at the county (district) level comprehensively determine the treatment and management of the patients and close the case based on the information reported by the primary medical and health institutions and the information of the patients' treatment and follow-up visits.

17.1.8.3 Inpatient Management

1. The designated medical institutions shall adopt the method of "medical personnel management" for inpatients.
2. Areas where conditions permit should implement hospital isolation and treatment of infectious pulmonary tuberculosis patients. Hospitalization of patients with rifampicin-resistant tuberculosis placed in relatively independent drug-resistant wards.
3. After leaving the hospital, the patients should follow the outpatient treatment.

17.1.8.4 Management of Close Contacts

Tuberculosis Screening

Tuberculosis screening is divided into two situations: contacts under the age of 15, screening for suspected symptoms of tuberculosis and TST testing at the same time (IGRA can be used in areas with contraindications or conditions), those with suspected symptoms of tuberculosis or those with strong positive TST test/IGRA positive patients must have a chest X-ray. For those who need differential diagnosis, further examinations such as CT can be used. Contacts aged 15 years and above must be screened for suspicious symptoms of pulmonary tuberculosis, TST testing (IGRA can be used in areas with contraindications or conditions), and chest X-ray examination. For those who need differential diagnosis, further examinations such as CT can be used. Suspected symptoms of pulmonary tuberculosis, strong positive TST test/strong positive IGRA, and abnormal chest X-ray films should be examined for etiology; Pathogenic positive should be further tested for bacterial species identification and drug susceptibility testing. Etiologically positive specimens, nucleic acids, and strains should be retained for review of results and strain homology testing.

Detection of Latent Infection

There is currently no gold standard for the diagnosis of LTBI. The 2020 edition of the guidelines [26] issued by WHO recommends TST or gamma-interferon release assay (IGRA) for the detection of LTBI. Both are diagnosed by LTBI by detecting the host's cellular immune response to MTB antigens, and positive results indicate MTB infection. TST is simple to operate and widely used in the screening of LTBI, but TST cross-reacts with BCG and non-tuberculous mycobacteria, which has certain limitations. The presence of IGRA has reduced some TST-positive results due to BCG vaccination and reduced overdiagnosis of LTBI. The sensitivity and specificity of IGRA are good, but there is greater heterogeneity in different immunodeficiency populations, depending on the degree and status of the subject's immunodeficiency.

Objects of Preventive Treatment

1. Children under 5 years old who are in close contact with etiologically positive pulmonary tuberculosis patients should be given preventive treatment even if there is no LTBI test result; children aged ≥5 years old, if LTBI test cannot be performed, it is recommended to be given preventive treatment if possible.
2. HIV-infected patients

   WHO strongly recommends that HIV-infected adults and adolescents receive preventive treatment as part of comprehensive anti-HIV therapy. Regardless of the degree of immunosuppression, pregnant women, patients already on antiretroviral therapy, pregnant women and people who have already received anti-TB treatment should still receive preventive treatment even when LTBI testing is not possible. Meanwhile, for HIV-infected infants who have been in close contact with etiologically positive pulmonary TB patients <12 months, and who live in an environment with a high risk of TB transmission and are ≥12 years of age prophylactic treatment is recommended for HIV-infected infants (regardless of whether they are close contacts or not) at 6 months of age.
3. Close contact with MDR-TB patients with newly latent infection

   For high-risk household close contacts of a patient with MDR-TB, prophylaxis would be considered based on an individualized risk assessment and sound clinical judgment sex therapy.
4. Other high-risk population

   Patients need tumor necrosis factor therapy, long-term dialysis therapy, organ or bone marrow transplantation. Patients with silicosis and long-term use of glucocorticoids or other immunosuppressants are recommended LTBI detection and preventive treatment.

Management During Prophylaxis

Close monitoring of adverse events and monitoring of treatment adherence in the MDR-TB population receiving prophylactic therapy is necessary. Types of adverse reactions depend on the drug used, monitoring of adverse events can be carried out according to the WHO Safety Management and Monitoring Protocol for Drugs Against Active Tuberculosis. Evidence of the efficacy and safety of preventive treatment for MDR-TB is currently particularly needed. The guidelines reiterate that, based on clinical practice and national guidelines, intensive surveillance for active TB for at least 2 years after exposure to MDR-TB prophylaxis is required. Interactions between MDR-TB preventive therapy drugs and antiretroviral drugs, immunosuppressants, and other drugs should also be considered. The success of LTBI therapy to prevent TB depends on selecting a patient-appropriate individualized treatment regimen, monitoring for potential adverse clinical events, and utilizing strategies to promote adherence. There is a need for treatment options that are safer, less expensive, and easier to complete and should be combined with interventions. If any of the following situations occur, the drug should be discontinued immediately: completing the prescribed course of treatment, severe adverse drug reactions during the course of treatment resulting in the inability to continue taking the drug, irregular taking of the drug due to various reasons, or failure to complete the entire course of treatment and during the period of taking the drug active TB lesions anywhere on the body.

Medical Observation

TST Test Strong Positive/IGRA Positive

If TST test positive/IGRA positive patients are unwilling to receive preventive treatment, chest X-ray examinations should be performed at the end of 3 months, the end of June, the end of December, and the end of 24 months after the first screening.

TST Test Moderately Positive and Generally Positive

When there is a sporadic outbreak of 3 or more epidemiologically linked cases, it is recommended to test moderately positive and generally positive TST in repeat chest X-ray after 3 months.

TST Test Negative/IGRA Negative

In the event of a school TB public health emergency, repeat TST testing or IGRA testing should be performed after 3 months, and chest X-rays should be performed for positive converts.

In the event of a sporadic outbreak of 3 or more epidemiologically linked cases, a repeat chest X-ray after 3 months is recommended for those with moderately positive and generally positive TST tests.

17.2 Prognostic Determinants

17.2.1 Influence Factors

17.2.1.1 Immunocompromised

Immunocompromised patients had a shorter median survival time. Among them, HIV seropositivity was significantly associated with death and was an important risk factor for death during treatment in MDR-TB patients. When HIV infects the body, it will damage the body's immune system, inhibit the function of lymphocytes, especially CD4+ T lymphocytes and macrophages in the body, resulting in a continuous decrease in the number of lymphocytes. The ability to respond to mycobacterium tuberculosis antigens is destroyed, leading to HIV endogenous relapse or exogenous reinfection of tuberculosis in an infected person. Once a tuberculosis patient is infected with HIV, the decline of the immune function of the body will also make the tuberculosis disease develop rapidly, making the disease progress, worsen, and quickly lead to death [38].

17.2.1.2 Age and Appropriate Treatment

The risk of death increases with age in MDR-TB patients, nearly doubling for every 10-year increase in age. With increasing age, various functions of the body decline, and complications are prone to occur, resulting in decreased survival time and increased mortality. Patients who received appropriate treatment had a longer median survival time and a lower chance of death. A key factor contributing to increased mortality is whether the time from MDR-TB diagnosis to initiation of treatment is more than 1 month. Patients who delayed treatment by more than 1 month had a shorter mean survival time than those who received normal treatment. In addition, antiretroviral therapy has a positive effect on prolonging the survival time of patients with HIV and drug-resistant TB co-infection [39].

17.2.1.3 Nutritional Status and Clinical Complications

When MDR-TB patients suffer from certain clinical complications at the same time, it will affect the survival time, such as anemia, malnutrition, diabetes, etc. People with diabetes are not only more prone to developing TB, they may also be at increased risk of developing MDR-TB. In the state of anemia and malnutrition, various functions of the patient's body will be lower than normal levels, resulting in a shortened survival time of MDR-TB patients [40].

17.2.1.4 Other Factors

Other important factors affecting the survival time of MDR-TB patients include smoking, alcohol abuse, low education, unemployment, resistance to second-line drugs, number of people resistant to first-line drugs at the time of initiation of treatment, and living in rural areas with poor sanitation [41].

17.2.2 Prognosis

The 2017 GBD data showed that the global standardized mortality rates of MDR-TB and XDR-TB were 1.6/100,000 and 0.2/100,000, respectively, but the incidence of MDR/Rifampicin resistance in China ranks second in the world [42]. WHO summarized data from 13,273 MDR/RR-TB patients from 55 studies in 38 countries and conducted a meta-analysis and found that the treatment success rate of the Bdq-containing all-oral short-course regimen (73%) was significantly higher than that of the standardized short-course treatment regimen containing injections (60%). The study also showed that the BPaL regimen had a success rate of nearly 90% and had a good overall safety profile among the patients with XDR-TB and poorly treated MDR-TB [26].

References

1. World Health Organization. Global tuberculosis report 2021[EB/OL]. [2021-10-14]. https://www.who.int/publications/digital/global-tuberculosis-report-2021.
2. Gao J, Mei J. Transmission is the main reason for the high drug resistance rate of TB in China. Chin J Antituberculosis. 2015;37(11):1091–6.
3. Mitchison D, Da Vies G. The chemotherapy of tuberculosis: past, present and future[J]. Int J Tuberc Lung Dis. 2012;16(6):724–32.
4. Shah NS, Auld SC, Brust J, et al. Transmission of extensively drug-resistant tuberculosis in South Africa[J]. N Engl J Med. 2017;376(3):243.
5. Shen X, Deriemer K, Yuan ZA, et al. Drug-resistant tuberculosis in Shanghai, China, 2000-2006: prevalence, trends and risk factors[J]. Int J Tuberc Lung Dis. 2009;13(2):253.
6. Yang C, Shen X, Peng Y, et al. Transmission of Mycobacterium tuberculosis in China: a population-based molecular epidemiologic study. Clin Infect Dis. 2015;61(2):219–27.
7. Ministry of Health of the People's Republic of China. National baseline survey report on drug resistance of tuberculosis [M]. Beijing: People's Medical Publishing House; 2010.
8. Li X, Zhang Y, Shen X, et al. Transmission of drug-resistant tuberculosis among treated patients in Shanghai, China[J]. Infect Dis. 2007;195(6):864–9.
9. Kendall EA, Azman AS, Cobelens FG, et al. MDR-TB treatment as prevention: The projected population-level impact of expanded treatment for multidrug-resistant tuberculosis[J]. PLoS One. 2017;12(3):e0172748.
10. Zhao P, Fang F, Yu Q, et al. Evaluation of BACTEC MGIT 960 system for testing susceptibility of Mycobacterium tuberculosis to first-line drugs in China[J]. PLoS One. 2014;9(9):e99659.
11. Abuali MM, Katariwala R, LaBombardi VJ. A comparison of the Sensititre® MYCOTB panel and the agar proportion method for the susceptibility testing of Mycobacterium tuberculosis[J]. Eur J Clin Microbiol Infect Dis. 2012;31(5):835–9.
12. Lee J, Armstrong DT, Sengooba W, et al. Sensititre MYCOTB MIC plate for testing Mycobacterium tuberculosis susceptibility to first- and second-line drugs[J]. Antimicrob Agents Chemother. 2014;58(1):11–8.
13. Yu X, Ma YF, Jiang GL, et al. Sensititre® MYCOTB MIC plate for drug susceptibility testing of Mycobacterium tuberculosis complex isolates[J]. Int J Tuberc Lung Dis. 2016;20(3):329–34.
14. Xia H, Zheng Y, Zhao B, et al. Assessment of a 96-well plate assay of quantitative drug susceptibility testing for Mycobacterium tuberculosis complex in China[J]. PLoS One. 2017;12(1):e0169413.
15. Hall L, Jude KP, Clark SL, et al. Evaluation of the sensititre MycoTB plate for susceptibility testing of the Mycobacterium tuberculosis complex against first- and second-line agents[J]. J Clin Microbiol. 2012;50(11):3732–4.
16. Steingart KR, Schiller I, Horne DJ, et al. Xpert® MTB/RIF assay for pulmonary tuberculosis and rifampicin resistance in adults[J]. Cochrane Database Syst Rev. 2014;21(1):CD009593.
17. Zhao B, Ou X, Xia H, et al. Application evaluation of XpertMtb/RIF detection technology in the diagnosis of tuberculosis[J]. Chin J Antituberculosis. 2014;6:462–6.
18. Tao C, Yuxiang W, Junfeng Z, et al. Diagnostic reliability of Xpert MTB/RIF with rifampicin resistance detected at very low bacte-

rial level: a retrospective analysis[J/CD]. Electron J Emerg Inf Dis. 2021;6(4):319–22.
19. Chen X, He G, Wang S, et al. Evaluation of whole-genome sequence method to diagnose resistance of 13 anti-tuberculosis drugs and characterize resistance genes in clinical multi-drug resistance Mycobacterium tuberculosis isolates From China[J]. Front Microbiol. 2019;10:1741.
20. Allix-Béguec C, Arandjelovic I, et al. Prediction of susceptibility to first-line tuberculosis drugs by DNA sequencing[J]. N Engl J Med. 2018;379(15):1403–15.
21. Nimmo C, Doyle R, Burgess C, et al. Rapid identification of a Mycobacterium tuberculosis full genetic drug resistance profile through whole genome sequencing directly from sputum[J]. Int J Infect Dis. 2017;62:44–6.
22. Phelan J, O'Sullivan DM, Machado D, et al. The variability and reproducibility of whole genome sequencing technology for detecting resistance to anti-tuberculous drugs[J]. Genome Med. 2016;8(1):132.
23. Dheda K, Gumbo T, Maartens G, et al. The epidemiology, pathogenesis, transmission, diagnosis, and management of multidrug-resistant, extensively drug-resistant, and incurable tuberculosis[J]. Lancet Respir Med. 2017;5(4):291–360.
24. Zignol M, Cabibbe AM, Dean AS, et al. Genetic sequencing for surveillance of drug resistance in tuberculosis in highly endemic countries: a multi-country population-based surveillance study[J]. Lancet Infect Dis. 2018;18(6):675–83.
25. China Tuberculosis Prevention Association. Guidelines for chemotherapy of drug-resistant tuberculosis (2019 abbreviated version) [J]. Chin J Tuberculosis Prevent. 2019;41(10):48.
26. WHO. WHO consolidated guidelines on tuberculosis: module 4: treatment drug-resistant tuberculosis treatment[EB/OL]. Geneva: World Health Organization; 2020. https://apps.who.int/iris/handle/10665/332397.
27. Zhang L, Liu Y, Gao J, et al. Interpretation of WHO 2020 "Integrated tuberculosis guidelines module 4: treatment of drug-resistant tuberculosis"[J]. Chin J Tuberculosis Respir Med. 2021;44(4):349–53.
28. Sterling TR, Villarino ME, Borisov AS, et al. Three months of rifapentine and isoniazid for latent tuberculosis infection[J]. N Engl J Med. 2011;365(23):2155–66.
29. Centers for Disease Control and Prevention (CDC). Recommendations for use of an isoniazid-rifapentine regimen with direct observation to treat latent Mycobacterium tuberculosis infection[J]. MMWR Morb Mortal Wkly Rep. 2011;60(48):1650–3.
30. Bamrah S, Brostrom R, Dorina F, et al. Treatment for LTBI in contacts of MDR-TB patients, Federated States of Micronesia, 2009-2012[J]. Int J Tuberc Lung Dis. 2014;18(8):912–8.
31. Marks SM, Mase SR, Bamrah MS. Systematic review, meta-analysis, and cost-effectiveness of treatment of latent tuberculosis to reduce progression to multidrug-resistant tuberculosis[J]. Clin Infect Dis. 2017;64(12):1670–7.
32. Nicholson A, Becerra MC, Seddon JA, et al. Global consultation on best practices in the delivery of preventive therapy for household contacts of patients with drug-resistant tuberculosis.
33. Nardell EA. Transmission and institutional infection control of tuberculosis[J]. Cold Spring Harb Perspect Med. 2015;6:a018192.
34. Matsie A, Dharmadhikari AS, et al. Institutional tuberculosis transmission. controlled trial of upper room ultraviolet air disinfection: a basis for new dosing guidelines[J]. Am J Respir Crit Care Med. 2015;192(4):477–84.
35. Yanai H, Limpakarnjanarat K, Uthaivoravit W, et al. Risk of Mycobacterium tuberculosis infection and disease among health care workers, Chiang Rai, Thailand[J]. Int J Tuberc Lung Dis. 2003;7(1):36–45.
36. Welbel SF, French AL, Bush P, et al. Protecting health care workers from tuberculosis: a 10-year experience[J]. Am J Infect Control. 2009;37(8):668–73.
37. Behrman AJ, Shofer FS. Tuberculosis exposure and control in an urban emergency department[J]. Ann Emerg Med. 1998;31(3):370–5.
38. Drobniewski F, Eltringham I, Graham C, et al. A national study of clinical and laboratory factors affecting the survival of patients with multiple drug resistant tuberculosis in the UK[J]. Thorax. 2002;57(9):810–6.
39. Zemedu TG, Bayray A, Weldearegay B. Survival and predictors of mortality among patients under multidrug resistant tuberculosis treatment in Ethiopia[J]. Int J Pharm Sci Res. 2013;4(2):776–87.
40. Johnston JC, Shahidi N, Sadatsafavi M, et al. Treatment outcomes of multidrug-resistant tuberculosis: a systematic review and meta-analysis[J]. PLoS One. 2009;4(9):e6914.
41. Balabanova Y, Ignatyeva O, Fiebig L, et al. Survival of patients with multidrug-resistant TB in Eastern Europe: what makes a difference?[J]. Thorax. 2016;71(9):854–61.
42. GBD 2017 Causes of Death Collaborators. Global, regional, and national age-sex-specific mortality for 282 causes of death in 195 countries and territories, 1980-2017: a systematic analysis for the Global Burden of Disease Study 2017[J]. Lancet. 2018;392(10159):1736–88.

GPSR Compliance

The European Union's (EU) General Product Safety Regulation (GPSR) is a set of rules that requires consumer products to be safe and our obligations to ensure this.

If you have any concerns about our products, you can contact us on ProductSafety@springernature.com

In case Publisher is established outside the EU, the EU authorized representative is:

Springer Nature Customer Service Center GmbH
Europaplatz 3
69115 Heidelberg, Germany

Batch number: 08049556

Printed by Printforce, the Netherlands